REHABILITATION TECHNIQUES
IN SPORTS MEDICINE

REHABILITATION TECHNIQUES IN SPORTS MEDICINE

WILLIAM E. PRENTICE, Ph.D., A.T.,C., P.T.

Associate Professor of Physical Education
Coordinator of the Sports Medicine Specialization
Department of Physical Education
Assistant Clinical Professor of Physical Therapy
Department of Medical Allied Health Professions
The University of North Carolina,
Chapel Hill, North Carolina
Director of Sports Medicine Education and Fellowship Programs,
HEALTHSOUTH Rehabilitation Corporation,
Birmingham, Alabama

with *340 illustrations*

TIMES MIRROR / MOSBY
COLLEGE PUBLISHING

St. Louis • Boston • Los Altos • Toronto   1990

Editor: Pat Coryell
Editorial Assistant: Loren Stevenson
Production Editor: Radhika Rao Gupta
Cover Designer: Susan E. Lane
Production/Editing: Editing, Design & Production, Inc.

Cover photograph © 1988 Tim Davis

Printed in the United States of America

Library of Congress Cataloging-in-Publication Data

Rehabilitation techniques in sports medicine/[edited by] William E.
    Prentice
        p.   cm.
    Includes bibliographical references.
    ISBN 0-8016-6147-1
    1. Sports—Accidents and injuries—Patients—Rehabilitation.
    2. Physical therapy.   I. Prentice, William E.
    [DNLM: 1. Athletic Injuries—rehabilitation.   2. Athletic
Injuries—therapy.   3. Physical Therapy—methods.   QT 260 R345]
    RD97.R44   1990
    617.1'027—dc20
    DNLM/DLC
    for Library of Congress   89-20565
                                                                            CIP

C/VH/VH 9 8 7 6 5 4 3 2   01/D/018

Contributors

Gerald W. Bell, Ed.D., P.T., A.T.,C.,R.

Coordinator of Athletic Training
Director, Sports Injury Research
Assistant Professor, Kinesiology/Rehabilitation
  Education
University of Illinois
Urbana, Illinois

Donald A. Chu, Ph.D., P.T., A.T.,C.

Director, Ather Sports Injury Clinic
Dublin, California

John Marc Davis, P.T., A.T.,C.

Physical Therapist/Athletic Trainer
Division of Sports Medicine
The University of North Carolina
Chapel Hill, North Carolina

Bernard DePalma, M.Ed., P.T., A.T.,C.

Head Athletic Trainer
Cornell University
Ithaca, New York

Danny T. Foster, M.A., A.T.,C.

Associate Director of Athletic Training Services
Curriculum Director of Athletic Training Education
The University of Iowa
Iowa City, Iowa

Joe Gieck, Ed.D., P.T., A.T.,C.

Associate Professor, Department of Human Services,
  Curry School of Education
Assistant Clinical Professor, Department of
  Orthopaedics and Rehabilitation
Head Athletic Trainer
The University of Virginia
Charlottesville, Virginia

Charles L. Henry, M.S., P.T.

Director of Clinical Services
Augusta Rehabilitation Inc.
Augusta, Georgia

Stewart L. (Skip) Hunter, P.T., A.T.,C.

Coordinator of Sports Medicine Programs
Carolinas Spine and Rehabilitation Center
Charlotte, North Carolina

Scott M. Lephart, Ph.D., A.T.,C.

Director, Athletic Training/Sports Medicine Program
Assistant Professor, School of Education
University of Pittsburgh
Pittsburgh, Pennsylvania

Julie Ann Moyer, Ed.D., P.T., A.T.,C.

Clinical Assistant Professor
Thomas Jefferson University, Philadelphia, Pennsylvania
Adjunct Professor
University of Delaware
  Newark, Delaware
Adjunct Professor
Delaware Technical and
  Community College
  Wilmington, Delaware
Director, Pike Creek Sports Medicine-Physical Therapy,
  Wilmington, Delaware

Gregory A. Ott, P.T., A.T.,C.

Coordinator of Athletic Training Services
Head Athletic Trainer
West Virginia University
Morgantown, West Virginia

David H. Perrin, Ph.D., A.T.,C.

Director, Graduate Athletic Training Program
Assistant Professor, Curry School of Education
The University of Virginia
Charlottesville, Virginia

William E. Prentice, Ph.D., P.T., A.T.,C.
Associate Professor of Physical Education
Assistant Clinical Professor of Physical Therapy
Coordinator of the Sports Medicine Program
The University of North Carolina
Chapel Hill, North Carolina
Director, Sports Medicine Education and Fellowship
    Programs
HEALTHSOUTH Rehabilitation Corporation
Birmingham, Alabama

Rich Reihl, M.A., A.T.,C.
National Teams Athletic Trainer
United States Soccer Federation
Colorado Springs, Colorado

Preface

One of the primary goals of every sports medicine professional is to create a playing environment for the athlete that is as safe as it can possibly be. Despite that effort, the nature of athletic participation dictates that injuries will eventually occur. Fortunately, few of the injuries that occur in an athletic setting are life-threatening. The majority of athletic injuries are not serious and lend themselves to rapid rehabilitation. When injuries do occur, the focus of the sports therapist shifts from injury prevention to injury treatment and rehabilitation.

The process of rehabilitation begins immediately following injury. Initial first-aid and management techniques can have a substantial impact on the course and ultimate outcome of the rehabilitative process. Thus, in addition to possessing a sound understanding of how injuries can be prevented, the sports therapist must also be competent in providing correct and appropriate initial care when injury does occur.

In a sports medicine setting, the athletic sports therapist generally assumes the primary responsibility for design, implementation, and supervision of the rehabilitation program for the injured athlete.

Designing programs for rehabilitation is relatively simple and involves three basic short-term goals: 1) controlling pain, 2) maintaining or improving flexibility, and 3) returning to or increasing strength. The long-term goal is to return the injured athlete to practice or competition as quickly and as safely as possible. This is the easy part of supervising a rehabilitation program. The difficult part is knowing exactly when and how to change the rehabilitation protocols to accomplish both long- and short-term goals as effectively as possible.

The approach to rehabilitation in a sports medicine environment is considerably different from that of most other rehabilitation settings. The competitive nature of athletics necessitates an aggressive approach to rehabilitation. Since the competitive season in most sports is relatively short, the athlete does not have the luxury of being able to sit around and do nothing until the injury heals. The goal is to return to activity as soon as is safely possible. Thus, the sports therapist who is supervising the rehabilitation program must perform a balancing act, walking along the thin line between not pushing the athlete hard enough or fast enough and being overly aggressive. In either case, a mistake in judgment on the part of the sports therapist may hinder the athlete's return to activity.

Decisions as to when and how to alter and progress a rehabilitation program should be formulated within the framework of the healing process. The sports therapist must possess a sound understanding of both the sequence and time frames for the various phases of healing, realizing that certain physiological events must occur during each of the phases. Anything that is done during a rehabilitation program that interferes with this healing process is likely to increase the length of time required for rehabilitation and slow return to full activity. The healing process must have an opportunity to accomplish what it is supposed to. At best the sports therapist can try and create an environment that is conducive to the healing process. There is little that can be done to speed up that process physiologically, but there are many things that may be done during rehabilitation to impede healing.

The sports therapist has many tools at his or her disposal that can facilitate the rehabilitative process. How those tools are used is often a matter of individual preference and experience. Additionally, each individual patient is a little different and his or her response to various treatment protocols is somewhat variable. Thus, it is impossible to "cookbook" specific protocols that can be followed like a recipe. In fact, use of rehabilitation "recipes" should be strongly discouraged. Instead the sports therapist must develop a broad theoretical knowledge base from which specific techniques of rehabilitation may be selected and applied to each individual patient.

I hope that this text will aid in the clinical decision-making process, serving as a guide and a reference for the sports medicine professional overseeing programs of rehabilitation.

The following are a number of reasons why this text should be adopted for use.

COMPREHENSIVE COVERAGE OF REHABILITATION TECHNIQUES USED IN A SPORTS MEDICINE SETTING

The purpose of this text is to provide the sports therapist with a comprehensive guide to the design, implementation, and supervision of rehabilitation programs for sport-related injuries. It is intended for use in advanced courses in sports medicine, which deal with the practical application of theory in a clinical setting.

The text is essentially divided into two sections. The first eight chapters discuss the various techniques and theories on which rehabilitation protocols should be based. Chapter 1 discusses the healing process relative to the pathophysiology of various types of sport-related injuries. The sports therapist must base the entire rehabilitation program on what is occurring in the healing process. Chapter 2 discusses the short-term and long-term goals of a sports injury rehabilitation program. Chapter 3 provides an overview of reconditioning techniques and the theory underlying therapeutic exercise, which must be applied in all rehabilitation protocols. Chapter 4 emphasizes the importance of including techniques of manual therapy during rehabilitation. Chapter 5 describes the method of injury evaluation that is essential to the appropriate progression of rehabilitation programs. If the sports therapist cannot accurately evaluate the status of an injury to determine the appropriate stage of healing, chances are that alteration or progression of the rehabilitation protocol may be inappropriate. Chapter 6 discusses how the sports therapist should deal with the psycholog-

ical rehabilitation of the injured athlete. Arguably, psychological rehabilitation may be at least as critical as physiological rehabilitation in achieving the long-term goals. Chapter 7 identifies the various types of therapeutic modalities available to the sports therapist, explaining how and when they are most effectively used to facilitate the healing process. Chapter 8 discusses how various medications may be used to assist the rehabilitative process as well as indications and contraindications for their use in an athletic environment.

Chapters 9 through 17 discuss the practical application of the theory that forms the basis for rehabilitation as presented in the first half of the text relative to specific regional anatomical areas. Included are chapters on the rehabilitation of injuries to the spine, the shoulder, the elbow, the wrist and hand, the hip and thigh, the knee, the lower leg, the ankle, and finally, the foot. Each chapter briefly identifies the pathophysiology of the various injuries, followed by a discussion of potential techniques of rehabilitation, which may be applied to the different phases of the healing process.

TIMELY AND USEFUL

As the art and science of sports medicine becomes more sophisticated and specialized, the need arises for textbooks that deal with specific aspects of sports injury management. Rehabilitation is certainly one of the major areas of responsibility for the sports therapist.

For the classroom instructor there are a number of texts that present a general overview of the various aspects of sports medicine. However, in the past many instructors have relied on a collection of handout materials that dealt with information specific to rehabilitation techniques to be used in advanced courses. The contributing authors have attempted to combine their expertise and knowledge to produce a single text that encompasses all aspects of rehabilitation in a sports medicine setting.

This text on rehabilitation techniques fills a void that has existed for some time. It is intended for the student of sports medicine who is interested in gaining more in-depth exposure to the theory and practice of rehabilitation techniques in a sports medicine environment.

RESEARCH-BASED MATERIAL

Compared with some of the other health care specializations, sports medicine is still in its infancy. Its growth dictates the necessity for expanding our research efforts to identify new and more effective methods and techniques for dealing with sports-related injury. A sincere effort has been made by the contributing authors to present the most recent information on the various aspects of injury rehabilitation available from the literature.

Additionally, this manuscript has been critically reviewed by selected athletic trainers and physical therapists who are well-respected clinicians, educators, and researchers in this field to further ensure that the material presented is accurate and current.

PERTINENT TO SPORTS MEDICINE

There are many texts currently available that deal with the subject of rehabilitation of injury in various patient populations. However, this text concentrates exclusively on the application of rehabilitation techniques in a sport-related setting. The emphasis on sports medicine makes this text uncommon and valuable.

PEDAGOGICAL AIDS

The aids provided in this text to assist the student in its use include:

Objectives

These are listed at the beginning of each individual chapter to emphasize the concepts to be presented.

Figures and Tables

The numerous figures and tables included throughout the text graphically depict various rehabilitation techniques and other important points.

Summary

Each chapter has a summary that outlines the major points presented.

References

A comprehensive list of up-to-date references is included at the end of each chapter to provide additional information relative to a specific area.

ACKNOWLEDGMENTS

The preparation of the manuscript for a textbook is a long-term and extremely demanding effort that requires input and cooperation on the part of many different individuals.

I would like to personally thank each of the contributing authors. They were asked to contribute to this text because I have tremendous respect for them both personally and professionally. These individuals have distinguished themselves as educators and clinicians dedicated to the field of sports medicine. I am exceedingly grateful for their input.

In addition, I would like to acknowledge the efforts of Gerald Spadaccini and Cheryl Lissy (Chapter 2), Donna Beatty and Ann Smith (Chapter 10), Jim Case (Chapter 13), and Dr. Michael Gross (Chapter 17) for their assistance in the preparation of those chapters.

Loren Stevenson, my Developmental Editor at Mosby, has been persistent and diligent in the completion of this text. She has patiently and quietly encouraged me and I certainly have appreciated her support.

Annette Hall, of Editing, Design & Production, Inc., has taken care of the production details and has been invaluable in establishing consistency.

The following individuals have invested a significant amount of time and energy as reviewers for this manuscript and I appreciate their efforts.

Susan Hillman, M.A., M.S., A.T.,C., P.T.
University of Arizona

Sherry Bovinet, Ph.D., A.T.,C.
Keene State College

Gordon Stoddard, M.Ed., A.T.,C.
University of Wisconsin-Madison

Richard F. Irvin, Ed.D., A.T.,C.
Oregon State University

Earlene Durrant, Ed.D., A.T.,C.
Brigham Young University

Finally, and most important, this is for Tena, Brian, and Zachary, who make it all worth it.

William E. Prentice

Contents

1 **Pathophysiology of Musculoskeletal Injuries and the Healing Process,** 1

WILLIAM E. PRENTICE

GERALD W. BELL

Tissue Types, 1
Musculoskeletal Injuries, 6
Initial Management of Injuries, 13
Understanding the Healing Process, 15
Tendon Healing, 20
Bone Healing, 20
Nerve Tissue Regeneration, 21
Muscle Injury, 21
Summary, 21

2 **Rehabilitation Goals in Sports Medicine,** 24

JULIE ANN MOYER

Injury Prevention, 24
Initial Evaluation, Treatment, and
   Rehabilitation, 27
Factors That Influence Rehabilitation
   Goals, 32
Summary, 33

3 **Techniques of Reconditioning in Rehabilitation,** 34

WILLIAM E. PRENTICE

Improving Muscular Strength and
   Endurance, 35
Improving Flexibility, 47
The Relationship of Strength and
   Flexibility, 52
Maintenance of Cardiorespiratory
   Endurance, 52
Summary, 59

4 **Techniques of Manual Therapy,** 62

WILLIAM E. PRENTICE

Pain in Musculoskeletal Dysfunction, 62
Motion Assessment, 63
Philosophies in Manual Therapy, 65
Physiological Versus Accessory Motion, 65
Mobilization Techniques, 65
Traction Techniques, 67
Contraindications to Mobilization, 67
Proprioceptive Neuromuscular Facilitation
   Techniques, 68
Summary, 84

5 **The Evaluation Process in Rehabilitation,** 87

DAVID H. PERRIN

Preparticipation Examination, 87
On-Field Evaluation, 91
Off-Field Evaluation, 93
Documentation of Findings, 104
Summary, 105

6 **Psychological Considerations of Rehabilitation,** 107

JOE GIECK

The Injury-Prone Athlete, 108
Attitudes Setting Up Injury, 109
Phases of Injury, 111
It Is the Athlete's Injury, 112
Irrational Thinking, 112
Strategies for Gaining Control, 114
Interpersonal Relationships of the
   Athlete and the Sports Therapist, 115
Adherence to the Rehabilitation Process,
   116

Coping with Injury, 117
Goals, 119
Problems in the Rehabilitation Process, 120
Rehabilitation Personnel, 121
Conclusion, 121
Summary, 121

7 **Therapeutic Modalities in Rehabilitation,** 123
WILLIAM E. PRENTICE
CHARLES L. HENRY

Electrical Stimulating Currents, 123
Ultrasound, 129
Infrared Modalities, 130
Intermittent Compression, 132
Low-Power Laser, 133
Treatment of Acute Injury, 134
Treatment of Chronic Injury, 136
Indications and Contraindications, 137
Summary, 137

8 **Pharmacological Considerations in a Rehabilitation Program,** 140
WILLIAM E. PRENTICE

Common Medications, 141
Administering Versus Dispensing of Medication, 148
Drug Testing, 149
Summary, 149

9 **Rehabilitation of Low Back Injuries,** 151
DONALD A. CHU

The Examination, 152
Treatment, 161
Common Lumbosacral Injuries in Athletes, 164
Conclusion, 166
Back Rehabilitation Protocol, 166
Summary, 183

10 **Rehabilitation of Shoulder Injuries,** 186
GREGORY OTT

Rehabilitation Techniques, 187
Rehabilitation Programs, 207
Summary, 229

11 **Rehabilitation of Elbow Injuries,** 232
DANNY T. FOSTER

Inflammations, 232
Medications, 235
Joint Structures and Musculotendinous Unit Injuries, 235
Summary, 246

12 **Rehabilitation of Hand and Wrist Injuries,** 249
SCOTT M. LEPHART

Wrist Injuries, 249
Rehabilitation of Wrist Injuries, 252
Hand Injuries, 254
Rehabilitation of the Hand, 259
Summary, 263

13 **Rehabilitation of Hip and Thigh Injuries,** 265
BERNHARD DEPALMA

Hip Pointer, 265
Injury to the Iliac Spine, 268
Piriformis Syndrome Sciatica, 269
Bursitis of the Hip, 273
Pubic Injuries, 275
Hip Dislocation, 278
Hamstring Injuries, 279
Femoral Fractures, 285
Quadriceps Muscle Strain, 286
Quadriceps Contusion, 289
Myositis Ossificans, 292
Summary, 292

14   **Rehabilitation of Knee Injuries,** 294

J. MARC DAVIS

General Principle of Rehabilitation, 295
Phases of Rehabilitation, 297
Knee Injury, 298
UNC Sports Medicine/Physical Therapy
    Return to Activity Progressive Running
    Program, 312
Summary, 314

15   **Rehabilitation of Lower Leg Injuries,** 316

RICH RIEHL

Reconditioning Exercises, 316
Strengthing Exercises, 317
Cardiovascular Fitness, 320
Restoration of Smooth, Coordinated
    Movement, 320
Maintenance, 320
Injuries to the Lower Extremity, 321
Shin Splint Syndromes, 324
Retrocalcaneobursitis, 326
Compartment Syndromes, 326
Stress Fractures, 328
Summary, 329

16   **Rehabilitation of Ankle Injuries,** 331

STEWART L. (SKIP) HUNTER

Mechanisms of Injury, 331
Treatment and Rehabilitation of Ankle
    Sprains, 332
Summary, 339

17   **Rehabilitation of Foot Injuries,** 342

STEWART L. (SKIP) HUNTER

The Subtalar Joint, 342
The Midtarsal Joint, 343
Causes of Pronation, 344
Identification of Pronators, 347
Orthotics, 347
Shoe Selection, 352
Pathologies of the Foot, 353
Summary, 356

Pathophysiology of Musculoskeletal Injuries and the Healing Process

William E. Prentice and Gerald W. Bell

1

OBJECTIVES

Following completion of the chapter, the student should be able to:

■ Identify the four types of tissue in the human body.

■ Discuss the etiology and pathology of various musculoskeletal injuries.

■ Explain the importance of initial first aid and injury management of these injuries and their impact on the rehabilitation process.

■ Describe the pathophysiology of the healing process.

■ Identify those factors that may impede the healing process.

■ Discuss the healing process relative to tendon, bone, nerve, and muscle.

Rehabilitation of sport-related injuries requires some knowledge and understanding of the etiology and pathology involved in various types of musculoskeletal injuries that may occur. When injury does occur, the sports therapist is charged with the responsibility of designing, implementing, and supervising the rehabilitation program. Rehabilitation protocols and progressions must be based primarily on the physiological responses of the tissues to injury. Thus the sports therapist must understand the healing process to be effective in supervising the rehabilitative process. This chapter discusses the healing process relative to the various musculoskeletal injuries that may be encountered in a sports medicine setting.

TISSUE TYPES

There are four types of fundamental tissues in the human body: epithelial, muscular, nervous, and connective (Table 1-1). According to Guyton, all tissues of the body can be defined as soft tissue except bone.[18] Cailliet, however, more technically defines **soft tissue** as the matrix of the human body comprised of cellular elements within a ground substance. Furthermore, Cailliet believes that soft tissue is the most common site of functional impairment of the musculoskeletal system.[5] Therefore, most sports-related injuries occur to the soft tissues. With this in mind, soft tissue structure is explained and bone structure is briefly described in this chapter.

Epithelial Tissue

The first fundamental tissue is epithelial tissue (Fig. 1-1). This specific tissue covers all internal and external body surfaces and therefore encompasses such structures as the skin, the outer layer of the internal organs, and the inner lining of the blood vessels and glands. A basic purpose of epithelial tissue, as presented by Fahey, is to protect as well as form structure for other tissues and organs.[11] In addition, this tissue functions in absorption (for example, in the digestive tract)

1

TABLE 1-1

Tissues

Tissue	Location	Function
EPITHELIAL		
Simple squamous	Alveoli of lungs	Absorption by diffusion of respiratory gases between alveolar air and blood
	Lining of blood and lymphatic vessels	Absorption by diffusion, filtration, and osmosis
Stratified squamous	Surface of lining of mouth and esophagus	Protection
	Surface of skin (epidermis)	Protection
Simple columnar	Surface layer of lining of stomach, intestines, and parts of respiratory tract	Protection; secretion; absorption
Stratified transitional	Urinary bladder	Protection
CONNECTIVE (most widely distributed of all tissues)		
Areolar	Between other tissues and organs	Connection
Adipose (fat)	Under skin	Protection
	Padding at various points	Insulation; support; reserve food
Dense fibrous	Tendons; ligaments	Flexible but strong connection
Bone	Skeleton	Support; protection
Cartilage	Part of nasal septum; covering articular surfaces of bones; larynx; rings in trachea and bronchi	Firm but flexible support
	Disks between vertebrae	
	External ear	
Blood	Blood vessels	Transportation
MUSCLE		
Skeletal (striated voluntary)	Muscles that attach to bones	Movement of bones
	Eyeball muscles	Eye movements
	Upper third of esophagus	First part of swallowing
Cardiac (striated involuntary)	Wall of heart	Contraction of heart
Visceral (nonstriated involuntary or smooth)	In walls of tubular viscera of digestive, respiratory, and genitourinary tracts	Movement of substances along respective tracts
	In walls of blood vessels and large lymphatic vessels	Changing of diameter of blood vessels
	In ducts of glands	Movement of substances along ducts
	Intrinsic eye muscles (iris and ciliary body)	Changing of diameter of pupils and shape of lens
	Arrector muscles of hairs	Erection of hairs (gooseflesh)
NERVOUS		
	Brain; spinal cord; nerves	Irritability; conduction

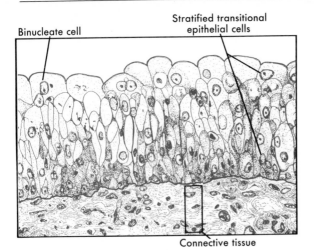

Binucleate cell

Stratified transitional epithelial cells

Connective tissue

Fig. 1-1. Epithelial cells exist in several layers.

and secretion (as in glands). A principal physiological characteristic of epithelial tissue is that it contains no blood supply per se, so it must depend upon the process of diffusion for nutrition, oxygenation, and elimination of waste products. Most sports-related injuries to this type of tissue are traumatic, including abrasions, lacerations, punctures, and avulsions. Other injuries to this tissue may include infection, inflammation, or disease.

Connective Tissue

A second tissue type is connective tissue. This complex tissue is comprised of tendons, ligaments, adipose tissue, cartilage, blood, lymph, and bone. Connective tissue is the framework for most organs; it supports and protects the body. Fat connective tissue, that is, adipose tissue, has the primary functions of energy storage and metabolism. A tendon connects muscle to bone; the Achilles tendon connecting the gastrocnemius muscle to the calcaneus is one of the largest tendons of the body. An aponeurosis is a flattened, sheetlike tendon. Another type of connective tissue is the ligament, which functions to connect bone to bone. Cartilage is a firm connective tissue with great structure. It is found within the knee joint, where it acts as a shock absorber and distributor of forces, and in the nose and ear. Bone, the densest of all connective tissue, is discussed in a later section. The final

component of the connective tissue category is blood and lymph. Although this component does not function in structure, it is essential for the nutrition, cleansing, and physiology of the body.

The principle cell of the connective tissue is the fibroblast, which produces collagen and elastin. Collagen is a major structural protein that forms strong, flexible, inelastic structures. Elastin, however, produces highly elastic tissues. Examples of collagen tissues are tendons, ligaments, and resistant membranes, whereas elastin primarily forms the walls of blood vessels, especially the larger arteries. Other cells in connective tissue include macrophages, mast cells, plasma cells, and white blood cells. With connective tissue playing such a major role throughout the human body, that it is the location of most sports-related injuries is not surprising. These injuries include all sprains and strains, as well as a significant number of contusions, inflammations, traumas, overuse syndromes, infections, and ruptures.

Muscle Tissue

Muscle tissue is often considered to be a type of connective tissue, but here it is treated as the third of the fundamental tissues. Muscular tissue is designed to contract and thus provide movement of other tissues and organs. The three types of muscles are smooth (involuntary), cardiac, and skeletal (voluntary). Smooth muscle is found within the viscera, where it forms the walls of the internal organs, and within many hollow chambers.

Cardiac muscle is found only in the heart and is responsible for its contraction. A significant characteristic of the cardiac muscle is that it contracts as a single fiber, unlike smooth and skeletal muscles, which contract as separate units. The importance of this characteristic is that it forces the heart to work as a single unit, continuously; therefore, if one portion of the muscle should die (as in myocardial infarction), the entire contraction of the heart does not cease.

Skeletal or voluntary muscle is the striated muscle within the body responsible for the movement of bony levers (Fig. 1-2). These muscles of the skeleton are composed of detailed filaments with a unique and complex physiology.

All muscles are composed of the cellular unit

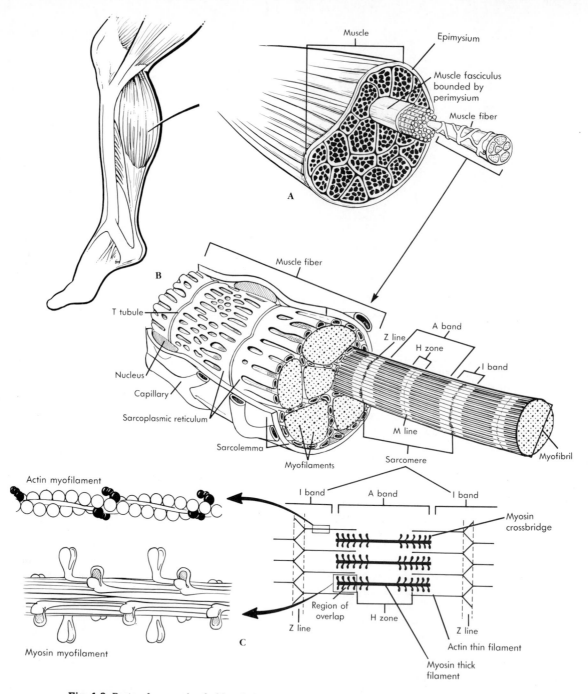

Fig. 1-2. Parts of a muscle. **A,** Muscle is composed of muscle fasciculi, which can be seen by the unaided eye as striations in the muscle. The fasciculi are composed of bundles of individual muscle fibers (muscle cells). **B,** Each muscle fiber contains myofibrils in which the banding patterns of the sarcomeres are seen. **C,** The myofibrils are composed of actin myofilament and myosin myofilaments, which are formed from thousands of individual actin and myosin molecules.

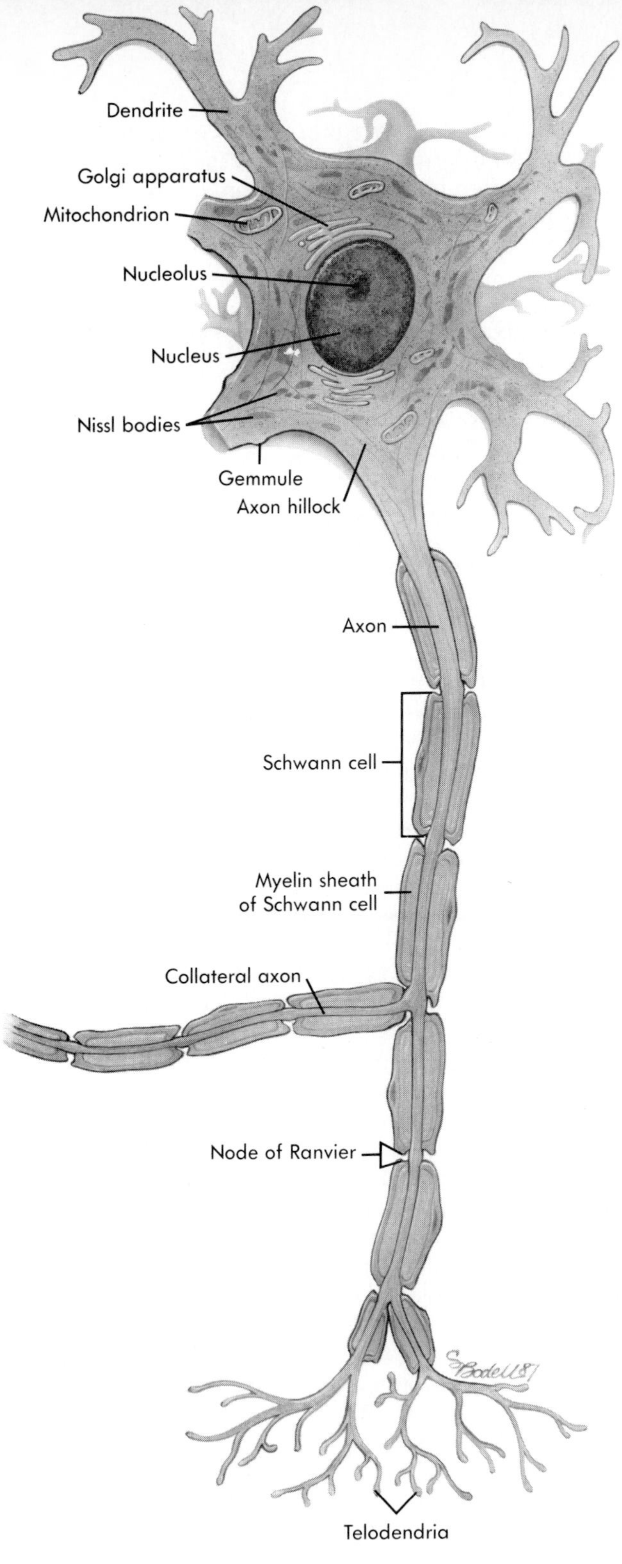
Dendrite
Golgi apparatus
Mitochondrion
Nucleolus
Nucleus
Nissl bodies
Gemmule
Axon hillock
Axon
Schwann cell
Myelin sheath
of Schwann cell
Collateral axon
Node of Ranvier
Telodendria

Fig. 1-3. Structural features of a nerve cell.

referred to as a **muscle fiber.** Muscle fibers are grouped into bundles that are then termed **fasciculi.** Of the various types of muscle fibers, the three to be discussed here are:

1. Slow twitch, type I
2. Intermediate fibers, type IIA
3. Fast twitch, type IIB

These fibers are differentiated by their biochemistry, fuel or substrate preference, strength, fatigability, and blood supply. Slow-twitch, type I fibers, for instance, are low-intensity, high-endurance fibers, specifically high oxidative and low glycolytic, whereas fast-twitch, type IIB fibers are high intensity with rapid fatigability, and therefore have high glycolytic and low oxidative properties. Muscular injuries involve contusions, strains, myositis ossificans, infections, and inflammations.

Nerve Tissue

The final fundamental tissue is nerve tissue (Fig. 1-3). This tissue provides sensitivity and communication from the central nervous system (brain and spinal cord) to the muscles, sensory organs, various systems, and the periphery. The basic nerve cell is the neuron. A nerve itself is a bundle of nerve cells held together by some connective tissue, usually a lipid-protein layer called **myelin.** Neurology is an extremely complex science, and only a brief presentation of its relation to sports-related injuries is covered here. Most often, nerves are involved in contusions and inflammations. More serious injuries involve the crushing of a nerve or complete division (severing). This type of injury may produce the serious consequences of a life-long physical disability such as paraplegia or quadriplegia and should therefore not be overlooked in any circumstance.

Bone Tissue

Bone is a type of connective tissue consisting of both living cells and minerals deposited in a matrix (Fig. 1-4). The two types of bone material are **cancellous** or spongy bone and **cortical** or compact bone. Cancellous bone contains a series of air spaces referred to as *trabeculae,* whereas cortical bone is relatively solid. Bone has a rich blood supply that certainly facilitates the healing process following injury.

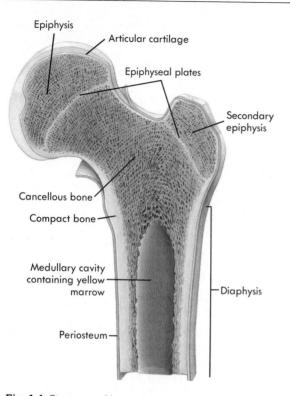

Fig. 1-4. Structure of bone shown in cross-section.

Bone has the functions of support, movement, and protection. Furthermore, bone stores and releases calcium into the bloodstream and manufactures red blood cells.

MUSCULOSKELETAL INJURIES
Fractures

Fractures are extremely common injuries among the athletic population. They can be generally classified as being either simple or compound. A simple fracture, also sometimes called a *closed* fracture, involves little or no displacement of the bones; a compound or open fracture involves enough displacement of the fractured ends that the bone actually disrupts the cutaneous layers and breaks through the skin. Both fractures can be relatively serious if not managed properly, but an increased possibility of infection exists in a compound fracture.

The varieties of fractures that can occur include green-stick, transverse, oblique, spiral, comminuted, impacted, avulsive, and stress fractures. A **green-stick** fracture (Fig. 1-5, *A*) occurs most often in children whose bones are still growing and have not yet had a chance to calcify and harden. It is called a green-stick fracture because of the resemblance to the splintering that occurs to a tree twig that is bent to the point of breaking. Because the twig is green, it splinters but can be bent without causing an actual break. A physician may or may not elect to splint or cast a green-stick fracture, depending on where the injury has occurred.

A **transverse** fracture (Fig. 1-5, *B*) involves a crack perpendicular to the longitudinal axis of the bone that goes all the way through the bone. Displacement may occur; however, because of the shape of the fractured ends, the soft tissue (such as muscles, tendons, and fat) that surrounds it sustains relatively little damage.

An **oblique** fracture (Fig. 1-5, *C*) results in a diagonal crack across the bone and two very jagged, pointed ends that, if displaced, can potentially cause a good bit of soft tissue damage. Oblique and spiral fractures are the two types most likely to result in compound fractures.

A **spiral** fracture (Fig. 1-5, *D*) is similar to an oblique fracture in that the angle of the fracture is diagonal across the bone. In addition, an element of twisting or rotation causes the fracture to spiral along the longitudinal axis of the bone. Spiral fractures used to be fairly common in ski injuries occurring just above the top of the boot when the bindings on the ski failed to release when the foot was rotated. These injuries are now less common due to improvements in equipment design.

A **comminuted** fracture (Fig. 1-5, *E*), also sometimes called a **blowout fracture,** is a serious problem that may require an extremely long time for rehabilitation. In the comminuted fracture, multiple fragments of bone must be surgically repaired and fixed with screws and wires. If a fracture of this type occurs to a weight-bearing bone, as in the leg, a permanent discrepancy in leg length may develop.

In an **impacted** fracture (Fig. 1-5, *F*), one end of the fractured bone is driven up into the other end. As with the comminuted fracture, correcting discrepancies in the length of the extremity may require long periods of intensive rehabilitation.

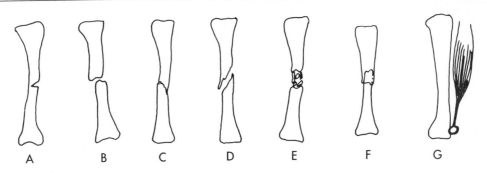

Fig. 1-5. Fractures of bone: **A,** green-stick; **B,** transverse; **C,** oblique; **D,** spiral; **E,** comminuted; **F,** impacted; and **G,** avulsion.

An **avulsion** fracture (Fig. 1-5, *G*) occurs when a fragment of bone is pulled away at the bony attachment of a muscle, tendon, or ligament. Avulsion fractures are common in the fingers and some of the smaller bones but can also occur in larger bones whose tendinous or ligamentous attachments are subjected to a large amount of force.

In most instances, fracture of a bone requires immobilization for some period of time. In general, fractures of the long bones of the arm and leg require approximately 6 weeks of casting, and the smaller bones may require as little as 3 weeks of either casting or splinting. In some instances, for example, the four small toes, immobilization may not be required for healing. Of course, any complications may lengthen the time required for casting as well as rehabilitation.

In order for a fracture to heal, bone-producing cells called *osteoblasts* must lay down a bony callus over the fracture site during the period of immobilization. Once the cast is removed, the bone must be subjected to normal stresses and strains so that tensile strength may be regained before the healing process is complete.

Perhaps the most common fracture resulting from physical activity is the stress fracture. Unlike the other types of fractures that have been discussed, the stress fracture results from overuse rather than acute trauma. Common sites for stress fractures include the weight-bearing bones of the leg and foot.

In either case, repetitive forces transmitted through the bones produce irritations at specific areas. The pain usually begins as a dull ache that becomes progressively painful day after day. Initially pain is most severe during activity. However, when a stress fracture actually develops, pain becomes worse after the activity is stopped.

The biggest problem with a stress fracture is that often it does not show up on an x-ray until the osteoblasts begin laying down bone, at which point a small white line appears. If a stress fracture is suspected, the athlete ought to stop strenuous activity for a period of at least 14 days. Stress fractures do not usually require casting but may become normal fractures that must be immobilized if not handled correctly.

The only definitive technique for determining if a fracture does exist is to x-ray it. If a fracture does occur, it should be managed and rehabilitated by a qualified orthopedist, sports therapist, and/or physical therapist.

Dislocations and Subluxations

A dislocation occurs when at least one bone in an articulation is forced out of its normal and proper alignment and stays out until it is either manually or surgically put back into place or reduced. Dislocations most commonly occur in the shoulder joint, elbow, and fingers, but they can occur wherever two bones articulate.

A subluxation is like a dislocation except that in this situation a bone pops out of its normal articulation but then goes right back into place. Subluxations most commonly occur in the shoulder joint, as well as in the knee cap in females.

Dislocations should never be reduced immediately, regardless of where they occur. The sports therapist ought to take the athlete to a hospital where x-rays can be taken to rule out

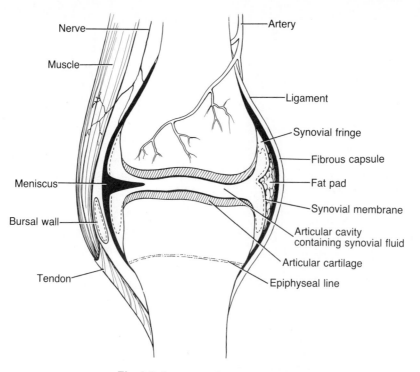

Fig. 1-6. Structure of a synovial joint.

fractures or other problems prior to reduction. Inappropriate techniques of reduction may only exacerbate the problem.

Ligament Sprains

A sprain involves damage to a ligament that provides support to a joint. A ligament is a tough, relatively inelastic band of tissue that connects one bone to another.

Before discussing injuries to joints, a review of joint structure is in order (Fig. 1-6). All joints are composed of two or more bones that articulate with one another to allow motion in one or more places. The articulating surfaces of the bone are lined with a very thin, smooth, cartilaginous covering called a **hyaline cartilage.** All joints are entirely surrounded by a thick ligamentous joint capsule. The inner surface of this joint capsule is lined by a very thin synovial membrane that is highly vascularized and innervated. The synovial membrane produces synovial fluid, the functions of which include lubrication, shock absorption, and nutrition of the joint.

Some joints contain a thick fibrocartilage called a **meniscus.** The knee joint, for example, contains two wedge-shaped menisci that deepen the articulation and provide shock absorption in that joint.

Finally, the main structural support and joint stability is provided by the ligaments, which may be either thickened portions of a joint capsule or totally separate bands. The anatomical positioning of the ligaments determines in part what motions a joint can make.

If stress is applied to a joint that forces motion beyond its normal limits or planes of movement, injury to the ligament is likely (Fig. 1-7). The severity of damage to the ligament is classified in many different ways; however, the most commonly used system involves three degrees of ligamentous sprain.

First-degree sprain: There is some stretching or perhaps tearing of the ligamentous fibers with little or no joint instability. Mild pain, little swelling, and joint stiffness may be apparent.

Second-degree sprain: There is some tearing

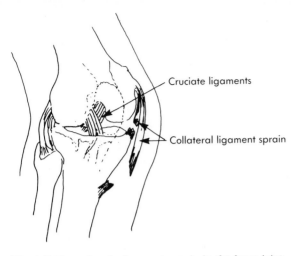

Fig. 1-7. Example of a ligament sprain in the knee joint.

and separation of the ligamentous fibers and moderate instability of the joint. Moderate to severe pain, swelling, and joint stiffness should be expected.

Third-degree sprain: There is total rupture of the ligament, manifested primarily by gross instability of the joint. Severe pain may be present initially, followed by little or no pain due to total disruption of nerve fibers. Swelling may be profuse and thus the joint tends to become very stiff some hours following the injury. A third-degree sprain with marked instability usually requires surgical repair. Frequently the force producing the ligament injury is so great that other ligaments or structures surrounding the joint may also be injured.

Rehabilitation of third-degree sprains involving surgery is a long-term process. For example, a rehabilitation program following knee surgery may last for 12 to 15 months before normal functional activity returns.

The biggest problem in the rehabilitation of first- and second-degree sprains is restoring stability to the joint. Once a ligament has been stretched or partially torn, inelastic scar tissue forms and prevents the ligament from regaining its original tension. Thus to restore stability to the joint, the other structures that surround that joint, primarily muscles and their tendons, must be strengthened. The increased muscle tension provided by strength training can have some effect on improving stability of the injured joint.

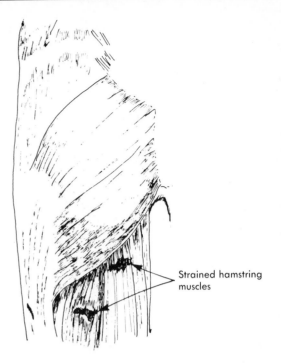

Fig. 1-8. A muscle strain results in tearing or separation of fibers.

Muscle Strains

The muscle is basically composed of separate fibers that are capable of simultaneous contraction when stimulated by the central nervous system. Each muscle is attached to bone at both proximal and distal ends by strong, relatively inelastic tendons that cross over joints.

If a muscle is overstretched or forced to contract against too much resistance, damage occurs to the muscle fibers. This separation or tearing of muscle fibers is referred to as a *strain* (Fig. 1-8). Muscle strains, like ligament sprains, are subject to various classification systems. The following is a simple system of classification of muscle strains:

First-degree strain: Some muscle fibers have been stretched or actually torn. Active motion produces some tenderness and pain. Movement is painful, but full range of motion is usually possible.

Second-degree strain: Some muscle fibers have been torn, and active contraction of the muscle is extremely painful. Usually a palpable depression or divot exists somewhere in the muscle belly at the spot where the muscle fibers have been torn. Some swelling may occur because of capillary bleeding.

Third-degree strain: There is a complete rupture of a muscle in the muscle belly, in the area where muscle becomes tendon, or at the tendinous attachment to the bone. The athlete has significant impairment to or perhaps total loss of movement. Pain is intense initially but diminishes quickly because of complete separation of the nerve fibers.

Muscle strains can occur in any muscle and usually result from some uncoordinated activity between synergistic muscle groups. Third-degree strains are most common in the biceps tendon of the upper arm or in the Achilles heelcord in the back of the calf. When either of these tendons rupture, the muscle tends to bunch toward its proximal attachment. Third-degree strains involving large tendons that produce great amounts of force must be surgically repaired. Smaller musculotendinous ruptures, such as those that occur in the fingers, may heal by immobilization with a splint.

Regardless of the severity of the strain, the time required for rehabilitation is fairly lengthy. In many instances, rehabilitation time for a muscle strain is no longer than for a ligament sprain. These incapacitating muscle strains occur most frequently in the large, force-producing hamstring and quadriceps muscles of the lower extremity. The treatment of hamstring strains requires a healing period of 6 to 8 weeks and a considerable amount of patience. Trying to return to activity too soon frequently causes reinjury to the area of the muscle that has been strained, and the healing process must begin again.

Muscle Soreness

Overexertion in strenuous muscular exercise often results in muscular pain. Everyone at one time or another has experienced muscle soreness, usually resulting from some unaccustomed physical activity. Muscle soreness differs from a muscle strain in that soreness generally does not involve damage to the muscle fibers.

One type of muscle pain accompanies fatigue.

It is transient, occurs during and immediately after exercise, and can be attributed to the buildup of a product of anaerobic metabolism called **lactic acid.** Lactic acid accumulates in the muscle because of insufficient oxygen supply to the working muscle tissues and thus stimulates pain receptors in the area. In addition, fluid collects in the muscles during increased activity because of an increase in hydrostatic pressure, which results in swelling. The muscle becomes shorter and thicker and thus more resistant to stretching. Therefore, when a muscle is stretched, a sensation of stiffness may last for some time and is a symptom of the second type of muscle pain. An appropriate cool-down period can facilitate the removal of lactic acid and thus reduce the acute effects of muscular exertion.

The second type of muscle soreness involves delayed muscle pain that appears approximately 12 hours after injury. It becomes most intense after 24 to 48 hours and then gradually subsides so that the muscle becomes symptom free after 4 to 6 days. This second type of pain may best be described as a syndrome of delayed muscle pain caused by muscle spasm leading to increased muscle tension, edema formation, increased stiffness, and resistance to stretching.

Delayed muscle pain has been hypothesized to be caused by the tonic, localized spasm of motor units, varying in number with the severity of pain. This theory, known as the **spasm theory,** can be explained on the basis that exercise causes varying degrees of ischemia in the working muscles. This ischemia causes pain, which results in reflex tonic muscle contraction that increases and prolongs the ischemia. Consequently a cycle of increasing severity is begun. To eliminate this muscle soreness, this cycle must be broken by allowing the muscle to rest over a period of days. Treatment of muscle soreness usually also involves static or PNF stretching activity. As with other conditions discussed in this chapter, ice is important as a treatment for muscle soreness, particularly within the first 48 to 72 hours.

Tendonitis

Of all the overuse problems associated with physical activity, tendonitis is probably the most common. During muscle activity a tendon must move or slide on other structures around it whenever the muscle contracts. If a particular movement is performed repeatedly, the tendon becomes irritated and inflamed. This inflammation is manifested by pain on movement, redness, swelling, possibly some warmth, and usually crepitus. Crepitus is a crackling sound similar to the sound produced by rolling hair between the fingers by the ear. Crepitus is usually caused by the tendon's adhering to the surrounding structure as it slides back and forth. This adhesion is caused primarily by the chemical products of inflammation that accumulate on the irritated tendon.

As indicated later in this chapter, the inflammatory process is an essential part of healing. Inflammation is supposed to be an acute process that has an end point after its function in the healing process has been fulfilled. However, if the source of irritation (that is, the repetitive movements that cause stress to the tendon) is not removed, then the inflammatory process becomes chronic rather than acute. When this occurs, tendonitis may become disabling.

The key to the treatment of tendonitis is rest. If the repetitive motion causing irritation to the tendon is eliminated, chances are the inflammatory process allows the tendon to heal. Unfortunately, an athlete who is seriously involved with some physical activity may have difficulty abstaining for 2 weeks or more while the tendonitis subsides. An alternative activity such as bicycling or swimming is advisable to maintain fitness levels to a certain degree while allowing the tendon a chance to heal.

Tendonitis most commonly occurs in the Achilles tendon in the back of the lower leg in runners or in the muscle tendons of the shoulder joint in swimmers, although it can certainly flare up in any tendon in which overuse and repetitive movements occur.

Tenosynovitis

Tenosynovitis is very similar to tendonitis in that the muscle tendons are involved in inflammation. However, many tendons are subject to an increased amount of friction due to the tightness of the space through which they must move. In these areas of high friction, tendons are usually surrounded by synovial sheaths that are in effect

bursae that reduce friction on movement. If the tendon sliding through these bursal sheaths is subjected to overuse, inflammation is likely to occur. The inflammatory process produces by-products that are sticky and tend to cause the sliding tendon to adhere to the synovial sheath surrounding it.

Symptomatically, tenosynovitis is very similar to tendonitis, with pain on movement, tenderness, swelling, and crepitus. Movement may be more limited with tenosynovitis because the space provided for the tendon and its synovial covering is more limited.

Tenosynovitis occurs most commonly in the long flexor tendons of the fingers as they cross over the wrist joint and in the biceps tendon around the shoulder joint.

Treatment for tenosynovitis is the same as for tendonitis. Because both conditions involve inflammation, mild antiinflammatory drugs such as aspirin may be helpful in chronic cases.

Bursitis

In many areas, particularly around joints, friction occurs between tendons and bones, skin and bone, or two muscles. Without some mechanism of protection in these high-friction areas, chronic irritation would be likely.

Bursae are small, fibrous sacs lined with synovial membrane that contain small amounts of synovial fluid. These small bags of synovium permit motion of these structures without friction.

If excessive movement or perhaps some acute trauma occurs around these bursae, they become irritated and inflamed and begin producing large amounts of synovial fluid. The longer the irritation continues or the more severe the acute trauma, the more fluid is produced. As the fluid continues to accumulate in a limited space, pressure tends to increase and cause irritation of the pain receptors in the area.

Bursitis can be an extremely painful condition that has the capability of severely restricting movement, especially if it occurs around a joint. Synovial fluid continues to be produced until the movement or trauma producing the irritation is eliminated.

A bursa sac that occasionally completely surrounds a tendon to allow more freedom of movement in a tight area is referred to as a **synovial sheath.** Irritation of this synovial sheath may restrict tendon motion.

All joints have many bursae surrounding them. The three bursae most commonly irritated as a result of various types of physical activity are the subacromial bursa in the shoulder joint under the clavicle, the olecranon bursa on the tip of the elbow, and the prepatellar bursa on the front surface of the patella. All three of these bursae have been known to produce large amounts of synovial fluid that affects motion at their respective joints.

Contusion

A contusion is synonymous with the term **bruise.** The mechanism that produces it is a blow from some external object that causes soft tissues (such as skin, fat, and muscle) to be compressed against the hard bone underneath. If the blow is hard enough, capillaries rupture and allow bleeding into the tissues. The bleeding, if superficial enough, causes a bluish purple discoloration to the skin that persists for several days. The contusion may be very sore to the touch. If damage has occurred to muscle, pain may be elicited on active movement. In most cases the pain ceases within a few days, and discoloration disappears in usually 2 to 3 weeks.

The major problem with contusions occurs where an area is subjected to repeated blows. If the same area or more specifically a muscle is bruised over and over again, small calcium deposits may begin to accumulate in the injured area. These pieces of calcium may be found between several fibers in the muscle belly, or calcium may form a spur that projects from the underlying bone. These calcium formations, which may significantly impair movement, are referred to as **myositis ossificans.**

The key to preventing myositis ossificans occurring from repeated contusion is protection of the injured area by padding. If the area is properly protected following the first contusion, myositis ossificans may never develop. Protection, along with rest, may frequently allow the calcium to be reabsorbed and eliminate any need for surgical intervention.

The two areas that seem to be the most vulnerable to repeated contusions during physical activity are the quadriceps muscle group on the front of the thigh and the biceps muscle on the front of the upper arm. The formation of myositis ossificans in either of these or any other areas may be detected by x-rays.

Osteoarthrosis

This condition needs to be mentioned because it is a degenerative condition of both bone and cartilage in and about the joint. **Arthritis** should be defined as primarily an inflammatory condition with possible secondary destruction. **Arthrosis** is primarily a degenerative process with destruction of cartilage, remodeling of bone, and possible secondary inflammatory components.

Cartilage fibrillates, that is, releases fibers or groups of fibers and ground substance into the joint. Peripheral cartilage that is not exposed to weight-bearing and/or compression-decompression mechanisms is particularly likely to fibrillate. Fibrillation is typically found in the degenerative process associated with poor nutrition or disuse. This process can then extend even to weight-bearing areas with progressive destruction of cartilage proportional to stresses applied on it. When forces are increased, thus increasing stress, osteochondral or subchondral fractures can occur. Concentration of stress on small areas may produce pressures that overwhelm the tissue's capabilities. Typically, lower limb joints have to handle greater stresses, but their surface area is typically larger than the surface area of upper limbs. The articular cartilage is protected to some extent by the synovial fluid, which acts as a lubricant. It is also protected by the subchondral bone, which responds to stresses in an elastic fashion. It is more compliant than compact bone, and microfractures may be a means of force absorption. Trabeculae may fracture or may be displaced due to pressures applied on the subchondral bone. In compact bone, fracture may be a means of defense to dissipate force. In the joint also, forces may be absorbed by joint movement and eccentric contraction of muscles. Typically in joints the surfaces are congruent. If they are not, certain areas concentrate the forces being applied, which favors joint degeneration. Osteophytosis is a response of bone to increase its surface area. Typically people describe these as "bone spurs." Chondromalacia is the nonprogressive transformation of cartilage with irregular surfaces and areas of softening. Typically it occurs in non-weight-bearing areas at first and may progress to areas of excessive stress.

In athletes, certain joints may be more susceptible to a response resembling osteoarthrosis. The proportion of body weight resting on the joint, the pull of musculotendinous tissue, and any significant external force applied to the joint are predisposing factors. Altered joint mechanics due to laxity or previous trauma are also factors that come into play. The intensity of forces may be great, as in the hip, where the above-mentioned factors can produce pressures or forces that may be four times that of body weight and up to ten times that of body weight on the knee. Typically muscle forces generate more stress than body weight itself.

Particular injuries are conducive to osteoarthritic changes such as subluxation and dislocation of the patella, osteochondritis dissecans, recurrent synovial effusion, and hemarthrosis. Also, ligamentous injuries may bring about a breakage in proprioceptive mechanisms, loss of adequate joint alignment, and meniscal damage in the knees with removal of the injured meniscus. Other factors that have an impact are loss of full range of motion, poor muscular power and strength, and altered biomechanics on the joint. Different joints are affected in different sports: the knee and ankle in European football, the hand in boxing, the shoulder and elbow in baseball, and the patella in cycling. This list is not exhaustive. In sport participation, however, spurring and spiking of bone are not synonymous with osteoarthrosis if the joint space is maintained and the cartilage lining is intact. It may simply be an adaptation to the increased stress of physical activity.

INITIAL MANAGEMENT OF INJURIES

Initial first aid and management techniques are perhaps the most critical part of any rehabilitation program. The initial management unquestionably has a significant impact on the course of the rehabilitative process. Regardless of the type of injury, the one problem they all have in common is swelling. Swelling may be caused by any number of factors, including bleeding, production of synovial fluid, an accumulation of inflammatory by-products, edema (which is nothing more than an accumulation of body fluid), or a combination of several factors. No matter which mechanism is involved, swelling produces an increased pressure in the injured area, and increased pressure causes pain. Swelling is most likely during the first 72 hours after an injury. Once swelling has occurred, the healing process is significantly retarded. The injured area cannot return to normal until all the swelling is gone.

Therefore, everything that is done in terms of first aid management of any of these conditions should be directed toward controlling the swelling. If the swelling can be controlled initially in the acute stage of injury, the time required for rehabilitation is likely to be significantly reduced.

To control and severely limit the amount of swelling, the RICE principle—rest, ice, compression, and elevation—can be applied (Fig. 1-9). Each factor plays a critical role in limiting swelling, and all should be used simultaneously.

Rest

Rest following any type of injury is an extremely important component of any treatment program. Once an anatomic structure is injured, it immediately begins the process of healing. If the injured structure is not rested and is subjected to external stress and strains, the healing process

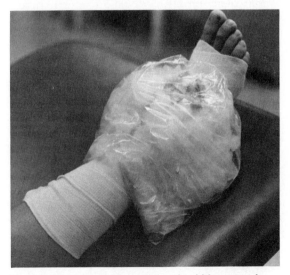

Fig. 1-9. Musculoskeletal injuries should be treated initially with ice, compression, and elevation.

never really gets a chance. Consequently, the injury does not get well, and the time required for rehabilitation is markedly increased. The number of days necessary for resting varies with the severity of the injury, but most minor injuries should rest for approximately 72 hours before an active rehabilitation program is begun.

Ice

In acute injury the use of cold is the initial treatment of choice for most conditions involving injuries to the musculoskeletal system. It is most commonly used immediately after injury to decrease pain and promote local vasoconstriction, thus controlling hemorrhage and edema. It is also used in the acute phase of inflammatory conditions such as bursitis, tenosynovitis, and tendonitis in which heat may cause additional pain and swelling. Cold is also used to reduce the reflex muscle spasm and spastic conditions that accompany pain. Its analgesic effect is probably one of its greatest benefits. One explanation of the analgesic effect is that cold decreases the velocity of nerve conduction, although it does not entirely eliminate it. Cold may also bombard central pain receptor areas with so many cold impulses that pain impulses are lost. With ice treatments, the athlete reports an uncomfortable sensation of cold, followed by burning, an aching sensation, and finally complete numbness.

Because of the low thermal conductivity of underlying subcutaneous fat tissues, applications of cold for short periods are ineffective in cooling deeper tissues. For this reason longer treatments of 20 to 30 minutes are recommended. Cold treatments are generally believed to be more effective in reaching deep tissues than most forms of heat. Cold applied to the skin is capable of significantly lowering the temperature of tissues at a considerable depth. The extent of this lowered tissue temperature depends on the type of cold applied to the skin, the duration of its application, the thickness of the subcutaneous fat, and the region of the body to which it is applied. Ice should be applied to the area for at least 72 hours after an acute injury.

Compression

Compression is equally as important as ice for controlling swelling. The purpose of compression

is to reduce the amount of space available for swelling by applying pressure around an injured area. The best way of applying pressure is to use an elastic wrap (such as an Ace bandage) to apply firm but even pressure around the injury.

Because of the pressure buildup in the tissues, having a compression wrap in place for a long time may become painful. However, the wrap must be kept in place despite significant pain because it is so important in the control of swelling. The compression wrap should be left in place for at least 72 hours after an acute injury. In many chronic overuse problems, such as tendonitis, tenosynovitis, and particularly bursitis, the compression wrap should be worn until the swelling is almost entirely gone.

Elevation

The fourth factor that assists in controlling swelling is elevation. The injured part, particularly an extremity, should be elevated to eliminate the effects of gravity on blood pooling in the extremities. Elevation assists venous drainage of blood and other fluids from the injured area back to the central circulatory system. The greater the degree of elevation, the more effective the reduction in swelling. For example, in an ankle sprain, the leg should be placed in such a position that the ankle is virtually straight up in the air. The injured part should be elevated as much as possible during the first 72 hours.

The appropriate technique for initial management of the acute injuries discussed in this chapter, regardless of where they occur, would be the following:

1. Apply a compression wrap directly over the injury. Wrapping should be from distal to proximal. Tension should be firm and consistent. Wetting the elastic wrap to facilitate the passage of cold from ice packs may be helpful.
2. Surround the injured area entirely with ice bags and secure them in place. Ice bags should be left on for 45 minutes initially and then 1 hour off and 30 minutes on as much as possible over the next 24 hours. During the following 48-hour period, ice should be applied as often as possible.
3. The injured part should be elevated as much as possible during the initial 72-hour

period after injury. Keeping the injury elevated while sleeping is particularly important.

4. Allow the injured part to rest for approximately 72 hours following the injury.

UNDERSTANDING THE HEALING PROCESS

Rehabilitation programs must be based on the framework of the healing process. The sports therapist must have a sound understanding of the healing process not only in terms of the sequence of the various stages of healing that take place but also with regard to the approximate time lines for each stage. Basically the healing process consists of the inflammatory phase, the fibroblastic phase, and the maturation phase. The healing process is a continuum. Phases of the healing process overlap one another and have no definitive beginning or end points.

Inflammatory Phase

Once a tissue is injured, the process of healing begins immediately (Fig. 1-10, *A*). The destruction of tissue produces direct injury to the cells of the various soft tissues discussed previously. Cellular injury results in altered metabolism and the liberation of materials that initiate the inflammatory process. It is characterized by redness, swelling, tenderness, and increased temperature.

Inflammation is a process by means of which leukocytes and other phagocytic cells and exudate accumulate in the injured tissue in order to protect the area from further injury. This reaction is generally protective, tending to localize or dispose of injury by-products (for example, blood, damaged cells) through phagocytosis and thus setting the stage for repair. Locally vascular effects, disturbances of fluid exchange, and migration of leukocytes from the blood to the tissues occur.

The vascular reaction involves vascular spasm, formation of a platelet plug, blood coagulation, and growth of fibrous tissue. The immediate response to damage is a vasoconstriction of the vascular walls that last for approximately 5 to 10 minutes. This spasm presses the opposing endothelial linings together to produce a local anemia that is rapidly replaced by hyperemia of the area due to dilation. This increase in

blood flow is transitory and gives way to slowing of the flow in the dilated vessels, which then progresses to stagnation and stasis. The initial effusion of blood and plasma lasts for 24 to 36 hours.

Histamine released from the injured mast cells causes vasodilation and increased cell permeability, owing to swelling of endothelial cells, and then separation between the cells. Increased cell permeability locally affects passage of the fluid and cells through cell walls to form exudate. Therefore, vasodilation and active hyperemia are important in exudate formation and supplying leukocytes to the injured area. By and large, exudate is plasma from blood.

Platelets do not normally adhere to the vascular wall. However, injury to a vessel disrupts the endothelium and exposes the collagen fibers. Platelets adhere to the collagen fibers to create a sticky matrix on the vascular wall, to which additional platelets and leukocytes adhere and eventually form a plug. These plugs obstruct local lymphatic fluid drainage and thus localize the injury response.

The event that precipitates clot formation is the conversion of fibrinogen to fibrin. This transformation occurs due to a cascading effect beginning with the release of a protein molecule called **thromboplastin** from the damaged cell. Thromboplastin causes prothrombin to be changed into thrombin, which in turn causes the conversion of fibrinogen into a very sticky fibrin clot that shuts off blood supply to the injured area. Clot formation begins around 12 hours following injury and is completed by 48 hours.

As a result of a combination of these factors, the injured area becomes walled off during the inflammatory stage of healing. The leukocytes phagocytize most of the foreign debris toward the end of the inflammatory stage.

Fibroplastic Phase

During the fibroplastic stage of healing, proliferative and reparative activity leading to scar formation follows the vascular and exudative phenomena of inflammation and to some extent occur simultaneously (Fig. 1-10, *B*). The period of scar formation referred to as *fibroplasia* begins within the first few hours following injury and lasts for as long as 4 weeks. During this phase, fibroblasts and endothelial budding of capillaries

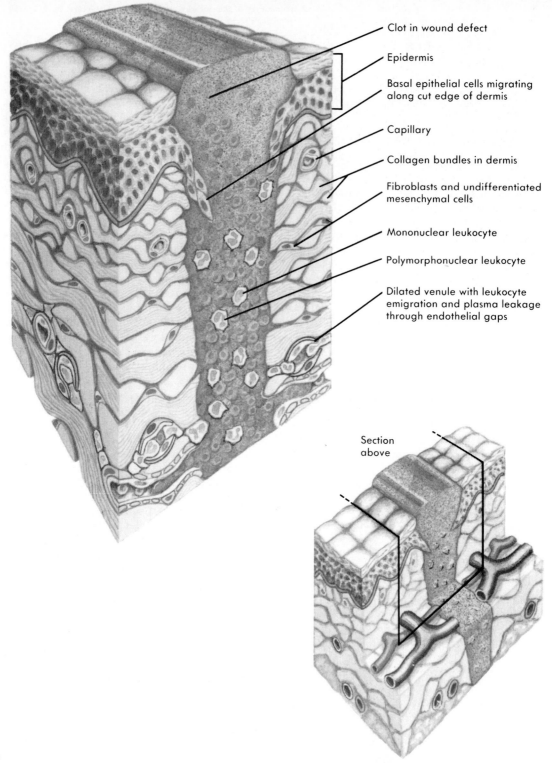

Clot in wound defect

Epidermis

Basal epithelial cells migrating along cut edge of dermis

Capillary

Collagen bundles in dermis

Fibroblasts and undifferentiated mesenchymal cells

Mononuclear leukocyte

Polymorphonuclear leukocyte

Dilated venule with leukocyte emigration and plasma leakage through endothelial gaps

Section above

A

Fig. 1-10. The healing process: **A,** inflammatory phase.

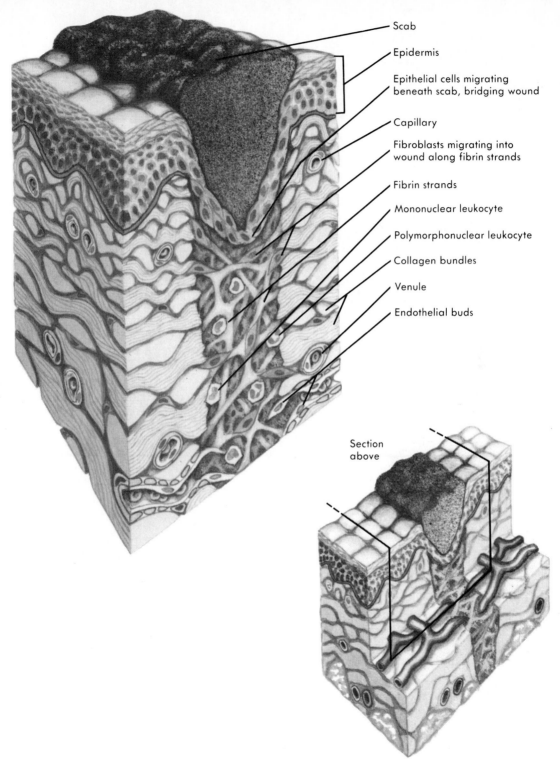

Scab

Epidermis

Epithelial cells migrating
beneath scab, bridging wound

Capillary

Fibroblasts migrating into
wound along fibrin strands

Fibrin strands

Mononuclear leukocyte

Polymorphonuclear leukocyte

Collagen bundles

Venule

Endothelial buds

Section
above

B

Fig. 1-10, cont'd. B, Fibroplastic phase.

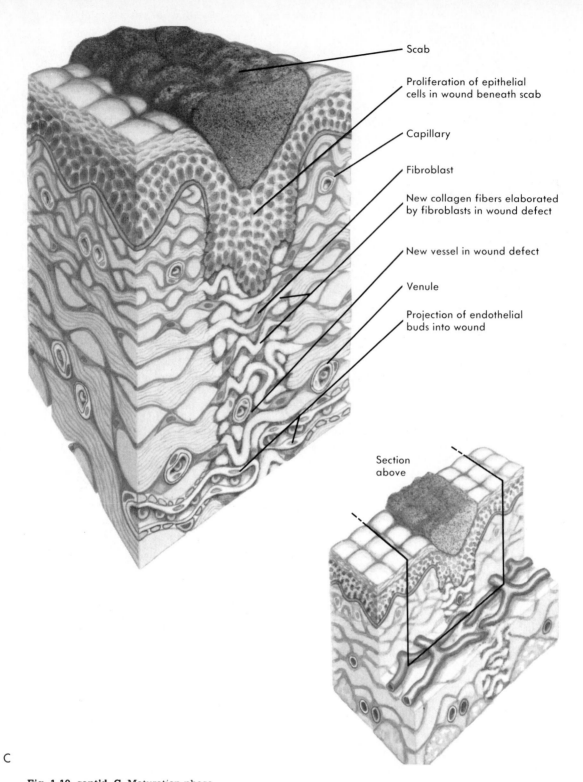

Scab

Proliferation of epithelial cells in wound beneath scab

Capillary

Fibroblast

New collagen fibers elaborated by fibroblasts in wound defect

New vessel in wound defect

Venule

Projection of endothelial buds into wound

Section above

C

Fig. 1-10, cont'd. C, Maturation phase.

invade the wound. In addition, the formation of granulation tissue occurs with the breakdown of the fibrin clot. Granulation tissue is a highly vascularized, reddish granular mass of connective tissue that fills in the gaps during the healing process.

Fibroblastic cells synthesize the mucopolysaccharides and glycoproteins which form the ground substance of connective tissue. On about the third day, they also begin producing collagen fibers that are deposited in a random fashion throughout the forming scar. As the collagen continues to proliferate, the tensile strength of the wound rapidly increases in proportion to the rate of collagen synthesis. As the tensile strength increases, the number of fibroblasts diminishes to signal the beginning of the maturation phase.

Maturation Phase

The maturation phase of healing is a long-term process (Fig. 1-10, *C)*. This phase features a realignment or remodeling of the collagen fibers that make up the scar tissue according to the tensile forces to which that scar is subjected. Ongoing breakdown and synthesis of collagen occur with a steady increase in the tensile strength of the scar matrix. The collagen fibers realign in a position of maximum efficiency parallel to the lines of tension. The tissue gradually assumes normal appearance and function, although a scar is rarely as strong as the normal injured tissue. Usually by the end of approximately 3 weeks, a firm, strong, contracted, nonvascular scar exists. The maturation phase of healing may require several years to be totally complete.

Tissue Repair

Tissue repair may occur either through regeneration of tissue or by replacement. Regeneration results in complete restitution in both appearance and function of the destroyed tissue. In replacement, a different type of tissue develops and eventually results in a scar and also in a decrease in tissue function. Most wounds heal through some combination of these two processes.

Factors That Impede Healing

EDEMA. The increased pressure caused by swelling retards the healing process, causes separation of tissues, and impedes nutrition in the injured part. Edema is best controlled and managed during the initial first aid management period as described previously.

HEMORRHAGE. Bleeding occurs with even the smallest amount of damage to the capillaries. Bleeding produces the same negative effects on healing as does the accumulation of edema, and its presence produces additional tissue damage and thus exacerbation of the injury.

SEPARATION OF TISSUE. Mechanical separation may result from the force of the injury, tissue separation may occur due to the presence of tissue between the torn ends of tissue, or lack of proper immobilization may cause tissue separation. The results are the same in that healing takes longer due to the widened gap that must be bridged by granulation tissue, and a larger scar develops.

MUSCLE SPASM. Muscle spasm causes traction on the torn tissue, separates the two ends, and prevents approximation. Both local and generalized ischemia may result from spasm.

ATROPHY. Wasting away of muscle tissue begins immediately with injury. Strengthening and early mobilization of the injured structure retards atrophy.

CORTICOSTEROIDS. Use of corticosteroids in the treatment of inflammation is controversial. Steroid use in the early stages of healing has been demonstrated to inhibit fibroplasia, capillary proliferation, collagen synthesis, and increases in tensile strength of the healing scar. Their use in the later stages of healing and with chronic inflammation is debatable.

KELOIDS AND HYPERTROPHIC SCARS. Keloids occur when the rate of collagen production exceeds the rate of collagen breakdown during the maturation phase of healing. This process leads to hypertrophy of scar tissue, particularly around the periphery of the wound.

INFECTION. Perhaps the most common deterrent to the healing process is infection. Any injury to soft tissue has the potential to become infected. Infection must be controlled before the healing process can advance to the latter stages.

HUMIDITY, CLIMATE, AND OXYGEN TENSION. Humidity significantly influences the process of epithelization. Occlusive dressings stimulate the epithelium to migrate twice as fast without crust or scab formation. The formation of a scab occurs with dehydration of the wound and traps wound drainage, which promotes infection. Keeping the wound moist provides an advantage for the necrotic debris to go to the surface and be shed.

Oxygen tension relates to the neovascularization of the wound, which translates into optimal saturation and maximal tensile strength development. Circulation to the wound can be affected by ischemia, venous stasis, hematomas, and vessel trauma.

HEALTH, AGE, AND NUTRITION. The elastic qualities of the skin decrease with aging. Degenerative diseases such as diabetes and arteriosclerosis also become a concern of the older athlete and may affect wound healing. Nutrition is important for wound healing. In particular, vitamin C (scurvy), vitamin K (clotting), vitamins A and E (collagen synthesis), zinc for the enzyme systems, and amino acids play critical roles in the healing process.

TENDON HEALING

Unlike most soft tissue healing, tendon injuries pose a particular problem in rehabilitation. The injured tendon requires both dense fibrous union of the separated ends and extensibility and flexibility at the site of attachment. Thus an abundance of collagen is required to achieve good tensile strength. Unfortunately, collagen can form adhesions to the surrounding tissues that interfere with the gliding that is essential for smooth motion. Fortunately, over a period of time the scar tissue of the surrounding tissues becomes elongated in its structure because of a breakdown in the cross-links between fibrin units and thus allows the necessary gliding motion. A tendon injury that occurs where the tendon is surrounded by a synovial sheath can potentially be devastating.

A typical time frame for tendon healing would be that during the second week the healing tendon adheres to the surrounding tissue to form a single mass. During the third week, the tendon separates to varying degrees from the surrounding tissues. However, the tensile strength is not sufficient to permit a strong pull on the tendon for at least 4 to 5 weeks, the danger being that a strong contraction can pull the tendon ends apart.

BONE HEALING

Healing of injured bone tissue is similar to soft tissue healing in that all phases of the healing process may be identified, although bone regeneration capabilities are somewhat limited. However, the functional elements of healing differ significantly from those of soft tissue. Tensile strength of the scar is the single most critical factor in soft tissue healing, whereas bone has to contend with a number of additional forces including torsion, bending, and compression. Trauma to bone may vary from contusions of the periosteum to simple, nondisplaced fractures to severely displaced compound fractures that also involve significant soft tissue damage.

In a fracture, hemorrhaging from the marrow is contained by the periosteum and the surrounding soft tissue in the region of the fracture. The fibrin strands within the clot serve as the framework for proliferating vessels along with fibroblasts and osteogenic cells called *osteoblasts* during the repair phase. Mechanical disturbance of the periosteum activates these osteoblasts to proliferate. Osteoblasts produce new periosteal bone along the outer surface of the shaft. It acts as an anchor for the callus, which is essentially a fibrous matrix of collagen. At first the callus is soft and firm because it is composed primarily of fibrin. The callus becomes firm and more rubbery as cartilage begins to predominate. Finally the callus crystalizes into bone, at which point remodeling of the bone begins. The size of the callus is proportional both to the damage and to the amount of irritation to the fracture site during the healing process.

The remodeling process is similar to the growth process of bone in that the fibrous cartilage is gradually replaced by fibrous bone and then by more structurally efficient lamellar bone. Remodeling involves an ongoing process during which osteoblasts lay down new bone and osteoclasts remove and break down bone according to the forces placed upon the healing bone.

The time required for bone healing is variable

and based on a number of factors such as severity of the fracture, site of the fracture, extensiveness of the trauma, and age of the patient. Normal periods of immobilization range from as short as 3 weeks for the small bones in the hands and feet to as long as 8 weeks in the long bones of the upper and lower extremities. The healing process is certainly not complete when the splint or cast is removed. Osteoblastic and osteoclastic activity may continue for 2 to 3 years following severe fractures.

NERVE TISSUE REGENERATION

Specialized tissue such as nerve cells cannot regenerate once the nerve cell dies. In an injured peripheral nerve, however, the nerve fiber can regenerate significantly if the injury does not affect the cell body. The proximity of the axonal injury to the cell body can significantly affect the time required for healing. The closer an injury is to the cell body, the more difficult the regenerative process.

For regeneration to occur, an optimal environment for healing must exist. In the case of a severed nerve, surgical intervention can markedly enhance regeneration. Injury to a nerve axon causes a short-term degeneration of the myelin sheath distal to the injury and to some extent in a proximal direction as well. After the initial degeneration of the axon, some progressive enlargement of the cell body and the proximal axon segment occurs, with a concomitant increase in metabolism and protein production by the nerve cell body to facilitate the regenerative process. The distal axon is simultaneously undergoing wallerian degeneration, in which the myelin and axon degenerate. Schwann cells in the distal axon begin growing initially toward the proximal axon and eventually unite the proximal and distal segments. They also begin to multiply and phagocytize the degenerated axon and myelin sheath in the distal direction. Axon regeneration occurs by forming buds from the proximal segment which migrate distally along Schwann cell tubes. Myelin sheaths form around the axon. Axon regeneration can be obstructed by scar formation due to excessive fibroplasia. Axon regeneration progresses at a rate of approximately 2.5 cm per day and tends to slow down as it reaches its termination.

MUSCLE INJURY

Injuries to muscle tissue heal in one of two ways. Mild contusions or strains may cause only slight damage to the capillaries. Bleeding would be the result of this damage but not because of actual derangement of the muscle fiber. The elastic quality of muscle helps to keep these injuries at a minimum in terms of degree of damage. A muscle is more elastic when contracted than in the relaxed state.

If the trauma is severe enough to destroy some fibers, they may heal by proliferation of new fibers, as some regeneration is possible in muscle tissue. If the torn ends are in apposition, first intention healing occurs.

Separation of tissue owing to severe strain or tear owing to force of impact or excessive hemorrhage requires an ingrowth of granulation tissue and approximately 3 weeks for healing. Reinjury with additional hemorrhage is common and may result in myositis ossificans (bony deposits in muscle).

Although the dangers of swelling in muscle are not mentioned as often as such problems with joint injuries, adequate first aid is of the highest importance in caring for the muscle injury. Practicing first intention healing whenever possible can make the athlete ready for competition with less disability.

SUMMARY

1. The four fundamental types of tissue in the human body are epithelial, muscular, nervous, and connective tissues.
2. Fractures may be classified as either greenstick, transverse, oblique, spiral, comminuted, impacted, avulsive, or stress.
3. Dislocations and subluxations involve disruption of the joint capsule and ligamentous structures surrounding the joint.
4. Ligament sprains involve stretching or tearing the fibers that provide stability at the joint.
5. Muscle strains involve a stretching or tearing of muscle fibers of their tendons and cause impairment to active movement.
6. Muscle soreness results in spasms, which are caused by ischemia in working muscles.
7. Tendonitis, an inflammation of a muscle ten-

don that causes pain on movement, usually occurs because of overuse.

8. Tenosynovitis is an inflammation of the synovial sheath through which a tendon must slide during motion.

9. Bursitis is an inflammation of the synovial membranes located in areas where friction occurs between various anatomic structures.

10. Repeated contusions may lead to the development of myositis ossificans.

11. All injuries should be initially managed with rest, ice, compression, and elevation for the purpose of controlling swelling and thus reducing the time required for rehabilitation.

12. The three distinct phases of the healing process are inflammation, fibroplasia, and maturation, which occur in sequence but overlap one another in a continuum.

13. Factors that may impede the healing process include edema, hemorrhage, separation of tissue, muscle spasm, atrophy, corticosteroids, hypertrophic scars, infection, climate and humidity, age, health, and nutrition.

14. Some special considerations must be given to the healing process with regard to tendon, bone, nerve, and muscle.

REFERENCES

1 Arnheim DD: Modern principles of athletic training, ed 7, St Louis, 1989, Times Mirror/Mosby College Publishing.

2 Beck EW: Mosby's atlas of functional human anatomy, St Louis, 1982, The CV Mosby Co.

3 Booher JM and Thibodeau GA: Athletic injury assessment, ed 2, St Louis, 1989, Times Mirror/Mosby College Publishing.

4 Bryant MW: Wound healing, CIBA Clinical Symposia 29(3):2–36, 1977.

5 Cailliet, R: Soft tissue pain and disability, ed. 2, Philadelphia, 1988, FA Davis Co.

6 Carley PJ and Wainapel SF: Electrotherapy for acceleration of sound healing: low intensity direct current, Arch Phys Med Rehabil 66:443–446, 1985.

7 Carrico TJ, Mehrhof AI, and Cohen IK: Biology and wound healing, Surg Clin North Am 64(4):721-734, 1984.

8 Cheng N and others: The effects of electrocurrents on A.T.P. generation, protein synthesis and membrane transport, J Orth Related Research, 171:264–272, 1982.

9 Cyriax J: Textbook of orthopaedic medicine, ed 9, vol 2, Baltimore, 1977, Williams & Wilkins.

10 Derscheid GL and Garrick JG: Medial collateral ligament injuries in football: nonoperative management of grade I and grade II sprains, Am J Sports Med 9(6):365–368, 1981.

11 Fahey TD: Athletic training: principles and practice, Palo Alto, Calif, 1986, Mayfield Publishing Co.

12 Fernandez A and Finlew JM: Wound healing: helping a natural process, Postgrad Med 74(4):311-318, 1983.

13 Frankel VH and Nordin M: Basic biomechanics of the skeletal system, Philadelphia, 1980, Lea & Febiger.

14 Glick JM: Muscle strains: prevention and treatment, Phys Sports Med 8(11):73–77, 1980.

15 Gould JA and Davies GJ, editors: Orthopaedic and sports physical therapy, St Louis, The CV Mosby Co.

16 Gradisar IA: Fracture stabilization and healing. In Gould JA and Davies GJ, editors: Orthopaedic and sports physical medicine, St Louis, 1985, The CV Mosby Co.

17 Gross A and others: Effectiveness of pulsating water jet lavage in treatment of contaminated crush wounds, Am J Surg 124:373-375, 1972.

18 Guyton AC: Textbook of medical physiology, Philadelphia, 1986, WB Saunders Co.

19 Hamilton R: Personal communication, 1981, Team Physician, DePaul University, Chicago.

20 Henning CE: Semilunar cartilage of the knee: function and pathology. In KB Pandolf, editor: Exercise and sport science review, New York, 1988, Macmillan Publishing Co.

21 Hettinga DL: Inflammatory response of synovial joint structures. In Gould JA and Davies, GJ, editors: Orthopaedic and sports physical therapy, St Louis, 1985, The CV Mosby Co.

22 Influencing repair and recovery, Am J Nurs 82:1550–1558, 1982.

23 Keene JS: Ligament and muscle tendon unit injuries. In Gould JA and Davies GJ, editors: Orthopaedic and sports physical therapy, St Louis, 1985, The CV Mosby Co.

24 Kissane JM: Anderson's pathology, ed 8, St Louis, 1985, The CV Mosby Co.

25 Knight KL: Cryotherapy: theory, technique and physiology, Chattanooga, Tenn, 1985, Chattanooga Corporation.

26 Lane NE and others: Aging, long-distance running, and the development of musculoskeletal disability, Am J Med 82:772–780, 1987.

27 Leonard PC: Building a medical vocabulary ed 2, Philadelphia, 1988, WB Saunders Co.

28 McMaster JH: The ABC's of sports medicine, Melbourne, Fla, 1982, RE Kreiger Publishing Co.

29 Marchesi VT: Inflammation and healing. In Kissane JM, editor: Anderson's pathology, ed 8, St Louis, 1985, The CV Mosby Co.

30 Messier SP and Pittala KA: Etiologic factors associated with selected running injuries, Med Sci Sport Exer 20(5):501–505, 1988.

31 Muckle DS: Outline of fractures and dislocations, Bristol, England, 1985, Wright Publishing.

32 Musacchia XJ and others: Disuse atrophy of skeletal muscle: animal models. In KB Pandolf, editor: Exercise and sport sciences review, New York, 1988, Macmillan Publishing Co.

33 Norkin C and Levangie P: Joint structure and function: a comprehensive analysis, Philadelphia, 1983, FA Davis Co.

34 Noyes FR: Functional properties of knee ligaments and

alterations induced by immobilization, Clin Orthop 123:210–242, 1977.

35 Owoeye I and others: Low-intensity pulsed galvanic current and the healing of tenotomized rat achilles tendons: a preliminary report using load-to-breaking measurements, Arch Phys Med Rehabil 68:415–418, 1987.

36 Panush RS and Brown DG: Exercise and arthritis, Sports Medicine 4:54–64, 1987.

37 Prentice WE, editor: Therapeutic modalities in sports medicine, St Louis, 1986, Times Mirror/Mosby College Publishing.

38 Riley WB: Wound healing, Am Fam Physician 24:5, 1981.

39 Robbins SL, Cotran RS, and Kumar V: Pathologic basis of disease, ed 3, Philadelphia, 1984, WB Saunders Co.

40 Roy S and Irvin R: Sports medicine, prevention, evaluation, management and rehabilitation, Englewood Cliffs, NJ, 1983, Prentice-Hall.

41 Rywlin AM: Hemopoietic system. In Kissane JM, editor: Anderson's pathology, ed 8, St Louis, 1985, The CV Mosby Co.

42 Seller RH: Differential diagnosis of common complaints, Philadelphia, 1986, WB Saunders Co.

43 Stanish WD and Gunnlaugson B: Electrical energy and soft tissue injury healing, Sportcare and Fitness 9:12, 1988.

44 Stanish WD and others: The use of electricity in ligament and tendon repair, Phys Sports Med 13:8, 1985.

45 Stewart J: Clinical anatomy and physiology, Miami, 1986, Medmaster.

46 Stone MH: Implications for connective tissue and bone alterations resulting from rest and exercise training, Med Sci Sport Exer 20(5):S162–168, 1988.

47 Wallace L: New perspectives in rehabilitation and preventative health care services: M.E.N.S. therapy, procedures manual, Lyndhurst, Ohio, 1986, Ohio Physical Therapy.

48 Wallace L: M.E.N.S. therapy and the shoulder impingement syndrome: brief study, Contemporary PT 1(3)2, 1988.

49 Wells PE, Frampton V, and Bowsher D: Pain management in physical therapy, Norwalk, Conn, 1988, Appleton and Lange.

50 Whiteside JA, Fleagle SB, and Kalenak A: Fractures and refractures in intercollegiate athletes: an eleven year experience, Am J Sports Med 9(6):369–377, 1981.

51 Woodman R and Pare L: Evaluation and treatment of soft tissue lesions of the ankle and foot using the Cyriax approach, Phys Ther 62:1144–1147, 1982.

Rehabilitation Goals in Sports Medicine

2

Julie Ann Moyer

OBJECTIVES

Following completion of this chapter, the student will be able to:

- Describe the two primary rehabilitation goals of sports medicine.

- Discuss factors involved with the prevention of athletic injuries.

- Describe immediate, short-, and long-term rehabilitation goals and general treatment management programs.

A rehabilitative goal is an end that one tries to achieve via therapeutic intervention. These goals are used to direct the treatment management programs and are established after a thorough initial evaluation and subsequent reevaluations. The two primary rehabilitative goals in sports medicine are: (1) the prevention of injuries to athletes and (2) the safe return of an injured athlete to the previous level of competition as quickly as possible.

INJURY PREVENTION
Physical Conditioning

The primary goal in rehabilitation, injury prevention, can be aided by proper physical conditioning. Off-season conditioning is essential for an athlete seeking maximal in-season performance.[19,20] Off-season conditioning (1) decreases the athlete's risk of acquiring an injury; (2) decreases the rehabilitation time once an injury has occurred; (3) promotes excellence; (4) maintains an athlete's previous education of task performance; and (5) provides for a close, positive bond between the athlete and the sport, thus aiding in the athlete's mental well-being and sport enjoyment.[9]

The first 4 weeks of a season are the most dangerous, because the participants are gener-ally out of condition.[14] Therefore, the major goal of off-season conditioning is to achieve the highest level of fitness possible and thus enter the season in a conditioned rather than an unconditioned state. This is best accomplished by structuring a well-balanced conditioning program that can be performed as effectively yet efficiently as possible. This program should include seven major phases: (1) the warm-up primarily performed to prepare the cardiovascular system for stress, (2) stretching to promote proper range of motion, (3) strengthening exercises, (4) endurance activities, (5) sport-specific or functional activities to meet the special demands and skills a particular sport requires, (6) cool-down, and (7) relaxation techniques to aid in the recovery from fatigue and promote stress reduction (Figs. 2-1 through 2-3). The off-season gives the sports therapist an opportunity to rehabilitate injuries incurred during inseason participation.

Preparticipation Physical

A physical examination should be mandatory before, and specific to, participation at all levels and ages of sports participation (Fig. 2-4). The exam determines if the athlete is physically capable of withstanding the stresses of the sport and helps

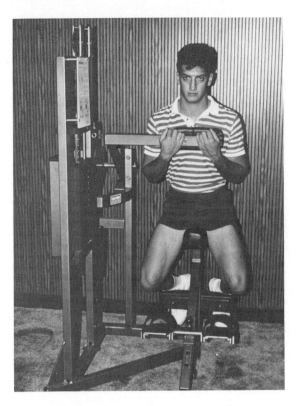

Fig. 2-1. Strengthening exercises are one phase of a seven-step conditioning program.

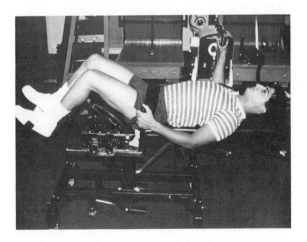

Fig. 2-2. The Cybex machine provides a means of performing isokinetic exercises.

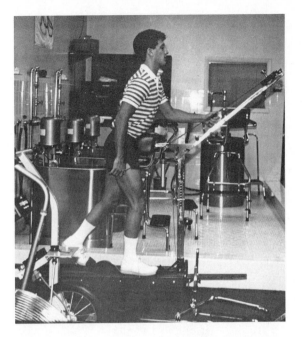

Fig. 2-3. Aerobic conditioning is an important part of injury prevention and rehabilitation.

to reveal imbalances and weaknesses that may be corrected via rehabilitation.

Ideally the examination should be performed 4 to 6 weeks before the start of the season to give the physician a good indication of the athlete's level of health and, if necessary, give the sports therapist adequate time to adopt goals and develop a rehabilitation program.

The eight major parts of a sports examination are (1) past medical history and current medical information; (2) measurements including range of motion, body type, strength, percent body fat, girth, posture, level of maturation, and cardiovascular fitness; (3) orthopedic examination; (4) eye examination; (5) dental screening; (6) laboratory tests; (7) and review of the examination by a physician in order to allow, disallow, or restrict athletic participation.[25]

Nutrition and Diet

Nutrition is an important component of in-season and off-season conditioning. A good nutritional program should consist of low-fat, high-fiber, well-balanced foods from the four major food

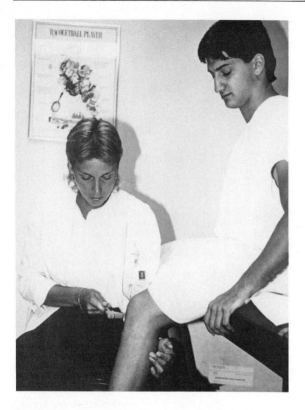

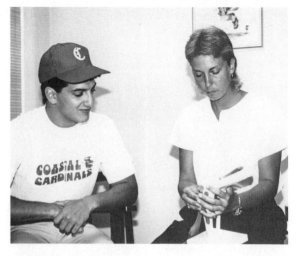

Fig. 2-5. Education of the athlete assists in the prevention and treatment of injuries.

Fig. 2-4. The preparticipation physical examination should be mandatory before, and specific to, participation at all levels and ages of sports.

groups: milk, fruits and vegetables, breads and cereals, and meat. The average ratios of these foods are 60% carbohydrate, 25% fat, and 15% protein.[30] Nutritional supplements such as protein, vitamins, and minerals are expensive and are often not necessary if the athlete's diet is nutritionally well balanced.

The major difference between in-season and off-season nutritional conditioning is caloric intake. The caloric intake of individuals is very dependent upon activity level. The average sedentary person may require about 1500 calories per day, whereas moderately training athletes average 3000 calories per day and intensely training endurance athletes may require over 5000 calories per day.

During a lowered training level such as off-season conditioning, the athlete's basal metabolic rate (BMR) lowers. The BMR is the lowest amount of energy needed to keep the body run-

ning during waking hours. When the BMR lowers, fewer calories are burned by the athlete; the potential of increased body fat exists. Therefore, most off-season conditioning programs should include caloric restrictions.

Education

Education is the best form of preventive medicine. The educated athlete studies off-season conditioning programs, biomechanics, diet and nutrition, equipment fitting, sports psychology, injury prevention techniques, and injury treatment procedures (Fig. 2-5). The educated athlete also becomes familiar with the rules and regulations of the sport, especially as they relate to drug control and banned substances. Knowledge and understanding of all these concepts aid the athlete in the prevention and treatment of injuries.

Safe Playing Environment and Equipment

The sports medicine practitioner has the responsibility of carefully inspecting all playing facilities to ensure that they are safe for play. Weather conditions should also be monitored with recommendations made to the coach or athletic director. Such weather conditions include heat, cold, rain, and lightning.

The most common types of disorders associated with heat are heat cramps, heat exhaustion, and heat stroke. These serious heat-related problems primarily occur when the temperature outside goes above 87° F and the body begins to absorb heat at a faster rate than heat is expelled by means such as perspiration and evaporation. When this occurs, the athlete is at risk of overheating.

Lightning is another serious weather occurrence that must be treated with respect. As with all potential injuries, the best treatment is prevention. The rule of thumb when playing during lightning is if you can count 15 seconds or less between the time you see lightning and the time you hear thunder, the athletic competition should be postponed (1 mile = 5 seconds; lightning can strike up to 3 miles away).[20]

Injuries can be prevented with appropriate clothing and equipment[19] (Fig. 2-6). Also, the correct fitting of the equipment is essential. Protective clothing and equipment not only are used to protect the athlete from acquiring an injury but also can be used to give further protection to an injury already sustained.

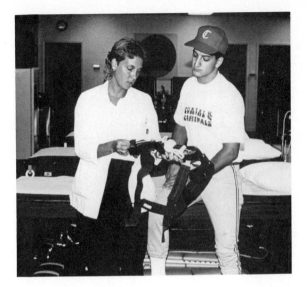

Fig. 2-6. Proper instruction for wear and care is essential when utilizing protective equipment.

INITIAL EVALUATION, TREATMENT, AND REHABILITATION
Rehabilitation

The second primary goal of rehabilitation is the safe return of injured athletes to their prior level of competition as quickly as possible. This is best achieved by a thorough initial evaluation, proper immediate treatment, and a comprehensive rehabilitation program (Fig. 2-7). Rehabilitation in sports medicine should involve a multidisciplinary team approach including athletic trainers, sports therapists, physicians, coaches, and athletes.

The most efficient and effective form of rehabilitation is therapeutic exercise (see Chapter 3). Appropriate therapeutic exercise helps the athlete achieve the goals of increased strength, increased power, improved proprioception and kinesthesia, increased range of motion, improved cardiovascular and musculoskeletal endurance, and relaxation. Increased coordination, decreased biomechanical and anatomical deficits, improved balance, maximized function, and minimized swelling can also be assisted through the

use of exercise. Exercise also helps to minimize damage that results from disuse such as muscle atrophy and that from osteoporosis as well.

For these goals to be achieved four principles must be observed. First of all, therapeutic exercises must be adapted based upon the individualized needs of the athlete. Second, the initial exercise program should not aggravate the disorder. Third, the exercises should be performed in orderly, progressive steps (Table 2-1). Last, the exercise program should be well rounded: (1) use a wide variety of exercise techniques; (2) constantly change the exercise program in order to avoid boredom; (3) make sure the uninvolved areas of the body remain conditioned so the risk of acquiring other injuries is reduced when the athlete returns to competition; (4) set realistic goals for and with the athlete, with constant reevaluation and modification of the goals and treatment program; and (5) have the athlete actively enrolled in a home therapy program as well as the outpatient physical therapy and athletic training room program.

Immediate, Short-Term, and Long-Term Goals

Rehabilitation goals (after insult) may be divided into three main stages: immediate, short-term, and long-term goals (Table 2-2). Collectively

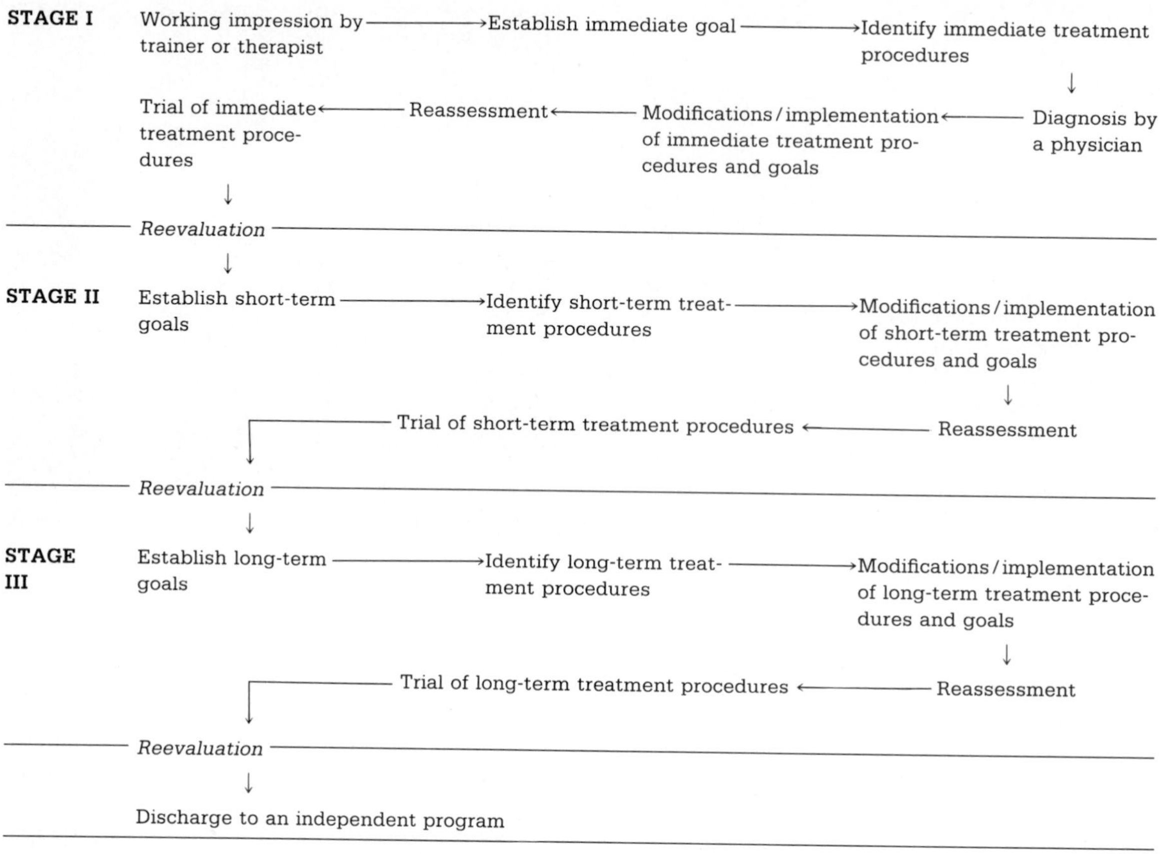

STAGE I   Working impression by ───────→Establish immediate goal ───────→Identify immediate treatment
           trainer or therapist   procedures

                                                                                       ↓

           Trial of immediate←─────── Reassessment←─────── Modifications/implementation←─────── Diagnosis by
           treatment proce-   of immediate treatment pro-   a physician
           dures   cedures and goals

                    ↓

──────── *Reevaluation* ──

                    ↓

STAGE II   Establish short-term ───────────→Identify short-term treat- ───────────→Modifications/implementation
           goals   ment procedures   of short-term treatment pro-
                                                                                     cedures and goals

                                                                                              ↓

                        ┌──────────── Trial of short-term treatment procedures ←─────────── Reassessment
                        │
──────── *Reevaluation* ↓ ───

                    ↓

STAGE   Establish long-term ───────────→Identify long-term treat- ───────────→Modifications/implementation
III   goals   ment procedures   of long-term treatment proce-
                                                                                   dures and goals

                                                                                            ↓

                        ┌──────────── Trial of long-term treatment procedures ←─────────── Reassessment
                        │
──────── *Reevaluation* ↓ ───

                    ↓

           Discharge to an independent program

Fig. 2-7. Goal setting and treatment sequencing.

TABLE 2-1

Sample of Progressive, Resistive Knee Exercise Stages by Davies

Stage	Exercise	Specifics
I	Submaximal, multiple-angle isometrics	10 sets of 10 repetitions, a 10-sec contraction, performed at 10 angles
II	Maximal, multiple-angle isometrics	
III	Submaximal, short-arc isokinetics	Primarily intermediate contractile velocity speeds at 60–180 deg/sec, using a velocity spectrum rehabilitation program (10 repetitions at every 30 deg/sec)
IV	Short-arc isotonics	Used with or in place of maximal, short-arc isokinetics
V	Maximal, short-arc isokinetics	
VI	Submaximal, full-range isokinetics	Primarily fast contractile velocity speeds at 180–300 deg/sec, using a velocity spectrum rehabilitation program
VII	Maximal, full-range of motion isokinetics	

Adapted from Reference 3.

TABLE 2-2
Rehabilitation Stages, Goals, and General Treatment Methods

Stage	Goal	General Treatment Methods
I. Immediate goals	Protection from further damage Resistive activity Control/minimize pain and swelling	Protective padding and strapping Splints, braces, immobilizers Ice Compression wrap tape, and other devices Elevate the injured area
II. Short-term goals	Assist the healing process and enable the symptoms and level of dysfunction to subside Maintain normal function of uninvolved body parts	Therapeutic modalities: cold agents, heat/diathermy, electric stimulation, intermittent compression devices, massage, taping/padding/immobilization as indicated Therapeutic exercises: isometric-PROM-AAROM-AROM of injured area, general vigorous exercise regime to uninvolved body parts, psychological exercises, education of the athlete
III. Long-term goals	Achieve normal strength, power, muscular and cardio-vascular endurance, agility, anatomical alignment, sensory feedback (proprioception, stereognosis), balance, timing, coordination, biomechanical motions, psychological conditioning Discharge to an independent program	Therapeutic modalities: to a lesser extent than stage I. Therapeutic exercise: PROM-AAROM-AROM, hydro/aquatherapy, psychological training, isometrics, isotonics (concentric and eccentric), isokinetics, PNF techniques, cardiovascular and muscular endurance activities, progressive sport-specific activities Education of the athlete

PROM: Passive range of motion.
AROM: Active range of motion.
AAROM: Active-assisted range of motion.

these rehabilitation goals provide a guideline to get the athlete back to the highest level of function in the shortest amount of time that is safely feasible. Establishing appropriate rehabilitation goals is often the most difficult aspect of the rehabilitative program.

The goals must specifically state the projected rehabilitation outcome at the end of each stage (Fig. 2-8). The goals should also be used to progress the athlete sequentially through the rehabilitation program from the time of injury insult until optimal level of function is achieved.

IMMEDIATE GOALS. Stage I of postinjury goal setting begins at the time of injury insult. The immediate rehabilitative goal is established at the time of injury and is based upon a quick but relatively thorough on-the-field evaluation and working impression by the sports therapist, along with an immediate diagnosis by the sports physician if available and indicated.

Following the evaluation, a conservative immediate goal must be established, along with the treatment management to accomplish this goal.

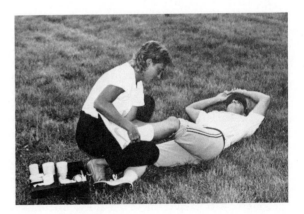

Fig. 2-8. The NATA-certified athletic trainer provides immediate on-the-field care of injured athletes.

This immediate goal setting and treatment implementation may range from protective padding for reentry into the competition to emergency care and transportation to a hospital with appropriate referrals to a physician specialist such as a neurologist or orthopedic surgeon.

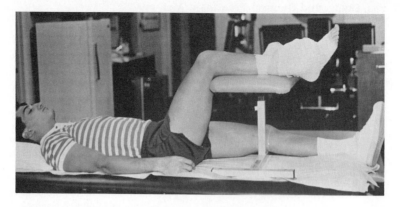

Fig. 2-9. PRICE is the most commonly used acronym in the immediate treatment of injuries.

One of the most frequently used immediate treatment management acronyms is PRICE: *Pro*tection, *R*estricted activity, *I*ce, *C*ompression, and *E*levation (Fig. 2-9). Protection means protecting the injured area from further insult, which may be performed in a variety of ways, including padding and strapping. With more serious injuries, or when there is doubt as to the severity of an injury, protection may also include slings, splints, and assistive ambulatory devices.

Restricted activity is probably the most controversial aspect of the PRICE treatment program. It is used to protect an injury from further damage. Restricted activity in the form of rest may be indicated for some serious injuries; however, prolonged immobilization may lead to a decreased functional length of musculotendinous tissue and decreased sport performance. Therefore, the term *restricted activity* is preferred to *rest.* Restricted activity allows the athlete to participate at the maximally safe level.

Ice application produces a decrease in metabolic production and therefore lowers the cell's oxygen and nutrient requirements. In turn, this produces a decrease in blood flow, decreased edema, and decreased muscular fatigue. Decreased pain is also noted. Cold application may be provided in many ways, including ice packs, ice massage, cold whirlpool (approximately 55° F), inflatable splints with refrigerant gas, and ice towels.

Compression may be performed with tape, wraps, compression sleeves, exercise, massage, or intermittent compression devices. The pur-

pose of compression is to enhance lymphatic and venous return, normalize osmotic pressure, minimize fluid accumulation in the intercellular space, and hence minimize swelling and edema at the injury site.

Elevation of the injured part also assists in this process and is accomplished via gravity by raising the injured part higher than the heart.

SHORT-TERM GOALS. The establishment of short-term goals signifies the beginning of stage II rehabilitation. After the immediate treatment program has been implemented, and when the environment allows (return to the out-patient clinic or training room), the athlete must be reevaluated so that short-term treatment goals and procedures may be developed. These treatment procedures and short-term goals are primarily concerned with assisting the healing process and enabling the subsidence of the symptoms associated with the injury, such as pain, swelling, and decreased function. These symptoms may be minimized with the assistance of therapeutic modalities (see Chapter 6), therapeutic exercises (see Chapter 3), and education of the athlete.

Hot and cold applications, shortwave and microwave diathermy, phonophoresis and iontophoresis, radiation, ultrasound, electrical stimulation, and intermittent compression devices are all examples of physical modalities that may be used to achieve these short-term goals (Figs. 2-10 and 2-11). Other physical measures that are also helpful are massage, joint mobilization, constant passive motion devices, and traction.

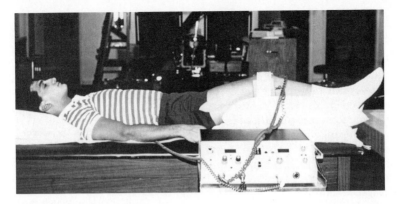

Fig. 2-10. Therapeutic modalities such as high-volt electrical stimulation are an integral part of injury rehabilitation.

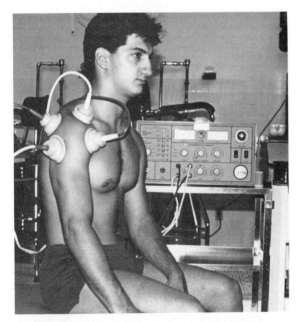

Fig. 2-11. Interferential therapy is another therapeutic modality that can be an integral part of injury rehabilitation.

Exercise is the most critical part of a rehabilitation program. The primary goals of therapeutic exercise during this stage of recovery are: (1) to maintain or promote normal function without aggravation to the injury and (2) to decrease swelling and edema via rhythmic isometric or active muscular contractions, thus assisting lymphatic return.

LONG-TERM GOALS. Stage III of rehabilitation begins with the establishment of long-term goals and ends when an optimal level of function is achieved. Therapeutic exercise plays an important part in the achievement of this long-term goal. Therapeutic exercise is used to increase strength, agility, speed, power, range of motion, sensory feedback, posture, endurance, coordination, balance, relaxation, and other psychological training skills.

The SAID principle (specific adaptations to imposed demands) must be reemphasized during the development of the long-term goals and treatment program. Rehabilitation must be adapted to the specific demands placed upon the athlete's body and on the injured part by the specific requirements of the sport and playing position.

As the long-term treatment program advances, a decision must be made as to whether or when a safe return to sport participation can take place. This decision is ultimately up to the sports physician, with the assistance of the sports therapist, coach, and athlete. Results of the reevaluation, along with understanding the specific physical demands of the athlete's individual sport and position, must be reviewed in order to determine whether the healing and functional level of the athlete are adequate for safe reentry in sports. Whenever in doubt concerning the degree of healing and safe return of the athlete, the health care professional must be conservative.

FACTORS THAT INFLUENCE REHABILITATION GOALS

Adherence to the SAID principle is a necessity for rehabilitation goals. Many athlete-specific factors can cause a health care practitioner to modify the rehabilitation goals. Such factors include type of sport, time remaining in the season, other sports of participation, game rules, outside sporting influences, psyche of the athlete, type and severity of the injury, stage of healing, and treatment techniques (see box).[25]

Different sports place different demands on an injury. For example, a shoulder injury to a soccer player does not produce as great a playing deficit as a shoulder injury to a baseball player. Likewise, the position played within the same sport is also influential; for example, a shoulder injury to a first baseman versus to a pitcher.

Time remaining in the season and other sport participations can produce modifications in the rehabilitation goals. If an injury occurs at the end of the season and there is no postseason championship play, the athlete may choose to be conservative and not strive for active participation in the last game. This may especially be the case if the athlete will soon be involved with another sport season.

Game rules also cause modifications in goals through protective padding and/or bracing restrictions and regulations regarding substitutions. Although outside sporting influences such as scholarship possibilities and coach or parental influence should not sway a health care practitioner's decision on the resumption of activity, those pressures do exist and should be weighed with extreme caution.

Sports psychology is an interesting but often overlooked aspect of athletic rehabilitation (see Chapter 5). Injury and illness produce a wide range of emotional reactions; therefore, the health care practitioner needs to understand and develop the individual psyche of each athlete. Athletes vary in terms of pain threshold, cooperation and compliance, competitiveness, denial of disability, depression, intrinsic and extrinsic motivation, anger, fear, guilt, and the ability to adjust to injury. Besides dealing with the mental aspect of the injury, sports psychology may also be used to improve total athletic performance

---

OUTLINE OF FACTORS THAT INFLUENCE REHABILITATION GOALS

1. **Type of sport**
   a. Demands that particular sport will make upon the injury
   b. Position played

2. **Time remaining in the season**
   a. Beginning versus the end of the season
   b. Postseason play and championships

3. **Other sports**
   a. Other sports in which the athlete participates
   b. Priorities of these sports

4. **Sport rules**
   a. As they relate to injuries and substitutions
   b. Protective equipment

5. **Outside sporting influence**
   a. Possibility of scholarships
   b. Parents' and/or coach's involvement with the injury

6. **Psyche of the athlete**
   a. Intrinsic and extrinsic motivation
   b. Cooperation and compliance
   c. Competitiveness
   d. Pain threshold

7. **Type of injury**
   a. Sprain versus contusion versus fracture
   b. Secondary injuries

8. **Severity of the injury**
   a. Amount and degree of dysfunction

9. **Type of treatment and rehabilitation**
   a. The requirement of surgical intervention including precautions, contraindications, and complications
   b. Speed in controlling initial pain and swelling
   c. Type of surgical procedure (e.g., meniscal repair versus meniscectomy)

---

through the use of techniques such as visualization, self-hypnosis, and relaxation.

The severity of the injury, along with the type of treatment and rehabilitation that is instituted, will influence immediate, short-term, and long-term goals. The amount of pain, swelling, and dysfunction, whether surgery (and the type of surgery) is required, and the existence of precautions, complications, or contraindications of treatment can all produce modifications in goal setting. Last, the stage of healing is a strong factor influencing rehabilitation goals and treatment management.

SUMMARY

1. The best way to treat a sports injury is to prevent the injury from occurring.
2. After an athlete has acquired an injury, a speedy but thorough initial evaluation must be performed so that appropriate, immediate rehabilitation goals and a treatment management program may be established.
3. Immediate goals are later followed by short-term and long-term rehabilitation goals.
4. The most efficient and effective form of rehabilitation is therapeutic exercise.
5. The rehabilitation goals after injury are based upon the safe return of an injured athlete to the previous level of competition as quickly as possible.

REFERENCES

1 Carlisle F: Effects of preliminary passive warming on swimming performance, Res Q 27:143–152, 1956.
2 Coplin TH: Isokinetic exercise: clinical usage, Ath Train 6(3):110–114, 1971.
3 Davies GJ: A compendium of isokinetics in clinical usage, La Crosse, Wis, 1984, S & S Publishers.
4 Gleim GW, Nicholas JA, and Webb JN: Isokinetic evaluation following leg injuries, Phys Sports Med 6:75–82, 1978.
5 Grose E: Depression of muscular fatigue curves by heat and cold, Res Q 29:19–31, 1958.
6 Hall VE, Muniz E, and Fitch B: Re-education of the strength of muscular contraction by application of moist heat to the overlying skin, Arch Phys Med Rehabil 28:493–499, 1947.
7 Heusner W: The theory of strength development, as reprinted by Isokinetics, Inc., ASCA Clinic, New Orleans, 1978.
8 Hislop HJ and Perrine JJ: The isokinetic concept of exercise, Phys Ther 47(2):114–117, 1967.
9 Hunter LY and Funk FJ: Rehabilitation of the injured knee, St Louis, 1984, The CV Mosby Co.
10 Johnson & Johnson: AthletiCare Newsletter (New Brunswick, N.J., Johnson & Johnson Consumer Products Co. Inc.) 2(2):1, 1986.
11 Johnson & Johnson: AthletiCare Newsletter (New Brunswick, N.J., Johnson & Johnson Consumer Products Co. Inc.) 2(4):1, 1986.
12 Johnson & Johnson: AthletiCare Newsletter (New Brunswick, N.J., Johnson & Johnson Consumer Products Co. Inc.) 3(2):1, 1987.
13 Johnson DJ and Leider FE: Influence of cold bath on maximum handgrip strength, Percept Mot Skill 44(1):323–326, 1977.
14 Klafs CE and Arnheim DD: Modern principles of athletic training, St Louis, 1977, The CV Mosby Co.
15 Kulund DN: The injured athlete, Philadelphia, 1982, JB Lippincott Co.
16 Lesmes GR and others: Muscle strength and power changes during maximal isokinetic training, Med Sci Sport 10(4):266–269, 1978.
17 Londeree BR: Strength testing, JPER 52:44–46, 1981.
18 Margaria R: The sources of muscular energy, Sci Am 226:84–91, 1972.
19 Mellion MB: Sports injuries & athletic problems, St Louis, 1988, Times Mirror/Mosby College Publishing.
20 Moffroid MT and Kusiak ET: The power struggle, Phys Ther 55:1098–1104, 1975.
21 Moyer JA: Playing in lightning is risky business, Softball News 6(7):2, 1988.
22 Nukuda A: Haultemperatur und Leistungfanigkeit in extremitaten bei starischer haltearbeit (1955), cited by Grose JE: Depression of muscular fatigue curves by heat and cold, Res Q 29:20, 1958.
23 Pipes TV: The acquisition of muscular strength through constant and variable resistance strength training, Ath Train 12(3):148–151, 1977.
24 Robins AC: The effect of hot and cold shower baths upon adolescents participating in physical education classes, Res Q 13:373–380, 1942.
25 Roy S and Irvin R: Sports medicine prevention, evaluation, management, and rehabilitation, Englewood Cliffs, N.J., 1983, Prentice-Hall Inc.
26 Sargeant AJ and Jones NL: Effect on power output of human muscle during short term dynamic exercise, Med Sci Sport 11:39, 1978.
27 Scudder GN: Torque curves produced at the knee during isometric and isokinetic exercise, Arch Phys Med Rehabil 61:68–73, 1980.
28 Sedwick AW and Whalen HR: The effect of passive warmup on muscular strength and endurance, Res Q 35:49–59, 1964.
29 Werner JK: Neuroscience: a clinical perspective, Philadelphia, 1980, WB Saunders Co.
30 Williams M and Stutzman L: Strength variation through the range of joint motion, Phys Ther 39:145–152, 1959.

Techniques of Reconditioning in Rehabilitation

3

William E. Prentice

OBJECTIVES

Following completion of this chapter, the student will be able to:

- Define strength and indicate its significance to health and skill of performance.

- Discuss the anatomy and physiology of skeletal muscle.

- Discuss the physiology of strength development and the factors that determine strength.

- Describe specific methods for improving muscular strength.

- Differentiate between muscle strength and muscle endurance.

- Define flexibility and describe its importance as a health-related component of fitness.

- Identify factors that limit flexibility.

- Differentiate between static and dynamic flexibility.

- Explain the difference between ballistic, static, and PNF stretching.

- Discuss the neurophysiological principles of stretching.

- Describe the oxygen transport system and the concept of maximal rate of oxygen utilization.

- Explain the relationships among heart rate, stroke volume, cardiac output, and rate of oxygen utilization.

- Describe the functions of the heart, blood vessels, and lungs in oxygen transport.

- Describe the principles of continuous, interval, fartlek, circuit, and par cours training and the potential of each technique for improving cardiorespiratory endurance.

- Describe the differences between aerobic and anaerobic activity.

T he sports therapist is responsible for designing, monitoring, and progressing programs of rehabilitation for injured athletes. The goals for a sports medicine rehabilitation program differ from goals for other patient populations. The athlete must return to competitive fitness levels, and the intensity of the rehabilitation must be adjusted appropriately during the course of the program.

The sports therapist has to have an understanding of the principles and techniques involved in reconditioning the injured athlete. The term **therapeutic exercise** is commonly used to refer to techniques of reconditioning. This chapter concentrates on principles and techniques for improving muscular strength and endurance, flexibility, and cardiorespiratory endurance.

IMPROVING MUSCULAR STRENGTH AND ENDURANCE

One of the primary rehabilitation program goals of any sports therapist is to return muscular strength and endurance to preinjury levels. By definition, **strength** is the maximal force that can be applied by a muscle during a single maximal contraction.

Maintenance of at least a normal level of general strength, as well as regaining strength lost in a given muscle or muscle group following injury, is important for the athlete during a rehabilitation period. Muscle weakness or imbalance can result in abnormal movement or gait and can impair normal functional movement. Thus strength training plays a critical role in injury rehabilitation programs.

Muscular strength is also related to **agility,** the ability of the body to change direction rapidly in a coordinated manner. Agility not only enhances athletic performance but also allows the athlete to avoid potentially injurious situations.

Muscular strength is closely associated with muscular endurance. Muscular endurance is the ability to perform repetitive muscular contractions against some resistance. As is noted later, as muscular strength increases, endurance tends to increase correspondingly. For example, a person can lift a weight 25 times. If muscular strength is increased by 10% through weight training, the maximal number of repetitions would probably be increased because the person can lift the weight more easily.

For most people, developing muscular endurance is more important than developing muscular strength because muscular endurance is more critical in carrying out the everyday activities of living. This fact becomes increasingly true with age. However, a tremendous amount of strength is necessary for anyone involved in some type of competition.

Most movements in sports are explosive and include elements of both strength and speed if they are to be effective. If a large amount of force is generated quickly, the movement can be referred to as a **power movement.** Without the ability to generate power, an athlete's performance capabilities are limited.[54]

Anatomy and Physiology of Skeletal Muscle Contraction

Skeletal muscle consists of (1) the muscle belly and (2) its tendons, which are collectively referred to as a **musculotendinous unit** (Fig. 3-1).

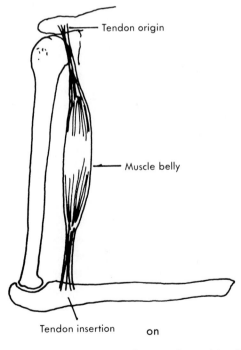

Tendon origin

Muscle belly

Tendon insertion   on

Fig. 3-1. The musculotendinous unit consists of the muscle belly and its tendon, which attaches the contractile portion of the muscle to the bone.

The muscle belly is composed of separate, parallel elastic fibers. Muscle fibers are composed of thousands of small protein fibers called **myofilaments,** as well as of a substantial amount of connective tissue that holds the fibers together. These myofilaments lie parallel to the long axis of the muscle fiber. The two types of myofilaments are **myosin,** a long, thick filament with fingerlike projections called **crossbridges,** and the thin **actin** filaments. When a muscle depolarizes, the actin filaments are pulled closer together by the myosin crossbridges, thus producing shortening of the muscles and movement at the joint that the muscle crosses (Fig. 3-2).[23]

The muscle tendon attaches muscle directly to bone. The muscle tendon is composed primarily of connective tissue and is relatively inelastic when compared with muscle fibers.

All skeletal muscles exhibit four characteristics: (1) the ability to change in length or stretch, which is **elasticity;** (2) the ability to shorten and return to normal length, which is **extensibility;** (3) the ability to respond to stimulation from the nervous system, which is **excitability;** and (4) the ability to shorten and contract in response to some neural command, which is **contractility.**

Muscles contract in response to stimulation by the central nervous system. An electrical impulse transmitted from the central nervous system through a single motor nerve to a group of muscle fibers causes a depolarization of those fibers. The motor nerve and the group of muscle fibers that it innervates are referred to collectively as a **motor unit.** An impulse coming from the central nervous system and traveling to a group of fibers through a particular motor nerve causes all the muscle fibers in that motor unit to depolarize and contract. This is referred to as the **all-or-none response** and applies to all skeletal muscles in the body.[23]

FAST-TWITCH VERSUS SLOW-TWITCH FIBERS. All fibers in a particular motor unit are either slow-twitch or fast-twitch fibers, each of which has distinctive metabolic as well as contractile capabilities. Slow-twitch fibers are also referred to as type I fibers. They are more resistant to fatigue than are fast-twitch fibers; however, the time required to generate force is much greater for slow-twitch fibers.[45]

Fast-twitch fibers are identified as type II fibers. They are capable of producing quick, forceful contractions but tend to fatigue more rapidly than do slow-twitch fibers. Fast-twitch fibers are capable of producing powerful contractions, whereas slow-twitch fibers produce a long-endurance type of force.

Slow-twitch fibers are relatively resistant to fatigue and are associated primarily with long-duration, aerobic-type activities. Fast-twitch fibers are useful in short-term, high-intensity activities, which mainly involve the anaerobic system.

Fast-twitch fibers have been subdivided into type IIa, which have a fast speed of contraction along with a moderate capacity for both aerobic and anaerobic activities, and type IIb fibers, which are almost exclusively anaerobic.

Within a particular muscle are both types of fibers, and the ratio varies with each person. The average is about 50% slow-twitch and 50% fast-twitch fibers. However, tremendous variations have been demonstrated in both different muscle groups and in different groups of athletes.[25] The percentages of each muscle fiber type are

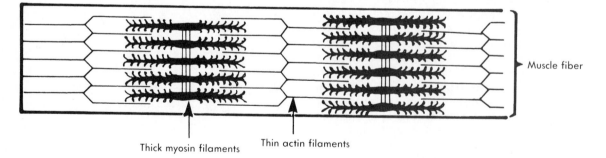

Thick myosin filaments   Thin actin filaments

Fig. 3-2. A muscle contracts or shortens when an electrical impulse from the central nervous system causes the myofilaments in a muscle fiber to move closer together.

by and large genetically determined and cannot be significantly altered through training.

Because this ratio is genetically determined, it may play a large role in determining ability for a given sport activity. Sprinters, for example, have a large percentage of fast-twitch fibers in relation to slow-twitch fibers.[15] One study has shown that they may have as much as 95% fast-twitch fibers in certain muscles. Conversely, marathon runners generally have a higher percentage of slow-twitch fibers.

Factors That Determine Muscular Strength

Muscular strength is closely related to the cross-sectional diameter of a muscle. The bigger a particular muscle, the stronger it is, and thus the more force it is capable of generating. The size of a muscle tends to increase in cross-sectional diameter with weight training. This increase in size is referred to as **hypertrophy.**[35] Conversely, a decrease in the size of a muscle is referred to as **atrophy.**

Strength is a function of the number and diameter of muscle fibers composing a given muscle. The number of fibers is an inherited characteristic; thus a person with a large number of muscle fibers to begin with has the potential to hypertrophy to a much greater degree than does someone with relatively fewer fibers.[26]

Strength is also directly related to the efficiency of the neuromuscular system and the function of the motor unit in producing muscular force. As indicated later in this chapter, initial increases in strength during a weight-training program can be attributed primarily to increased neuromuscular efficiency.

Strength in a given muscle is determined not only by the physical properties of the muscle itself but also by mechanical factors that dictate how much force can be generated through a system of levers to an external object.

The elbow joint is considered to be one of these lever systems, and the biceps muscle produces flexion of this joint (Fig. 3-3). The position of the attachment of the biceps muscle on the lever arm, in this case, the forearm, largely determines how much force this muscle is capable of generating. If person A has a biceps attachment that is closer to the fulcrum (the elbow joint) than person B, then person A must produce

a greater force with the biceps muscle to hold the weight at a right angle because the length of the lever arm is greater than with person B.

When the weight is held at an angle of 45 degrees (Fig. 3-4, *A*) or 150 degrees (Fig. 3-4, *C*), the contracting force of the biceps muscle required to hold the weight stationary is considerably less than it would be at 90 degrees. Thus if we move this weight through a full range of motion from extension to flexion, the amount of strength, or force, required to move the weight varies at different angles, forming a strength curve for that movement (Fig. 3-5).

A third critical factor in determining muscle strength is muscle length. Because strength curves vary for individual muscles, development of maximal force has an optimal length and tension. In general, a muscle is capable of generating its maximal force when it is in its midrange of movement. If the muscle is stretched beyond its normal length, it may be incapable of producing any muscular force, and injury is likely. In fact, the initial stretch of a muscle evokes a reflex called the **stretch reflex,** which does not allow the muscle to be lengthened. This stretch reflex is discussed in detail later in this chapter. The shorter the muscle becomes, the less force it is capable of generating. A muscle that is fully contracted is incapable of producing any additional muscular force past this point.

The ability to generate muscular force is also related to age. Both men and women seem to be able to increase strength throughout puberty

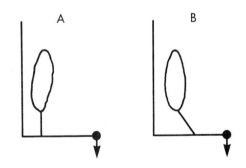

Fig. 3-3. The position of attachment of the muscle tendon on the lever arm can affect the ability of that muscle to generate force. **B** should be able to generate more force than **A** because the tendon attachment on the lever arm is closer to the resistance.

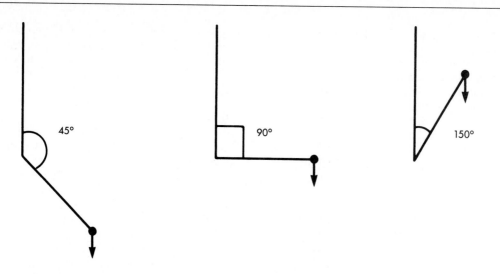

Fig. 3-4. Because of the mechanical factors, the force necessary to overcome resistance changes at different joint angles.

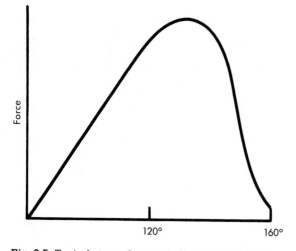

Fig. 3-5. Typical strength curve indicating changes in the amount of force required to move a resistance throughout a full range of motion.

and adolescence and reach a peak around 20 to 25 years of age, at which time this ability begins to level off and in some cases declines. After about age 25, a person generally loses an average of 1% of the maximal remaining strength each year. Thus, at age 65 people have only about 60% of their strength at age 25.[43]

This loss in muscle strength is definitely related to individual levels of physical activity. Those people who are more active and those who continue to train for strength considerably decrease this tendency toward declining muscle strength. In addition to retarding this decrease in muscular strength, exercise may also have an effect in slowing the decrease in cardiorespiratory endurance, flexibility, and so on. Thus, strength maintenance is important for all individuals, regardless of age or the level of competition.

Physiology of Strength Development

Weight training to improve muscular strength results in the increased size, or hypertrophy, of a muscle. What causes a muscle to hypertrophy? A number of theories have been proposed to explain this increase in muscle size.[21]

Some evidence exists that the number of muscle fibers increases due to fiber splitting in response to training.[26] However, this research has been conducted in animals and should not be generalized to humans. It is generally accepted that the number of fibers is genetically determined and does not seem to increase with training.

One hypothesis is that because the muscle is working harder in weight training, more blood is required to supply that muscle with oxygen and other nutrients, and thus the number of capillaries is increased. This hypothesis is only partially correct. No new capillaries are formed during strength training; however, a number of dormant capillaries may well become patent to meet this increased demand for blood supply.

A third theory to explain this increase in muscle size seems the most credible. Muscle fibers are composed primarily of small protein filaments, called **myofilaments,** which are the contractile elements in muscle. These actin and myosin myofilaments increase in both size and number as a result of strength training and cause the individual muscle fibers themselves to increase in cross-sectional diameter.[45] This effect is particularly true in men, although women also see some increase in muscle size.

Methods of Improving Strength

The three different methods of training for strength improvement are **isometric training, isotonic training,** and **isokinetic training.** Regardless of which method is used, one basic principle of training is extremely important. For a muscle to improve in strength, it must be forced to work at a higher level than that to which it is accustomed. In other words, the muscle must be overloaded. Without overload the muscle is able to maintain strength as long as training is continued against a resistance the muscle is accustomed to. However, no additional strength gains are realized. This maintenance of existing levels of muscular strength may be more important in weight-training programs that emphasize muscular endurance rather than strength gains. Certainly many individuals can benefit more in terms of overall health by concentrating on improving muscular endurance. However, to most effectively build muscular strength, weight training requires a consistent, increasing effort against progressively increasing resistance. If this principle of overload is applied, all three training methods will produce improvement of muscular strength over a period of time.

ISOMETRIC EXERCISE. An isometric exercise involves a muscle contraction in which the length of the muscle remains constant while tension develops toward a maximal force against an immovable resistance[44] (Fig. 3-6). The muscle should generate a maximal force for 5 seconds at a time, and this contraction should be repeated 5 to 10 times per day.

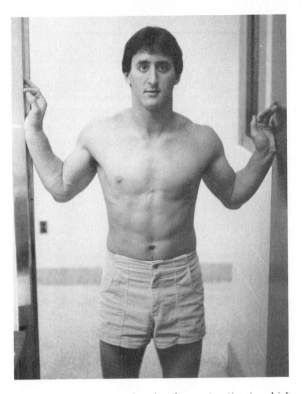

Fig. 3-6. Isometric exercises involve contraction in which the muscle generates increased tension but the length of the muscle does not change.

Isometric exercises were popular in the late 1960s and early 1970s. Several books were published that discussed a series of isometric exercises that could be done while sitting at a desk. The exercises included techniques such as putting the arms underneath the middle desk drawer and pushing up as hard as possible and pushing out on the inside of the chair space with the knees. These brief maximal isometric contractions were claimed to be capable of producing some rather dramatic increases in muscular strength. Indeed, these isometric exercises are capable of increasing muscular strength; unfortunately, strength gains are specific to the joint angle at which training is performed. At other angles the strength curve drops off dramatically because of a lack of motor activity at that angle. Thus arm strength is increased at the specific angle pressed against the desk drawer, but no corresponding increase in strength occurs at other positions in the range of motion.

Another major disadvantage of these isometric "sit at the desk" exercises is that they tend to produce a spike in blood pressure that can result in potentially life-threatening cardiovascular accidents.[20] This sharp increase in blood pressure results when the breath is held and intrathoracic pressure increases. Consequently, the blood pressure experienced by the heart increases significantly. This process has been referred to as the Valsalva effect. Breathing during the maximal contraction avoids or minimizes this effect and helps to prevent this increase in pressure.

Isometric exercises may be valuable in both training and conditioning programs as well as in injury rehabilitation programs. In certain instances an isometric contraction can greatly enhance a particular movement. For example, one of the exercises in power weight lifting is a squat. A **squat** is an exercise in which the weight is supported on the shoulders in a standing position. The knees are then flexed, and the weight is lowered to a three-quarter squat position, from which the lifter must stand completely straight once again.

Sometimes, at one particular angle in the range of motion, smooth movement through that specific angle is difficult because of insufficient strength. This joint angle is referred to as a **sticking point.** A power lifter typically employs an isometric contraction against some immovable resistance to increase strength at this sticking point. If strength can be improved at this joint angle, then a smooth, coordinated power lift can be performed through a full range of movement.

Isometric exercises are used frequently in injury rehabilitation or reconditioning. Several conditions or ailments that result from either trauma or overuse must be treated with strengthening exercise. Unfortunately, these problems may be exacerbated with full range-of-motion strengthening exercises. Isometric exercises may be more desirable until the injury has healed to the point at which the full-range activities can be performed. Generally, isometric exercises are used in the early stages of a rehabilitation program when full range-of-motion exercises are contraindicated.

ISOTONIC EXERCISE. A second method of weight training is more commonly used in improving muscular strength. **Isotonic exercise** involves a muscle contraction in which force is generated while the muscle is changing length.

Isotonic contractions are of two types. In a biceps curl, to lift the weight from the starting position, the biceps muscle must contract and shorten in length. This shortening contraction is referred to as a **concentric** (positive) contraction. If the biceps muscle does not remain contracted when the weight is being lowered, gravity causes this weight to fall back to the starting position. Thus to control the weight as it is being lowered, the biceps muscle must continue to contract while at the same time gradually lengthening. A contraction in which the muscle is lengthening while still applying force is called an **eccentric** (negative) contraction.

When training isotonically, utilizing both concentric and eccentric contractions is essential. Research has clearly demonstrated that the muscle must be overloaded and fatigued both concentrically and eccentrically for the greatest strength improvement to occur. However, the superiority of one method over the other for improving strength has not been clearly demonstrated. Eccentric training appears to be specific to strength gains only in eccentric strength. Eccentric contractions generate greater force than do concentric contractions. Thus eccentric contraction may be used to facilitate motion throughout the range for a weak muscle that cannot produce full-range activity through a concentric contraction. The value of eccentric training has been significantly emphasized in the recent research literature. Both types of contractions can be done with any type of isotonic equipment.

Various devices and machines can be classified as isotonic devices. Free weights, barbells, and dumbbells are the most common forms of isotonic equipment. Many manufacturers produce machines that would be considered isotonic, including Universal (Fig. 3-7), Nautilus, Eagle, Body Master, Keiser, Paramount, Continental, Pyramid, Sprint, Hydrafitness, Future, and Bull. Each type of isotonic device has advantages and disadvantages. The machines are relatively safe to use in comparison with free weights. For example, people doing bench presses with free weights have to have a "spotter" to avoid dropping the weights on their chests. The Nautilus and Universal equipment allow lifters to drop the

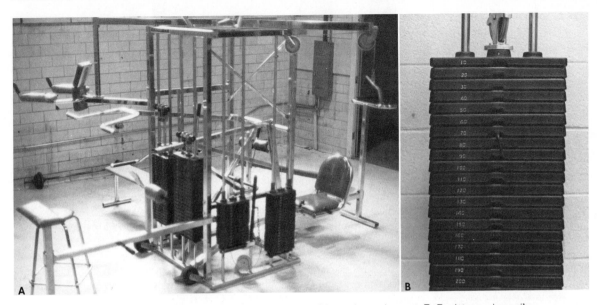

Fig. 3-7. A, Universal equipment is an example of isotonic equipment. **B,** Resistance is easily changed by simply changing the key in the stack of weights.

weight easily and safely without fear of injury.

Also increasing or decreasing the weight by moving a single weight key is a simple process with the machines, although changes can generally be made only in increments of 10 or 15 pounds. With free weights, iron plates must be added or removed from each side of the barbell. Regardless of which type of equipment is used, the same principles of isotonic training may be applied.

In a reconditioning program, when training is specifically for the development of muscular strength and endurance, both the concentric and eccentric contractions should be slow and controlled to avoid placing increased stress on the injured structures. Arthur Jones, the inventor of the Nautilus equipment, stresses the use of these positive and negative contractions in his training program, and this principle should be applied regardless of which brand of equipment is used.

People who have strength-trained using both free weights and one of the machines realize the difference in the amount of weight that can be lifted. Unlike the machines, free weights have no restricted motion and can thus move in many different directions, depending on the forces applied. With free weights, an element of muscular control on the part of the lifter to prevent the weight from moving in any other direction other than vertical will usually decrease the amount of weight that can be lifted.[68]

One problem often mentioned in relation to isotonic training involves changes that occur in the muscles' capabilities of moving the resistance throughout the range of motion. Regarding mechanical factors that determine levels of strength, the amount of force necessary to move a weight through a range of motion changes according to the joint angle and is greatest when the joint angle is somewhere in the midrange of motion (Fig. 3-4, *B*). In addition, once the inertia of the weight has been overcome and momentum has been established, the force required to move the resistance varies according to the force that the muscle can produce through the range of motion. Thus a disadvantage of any type of isotonic equipment is that loads encountered by the exercising muscle vary throughout the range of movement as a result of changes in the vertical components of gravity. If a load is applied, the ability of that muscle to move a resistance throughout a range is limited by the weakest point in that range or at its point of least mechanical advantage.

Nautilus has attempted to alleviate this problem of changing force capabilities by using a cam in its pulley system (Fig. 3-8, *B*). The cam has been individually designed for each piece of equipment so that the resistance is variable throughout the movement. It attempts to alter resistance so that the muscle can handle a greater load, but at the points where the joint angle or muscle length is mechanically disadvantageous, it reduces the resistance to muscle movement. Whether this design does what it claims is debatable. This change in resistance at different points in the range has been labeled **variable resistance.**

ISOKINETIC EXERCISE. The third method of strength training takes a different approach to the problem of changing force capabilities. An **isokinetic exercise** is one in which the length of the muscle is changing while the contraction is performed at a constant velocity. In theory, maximal resistance is provided throughout the range

of motion because the resistance moves only at some preset speed regardless of the force applied to it. Thus the key to isokinetic exercise is that the exercising limb can be loaded maximally throughout the range at some preset velocity because it is not limited by the weakest point in the range.

Several isokinetic devices are available commercially; the Ariel Computerized Exercise System, Cybex, Orthotron, KinCom, Biodex, Lido, MERAC, and Mini-Gym are all isokinetic devices (Fig. 3-9). In general they rely on hydraulic, pneumatic, or mechanical pressure systems to produce this constant velocity of motion.

Isokinetic strength training has gained a great deal of popularity in rehabilitation settings during recent years. Because the capability exists for training at specific speeds, comparisons have been made regarding the relative advantages of training at fast or slow speeds. The research lit-

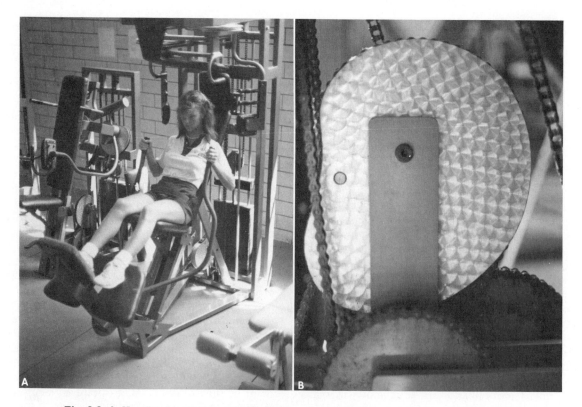

Fig. 3-8. A, Nautilus bench press station. **B,** The cam on the Nautilus is designed to equalize or accommodate resistance throughout the range of motion.

erature seems to indicate that strength increases from slow-speed training are relatively specific to the velocity used in training. Conversely, training at faster speeds seems to produce a more generalized increase in torque values at all velocities. Minimal hypertrophy was observed only while training at fast speeds affecting only type II or fast-twitch fibers.[17,51] An increase in neuromuscular efficiency owing to more effective motor unit firing patterns has been demonstrated with slow-speed training.[43]

A major disadvantage of the isokinetic devices is their cost. Most of these devices come with a microcomputer and are used primarily as diagnostic and rehabilitative tools in treatment.

Isokinetic devices are designed so that regardless of the amount of force applied against a resistance, they can be moved only at a certain speed. That speed is the same whether maximal force or only half the maximal force is applied. Consequently, when training isokinetically, exerting as much force as possible against the resistance is absolutely necessary for maximal strength gains to occur. This design limitation is one of the major disadvantages of an isokinetic strength-training program.

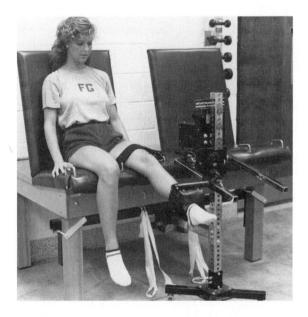

Fig. 3-9. The orthotron is an isokinetic device that provides resistance at a constant velocity.

Anyone who has been involved in a weight-training program knows how on some days finding the motivation to work out is difficult. Because isokinetic training requires a maximal effort, to "cheat" and not go through the workout at a high level of intensity is very easy. In an isotonic program, the athlete knows how much weight has to be lifted with how many repetitions. Thus isokinetic training is often more effective if a partner system is used primarily as a means of motivation toward a maximal effort from the athlete.

When isokinetic training is done properly with a maximal effort, it is theoretically possible that maximal strength gains are best achieved through the isokinetic training method in which the velocity and force of the resistance are equal throughout the range of motion.

Whether this changing force capability is in fact a deterrent to improving the ability to generate force against some resistance is debatable. In real life whether the resistance is changing does not matter. What is important is that enough strength is developed to move objects from one place to another. The amount of strength necessary for athletes is largely dependent on their life-styles and their level of competition.

SPECIFIC TECHNIQUES OF STRENGTH TRAINING. Specific techniques for improving muscular strength are controversial among sports therapists. A considerable amount of research has been done in the area of weight training to determine optimal techniques in terms of (1) the amount of weight to be used, (2) the number of repetitions, (3) the number of sets, and (4) the frequency of training.

The following recommendations are based on this research and are the principles that seem to be most widely accepted by strength-training experts. However, the healing process must dictate the specifics of any strength-training program. Regardless of specific techniques used, certainly to improve strength the muscle must be overloaded. The amount of weight used and the number of repetitions must be enough to make the muscle work at higher intensity than it is used to doing. This factor is the most critical in any strength-training program. The strength-training program must also be designed to meet the specific competitive needs of the athlete.

A number of programs have been proposed that look at the optimal amount of weight and repetitions for producing maximal gains in levels of muscular strength.

One of the first widely accepted strength-development programs to be used in a rehabilitation program was developed by DeLorme and was based on a repetition maximum of 10 (10 RM).[18] The amount of weight used is what can be lifted exactly 10 times (Table 3-1).

Zinovieff proposed the Oxford Technique, which, like DeLorme's program, was designed to be used in beginning, intermediate, and advanced levels of rehabilitation.[71] The only difference is that the percent of maximum was reversed in the three sets (Table 3-2).

MacQueen's technique[46] differentiates between beginning to intermediate and advanced levels, as is shown in Table 3-3.

Sander's program (Table 3-4) was designed to be used in the advanced stages of rehabilitation and was based on a formula that used a percentage of body weight to determine starting weights.[57] The percentages below represent median starting points for different exercises:

Barbell squat—45% of body weight
Barbell bench press—30% of body weight
Leg extension—20% of body weight
Universal bench press—30% of body weight
Universal leg extension—20% of body weight
Universal leg curl—10–15% of body weight
Universal leg press—50% of body weight
Upright rowing—20% of body weight

Knight applied the concept of progressive resistive exercise in rehabilitation. His DAPRE (daily adjusted progressive resistive exercise)

TABLE 3-1
DeLorme's Program

Set	Amount of Weight	Repetitions
1	50% of 10 RM	10
2	75% of 10 RM	10
3	100% of 10 RM	10

TABLE 3-2
The Oxford Technique

Set	Amount of Weight	Repetitions
1	100% of 10 RM	10
2	75% of 10 RM	10
3	50% of 10 RM	10

TABLE 3-3
MacQueen's Technique

Sets	Amount of Weight	Repetitions
3 (Beginning/intermediate)	100% of 10 RM	10
4–5 (Advanced)	100% of 2–3 RM	2–3

TABLE 3-4
The Sanders' Program

Sets	Amount of Weight	Repetitions
Total of 4 sets (3 times per week)	100% of 5 RM	5
Day 1—4 sets	100% of 5 RM	5
Day 2—4 sets	100% of 3 RM	5
Day 3—1 set	100% of 5 RM	5
2 sets	100% of 3 RM	5
2 sets	100% of 2 RM	5

TABLE 3-5
Knight's DAPRE Program

Set	Amount of Weight	Repetitions
1	50% of RM	10
2	75% of RM	6
3	100% of RM	Maximum
4	Adjusted working weight*	Maximum

*See Table 3-6.

TABLE 3-6
DAPRE Adjusted Working Weight

Number of Repetitions Performed During Third Set	Adjusted Working Weight During Fourth Set	Next Exercise Session
0–2	−5–10 lb	−5–10 lb
3–4	−0–5 lb	Same weight
5–6	Same weight	+5–10 lb
7–10	+5–10 lb	+5–15 lb
11	+10–15 lb	+10–20 lb

TABLE 3-7
Berger's Adjustment Technique

Sets	Amount of Weight	Repetitions
3	100% of RM	6–8

program (Tables 3-5 and 3-6) allows for individual differences in the rates at which patients progress in their rehabilitation programs.[39]

Berger has proposed a technique that is adjustable within individual limitations. His research suggests that optimal training involves selecting a weight sufficient to allow six to eight repetitions in each of the three sets (Table 3-7). If at least three sets of six repetitions cannot be completed, the weight is too heavy and should be reduced. If more than three sets of eight repetitions can be done, the weight is too light and should be increased.[9]

Berger also indicates that a particular muscle or muscle group should be exercised consistently every other day. Thus, weight training should be done at least three times per week but no more than four times per week.

Arthur Jones, inventor of the Nautilus machine, has suggested that if training is done properly with the Nautilus equipment (that is, using both positive and negative contractions), strength-training is necessary only twice each week, although this schedule has not been sufficiently documented.

TRAINING FOR MUSCULAR STRENGTH VERSUS MUSCULAR ENDURANCE. Muscular endurance was defined as the ability to perform repeated muscle contractions against resistance. Most weight-training experts believe that muscular strength and muscular endurance are closely related.[60] As one improves, the other tends to improve also.

Weight training for strength is generally thought to require heavier weights with a lower number of repetitions. Conversely, endurance training calls for relatively lighter weights with a greater number of repetitions.

Recommendations are that endurance training should consist of 3 sets of 10 to 12 repetitions.[8] Thus, suggested training regimens for both muscular strength and endurance are similar in terms of sets and numbers of repetitions. People who possess great levels of strength tend to exhibit greater muscular endurance when asked to perform repeated contractions against resistance.

STRENGTH TRAINING DIFFERENCES BETWEEN MALES AND FEMALES. Strength training is absolutely essential for an athlete. The approach to strength training is no different for the female athlete than for male athletes. However, some obvious physiologic differences exist between the sexes.

The average woman does not build significant muscle bulk through weight training. Significant muscle hypertrophy is dependent on the presence of a steroidal hormone known as **testosterone.** Testosterone is considered a male hormone, although some women possess some testosterone in their systems. Women with higher testosterone levels tend to have more masculine characteristics, such as increased facial and body hair, a deeper voice, and the potential to develop a little more muscle bulk.[45] For the average female athlete, developing large, bulky muscles through strength training is unlikely, although muscle tone may be improved. Muscle tone basically refers to the firmness or tension of the muscle during a resting state. The initial stages of a strength-training program are likely to produce dramatic increases in levels of strength very rapidly. For a muscle to contract, an impulse must be transmitted from the nervous system to the muscle. Each muscle fiber is innervated by a specific motor unit. By overloading a particular muscle, as in weight training, the muscle is forced to work more efficiently. Efficiency is achieved by getting more motor units to fire, which causes a stronger contraction of the muscle. Consequently, women often see extremely rapid gains in strength when a weight-training program is first begun. These tremendous initial strength gains, which can be attributed to improved neuromuscular system efficiency, tend to plateau, and minimal improvement in muscular strength is realized during a continuing strength-training program. These initial neuromuscular strength gains are also seen in men, although their strength continues to increase with appropriate training. Again, women who possess higher testosterone levels have the potential to increase their strength further because of the development of greater muscle bulk.

Differences in strength levels between males and females are best illustrated when strength is expressed in relation to body weight minus fat. The reduced strength/body weight ratio in women is the result of their percentage of body fat. The strength/body weight ratio may be significantly improved through weight training by decreasing the body fat percentage while increasing lean weight.

The absolute strength differences are considerably reduced when body size and composition are considered. Leg strength may actually be stronger in the female than in the male, although upper extremity strength is much greater in the male.[45]

IMPROVING FLEXIBILITY

Flexibility has been defined as the ability to move a joint or series of joints through a full, nonrestricted, pain-free range of motion. For the sports therapist, a return to or improvement on this preinjury range is an important goal of any rehabilitation program. An athlete who has a restricted range of motion will probably realize a decrease in performance capabilities. For example, a sprinter with tight, inelastic hamstring muscles probably loses some speed because the hamstring muscles restrict the ability to flex the hip joint and thus shorten stride length. Lack of flexibility may also result in uncoordinated or awkward movement patterns.

Most sports therapists would agree that good flexibility is essential to successful physical performance. Likewise, they also believe that maintaining good flexibility is important in prevention of injury to the musculotendinous unit, and they will generally insist that stretching exercises be included as part of the warm-up before engaging in strenuous activity.

Flexibility can be discussed in relation to movement involving only one joint, such as in the knees, or movement involving a whole series of joints, such as the spinal vertebral joints, which must all move together to allow smooth bending or rotation of the trunk.

Flexibility is specific to a given joint or movement. A person may have good range of motion in the ankles, knees, hips, back, and one shoulder joint. If the other shoulder joint lacks normal movement, however, then a problem exists that needs to be corrected before the person can function normally.

Factors That Limit Flexibility

A number of factors may limit the ability of a joint to move through a full, unrestricted range of motion. The bony structure may restrict the endpoint in the range. An elbow that has been fractured through the joint may lay down excess calcium in the joint space, causing the joint to lose its ability to extend fully. However, in many instances we rely on bony prominences to stop movements at normal endpoints in the range.

Fat may also limit the ability to move through a full range of motion. A person who has a large amount of fat on the abdomen may have severely restricted trunk flexion when asked to bend forward and touch the toes. The fat may act as a wedge between two lever arms and restrict movement wherever it is found.

Skin might also be responsible for limiting movement. For example, a person who has had some type of injury or surgery involving a tearing incision or laceration of the skin, particularly over a joint, has inelastic scar tissue formed at that site. The scar tissue is incapable of stretching with joint movement.

Connective tissue surrounding the joint, such as ligaments on the joint capsule, may be subject to contractures. Ligaments and joint capsules do have some elasticity; however, if a joint is immobilized for a period of time, these structures tend to lose some elasticity and actually shorten. This condition is most commonly seen after surgical repair of an unstable joint, but it can also result from long periods of inactivity.

A person may also have relatively slack ligaments and joint capsules. These people are generally referred to as loose-jointed. An example is a knee or elbow that hyperextends beyond 180 degrees (Fig. 3-10). Frequently an instability associated with loose-jointedness may present as great a problem in movement as ligamentous or capsular contractures.

Muscles and their tendons, along with their surrounding fascial sheaths, are most often responsible for limiting range of motion. When performing stretching exercises for the purpose of improving flexibility about a particular joint, athletes are attempting to take advantage of the highly elastic properties of a muscle. Over time the elasticity, that is, the length that a given muscle can be stretched, can be increased. People who have a good deal of movement at a particular joint tend to have highly elastic and flexible muscles.

With the exception of bony structure, all other factors that limit flexibility may be altered to increase range of joint motion. Fat loss is possible

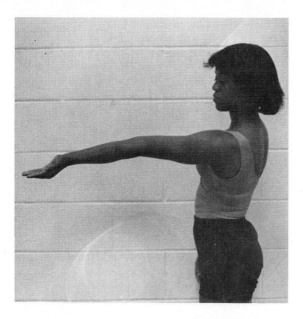

Fig. 3-10. Excessive joint motion, such as in the hyperextended elbow, can predispose a joint to injury.

through weight reduction, which removes a physical obstruction to movement.

Static and Dynamic Flexibility

Two types of flexibility must be considered for movement through a full range of motion. **Static flexibility** or **passive range of motion** refers to the degree to which a joint may be passively moved to the endpoints in the range of motion. No muscle contraction is involved with static flexibility.

Dynamic flexibility or **active range of motion** refers to the degree to which a joint can be moved by a muscle contraction, usually through the midrange of movement. Dynamic flexibility is not necessarily a good indicator of the stiffness or looseness of a joint because it applies to the ability to move a joint efficiently, with little resistance to motion.[35]

When a muscle contracts, it produces a joint movement through a specific range of motion. However, if passive pressure is applied to an extremity, it is capable of moving farther in the range of motion.

Dynamic flexibility is important in athletic performance. In sport activities an extremity must

be capable of moving through a nonrestricted range of motion. For example, a sprinter who cannot fully extend the knee joint in a normal stride is at a considerable disadvantage because stride length and thus speed are reduced significantly (Fig. 3-11).

Static flexibility is important for injury prevention. In many sports situations, a muscle is forced to stretch beyond its normal active limits. If the muscle does not have enough elasticity to compensate for this additional stretch, the musculotendinous unit may be injured.

Assessment of Flexibility

Accurate measurement of the range of joint motion is difficult. Various devices have been designed to accommodate variations in the size of the joints as well as the complexity of movements in articulations that involve more than one joint. Of these devices, the simplest and most widely used is the **goniometer** (Fig. 3-12), a large protractor with measurements in degrees. By aligning the two arms parallel to the longitudinal axis of the two segments involved in motion about a specific joint, relatively accurate measures of range of movement can be obtained. The goniometer has an important place in a rehabilitation setting, where it is essential to assess improvement in joint flexibility for the purpose of modifying rehabilitation programs. The sports therapist needs expertise and an in-depth understanding of goniometric techniques.

Stretching Techniques

Flexibility has been defined as the range of motion possible about a single joint or through a series of articulations. The maintenance of a full, nonrestricted range of motion has long been recognized as an essential component of a rehabilitation program. Flexibility is important not only for successful physical performance but also in the prevention of injury.[13]

The goal of any effective flexibility program should be to improve the range of motion at a given articulation by altering the extensibility of the musculotendinous units that produce movement at the joint. Exercises that stretch these musculotendinous units over a period of time increase the ROM possible about a given joint.[52]

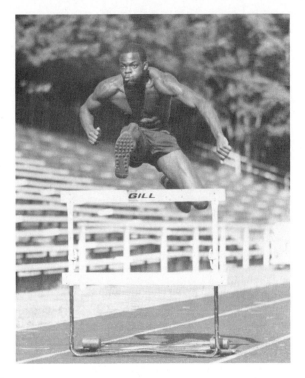

Fig. 3-11. Flexibility is an essential component of many sports-related activities.

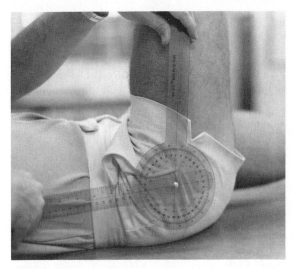

Fig. 3-12. Measurement of hip joint flexion using a goniometer.

Stretching techniques for improving flexibility have evolved over the years. The oldest technique for stretching is called **ballistic stretching;** it makes use of repetitive bouncing motions.

A second technique, known as **static stretching,** involves stretching a muscle to the point of discomfort and then holding it at the point for an extended time. This technique has been used for many years. Recently another group of stretching techniques known collectively as **proprioceptive neuromuscular facilitation (PNF),** involving alternating contractions and stretches, has also been recommended.[40]

Researchers have had considerable discussion about which of these techniques is most effective for improving range of motion.

AGONIST VERSUS ANTAGONIST MUSCLES. Before discussing the three different stretching techniques, defining the terms **agonist** and **antagonist** is essential. Most joints in the body are capable of more than one movement. The knee joint, for example, is capable of flexion and ex-

tension. Contraction of the quadriceps group of muscles on the front of the thigh causes knee extension, whereas contraction of the hamstring muscles on the back of the thigh produces knee flexion.

To achieve knee extension, the quadriceps group contracts while the hamstring muscles relax and stretch. The muscle that contracts to produce a movement, in this case the quadriceps, is referred to as the agonist muscle. Conversely, the muscle being stretched in response to contraction of the agonist muscle is called the antagonist muscle. In this example of knee extension, the antagonist muscle would be the hamstring group.

The relation of the agonist and antagonist muscles is essential to the understanding of the three stretching techniques.

BALLISTIC STRETCHING. On any spring or fall afternoon, people who are warming up to run by doing their stretching exercises typically use bouncing movements to stretch a particular muscle. This bouncing technique is more appropriately known as ballistic stretching, in which repetitive contractions of the agonist muscle are used to produce quick stretches of the antagonist muscle. The ballistic stretching technique, although apparently effective, has been virtually abandoned by most experts in the field because increased range of motion is achieved through a series of jerks or pulls on the resistant muscle tissue. If the forces generated by the jerks are greater than the tissues' extensibility, muscle injury may result. The stretch reflex is important in each of these stretching techniques.

STATIC STRETCHING. The static stretching technique is still an extremely effective and popular technique of stretching. It involves a contraction of the agonist muscle to stretch the antagonist muscle passively by placing it in a maximal position of stretch and holding it there for an extended time. Recommendations for the optimal time for holding this stretched position vary, ranging from as short as 3 seconds to as long as 60 seconds.[40] Data are inconclusive at present; however, 30 seconds appears to be a good time. The static stretch of each muscle should be repeated three or four times.

The extensive research done in comparing ballistic and static stretching techniques for the improvement of flexibility has shown that both static and ballistic stretching are effective in increasing flexibility and that no significant difference exists between the two. However, static stretching presents less danger of exceeding the extensibility limits of the involved joints because the stretch is more controlled. Ballistic stretching is apt to cause muscular soreness, whereas static stretching generally does not and is commonly used in injury rehabilitation of sore or strained muscles.[19]

PNF TECHNIQUES. The PNF techniques were first used by sports therapists for treating patients who had various types of neuromuscular paralysis. Only recently have PNF stretching exercises been used as a stretching technique for increasing flexibility. A disadvantage of the PNF technique is that it requires the athlete to have a partner to help with the stretching.[40]

Several different PNF techniques are currently being used for stretching, including slow-reversal-hold-relax, contract-relax, and hold-relax techniques. All involve some combination of alternating contraction and relaxation of both agonist and antagonist muscles (a 10-second pushing phase followed by a 10-second relaxing phase).

Using a hamstring-stretching technique as an example (Fig. 3-13), a variation of the slow-

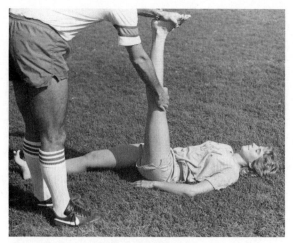

Fig. 3-13. A PNF technique (slow-reversal-hold) for stretching the hamstrings.

reversal-hold-relax technique would be done as follows. Lying on your back with the knee extended and the ankle flexed to 90 degrees, a partner passively flexes your leg at the hip joint to the point at which you feel slight discomfort in the muscle. At this point you begin pushing against your partner's resistance by contracting the hamstring muscle. After pushing for 10 seconds, the hamstring muscles are relaxed and the agonist quadriceps muscle is contracted while your partner applies passive pressure to stretch the antagonist hamstrings further. This pressure should move the leg to produce increased hip joint flexion. The relaxing phase lasts for 10 seconds, at which time you again push against your partner's resistance, beginning at this new joint angle. The push-relax sequence is repeated at least three times.[52]

The contract-relax and hold-relax techniques are variations on the slow-reversal-hold-relax method. In the contract-relax method, the hamstrings are isotonically contracted so that the leg actually moves toward the floor during the push phase. The hold-relax method involves an isometric hamstring contraction against immovable resistance during the push phase. During the relax phase, both techniques involve relaxation of hamstrings and quadriceps while the hamstrings are passively stretched. This same basic PNF technique can be used to stretch any muscle in the body.

Neurophysiological Basis of Stretching

All three stretching techniques are based on a neurophysiological phenomenon involving the stretch reflex (Fig. 4-5),[52] which is discussed in greater detail in Chapter 4. Every muscle in the body contains various types of receptors that when stimulated inform the central nervous system of what is happening with that muscle. The two receptors important in the stretch reflex are the **muscle spindle** and the **Golgi tendon organ.** Both types of receptors are sensitive to changes in muscle length. The Golgi tendon organs are also affected by changes in muscle tension and by the rate of this change.

When a muscle is stretched, the muscle spindles are also stretched, sending a volley of sensory impulses to the spinal cord that inform the central nervous system that the muscle is being stretched. Impulses return to the muscle from the spinal cord and cause the muscle to reflexly contract, thus resisting the stretch.[52]

If the stretch of the muscle continues for an extended period of time (at least 6 seconds), the Golgi tendon organs respond to the change in length and the increase in tension by firing off sensory impulses of their own to the spinal cord. The impulses from the Golgi tendon organs, unlike the signals from the muscle spindle, cause a reflex relaxation of the antagonist muscle. This reflex relaxation serves as a protective mechanism that allows the muscle to stretch through relaxation before the extensibility limits are exceeded and damage to the muscle fibers occurs.

With the jerking, bouncing motion of ballistic stretching, the muscle spindles are being repetitively stretched; thus, the muscle continuously resists further stretch. The ballistic stretch is not continued long enough to allow the Golgi tendon organs to have any relaxing effect.

The static stretch involves a continuously sustained stretch lasting from 6 to 60 seconds, which is sufficient time for the Golgi tendon organs to begin responding to the increase in tension. The impulses from the Golgi tendon organs have the ability to override the impulses coming from the muscle spindles and allow the muscle to relax reflexly after the initial reflex resistance to the change in length. Thus, lengthening the muscle and allowing it to remain in a stretched position for an extended period of time is unlikely to produce any injury to the muscle.

The effectiveness of the PNF techniques may be attributed in part to these same neurophysiological principles. The slow-reversal-hold technique discussed previously takes advantage of two additional neurophysiological phenomena.

The maximal isometric contraction of the antagonist muscle during the 10-second push phase again causes an increase in tension, which stimulates the Golgi tendon organs to effect a reflex relaxation of the antagonist even before the muscle is placed in a position of stretch. This relaxation of the antagonist muscle during contractions is referred to as **autogenic inhibition.**

During the relaxing phase, the antagonist is relaxed and passively stretched while maximal isotonic contraction of the agonist muscle pulls the extremity further into the agonist pattern. In any synergistic muscle group, a contraction of the agonist causes a reflex relaxation in the antagonist muscle, allows it to stretch, and protects it from injury. This phenomenon is referred to as **reciprocal inhibition** (Fig. 4-6).

With the PNF techniques, the additive effects of autogenic inhibition and reciprocal inhibition should theoretically allow the muscle to be stretched to a greater degree than is possible with either the static stretching technique or the ballistic technique.[52]

Practical Application of Stretching Techniques

Although all three stretching techniques have been demonstrated to improve flexibility, considerable debate continues as to which technique produces the greatest increases in range of movement. The ballistic technique is seldom recommended because of the potential for causing muscle soreness, and static stretching is perhaps the most widely used technique. It is a simple technique and does not require a partner. A fully nonrestricted range of motion can be attained through static stretching over time.

PNF stretching techniques are capable of producing dramatic increases in range of motion during one stretching session. Studies comparing static and PNF stretching suggest that PNF stretching is capable of producing greater improvement in flexibility over an extended training period.[52] The major disadvantage of PNF stretching is that a partner is required, although stretching with a partner may have some motivational advantages. More and more athletic teams seem to be adopting the PNF technique as the method of choice for improving flexibility.

THE RELATIONSHIP OF STRENGTH AND FLEXIBILITY

Strength training is often said to have negative effects on flexibility. For example, someone who develops large bulk through strength training is often referred to as *muscle-bound,* an expression with negative connotations in terms of that person's ability to move. People who have highly developed muscles are sometimes thought to have lost much of their ability to move freely through a full range of motion.

Occasionally a person develops so much bulk that the physical size of the muscle prevents a normal range of motion. Certainly strength training that is not properly done can impair movement; however, weight training, if done properly through a full range of motion, does not impair flexibility. Proper strength training probably improves dynamic flexibility and, if combined with a rigorous stretching program, can greatly enhance the powerful and coordinated movements that are essential for success in many athletic activities (Fig. 3-14).

MAINTENANCE OF CARDIORESPIRATORY ENDURANCE

Although strength and flexibility are commonly regarded as essential components in any injury rehabilitation program, relatively little consideration is given toward maintaining levels of cardiorespiratory endurance. An athlete spends a considerable amount of time preparing the cardiorespiratory system to be able to handle the increased demands made upon it during a competitive season. When injury occurs and the athlete is forced to miss training time, levels of cardiorespiratory endurance may decrease rapidly. Thus the sports therapist must design or substitute alternative activities that allow the indi-

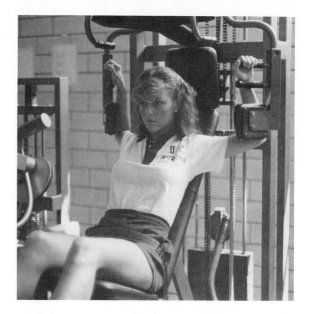

Fig. 3-14. Strength training through a full range of motion will not impair flexibility.

vidual to maintain existing levels of fitness during the rehabilitation period.

By definition, cardiorespiratory endurance is the ability to perform whole-body activities for extended periods of time. The cardiorespiratory system provides a means by which oxygen is supplied to the various tissues of the body. Without oxygen the cells within the human body cannot possibly function, and ultimately death will occur. Thus the cardiorespiratory system is the basic life-support system of the body.

Transport and Utilization of Oxygen

Basically, transport of oxygen throughout the body involves the coordinated function of four components: (1) the heart, (2) the lungs, (3) the blood vessels, and (4) the blood. The improvement of cardiorespiratory endurance through training occurs because of the increased efficiency of each of these four elements in providing necessary oxygen to the working tissues. The greatest rate at which oxygen can be taken in and utilized during exercise is referred to as **maximal oxygen consumption** ($VO_{2\,max}$).[3] The performance of any activity requires a certain rate of oxygen consumption that is about the same for all persons, depending on the present level of fitness. Generally the greater the rate or more intense the performance of an activity, the greater the oxygen consumption. Each person has an individual maximal rate of oxygen consumption. That person's ability to perform an activity (or to fatigue) is closely related to the amount of oxygen required by that activity and is limited by the person's maximal rate of oxygen consumption. The greater the percentage of maximal oxygen consumption required during an activity, the less time is available for the activity to be performed (Fig. 3-15).

The maximal rate at which oxygen can be utilized is a genetically determined characteristic; people inherit a certain range of $VO_{2\,max}$, and the more active a person is, the higher the existing $VO_{2\,max}$ will be in that range.[3,45] A training program can increase $VO_{2\,max}$ to its highest limit within a person's range. The $VO_{2\,max}$ is most often presented in terms of the volume of oxygen used relative to body weight per unit of time (ml/kg/min). A normal $VO_{2\,max}$ for most college-age athletes would fall somewhere in the range of 38 to 46 ml/kg/min.[5] A world-class male marathon runner may have a $VO_{2\,max}$ in the 70 to 80 ml/kg/min range.

Three factors determine the maximal rate at which oxygen can be utilized: (1) external respiration, involving the ventilatory process, or pulmonary function, which does not normally limit endurance, (2) gas transport, which is accomplished by the cardiovascular system (that is, the heart, blood vessels, and blood), and (3) internal respiration, which involves the use of oxygen by the cells to produce energy. Of these three factors the most limiting is generally the ability to transport oxygen through the system; thus the cardiovascular system limits the overall rate of oxygen consumption. A high $VO_{2\,max}$ within a person's inherited range indicates that all three systems are working well.

The detailed anatomy and physiology involved in the cardiorespiratory system are beyond the scope of this text. However, a basic discussion of the training effects and response to exercise that occur in the heart, blood vessels, blood, and lungs should make clear why the

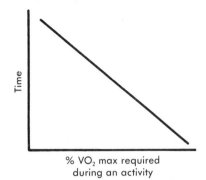

Fig. 3-15. The greater the percentage of $VO_{2\,max}$ required during an activity, the less time that activity can be performed.

training techniques to be discussed are so effective in improving cardiorespiratory endurance.

Exercise and the Cardiorespiratory System

THE HEART. The heart, the main pumping mechanism, circulates oxygenated blood throughout the body to the working tissues. The heart receives deoxygenated blood from the venous system and then pumps the blood through the pulmonary vessels to the lung, where carbon dioxide is exchanged for oxygen. The oxygenated blood then returns to the heart, from which it exits through the aorta to the arterial system and is circulated throughout the body, where it supplies oxygen to the tissues. As the body begins to exercise, the muscles utilize the oxygen at a much higher rate, and the heart must pump more oxygenated blood to meet this increased demand. The heart is capable of adapting to this increased demand through several mechanisms. Heart rate shows a gradual adaptation to an increased work load by increasing proportionally to the intensity of the exercise and plateaus at a given level after about 2 to 3 minutes (Fig. 3-16). The heart rate continues to increase linearly with the work load until it reaches some maximal rate. Maximal heart rate is age related and decreases with age.

Maximal heart rate is, in general, linearly related to maximal oxygen consumption. However, when the heart rate reaches its maximum, exercise can be continued for long periods of time

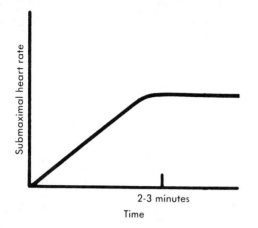

Fig. 3-16. For the heart rate to plateau at a given work load, 2 to 3 minutes are required.

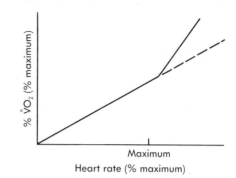

Fig. 3-17. Maximum heart rate is achieved at about the same time as $V_{O_2\,max}$.

without oxygen consumption's reaching its maximum[45] (Fig. 3-17). Thus, oxygen consumption also increases with increasing intensity of the work. Because of these direct linear relationships, the rate of oxygen consumption can be estimated by taking the heart rate.[19]

A second mechanism by which the heart is able to adapt to increased demands during exercise is to increase the stroke volume, the volume of blood being pumped out with each beat. The heart pumps out approximately 70 ml of blood per beat. Stroke volume can continue to increase only to the point at which not enough time remains between beats for the heart to fill up. This occurs at about 40% of maximal heart rate, and above this level increases in the volume of blood being pumped out per unit of time must be caused entirely by increases in heart rate (Fig. 3-18).

Stroke volume and heart rate together determine the volume of blood being pumped through the heart in a given unit of time. Approximately 5 liters of blood are pumped through the heart during each minute at rest. This cardiac output indicates how much blood the heart is capable of pumping in exactly 1 minute. Thus, cardiac output is the primary determinant of the maximal rate of oxygen consumption possible (Fig. 3-19). During exercise, cardiac output may increase as much as six times over its rate at rest.

Cardiac output = stroke volume × heart rate

A training effect that occurs with regard to

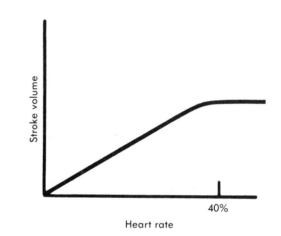

Fig. 3-18. Stroke volume plateaus at about 40% of maximal heart rate.

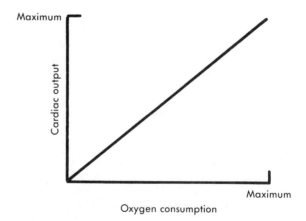

Fig. 3-19. Cardiac output limits $V_{O_2\,max}$.

cardiac output is that the stroke volume increases while exercise heart rate is reduced at a given standard exercise load. The heart becomes more efficient because it is capable of pumping more blood with each stroke. Because the heart is a muscle, it will hypertrophy to some extent, but this response is in no way a negative effect of training.

During exercise females tend to have a 5% to 10% higher cardiac output than males do at all intensities. This effect is likely due to a lower concentration of hemoglobin in the female, which is compensated for during exercise by an increased cardiac output.[4]

BLOOD FLOW. The amount of blood flowing to the various organs increases during exercise. However, the overall distribution of cardiac output changes. The percentage of total cardiac output to the nonessential organs is decreased, whereas it is increased to active skeletal muscle. The volume of blood flow to the myocardium increases substantially during exercise, even though the percentage of total cardiac output supplying the heart muscle remains unchanged. In skeletal muscle increased capillarization occurs, although whether new ones form or dormant ones become patent is not clear.

Blood pressure in the arterial system is determined by the cardiac output in relation to total peripheral resistance to blood flow. Overall, total peripheral resistance decreases and cardiac output increases. All these changes are adaptations to the increased demands of exercise.

HEMOGLOBIN. Blood transports oxygen throughout the system by binding it with hemoglobin. Found in red blood cells, **hemoglobin** is an iron-containing protein that has the capability of easily accepting or giving up molecules of oxygen as needed. Training for improvement in cardiorespiratory endurance produces an increase in total blood volume, with a corresponding increase in the amount of hemoglobin. The concentration of hemoglobin, or the hematocrit (percentage of the total blood volume occupied by red blood cells), in circulating blood increases with both brief and sustained periods of exercise.

LUNGS. As a result of training, some changes occur in lung volumes and capacities. The volume of air that can be inspired in a single maximal ventilation is increased. The diffusing capacity of the lungs is also increased, facilitating the exchange of oxygen and carbon dioxide. Pulmonary resistance to air flow is also decreased.

Effects on Work Ability

The level of cardiorespiratory endurance is in large part directly related to athletic performance. Fatigue is closely related to the percentage of $VO_{2\,max}$ that a particular workload demands. For example, Fig. 3-20 presents two persons, A and B. Person A has a $VO_{2\,max}$ of 50 ml/kg/min, whereas B has a $VO_{2\,max}$ of only 40 ml/kg/min. If both A and B are exercising at the same intensity, then A is working at a much lower percentage of $VO_{2\,max}$ than B is. Consequently, A should be able to sustain activity over a much longer period of time. Everyday activities may be impaired if the ability to utilize oxygen efficiently is impaired. Thus, improvement of cardiorespiratory endurance should be an essential component of any training program.

Regardless of the training technique used for the improvement of cardiorespiratory endurance, one principal goal remains the same: increasing the efficiency with which the cardiorespiratory system is able to supply a sufficient amount of oxygen to the working muscles. Without oxygen, the body is incapable of producing energy for an extended time.

Energy Systems

Various sports activities involve specific demands for energy. For example, sprinting and jumping are high-energy-output activities, requiring a relatively large production of energy for a short time. Conversely, long-distance running and swimming are mostly low-energy-output activities per unit of time and require energy production for a prolonged time. Other physical activities demand a blend of both high- and low-energy output. These various energy demands can be met by the different processes by which energy can be supplied to the skeletal muscles.

ATP: THE IMMEDIATE ENERGY SOURCE. **Adenosine triphosphate (ATP)** is the ultimate usable form of energy for muscular activity. It is produced in the muscle tissue from blood glucose or glycogen. Glucose is derived from the breakdown of dietary carbohydrates. Fats and proteins can also be metabolized to generate ATP.

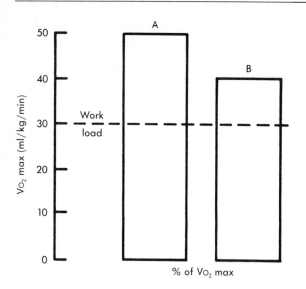

Fig. 3-20. Athlete A should be able to work longer than athlete B as a result of a lower percentage utilization of $Vo_{2\,max}$.

Glucose not needed immediately is stored as glycogen in the resting muscle and liver. Stored glycogen in the liver can later be converted back to glucose and transferred to the blood to meet the body's energy needs.

Once much of the muscle and liver glycogen is depleted, the body relies more heavily on fats stored in adipose tissue to meet its energy needs. The longer the duration of an activity, the greater the amount of fat being used, especially during the later stages of endurance events. During rest and submaximal exertion, both fat and carbohydrate are utilized as energy substrates in approximately a 60 : 40 ratio.[43]

Regardless of the nutrient source that produces ATP, it is always available in the cell as an immediate energy source. When all available sources of ATP are utilized, more must be regenerated for muscular contraction to continue.

ANAEROBIC VERSUS AEROBIC METABOLISM. Two major energy systems function in muscle tissue: anaerobic and aerobic metabolism. Each of these systems generates ATP.

During sudden outbursts of activity in intensive, short-term exercise, ATP can be rapidly metabolized to meet energy needs. After a few seconds of intensive exercise, however, the small stores of ATP are used up. The body then turns to glycogen as an energy source. Glycogen can

be metabolized within the muscle cells to generate ATP for muscle contractions. The breakdown of the glycogen molecule results in the formation of lactic acid. This process is referred to as **anaerobic glycolosis.**

Both ATP and muscle glycogen can be metabolized without oxygen. Thus this energy system involves **anaerobic metabolism** (occurring in the absence of oxygen).

As exercise continues, the body has to rely on the metabolism of carbohydrates (more specifically, glucose) and fats to generate ATP. This second energy system requires oxygen and is therefore referred to as **aerobic metabolism** (occurring in the presence of oxygen).

The degree to which the two major energy systems are involved is determined by the intensity and duration of the activity. For example, short bursts of muscle contraction, as in running or swimming sprints, utilize predominantly the anaerobic system. However, endurance events depend a great deal on the aerobic system. Most sports use a combination of both anaerobic and aerobic metabolism. A rehabilitation program should be designed to include both anaerobic and aerobic training. Neglect of either system during the rehabilitation period may prolong return to full activity.

Training Techniques for Improving Cardiorespiratory Endurance

The sports therapist must devise alternative training techniques for the injured athlete if existing levels of cardiorespiratory endurance are to be maintained or improved during a period of rehabilitation. For example, the distance runner who has sustained an ankle sprain is not able to continue with a running program. The sports therapist may substitute cycling or swimming as a means of maintaining cardiorespiratory endurance levels.

The different methods through which cardiorespiratory endurance may be maintained or even improved include (1) continuous or sustained training, (2) interval training, and (3) circuit training. To a large extent the amount of improvement possible is determined by initial levels of cardiorespiratory endurance.

CONTINUOUS TRAINING. Continuous training involves four considerations: (1) the mode or type of activity, (2) the frequency of the activity, (3) the duration of the activity, and (4) the intensity of the activity.

Mode. The type of activity used in continuous training must be aerobic. Basically, in an aerobic activity the amount of oxygen being supplied is sufficient to meet the demands of the working tissues. Conversely, in an anaerobic activity the intensity of the activity is too high for the system to keep up with oxygen demands; consequently an "oxygen debt" is incurred that must be "paid back" during a recovery period. Aerobic activities elevate the heart rate and maintain it at that level for an extended time. They generally involve repetitive, whole-body, large-muscle movements performed over an extended time. Examples of aerobic activities are running, jogging, walking, cycling, swimming, skipping rope, and cross-country skiing. The advantage of these aerobic activities as opposed to more intermittent activities, such as racquetball, squash, basketball, or tennis, is that aerobic activities are easy to regulate by either speeding up or slowing down the pace. Because the given intensity of the work load elicits a given heart rate, these aerobic activities allow the athlete to maintain heart rate at a specified or target level. Intermittent activities involve variable speeds and intensities that cause the heart rate to fluctuate considerably. Although these intermittent activities improve cardiorespiratory endurance, they are much more difficult to monitor in terms of intensity.

Frequency. Minimal improvement in cardiorespiratory endurance requires at least three sessions per week, and four or five sessions per week are necessary for the injured athlete to maintain some level of cardiovascular conditioning. A competitive athlete should be prepared to train as often as six times per week. Everyone should take off at least a day a week to give damaged tissues a chance to repair themselves.

Duration. For minimal improvement to occur, at least 20 minutes of continuous activity with the heart rate elevated to training levels is necessary. Generally, the greater the duration of the workout, the greater the improvement in cardiorespiratory endurance. The competitive athlete should train for at least 45 minutes.

Intensity. Of the four factors considered, the most critical is the intensity of training, even

though recommendations regarding training intensities vary. This statement is particularly true in the early stages of training when the body is forced to make a lot of adjustments to increased work load demands.

Because heart rate is linearly related to the intensity of the exercise as well as to the rate of oxygen consumption, identifying a specific work load (pace) that will make the heart rate plateau at the desired level is a relatively simple process. By monitoring heart rate, the sports therapist knows whether the pace is too fast or too slow to get the heart rate into a target range.

At several points heart rate is easily measured. The most reliable is the radial artery located on the radial side of the wrist. The pulse at the radial artery provides the most accurate measure of heart rate. Regardless of where the heart rate is taken, it should be monitored within 15 seconds after stopping exercise.

Another factor must be considered when measuring heart rate during exercise. The objective is to elevate the heart rate to a specified target rate and maintain it at that level during the entire workout. Heart rate can be increased or decreased by speeding up or slowing down the pace. Because the heart rate increases proportionately with the intensity of the work load and plateaus after 2 to 3 minutes of activity, the athlete should be actively engaged in the workout for 2 to 3 minutes before the pulse is measured.

Several formulas allow identification of a target training heart rate. This target zone is generally between 60% and 80% of maximal heart rate. Because maximal heart rate is age related and thought to be about 220 beats per minute, a relatively simple estimate of maximal heart rate is 220 minus the athlete's age. For a 20-year-old athlete, maximal heart rate would thus be about 200 beats per minute (220 − 20 = 200). To work at 70% of maximal rate, the target heart rate can be calculated by multiplying 0.7 × (220 − age). Again using a 20-year-old athlete as an example, target heart rate would be 140 beats per minute (0.7 × [220 − 20] = 140).

Another commonly used formula that takes into account the athlete's current level of fitness is the **Karvonen equation:**[37]

Target training HR = resting HR +
       (0.6 [maximum HR − resting HR])

A 20-year-old athlete with a resting pulse of 70 beats per minute, according to the Karvonen equation, would have a target training heart rate of 148 beats per minute (70 + 0.6 [200 − 70] = 148). Keep in mind that true resting heart rate should be monitored when the subject is lying down.

Regardless of the formula used, minimal improvement in cardiorespiratory endurance requires training with the heart rate elevated to at least 60% of its maximal rate.[3] Most authorities would agree that college-age students should train at around 85% of maximal rate, although no conclusive research supports this 85% maximal intensity.

In summary, when using the continuous training method, the activity selected must be aerobic and should be enjoyable. To see minimal improvement in cardiorespiratory endurance, training must be done for a period of 20 minutes three times per week with the heart rate elevated to an intensity of no less than 60% of its maximal rate. For the competitive athlete, however, training at this level does little more than maintain the existing levels of cardiorespiratory endurance.

INTERVAL TRAINING. Unlike continuous training, **interval training** involves intermittent activities. Interval training consists of alternating periods of relatively intense work and active recovery. It allows for performance of much more work at a more intense work load over a longer period of time than continuous work.[44]

Although working at an intensity of about 85% of maximal heart rate is most desirable in continuous training, obviously, sustaining activity at this high intensity over a 20-minute period would be extremely difficult. The advantage of interval training is that it allows work at this 85% or higher level for a short period of time followed by an active period of recovery with work at 30% to 45% of maximal heart rate.[22] Thus the intensity of the workout and its duration can be greater than with continuous training.

Most sports are anaerobic, involving short bursts of intense activity followed by a sort of active recovery period (for example, football, basketball, soccer, or tennis). Training with the interval technique allows a more sport-specific workout. With interval training the overload principle can make the training period much more intense.

In interval training, the **work period** is the amount of time that continuous activity is actually being performed, and the **rest period** is the time between work periods. A **set** is a group of combined work and rest periods, and a **repetition** is the number of work periods per set. **Training time** or **distance** refers to the rate or distance of the work period. The work/rest ratio indicates a time ratio for work versus rest.

An example of interval training would be an injured soccer player training on a stationary bicycle ergometer. An interval workout would involve pedaling at maximum speed for 30 seconds with a 60-second active recovery period between repetitions. During this training session the soccer player's heart rate would probably increase to 85% to 90% of maximal level during the "sprint" and fall to the 30% to 45% level during the recovery period.

Older athletes should exercise some caution when using interval training as a method for improving cardiorespiratory endurance. The intensity levels attained during the active periods may be too high for the untrained individual.

CIRCUIT TRAINING. Whether **circuit training** should be included as a technique for improving cardiorespiratory endurance is a matter of some controversy, although the use of circuit training during a rehabilitation program is of great value to the injured athlete. Circuit training employs a series of exercise stations that consist of weight training, flexibility, calisthenics, and brief aerobic exercises. Circuit training involves moving rapidly from one station to the next and performing whatever exercise is to be done at that station within a specified time period. A typical circuit consists of 8 to 12 stations repeated 3 times.

The primary reason that circuit training is often not considered an acceptable technique for improving cardiorespiratory endurance is that recovery periods tend to be too long between stations to keep the heart rate elevated to at least 60% of maximal level. Circuit training is most definitely an effective technique for improving strength and flexibility. Certainly if the pace or the time interval between stations is rapid and if work load is maintained at a high level of intensity, the cardiorespiratory system may benefit from this circuit. However, no research evidence shows that circuit training is very effective in improving cardiorespiratory endurance. It should be and is most often used as a technique for developing and improving muscular strength and endurance.

If a circuit training routine is performed according to the above guidelines, some improvement of cardiorespiratory endurance will occur.

ADDITIONAL TECHNIQUES. For those athletes who are capable of weight bearing, two additional techniques for maintaining cardiorespiratory endurance may be useful.

Fartlek. Fartlek is a training technique that is a type of cross-country running originated in Sweden. Fartlek literally means "speed play." It is similar to interval training in that the athlete must run for a specified period of time; however, specific pace and speed are not identified. The course for a fartlek workout should be some type of varied terrain with some level running, some uphill and downhill running, and some running around obstacles such as trees or rocks. The object is to put surges into a running workout and to vary the length of the surges according to individual purposes.

One big advantage of fartlek training is that because the terrain is always changing, the run may prevent boredom and may actually turn out to be relaxing.

Again, if fartlek training is going to improve cardiorespiratory endurance, it must elevate the heart rate to at least minimal training levels. Fartlek may best be utilized as an off-season conditioning activity or as a change-of-pace activity to counteract the boredom of training with the same activity day after day.

Par cours. Par cours is a technique for improving cardiorespiratory endurance that combines continuous training and circuit training. This technique involves jogging a short distance from station to station and performing a designated exercise at each station according to guidelines and directions provided on an instruction board located at that station. Par cours circuits provide an excellent means for gaining some aerobic benefits while incorporating some of the benefits of calisthenics. Par cours circuits are found most typically in parks or recreational areas within metropolitan areas.

SUMMARY

1. Strength may be defined as the maximal force that can be generated by a muscle during a single maximal contraction.
2. The ability to generate force is dependent on the physical properties of the muscle itself as well as the mechanical factors that dictate how much force can be generated through the lever system to an external object.
3. Muscular power involves the speed with which a forceful muscle contraction is performed.
4. Hypertrophy of a muscle is caused by increases in the size of the protein myofilaments, which result in an increased cross-sectional diameter of the muscle.
5. Three training techniques can improve muscular strength: isometric training, isotonic training, and isokinetic training.
6. In an isometric contraction, the muscle increases its tension while the length remains constant.
7. In an isotonic contraction, the muscle generates force while changing in length.
8. An isokinetic movement is one in which the length of the muscle is changing but the contraction is performed at a constant velocity.
9. Muscular endurance is the ability to perform repeated isotonic or isokinetic muscle contractions or to sustain an isometric contraction. Muscular endurance tends to improve with muscular strength; thus training techniques for these two components are similar.
10. Flexibility is the ability to move a joint or a series of joints smoothly through a full range of motion.
11. Flexibility may be limited by fat or by defects in bone structure, skin, connective tissue, ligaments, or muscles and tendons.
12. Static flexibility refers to the degree to which a joint may be passively moved to the endpoints in the range of motion, whereas dynamic flexibility refers to movement through the midrange of motion resulting from active contraction.
13. Measurement of joint flexibility is accomplished through the use of a goniometer.
14. An agonist muscle is one that contracts to

produce joint motion; the antagonist muscle is stretched with contraction of the agonist.

15. Ballistic, static, and proprioceptive neuro-muscular facilitation (PNF) techniques have all been used as stretching techniques for improving flexibility.

16. Each of these stretching techniques is based on the neurophysiologic phenomena involving the muscle spindles and Golgi tendon organs.

17. PNF techniques appear to be the most effective in producing increases in flexibility.

18. Strength training, if done correctly through a full range of motion, will probably improve flexibility.

19. Cardiorespiratory endurance involves the coordinated function of the heart, lungs, blood, and blood vessels to supply sufficient amounts of oxygen to the working tissues.

20. The best indicator of how efficiently the cardiorespiratory system functions is the maximal rate at which oxygen can be utilized by the tissues.

21. Heart rate is directly related to the rate of oxygen consumption. The intensity of the work in terms of a rate of oxygen utilization can be predicted by monitoring heart rate.

22. Aerobic exercise involves a sufficient amount of oxygen available to supply the demands of the working tissues. In anaerobic activity, oxygen is being utilized more quickly than it can be supplied; thus an oxygen debt is incurred that must be repaid before working tissue can return to its normal resting state.

23. Continuous or sustained training for improvement of cardiorespiratory endurance involves selecting an activity that is aerobic in nature and training at least three times per week for a time period of no less than 20 minutes with the heart rate elevated to at least 60% of maximal rate.

24. Interval training involves alternating periods of relatively intense work followed by active recovery periods. Interval training allows performance of more work at a relatively higher work load than continuous training does.

25. Circuit training involves a series of exercise stations consisting of weight training, flexibility, and calisthenic exercises; the athlete moves rapidly from one station to the next.

REFERENCES

1 Allsen E: Circulorespiratory endurance, J Phys Ed Rec Dance 52:36, 1981.

2 American Medical Association Council on Scientific Affairs: Indication and contraindications for exercise testing, JAMA 246:1015, 1981.

3 Astrand PO and Rodahl K: Textbook of work physiology, New York, 1986, McGraw-Hill Book Co.

4 Bar-Or O: Cardiac output of 10 to 13-year-old boys and girls during submaximal exercise, J Appl Physiol 30:219, 1971.

5 Basmajian J: Therapeutic exercise, Baltimore, 1978, Williams & Wilkins.

6 Bealieu JE: Developing a stretching program, Physician Sports Med 9(11):59, 1981.

7 Bealieu JE: Stretching for all sports, Pasadena, Calif, 1980, Athletic Press.

8 Berger R: Conditioning for men, Boston, 1973, Allyn & Bacon.

9 Berger R: Effect of varied weight training programs on strength, Res Quart 33:168, 1962.

10 Brooks GA and Fahey TD: Exercise physiology, New York, 1984, John Wiley & Sons.

11 Chapman EA, deVries HA, and Swezey R: Joint stiffness: effect of exercise on young and old men, J Gerontol 27:218, 1972.

12 Cooper KH: The aerobics program for total well being, New York, 1982, Bantam Books.

13 Corbin C and Noble L: Flexibility, J Phys Ed Rec 51:23, 1981.

14 Cornelius WL: Two effective flexibility methods, Athletic Training 16(1):23, 1980.

15 Costill D and others: Skeletal muscle enzymes and fiber compositions in male and female track athletes, J Appl Physiol 40:149, 1976.

16 Couch J: Runners world yoga book, Mountain View, Calif, 1979, World Publications.

17 Coyle E and others: Specificity of power improvements through slow and fast isokinetic training, J Appl Physiol 51:1437, 1981.

18 DeLorme T and Wilkins A: Progressive resistance exercise, New York, 1951, Appleton-Century-Crofts.

19 DeVries H: Physiology of exercise for physical education and athletics, Dubuque, Iowa, 1986, Wm C Brown Group.

20 Donald K and others: Cardiovascular responses to sustained (static) contractions. In Physiology of muscular exercise, American Heart Association Monograph, Nov 15, 1967.

21 Etheridge G and Thomas T: Physiological and biomedical changes of human skeletal muscle induced by different strength training programs, Med Sci Sports Exerc 14:141, 1982.

22 Fox E and Mathews D: The physiological basis of physical education and athletics, Philadelphia, 1981, WB Saunders.

23 Gettman L: Circuit weight training: a critical review of its physiological benefits, Physician Sports Med 9(1):44, 1981.

24 Gettman L, Ward P, and Hagan R: A comparison of com-

bined running and weight training with circuit weight training, Med Sci Sports Exerc 14:229, 1982.

25 Gollnick P and Sembrowich W: Adaptations in human skeletal muscle as a result of training. In Amsterdam EA, editor: Exercise in cardiovascular health and disease, New York, 1977, Yorke Medical Books.

26 Gonyea W: Role of exercise in inducing increases in skeletal muscle fiber number, J Appl Physiol 48:421, 1980.

27 Greer N and Katch F: Validity of palpation recovery pulse rate to estimate exercise heart rate following four intensities of bench step exercise, Res Quart Exerc Sport 53:340, 1982.

28 Gregory L: Some observations on strength training and assessment, J Sports Med Phys Fitness 21:130, 1981.

29 Hage P: Exercise guidelines: which to believe? Physician Sports Med 10:23, 1982.

30 Herling J: It's time to add strength training to our fitness programs, JOHPER 79:17, 1981.

31 How Fit Are You? University of California, Berkeley, Wellness Letter 1(9):7, 1985.

32 Humphrey LD: Flexibility, J Phys Ed Rec Dance 52:41, 1981.

33 Hutinger P: How flexible are you? Aquatic World Magazine, January 1974.

34 Ishii DK: Flexibility strexercises for co-ed groups, Scholastic Coach 45:31, 1976.

35 Jensen C and Fisher G: Scientific basis of athletic conditioning, Philadelphia, 1979, Lea & Febiger.

36 Johnson P, Updike W, Schaefer M, and Stolberg D: Sport exercise and you, New York, 1975, Holt, Rinehart & Winston.

37 Karvonen MJ, Kentala E, and Mustala O: The effects of training on heart rate: a longitudinal study, Anna Med Exp Biol 35:305, 1957.

38 Kickson J, Wilmore J, Constable S, and Buono M: Characterization of standardized weight training exercise, Med Sci Sports Exerc 14:169, 1982.

39 Knight K: Knee rehabilitation by the daily adjustable progressive resistive exercise technique, Am J Sports Med 7:336, 1979.

40 Knott M and Voss P: Proprioceptive neuromuscular facilitation, New York, 1965, Harper & Row, Publishers Inc.

41 Lamb DR: Anabolic steroids. In Williams MH, editor: Ergogenic aids in sport, Champaign, Ill, 1983, Human Kinetics Publishers Inc.

42 Londeree B and Moeschberger M: Effect of age and other factors on maximal heart rate, Res Quart Exerc Sport 53:297, 1982.

43 McArdle W, Katch F, and Katch V: Exercise physiology, energy, nutrition, and human performance, Philadelphia, 1986, Lea & Febiger.

44 MacDougall D and Sale D: Continuous vs interval training: a review for the athlete and coach, Can J Appl Sport Sci 6:93, 1981.

45 McGlynn GH: A reevaluation of isometric training, J Sports Med Phys Fitness 12:258, 1972.

46 MacQueen I: Recent advances in the technique of progressive resistance, Br Med J 11:1193, 1954.

47 Mead W and Hartwig R: Fitness evaluation and exercise prescription, J Fam Pract 13:1039, 1981.

48 Morgan WP: Psychophysiology of self-awareness during vigorous physical activity, Res Quart Exerc Sport 52:385, 1981.

49 Noble BJ: Physiology of exercise and sport, St Louis, 1986, Times Mirror/Mosby College Publishing.

50 O'Shea JP: Power weight training and the female athlete, Physician Sports Med 9(6):109, 1981.

51 Pipes T and Wilmore J: Isokinetic versus isotonic strength training in adult men, Med Sci Sports 7:262, 1975.

52 Prentice W: A comparison of static and PNF stretching for improvement of hip joint flexibility, Athletic Training 18(1):56, 1983.

53 President's Council on Physical Fitness and Sports: Adult fitness manual, Washington, DC, 1980, U.S. Government Printing Office.

54 President's Council on Physical Fitness and Sports: Weight training.

55 Rasch P and Burke R: Kinesiology and applied anatomy, Philadelphia, 1974, Lea & Febiger.

56 Sale D and MacDougall D: Specificity in strength training: a review for the coach and athlete. Can J Appl Sports Sci 6:87, 1981.

57 Sanders M: Unpublished study on resistive training, St Johns University, Collegeville, Minn, 1978.

58 Sapega AA and others: Biophysical factors in range-of-motion exercise, Physician Sports Med 9(12):57, 1981.

59 Shephard RJ and Sidney KH: Exercise and aging. In Hutton R, editor: Exercise and sport science reviews, vol 7, Philadelphia, 1984, Franklin Institute Press.

60 Smith TK: Developing local and general muscular endurance, Athletic J 62:42, 1981.

61 Sobey E: Aerobic weight training, Runner's World 16(8):43, 1981.

62 Stone M and others: Physiological effects of a short-term resistive training program on middle-aged untrained men, Nat Strength Coaches Assoc J 4:16, 1982.

63 Strauss RH, editor: Sportsmedicine, Philadelphia, 1984, WB Saunders Co.

64 Tanigawa MC: Comparison of the hold relax procedure and passive mobilization on increasing muscle length, Phys Ther 52:725, 1972.

65 Verrill D and Pate R: Relationship between duration of static stretch in the sit and reach position and biceps femoris electromyographic activity, Med Sci Sports Exerc 14:124, 1982.

66 Weaver N: Ten easy exercises to prevent injuries, Runner's World 17(11):40, 1982.

67 Weltman A and Stamford B: Home aerobic exercise programs, Physician Sports Med 11:210, 1983.

68 Weltman A and Stamford B: Strength training: free weights vs machines, Physician Sports Med 10:197, 1982.

69 Wescott WL: Strength and fitness, Boston, 1982, Allyn & Bacon.

70 Wilmore JH: Training for sport and activity, Boston, 1982, Allyn & Bacon.

71 Zinovieff A: Heavy resistance exercise, the Oxford technique, Br J Physiol Med 14:129, 1951.

Techniques of Manual Therapy

4

William E. Prentice

OBJECTIVES

Following completion of this chapter, the student will be able to:

- Discuss the relationship of pain and musculoskeletal dysfunction.

- Discuss the differentiation between inert and contractile tissue and how lesions of these tissues are identified.

- Describe active, passive, capsular, noncapsular, and resisted movement patterns.

- Discuss different philosophical approaches to manual therapy.

- Differentiate between physiological and accessory movements.

- Discuss techniques of joint mobilization.

- Understand the neurophysiological basis of proprioceptive neuromuscular facilitation.

- Discuss the basic principles used in proprioceptive neuromuscular facilitation.

- Discuss specific stretching and strengthening techniques used in proprioceptive neuromuscular facilitation.

For the sports therapist to be effective in the treatment of acute and chronic musculoskeletal disorders, some basic knowledge of the techniques of manual therapy is essential. Certainly, the goal of treatment is to restore normal, pain-free movement.[8] The skillful sports therapist can analyze motion to determine how specific movements relieve or exacerbate the symptoms associated with an injury. The purpose of manual therapy is to restore optimal function of a body part following injury by decreasing pain, increasing or decreasing mobility, and using passive, active, or resistive exercise to affect movement.[1]

This chapter discusses various techniques of manual therapy, including assessment of various types of motions used to identify specific lesions, mobilization techniques, and techniques of proprioceptive neuromuscular facilitation (PNF).

PAIN IN MUSCULOSKELETAL DYSFUNCTION

The presence of pain following injury is a major concern for both the injured athlete and the sports therapist. Cyriax[8] believes that all pain arises from a specific lesion and that treatment must reach that lesion if it is to be helpful. Lesions may occur in joints and/or the soft tissues that surround them. Injury to either structure produces spasm or guarding that restricts joint movement. Lack of movement results in atrophy or contractures of muscle and other soft tissue.

Atrophy and soft tissue contracture further impair joint motion and thus create a cycle of increasing severity. Thus manual therapy addresses the relationship that exists between joints and soft tissue in specific treatment techniques.

Zohn and Mennell[35] emphasize the importance of rest from function but not movement. Motion is important if the tissue surrounding the injured joint is to maintain its normal active function. However, the injured structure must be free of its normal stressful function if healing is to take place.[21]

Pain may occur at any point throughout the range of motion. A **painful arc** is pain that occurs at some point in the midrange but disappears as the limb passes this point in either direction.[31] It occurs due to pinching or impingement of sensitive structures between two surfaces, which can be caused either by a biomechanical fault in the articulating bones or by swollen tissue pinched between two normally aligned bony surfaces. Painful arcs are most typically associated with active motion but can also occur in passive motions in which a tissue is being stretched. A classic example of a painful arc is in impingement of the supraspinatus muscle.

Pain that occurs at the endpoint in the range of movement is usually caused by shortening or contracture of the capsule and ligaments. This tightness in the capsule places the joint in a **close-packed** position that abnormally compresses structures surrounding the joint. This problem may be eliminated by stretching the capsule in a neutral pain-free position.[23]

MOTION ASSESSMENT

If a joint or soft tissue lesion exists, the patient is likely to complain of pain on movement. Cyriax has developed a method for locating and identifying a lesion by applying tension selectively to each of the structures that might potentially produce this pain.[8] Tissues are classified as being either contractile or inert. **Contractile** tissues include muscles and their tendons; **inert** tissues include bones, ligaments, joint capsules, fascia, bursae, nerve roots, and dura mater.

If a lesion is present in contractile tissue, pain occurs with active motion in one direction as well as with passive motion in the opposite direction.

Thus a muscle strain would cause pain on both active contraction and passive stretch. Contractile tissues are tested through the midrange by an isometric contraction against maximum resistance. The specific location of the lesion within the musculotendinous unit cannot be specifically identified by the isometric contraction.

A lesion of inert tissue elicits pain on active and passive movement in the same direction. A sprain of a ligament results in pain whenever that ligament is stretched, through either active contraction or passive stretching. Again, a specific lesion of inert tissue cannot be identified by looking at movement patterns alone. Other special tests must be done to differentiate injured structures.

Active Range of Motion

Movement assessment should begin with active motion. The sports therapist should evaluate the quality of movement, range of movement, motion in other planes, movement at varying speeds, and strength throughout the range but in particular at the endpoint. A complaint of pain on active motion does not distinguish contractile pain from inert pain. Thus, the sports therapist must proceed with an evaluation of both passive and resistive motion. An athlete who seems to be free of pain in each of these tests throughout a full range should be tested by applying passive pressure at the endpoint.

Passive Range of Motion

When passive range of motion is being assessed, the athlete must relax completely and allow the sports therapist to move the extremity in order to reduce the influence of the contractile elements. Particular attention should be directed toward the sensation of the athlete at the end of the passive range. The sports therapist should categorize the "feel" of the endpoints as:[8]

NORMAL ENDPOINTS
1. Soft tissue approximation—soft and spongy, a gradual painless stop (e.g., knee flexion)
2. Capsular feel—an abrupt, hard, firm endpoint with only a little give (e.g., endpoint of hip rotation)

3. Bone-to-bone—a distinct and abrupt endpoint where two hard surfaces come in contact with one another (e.g., elbow in full extension)
4. Muscular—springy feel with some associated discomfort (e.g., end of shoulder abduction)

ABNORMAL ENDPOINTS

1. Empty feel—movement is definitely beyond the anatomical limit, and pain occurs before the end of the range (e.g., a complete ligament rupture)
2. Spasm—involuntary muscle contraction that prevents motion because of pain; should also be called *guarding* (e.g., back spasms)
3. Loose—occurs in extreme hypermobility (e.g., previously sprained ankle)[22]
4. Springy block—a rebound at the endpoint (e.g., meniscus tear)

Throughout the passive range of movement, the sports therapist is looking for limitation in movement and the presence of pain. If the athlete reports pain before the end of the available range, this likely indicates acute inflammation, in which stretching and manipulation are both contraindicated as treatments. Pain occurring synchronous with the end of the range indicates that the condition is subacute and has progressed to some inert tissue fibrosis. During this stage, gentle stretching may be started. If no pain occurs at the end of the range, the condition is chronic and contractures have replaced inflammation. At this point, mobilization, stretching, and exercise are all indicated.[9]

Capsular Patterns of Motion

A lesion that exists in the joint capsule or the synovial lining characteristically limits active movement in proportion to the extent of the various motions possible about that particular joint. This limitation in active movement, referred to as a **capsular pattern,** occurs only in synovial joints. Each joint exhibits its own individual capsular pattern. For example, the hip exhibits gross limitation of flexion, abduction, and internal rotation; slight limitation of extension; and little or no limitation of external rotation.[6,8]

Noncapsular Patterns of Motion

In a **noncapsular pattern,** the limitation of motion does not follow the normal capsular pattern. It generally indicates the presence of a lesion outside the capsule. Cyriax has classified the following lesions as noncapsular.[8]

A **ligamentous adhesion** occurs following injury and may result in a movement restriction in one plane, with a full pain-free range in other planes.

Internal derangement involves a sudden onset of localized pain resulting from the displacement of a loose body within the joint. The mechanical block restricts motion in one plane while allowing normal, pain-free motion in the opposite direction. Movement restrictions may change as the loose body shifts its position in the joint space.

An **extraarticular lesion** results from adhesions occurring outside the joint. Movement in a plane that stretches that adhesion results in pain, whereas motion in the opposite direction is pain-free and nonrestricted.

Resisted Motions

The purpose of resisting movement is to evaluate the status of the contractile tissues. The athlete is asked to perform an isometric contraction near the midrange of movement to avoid a position that pinches other inert structures around the joint. Because muscular contraction is under neural control, lesions of the nervous system may affect the strength of muscular contraction. Cyriax has designed the following system for differentiating lesions through assessment of muscular contraction:[8]

1. Strong and painless: normal muscle
2. Strong and painful: minor lesion in some part of the muscle or tendon
3. Weak and painless: complete rupture of muscle or tendon or some nervous system disorder
4. Weak and painful: a gross lesion of contractile tissue
5. Pain on repetition: a single contraction is strong and painless but repetition produces pain, as would exist in some vascular disorder

6. All muscles painful: may indicate a serious emotional or psychological problem

PHILOSOPHIES IN MANUAL THERAPY

Several different treatment philosophies have been proposed for treating musculoskeletal dysfunction, all of which possess some degree of credibility.

The science of chiropractic maintains that disturbance of nerve function is responsible for the majority of illnesses and that these illnesses can be normalized by structural adjustments to the spine and other structures. In addition, some chiropractors also advocate physiotherapeutical, dietary, and sanitary intervention.[29]

Osteopathic medicine stresses the maintenance of normal structural integrity through traditional medical practice including medication and surgery and occasionally through joint manipulation. Osteopathic medicine is well accepted by members of the medical community.[31]

The orthopedist James Cyriax, an authority on techniques of manual therapy, purports that the majority of spinal pain is caused by a disruption of the vertebral disk and can be eliminated through traction and manipulation.[8,9]

The Scandinavian sports therapist Kaltenborn has developed a system of mobilization using arthrokinematic principles to treat dysfunction. He has classified spinal dysfunction as relating to either disk degeneration or facet dysfunction. Loss of mobility is treated through a technique that locates the level of the lesion, locks the joints above and below, and then manipulates the joint in the direction of the limitation.[13]

The Australian sports therapist Maitland treats dysfunction by using a series of graded oscillations.[17,18] Paris, a sports therapist from New Zealand, bases his approach on disorders of the facet and stresses both mobilization and manipulation in treatment.[22,23]

PHYSIOLOGICAL VERSUS ACCESSORY MOTION

Passive exercise may be either physiological or accessory. **Physiological motion** is achieved when an external force moves the body part throughout the range. **Accessory motion** occurs between articulating surfaces of a joint involved in physiological motion and is described by such terms as *gliding* or *rolling.* Physiological movement is voluntary, and accessory movements normally accompany physiological movement. The two occur simultaneously. Although accessory movements cannot occur independently, they may be produced by some external force. Physiological motion is certainly the most important aspect of movement. However, motion through a normal, pain-free range cannot occur without accessory movements.[4,17,18]

Physiological and accessory movement may be hypomobile, normal, or hypermobile.[6] Each joint has an anatomic limit to motion that is determined by both bony arrangement and surrounding soft tissue. In a hypomobile joint, motion stops at some point referred to as a **pathological point,** short of the anatomical limit due to pain, spasm, or tissue resistance.

A hypermobile joint moves beyond its anatomical limit due to laxity in the surrounding structures. A hypomobile joint should respond well to techniques of mobilization and manipulation. A hypermobile joint should be treated with strengthening exercises, stability exercises, and, if indicated, taping, splinting, or bracing.[23]

Sports therapists have commonly used passive physiological movement to improve range of motion. It has traditionally been accomplished by using either sustained (static) or oscillating (ballistic) stretches.

The concept of accessory movement is critical in manual therapy. Generally, techniques designed to improve accessory motion can be used for tight articular structures when primary resistance is encountered from the ligaments and capsule of the joint, can be done in any portion of the physiological range, can be done in any direction, cause less pain for the degree of range of motion gained, and are relatively safe to use.[1]

MOBILIZATION TECHNIQUES

The techniques of **joint mobilization** are used to improve joint mobility or to decrease joint pain by restoring accessory movements to the joint and thus allow full, nonrestricted, pain-free range of motion.[33]

Mobilization techniques may be used to attain a variety of treatment goals: reducing pain; decreasing muscle guarding; stretching or lengthening tissue surrounding a joint, in particular capsular and ligamentous tissue; reflexogenic effects that either inhibit or facilitate muscle tone or stretch reflex; and proprioceptive effects to improve postural and kinesthetic awareness.[1]

Movement throughout a range of motion can be quantified with various measurement techniques. Physiological movement is measured with a goniometer and composes the major portion of the range. Accessory motion is thought of in millimeters, although it is not measured precisely. Thus treatment techniques designed to improve accessory movement are generally small-amplitude movements, the amplitude being the distance that the joint is moved passively within its total range. Mobilization techniques utilize these small-amplitude oscillating motions within a specific part of the range. Typical treatment of a joint may involve a series of three to six mobilizations lasting up to 30 seconds, with one to three oscillations per second.[18]

Mobilization should be done with both the athlete and the sports therapist positioned in a comfortable and relaxed manner. The sports therapist should mobilize one joint at a time. The joint should be stabilized as near one articulating surface as possible, while moving the other with a firm, confident grasp (Fig. 4-1).

Maitland has described the total amount of both physiological and accessory motion available in one direction and categorized mobilization techniques into five gradations as follows:[18]

GRADE I. A small-amplitude movement at the beginning of the range of movement. Used when pain and spasm limit movement early in the range of motion.

GRADE II. A large-amplitude movement within the midrange of movement. Used when spasm limits movement sooner with a quick oscillation than with a slow one, or when slowly increasing pain restricts movement halfway into the range.

GRADE III. A large-amplitude movement up to the pathological limit in the range of movement. Used when pain and resistance from spasm, inert tissue tension, or tissue compression limit movement near the end of the range.

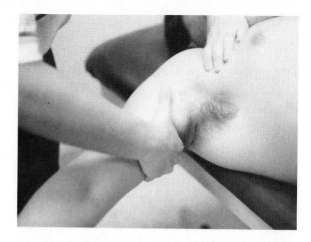

Fig. 4-1. In mobilization of the shoulder joint, the joint should be stabilized near the articulating surface while moving the other with a firm grip.

GRADE IV. A small-amplitude movement at the very end of the range of movement. Used when resistance limits movement in the absence of pain and spasm.

GRADE V. A small-amplitude, quick thrust delivered at the end of the range of movement, usually accompanied by a popping sound, which is called a *manipulation*. Used when minimal resistance limits the end of the range. Manipulation is most effectively accomplished by the velocity of the thrust rather than by the force of the thrust. Most authorities agree that manipulation should be used only by individuals trained specifically in these techniques because a great deal of skill and judgment is necessary for safe and effective treatment.

In Maitland's system, grades I and II are used primarily for treatment of pain, and grades III and IV are used for treating stiffness. Pain must be treated first and stiffness second.[18]

Fig. 4-2 shows the various grades of oscillation that are used in a joint with some limitation of motion. As the severity of the movement restriction increases, the point of limitation (PL) will move to the left away from the anatomic limit (AL) of motion. However, the relationships that exist among the five grades in terms of their positions within the range of motion remain the same. Mobilization should be done by stretching

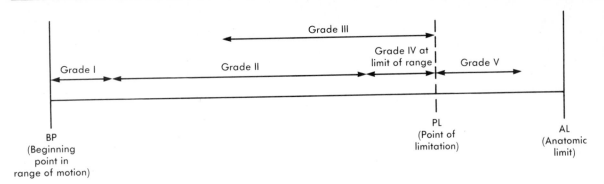

Fig. 4-2. Maitland's five grades of motion.[17,18] *PL* (point of limitation), *AL* (anatomic limit)

the joint in the direction of restricted accessory motion. However, Mangine has stated that the most effective treatment is in the direction opposite to the pain or the restriction and implies that pain should not be produced as a result of the treatment.[19]

Accessory motions can be classified as either spin, glide, or roll movements.[16] *Spin* movements involve rotation about a stationary axis. *Gliding* occurs involuntarily when two surfaces slide with respect to one another. Also called *translation,* it occurs only when two surfaces are congruent and flat or congruent and curved. *Rolling* occurs when two joint surfaces that are not congruent move on one another. One surface is concave, and the other is convex. In many joints, both rolling and gliding motions occur at some point in the range of motion (e.g., knee flexion and extension). The shape of the articulating surfaces usually dictates the direction of the mobilization being performed.

The direction of the technique used is the direction that produces the primary complaint of either pain or stiffness (Fig. 4-3). Usually in acute conditions it is the direction that reduces pain. In chronic conditions it is the direction that increases mobility and decreases stiffness. When the concave surface is stationary and the convex surface is moving, mobilization should be done in the opposite direction of the bone movement. If the convex articular surface is stationary and the concave surface is moving, the mobilization should be done in the same direction as the bone movement. If mobilization in the appropriate direction exacerbates complaints of pain or stiffness, the sports therapist should apply the tech-

nique in the opposite direction until the patient can tolerate the appropriate direction.[34]

TRACTION TECHNIQUES

Kaltenborn has proposed a system using traction as a means of mobilizing a joint. Whereas Maitland has divided motions within the full range into gradations, Kaltenborn[13] has labeled these gradations as stages and defined them as follows:

STAGE I *(Piccolo).* Traction that neutralizes pressure in the joint without actual separation of the joint surfaces. The purpose is to produce pain relief by reducing the "grinding" of articular surfaces during mobilization. This stage is analogous to a grade I mobilization.

STAGE II *(Take up the slack).* Traction that effectively separates the articulating surfaces and takes up the slack or eliminates play in the joint capsule. Stage II is used to relieve pain and is the same as a grade IV mobilization.

STAGE III *(Stretch).* Traction that involves actual stretching of the soft tissue surrounding the joint for the purpose of increasing mobility in a hypomobile joint. Kaltenborn's stages of mobilization are shown in Fig. 4-4.

CONTRAINDICATIONS TO MOBILIZATION

Techniques of mobilization and manipulation should not be used haphazardly. These techniques should generally not be used in cases of

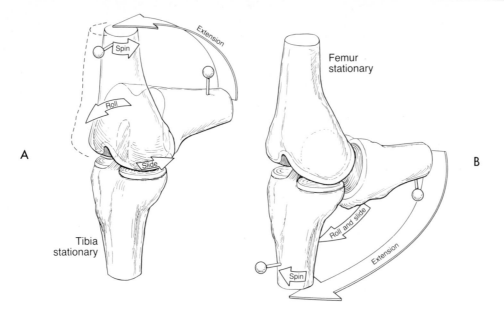

Fig. 4-3. Convex-concave rule: **A**, convex moving on concave; **B**, concave moving on convex.

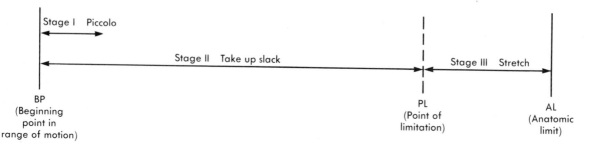

Fig. 4-4. Kaltenborn's stages of motion. *PL*, point of limitation, *AL*, anatomic limit.

inflammatory arthritis, malignancy, bone disease, neurological involvement, bone fracture, congenital bone deformities, and vascular disorders of the vertebral artery. Again, manipulation should be performed only by those sports therapists specifically trained in this procedure because some special knowledge and judgment is required for effective treatment.[34]

PROPRIOCEPTIVE NEUROMUSCULAR FACILITATION TECHNIQUES

Proprioceptive neuromuscular facilitation (PNF) is an approach to therapeutic exercise based on the principles of functional human anatomy and neurophysiology. It utilizes proprioceptive, cutaneous, and auditory input to produce functional improvement in motor output and can be a vital element in the rehabilitation process of many sports-related injuries. These techniques have been recommended for increasing strength as well as flexibility and range of motion.* This discussion should serve as a guide for the sports therapist using the principles and techniques of proprioceptive neuromuscular facilitation as a component of a rehabilitation program.

*References 7, 12, 20, 24, 26, 33.

The Neurophysiological Basis of PNF

The therapeutic techniques of facilitation were first used in the treatment of patients with paralysis and in the treatment of neuromuscular disorders. Most of the principles underlying modern therapeutic exercise techniques can be attributed to the work of Sherrington,[30] who first defined the concepts of facilitation and inhibition.

An impulse traveling down the corticospinal tract or afferent impulses traveling up from peripheral receptors in the muscle cause an impulse volley, which results in the discharge of a limited number of specific motor neurons as well as the discharge of additional surrounding (anatomically close) motor neurons in the so-called subliminal fringe area. An impulse causing the recruitment and discharge of additional motor neurons within the subliminal fringe is said to be facilitatory. Conversely, any stimulus that causes motor neurons to drop out of the discharge zone and away from the subliminal fringe is said to be inhibitory. Facilitation results in increased excitability, and inhibition results in decreased excitability of motor neurons.[21] Thus the function of weak muscles would be aided by facilitation, and muscle spasticity would be decreased by inhibition.[11]

Sherrington attributed the impulses transmitted from the peripheral stretch receptors via the afferent system as being the strongest influence on the alpha motor neurons. Therefore, the sports therapist should be able to modify the input from the peripheral receptors and thus influence the excitability of the alpha motor neurons. The discharge of motor neurons can be facilitated by peripheral stimulation, which causes afferent impulses to make contact with excitatory neurons and results in increased muscle tone or strength of voluntary contraction. Motor neurons can also be inhibited by peripheral stimulation, which causes afferent impulses to make contact with inhibitory neurons, thus resulting in muscle relaxation and allowing for stretching of the muscle.[30] To indicate any technique in which input from peripheral receptors is used for the purpose of either facilitation or inhibition PNF should be used.[11]

The principles and techniques of PNF described here are based primarily on the neurophysiological mechanisms involving the stretch reflex. The **stretch reflex** involves two types of receptors: (1) muscle spindles that are sensitive to a change in length as well as the rate of change in length of the muscle fiber, and (2) Golgi tendon organs that detect changes in tension (Fig. 4-5).

Stretching a given muscle causes an increase in the frequency of impulses transmitted to the spinal cord from the muscle spindle, which in turn produces an increase in the frequency of motor nerve impulses returning to that same muscle, thus reflexly resisting the stretch. However, the development of excessive tension within the muscle activates the Golgi tendon organs, whose sensory impulses are carried back to the spinal cord. These impulses have an inhibitory effect on the motor impulses returning to the muscles and thus cause that muscle to relax.

Two neurophysiological phenomena help to explain facilitation and inhibition of the neuromuscular systems. The first is known as **autogenic inhibition** and is defined as inhibition that is mediated by afferent fibers from a stretched muscle acting on the alpha motor neurons supplying that muscle, thus causing it to relax. When a muscle is stretched, motor neurons supplying that muscle receive both excitatory and inhibitory impulses from the receptors. If the stretch is continued for a slightly extended period of time, the inhibitory signals from the Golgi tendon organs eventually override the excitatory impulses and therefore cause relaxation. Because inhibitory motor neurons receive impulses from the Golgi tendon organs, while the muscle spindle creates an initial reflex excitation leading to contraction, the Golgi tendon organs apparently send inhibitory impulses that last for the duration of increased tension (resulting from either passive stretch or active contraction) and eventually dominate the weaker impulses from the muscle spindle. This inhibition seems to protect the muscle against injury from reflex contractions resulting from excessive stretch.

A second mechanism known as **reciprocal inhibition** deals with the relationships of the agonist and antagonist muscles (Fig. 4-6). The muscles that are contracting to produce joint motion are referred to as **agonists,** and the resulting movement is called an **agonistic pattern.** The

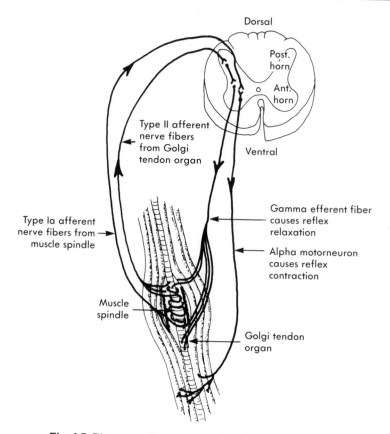

Fig. 4-5. Diagrammatic representation of the stretch reflex.

muscles that are stretching to allow the agonist pattern to occur are referred to as **antagonists.** Movement that occurs directly opposite to the agonist pattern is called the **antagonist pattern.**

When motor neurons of the agonist muscle receive excitatory impulses from afferent nerves, the motor neurons that supply the antagonist muscles are inhibited by the afferent impulses.[2] Thus contraction or extended stretch of the agonist muscle must elicit relaxation or inhibit the antagonist. Likewise, a quick stretch of the antagonist muscle facilitates a contraction of the agonist. For facilitating or inhibiting motion, PNF relies heavily on the actions of these agonist and antagonist muscle groups.

A final point of clarification should be made regarding both autogenic inhibition and reciprocal inhibition. The motor neurons of the spinal cord always receive a combination of inhibitory and excitatory impulses from the afferent nerves.

Whether these motor neurons will be excited or inhibited depends on the ratio of these two types of incoming impulses.

Several different approaches to therapeutic exercise based on the principles of facilitation and inhibition have been proposed. Among these are the Bobath Method 3, Brunnstrom Method 4, Rood Method 28, and the Knott and Voss Method 14, which they called proprioceptive neuromuscular facilitation. Although each of these techniques is important and useful, the PNF approach of Knott and Voss probably makes the most explicit use of proprioceptive stimulation.[14]

Rationale for Use

As a positive approach to injury rehabilitation, PNF is aimed at what the patient can do physically within the limitations of the injury. It is per-

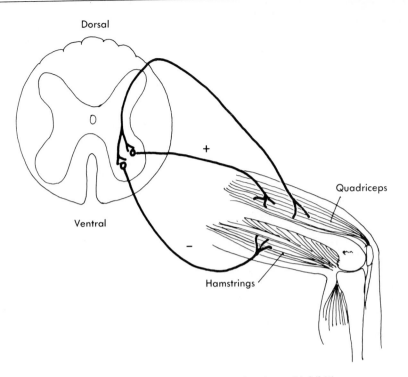

Fig. 4-6. Diagrammatic representation of reciprocal inhibition.

haps best utilized for the purpose of decreasing deficiencies in strength, flexibility, and coordination in response to demands that are placed on the neuromuscular systems.

The body tends to respond to the demands placed on it. The principles of PNF attempt to provide a maximal response for increasing strength, flexibility, and coordination. These principles should be applied with consideration of their appropriateness in achieving a particular goal.

That continued activity during a rehabilitation program is essential for maintaining or improving strength or flexibility is well accepted. Therefore, an intense program should offer the greatest potential for recovery.

The PNF approach is holistic, integrating sensory, motor, and psychological aspects of a rehabilitation program. It incorporates reflex activities from the spinal levels and upward, either inhibiting or facilitating them as appropriate.

The brain recognizes only gross joint movement and not individual muscle action. Moreover, the strength of a muscle contraction is di-

rectly proportional to the activated motor units. Therefore, to increase the strength of a muscle, the maximum number of motor units must be stimulated in order to strengthen the remaining muscle fibers.[12,14] This "irradiation" or overflow effect can occur when the stronger muscle groups help the weaker groups in completing a particular movement. This cooperation leads to the rehabilitation goal of return to optimal function.[2,14] The following principles of PNF should be applied to reach that ultimate goal.

Basic Principles of PNF

Margret Knott in her text on PNF[14] emphasized the importance of the principles rather than specific techniques in a rehabilitation program. These principles are the basis of PNF that must be superimposed on any specific techniques. Application of the following principles may assist in promoting a desired response in the patient being treated.

1. The patient must be taught the PNF patterns regarding the sequential move-

ments from starting position to terminal position. The sports therapist has to keep instructions brief and simplistic. The patterns should be used along with the techniques to increase the effects of the treatment.

2. When learning the patterns, the patient is often helped by looking at the moving limb. This visual stimulus offers the patient feedback for directional and positional control.

3. Verbal cues are used to coordinate voluntary effort with reflex responses. Commands should be firm and simple. Commands most commonly used with PNF techniques are "push" and "pull," which ask for an isotonic contraction; "hold," which implies an isometric contraction; and "relax."

4. Manual contact with appropriate pressure is essential for influencing direction of motion and facilitating a maximal response because reflex responses are greatly affected by pressure receptors. Manual contact should be firm and confident to give the patient a feeling of security. A movement response may be facilitated by hand positioning over the muscle being contracted to facilitate an increase in strength.

5. Proper mechanics and body positioning of the sports therapist are essential in applying pressure and resistance. The sports therapist should stand in a position that accommodates the diagonal movement pattern, with knees bent and close to the patient such that resistance can easily be applied throughout the range.

6. The amount of resistance given should facilitate a maximal response that allows smooth, coordinated motion. The appropriate resistance depends to a large extent on the capabilities of the patient. It may also change at different points throughout the range of motion. Maximal resistance may be used with those techniques that use isometric contractions to restrict motion to a specific point; it may also be used in isotonic contractions throughout a full range of movement.

7. Rotational movement is a critical component in all of the PNF patterns because maximal contraction is impossible without it.

8. Normal timing is the sequence of muscle contraction that occurs in any normal motor activity resulting in coordinated movement.[14] The distal movements of the patterns should occur first. The distal movement components should be completed by no later than halfway through the total PNF pattern. To accomplish this, appropriate verbal commands should be timed with manual commands. Normal timing may be used with maximal resistance or without resistance from the sports therapist.

9. Timing for emphasis is used primarily with isotonic contractions. This principle superimposes maximal resistance, at specific points in the range, upon the patterns of facilitation allowing overflow or irradiation to the weaker components of a movement pattern. Thus the stronger components are emphasized to facilitate the weaker components of a movement pattern.

10. Specific joints may be facilitated by using **traction** or **approximation**. Traction spreads apart the joint articulations, and approximation presses them together. Both techniques stimulate the joint proprioceptors. Traction increases the muscular response, promotes movement, assists isotonic contractions, and is used with most flexion antigravity movements. Traction must be maintained throughout the pattern. Approximation increases the muscular response, promotes stability, assists isometric contractions, and is used most with extension (gravity-assisted) movements. Approximation may be quick or gradual and may be repeated during a pattern.

11. Giving a quick stretch to the muscle prior to muscle contraction facilitates a muscle to respond with greater force through the mechanisms of the stretch reflex. It is most effective if all the components of a movement are stretched simultaneously.

However, this quick stretch may be contraindicated in many orthopedic conditions because the extensibility limits of a damaged musculotendinous unit or joint structure may be exceeded, thus exacerbating the injury.

Techniques of PNF

Each of the principles described above should be applied to the specific techniques of PNF. These techniques may be used in a rehabilitation program either for the purpose of strengthening or facilitating a particular agonistic muscle group or for stretching or inhibition of the antagonistic group. The choice of a specific technique depends on the deficits of a particular patient. Specific techniques or combinations of techniques should be selected on the basis of the patient problem.

STRENGTHENING TECHNIQUES. The following techniques are most appropriately used for the development of muscular strength, endurance, and coordination.

Repeated contraction is useful when a patient has weakness either at a specific point or throughout the entire range. It is used to correct imbalances that occur within the range by repeating the weakest portion of the total range. The patient moves isotonically against maximal resistance repeatedly until fatigue is evidenced in the weaker components of the motion. When fatigue of the weak components becomes apparent, a stretch at that point in the range should facilitate the weaker muscles and result in a smoother, more coordinated motion. Again, quick stretch may be contraindicated with some musculoskeletal injuries. The amount of resistance to motion given by the sports therapist should be modified to accommodate the strength of the muscle group. The patient is commanded to "push" by using the agonist both concentrically and eccentrically throughout the range.

Slow reversal involves an isotonic contraction of the antagonist followed immediately by an isotonic contraction of the agonist. The initial contraction of the antagonist muscle group facilitates the succeeding contraction of the agonist muscles. The slow reversal technique can be used for developing active range of motion of the agonists and normal reciprocal timing between the antagonists and agonists, which is critical for normal coordinated motion. The patient should be commanded to push against maximal resistance by using the antagonist and then to pull by using the agonist. The initial antagonistic push facilitates the succeeding agonist contraction.

Slow reversal-hold is an isotonic contraction of the agonist followed immediately by an isometric contraction, with a hold command given at the end of each active movement. The direction of the pattern is reversed by using the same sequence of contraction with no relaxation before shifting to the antagonistic pattern. This technique can be especially useful in developing strength at a specific point in the ROM.

Rhythmic stabilization uses an isometric contraction of the agonist, followed by an isometric contraction of the antagonist for the purpose of producing cocontraction and stability of the two opposing muscle groups. The command given is always "hold," and movement is resisted in each direction. Rhythmic stabilization results in an increase in the holding power to a point where the position cannot be broken. Holding should emphasize cocontraction of agonists and antagonists.

The rhythmic initiation technique involves a progression of initial passive, then active-assistive, followed by active movement through the agonist pattern. Movement is slow, goes through the available range of motion, and avoids activation of a quick stretch. It is used for patients who are unable to initiate movement and for patients who have a limited range of motion due to increased tone. It may also be used to teach the patient a movement pattern.

STRETCHING TECHNIQUES. The following techniques should be used for the purpose of increasing range of motion, relaxation, and inhibition.

Contract-relax is a stretching technique that moves the body part passively into the agonist pattern. The patient is instructed to push by contracting the antagonist isotonically against the resistance of the sports therapist. The patient then relaxes the antagonist while the therapist moves the part passively through as much range as possible to the point where limitation is again felt. This contract-relax technique is beneficial when range of motion is limited due to muscle tightness.

Hold-relax is very similar to the contract-relax technique. It begins with an isometric contraction of the antagonist against resistance, followed by a concentric contraction of the agonist muscle combined with light pressure from the sports therapist to produce maximal stretch of the antagonist. This technique is appropriate muscle tension on one side of a joint and may be used with either the agonist or antagonist.

Slow reversal-hold-relax technique begins with an isotonic contraction of the antagonist, which often limits range of motion in the agonist pattern, followed by an isometric contraction of the antagonist during the push phase. During the relax phase, the antagonists are relaxed while the agonists are contracting, causing movement in the direction of the agonist pattern and thus stretching the antagonist. This technique, like the contract-relax and hold-relax, is useful for increasing range of motion when the primary limiting factor is the antagonistic muscle group.

Because the goal of rehabilitation in most sports-related injuries is restoration of strength through a full, nonrestricted range of motion, several of these techniques are sometimes combined in sequence to accomplish this goal. Fig. 4-7 shows a PNF stretching technique in which the sports therapist is stretching the injured athlete.

PNF PATTERNS. The PNF patterns are concerned with gross movements as opposed to specific muscle actions. The techniques identified previously may be superimposed on any of the PNF patterns. The techniques of PNF are composed of both rotational and diagonal exercise patterns that are similar to the motions required in most sports and in normal daily activities.

The exercise patterns are three component movements: flexion-extension, abduction-adduction, and internal-external rotation. Human movement is patterned and rarely involves straight motion because all muscles are spiral in nature and lie in diagonal directions.

The PNF patterns described by Knott and Voss[14] involve distinct diagonal and rotational movements of upper extremity, lower extremity, upper trunk, lower trunk, and neck. The exercise

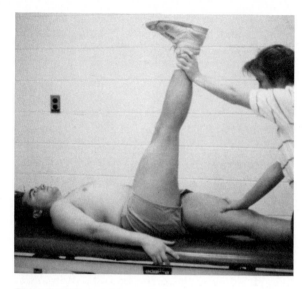

Fig. 4-7. PNF stretching technique.

pattern is initiated with the muscle groups in the lengthened or stretched position. The muscle group is then contracted, moving the body part through the range of motion to a shortened position.

The upper and lower extremities each have two separate patterns of diagonal movement for each part of the body, which are referred to as the **diagonal 1 (D1)** and **diagonal 2 (D2)** patterns. These two diagonal patterns are subdivided into D1 moving into flexion, D1 moving into extension, D2 moving into flexion, and D2 moving into extension.

Figs. 4-8 and 4-9 diagram the PNF patterns for the upper and lower extremities, respectively. The patterns are named according to the proximal pivots at either the shoulder or the hip (i.e., the glenohumeral joint or femoralacetabular joint).

Tables 4-1 and 4-2 describe specific movements in the D1 and D2 patterns for the upper extremities. Figs. 4-10 through 4-17 show starting positions and terminal positions for each of the diagonal patterns in the upper extremity.

Tables 4-3 and 4-4 describe specific movements in the D1 and D2 patterns for the lower extremities. Figs. 4-18 through 4-25 show the starting and terminal positions for each of the diagonal patterns in the lower extremity.

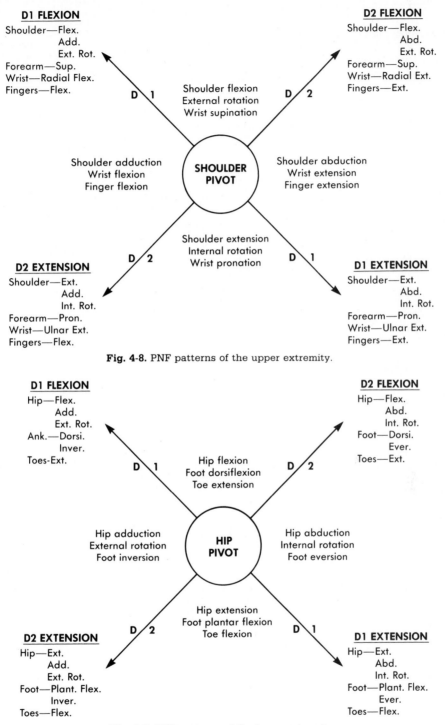

D1 FLEXION
Shoulder—Flex.
        Add.
        Ext. Rot.
Forearm—Sup.
Wrist—Radial Flex.
Fingers—Flex.

D2 FLEXION
Shoulder—Flex.
        Abd.
        Ext. Rot.
Forearm—Sup.
Wrist—Radial Ext.
Fingers—Ext.

Shoulder flexion
External rotation
Wrist supination

D 1   D 2

Shoulder adduction
Wrist flexion
Finger flexion

SHOULDER PIVOT

Shoulder abduction
Wrist extension
Finger extension

Shoulder extension
Internal rotation
Wrist pronation

D 2   D 1

D2 EXTENSION
Shoulder—Ext.
        Add.
        Int. Rot.
Forearm—Pron.
Wrist—Ulnar Ext.
Fingers—Flex.

D1 EXTENSION
Shoulder—Ext.
        Abd.
        Int. Rot.
Forearm—Pron.
Wrist—Ulnar Ext.
Fingers—Ext.

Fig. 4-8. PNF patterns of the upper extremity.

D1 FLEXION
Hip—Flex.
    Add.
    Ext. Rot.
Ank.—Dorsi.
      Inver.
Toes-Ext.

D2 FLEXION
Hip—Flex.
    Abd.
    Int. Rot.
Foot—Dorsi.
      Ever.
Toes—Ext.

Hip flexion
Foot dorsiflexion
Toe extension

D 1   D 2

Hip adduction
External rotation
Foot inversion

HIP PIVOT

Hip abduction
Internal rotation
Foot eversion

Hip extension
Foot plantar flexion
Toe flexion

D 2   D 1

D2 EXTENSION
Hip—Ext.
    Add.
    Ext. Rot.
Foot—Plant. Flex.
      Inver.
Toes—Flex.

D1 EXTENSION
Hip—Ext.
    Abd.
    Int. Rot.
Foot—Plant. Flex.
      Ever.
Toes—Flex.

Fig. 4-9. PNF patterns of the lower extremity.

TABLE 4-1
D1 Upper Extremity Movement Patterns

Body Part	Moving into Flexion		Moving into Extension	
	Starting Position (Fig. 4-10)	Terminal Position (Fig. 4-11)	Starting Position (Fig. 4-12)	Terminal Position (Fig. 4-13)
Shoulder	Extension Abduction Internal rotation	Flexion Adduction External rotation	Flexion Adduction External rotation	Extension Abduction Internal rotation
Scapula	Depression Retraction Downward rotation	Flexion Protraction Upward rotation	Elevation Protraction Upward rotation	Depression Retraction Downward rotation
Forearm	Pronation	Supination	Supination	Pronation
Wrist	Ulnar extension	Radial flexion	Radial flexion	Ulnar extension
Finger and thumb	Extension Abduction	Flexion Adduction	Flexion Adduction	Extension Abduction
Hand position*	Left and inside volar surface of hand Right hand underneath arm in cubital fossa of elbow		Left hand on back of elbow on humerus Right hand on dorsum of hand	
Verbal command	Pull		Push	

*For right arm.

TABLE 4-2
D2 Upper Extremity Movement Patterns

Body Part	Moving into Flexion		Moving into Extension	
	Starting Position (Fig. 4-14)	Terminal Position (Fig. 4-15)	Starting Position (Fig. 4-16)	Terminal Position (Fig. 4-17)
Shoulder	Extension Adduction Internal rotation	Flexion Abduction External rotation	Flexion Abduction External rotation	Extension Adduction Internal rotation
Scapula	Depression Protraction Downward rotation	Elevation Retraction Upward rotation	Elevation Retraction Upward rotation	Depression Protraction Downward rotation
Forearm	Pronation	Supination	Supination	Pronation
Wrist	Ulnar flexion	Radial extension	Radial extension	Ulnar flexion
Finger and thumb	Flexion Adduction	Extension Abduction	Extension Abduction	Flexion Adduction
Hand position*	Left hand on back of humerus Right hand on dorsum of hand		Left hand on volar surface of humerus Right hand on cubital fossa of elbow	
Verbal command	Push		Pull	

*For right arm.

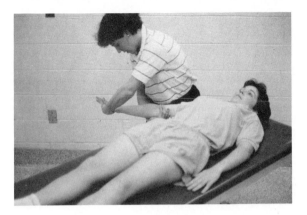

Fig. 4-10. D1 upper extremity movement pattern moving into flexion (starting position).

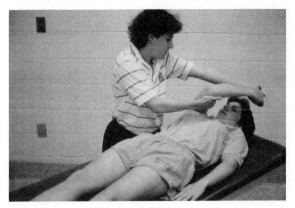

Fig. 4-11. D1 upper extremity movement pattern moving into flexion (terminal position).

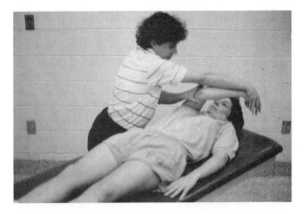

Fig. 4-12. D1 upper extremity movement pattern moving into extension (starting position).

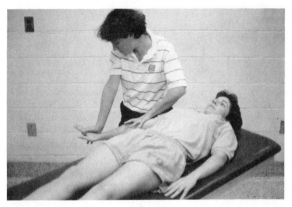

Fig. 4-13. D1 upper extremity movement pattern moving into extension (terminal position).

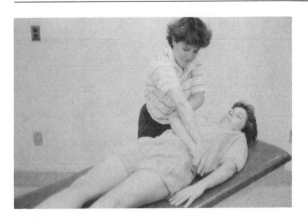

Fig. 4-14. D2 upper extremity movement pattern moving into flexion (starting position).

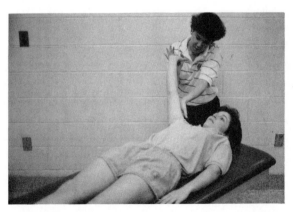

Fig. 4-15. D2 upper extremity movement pattern moving into flexion (terminal position).

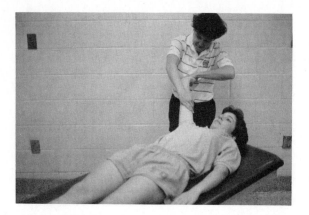

Fig. 4-16. D2 upper extremity movement pattern moving into extension (starting position).

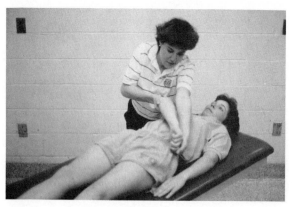

Fig. 4-17. D2 upper extremity movement pattern moving into extension (terminal position).

TABLE 4-3

D1 Lower Extremity Movement Patterns

Body Part	Moving into Flexion		Moving into Extension	
	Starting Position (Fig. 4-18)	Terminal Position (Fig. 4-19)	Starting Position (Fig. 4-20)	Terminal Position (Fig. 4-21)
Hip	Extended Abducted Internally rotated	Flexed Adducted Externally rotated	Flexed Adducted Externally rotated	Extended Abducted Internally rotated
Knee	Extended	Flexed	Flexed	Extended
Position of tibia	Externally rotated	Internally rotated	Internally rotated	Externally rotated
Ankle and foot	Plantar flexed Everted	Dorsi flexed Inverted	Dorsi flexed Inverted	Plantar flexed Everted
Toes	Flexed	Extended	Extended	Flexed
Hand position*	Right hand on dorsimedial surface of foot Left hand on anteromedial thigh near patella		Right hand on lateralplantar surface of foot Left hand on posteriorlateral thigh near popliteal crease	
Verbal command	Pull		Push	

*For right leg.

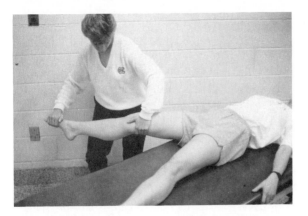

Fig. 4-18. D1 lower extremity movement pattern moving into flexion (starting position).

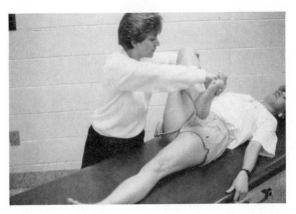

Fig. 4-19. D1 lower extremity movement pattern moving into flexion (terminal position).

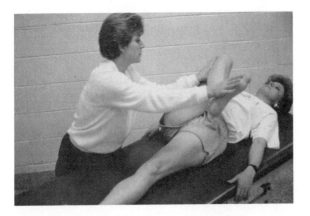

Fig. 4-20. D1 lower extremity movement pattern moving into extension (starting position).

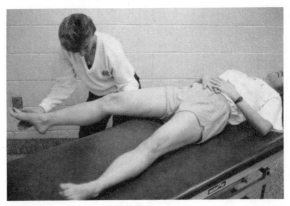

Fig. 4-21. D1 lower extremity movement pattern moving into extension (terminal position).

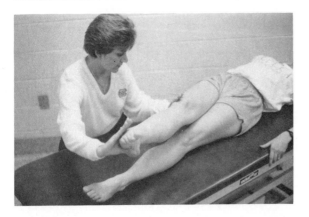

Fig. 4-22. D2 lower extremity movement pattern moving into flexion (starting position).

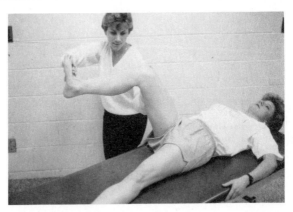

Fig. 4-23. D2 lower extremity movement pattern moving into flexion (terminal position).

TABLE 4-4
D2 Lower Extremity Movement Patterns

Body Part	Moving into Flexion		Moving into Extension	
	Starting Position (Fig. 4-22)	Terminal Position (Fig. 4-23)	Starting Position (Fig. 4-24)	Terminal Position (Fig. 4-25)
Hip	Extended Adducted Externally rotated	Flexed Abducted Internally rotated	Flexed Abducted Internally rotated	Extended Adducted Externally rotated
Knee	Extended	Flexed	Flexed	Extended
Position of tibia	Externally rotated	Internally rotated	Internally rotated	Externally rotated
Ankle and foot	Plantar flexed Inverted	Dorsi flexed Everted	Dorsi flexed Everted	Plantar flexed Inverted
Toes	Flexed	Extended	Extended	Flexed
Hand position*	Right hand on dorsilateral surface of foot Left hand on anterolateral thigh near patella		Right hand on medialplantar surface of foot Left hand on posteriormedial thigh near popliteal crease	
Verbal command	Pull		Push	

*For right leg.

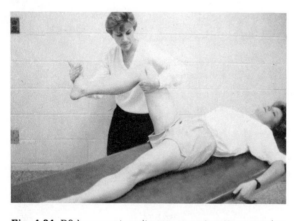

Fig. 4-24. D2 lower extremity movement pattern moving into extension (starting position).

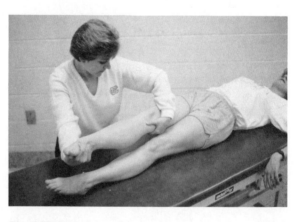

Fig. 4-25. D2 lower extremity movement pattern moving into extension (terminal position).

Table 4-5 describes the rotational movement of the upper trunk moving into extension (also called **chopping**) and moving into flexion (also called **lifting**). Figs. 4-26 and 4-27 show the starting and terminal positions of the upper extremity chopping pattern moving into flexion to the right. Figs. 4-28 and 4-29 show the starting and terminal positions for the upper extremity lifting pattern moving into extension to the right.

Table 4-6 describes rotational movement of the lower extremities moving into positions of flexion and extension. Figs. 4-30 and 4-31 show the lower extremity pattern moving into flexion to the left. Figs. 4-32 and 4-33 show the lower extremity pattern moving into extension to the left.

The neck patterns involve simply flexion and rotation to one side (Figs. 4-34 and 4-35) with extension and rotation to the opposite (Figs. 4-36 and 4-37). The patient should follow the direction of the movement with the eyes.

The principles and techniques of PNF, when used appropriately with specific patterns, can be an extremely effective tool for rehabilitation of sports-related injuries. They may be used as a method of strengthening weak muscles or muscle groups, as well as for improving the range of motion about an injured joint. Specific techniques selected for use should depend on individual patient needs and may be modified accordingly.

A final point of clarification should be made regarding both autogenic inhibition and reciprocal inhibition. The motor neurons of the spinal cord always receive a combination of inhibitory and excitatory impulses from the afferent nerves. Whether these motor neurons will be excited or inhibited depends on the ratio of these two types of incoming impulses.

The principles and techniques of PNF, when used appropriately with specific patterns, can be an extremely effective tool for rehabilitation of sports-related injury. They may be used as a method of strengthening weak muscles or muscle groups as well as for improving range of motion about an injured joint. Specific techniques selected for use should depend on individual patient needs and may be modified accordingly.

TABLE 4-5
Upper Trunk Movement Patterns

Body Part	Moving into Extension (Chopping)*		Moving into Flexion (Lifting)*	
	Starting Position (Fig. 4-26)	Terminal Position (Fig. 4-27)	Starting Position (Fig. 4-28)	Terminal Position (Fig. 4-29)
Right upper extremity	Flexion Adduction Internal rotation	Extension Abduction External rotation	Extension Adduction Internal rotation	Flexion Abduction External rotation
Left upper extremity (left hand grasps right forearm)	Flexion Abduction External rotation	Extended Adduction Internal rotation	Extension Abduction External rotation	Flexion Adduction Internal rotation
Trunk	Rotated and extended to left	Rotated and flexed to right	Rotated and flexed to left	Rotated and extended to right
Head	Rotated and extend to left	Rotated and flexed to right	Rotated and flexed to left	Rotated and extended to right
Hand position of therapist	Left hand on right anterolateral surface of forehead Right hand on dorsum of right hand		Right hand on dorsum of right hand Left hand on posterior lateral surface of head	
Verbal command	Pull down		Push up	

*Rotation is to the right.

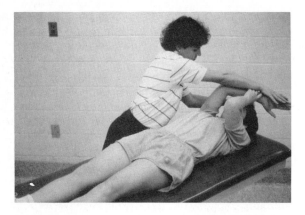

Fig. 4-26. Upper trunk pattern moving into extension or chopping (starting position).

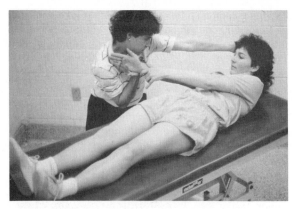

Fig. 4-27. Upper trunk pattern moving into extension or chopping (terminal position).

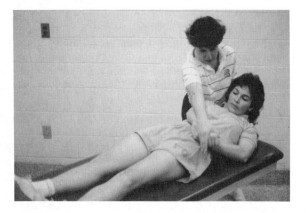

Fig. 4-28. Upper trunk pattern moving into flexion or lifting (starting position).

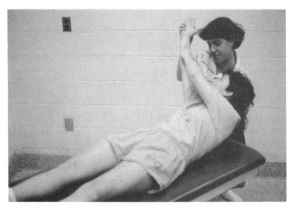

Fig. 4-29. Upper trunk pattern moving into flexion or lifting (terminal position).

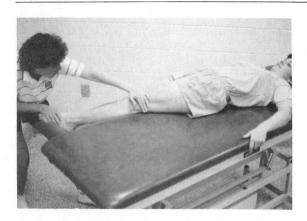

Fig. 4-30. Lower trunk pattern moving into flexion to the left (starting position).

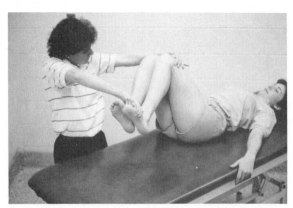

Fig. 4-31. Lower trunk pattern moving into flexion to the left (terminal position).

TABLE 4-6
Lower Trunk Movement Patterns

Body Part	Moving into Flexion*		Moving into Extension†	
	Starting Position (Fig. 4-30)	Terminal Position (Fig. 4-31)	Starting Position (Fig. 4-32)	Terminal Position (Fig. 4-33)
Right hip	Extension Abduction Externally rotated	Flexion Adduction Internally rotated	Flexion Adduction Internally rotated	Extension Abduction Externally rotated
Left hip	Extension Adduction Internally rotated	Flexion Abduction Externally rotated	Flexion Abduction Externally rotated	Extension Adduction Internally rotated
Ankles	Plantar flexed	Dorsiflexed	Dorsiflexed	Plantar flexed
Toes	Extended	Flexed	Flexed	Extended
Hand position of the therapist	Right hand on dorsum of feet Left hand on anterolateral surface of left knee		Right hand on plantar surface of foot Left hand on posterior lateral surface of right knee	
Verbal cues	Pull up and in		Push down and out	

*Rotation is to the left in flexion.
†Rotation is to the right in extension.

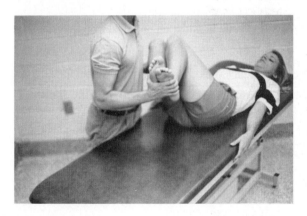

Fig. 4-32. Lower trunk pattern moving into extension to the left (starting position).

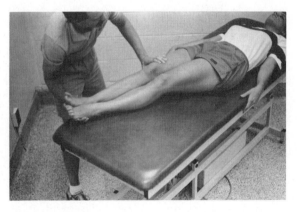

Fig. 4-33. Lower trunk pattern moving into extension to the left (terminal position).

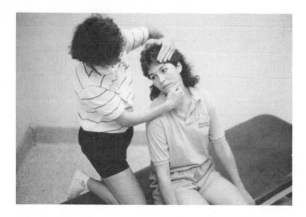

Fig. 4-34. Neck flexion and rotation to the left (starting position).

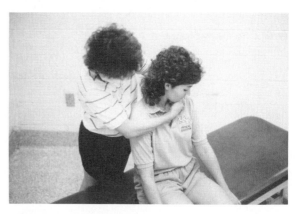

Fig. 4-35. Neck flexion and rotation to the left (terminal position).

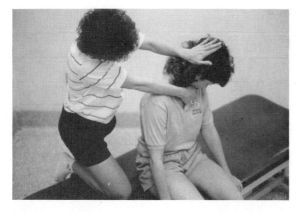

Fig. 4-36. Neck extension and rotation to the right (starting position).

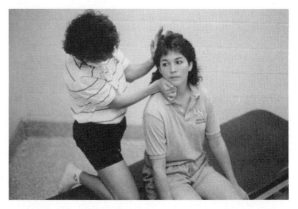

Fig. 4-37. Neck extension and rotation to the right (terminal position).

SUMMARY

1. Pain arises from a specific lesion affecting the soft tissue that surrounds the joint and may occur anywhere within the range of motion. Treatment must reach the involved structures to be effective.
2. The musculotendinous unit is classified as contractile tissue and bone, ligament, joint capsule, fascia, bursae, nerve roots, and dura mater as inert tissues.
3. A lesion in contractile tissue occurs in active motion in one direction and in passive motion in the opposite direction, whereas a lesion of inert tissue elicits pain on active and passive motion in the same direction.
4. The purpose of movement assessment is to determine specifically which anatomic structure is producing pain. The sports therapist must consider not only the type of motion that is producing pain but also other pertinent tests that help differentiate specific injuries.
5. Pain that occurs during active range of motion may indicate damage to either contractile of inert tissues.
6. Assessment of passive range should concentrate on the end point feel.
7. A lesion in the joint capsule tends to limit movement in a proportional way in each of the various movement patterns of that individual joint.
8. Noncapsular movement restriction may result from ligamentous adhesion, internal de-

rangement, or an extraarticular lesion.

9. Pain on resisted isometric contractions in the midrange eliminates capsular structures as a cause of pain.

10. Physiological and accessory motions occur simultaneously, and restriction of either can impair motion.

11. Mobilization techniques are used to increase joint mobility or decrease pain by restoring accessory movements to the joint.

12. Maitland has proposed a series of graded movements in the range of motion to treat pain and stiffness.

13. Kaltenborn uses various stages of traction to reduce pain and stiffness.

14. The PNF techniques may be used to increase both strength and range of motion and are based neurophysiologically on the stretch reflex.

15. The PNF techniques emphasize specific principles that may be superimposed on any of the specific techniques.

16. The PNF strengthening techniques include repeated contraction, slow-reversal, slow-reversal-hold, rhythmic stabilization, and rhythmic initiation.

17. The PNF stretching techniques include contract-relax, hold-relax, and slow-reversal-hold-relax.

18. The techniques of PNF are rotational and diagonal movements in the upper extremity, lower extremity, upper trunk, lower trunk, and the head and neck.

REFERENCES

1 Barak T, Rosen E, and Sofer R: Mobility: passive orthopedic manual therapy. In Gould J and Davies G, editors: Orthopedic and sports physical therapy, St Louis, 1985, CV Mosby Co.

2 Basmajian J: Therapeutic exercise, Baltimore, 1978, Williams & Wilkins.

3 Bobath B: The treatment of motor disorders of pyramidal and extrapyramidal by reflex inhibition and by facilitation of movement, Physiotherapy 41:146, 1955.

4 Brunnstrom S: Movement therapy in hemiplegia, New York, 1970, Harper & Row, Publishers Inc.

5 Cookson J: Orthopedic manual therapy: an overview, part II: the spine, J Am Phys Ther Assoc 59:259, 1979.

6 Cookson J and Kent B: Orthopedic manual therapy: an overview, part I: the extremities, J Am Phys Ther Assoc 59:136, 1979.

7 Cornelius W and Jackson A: The effects of cryotherapy and PNF on hip extension flexibility, Athletic Training 19(3):184, 1984.

8 Cyriax J: Textbook of orthopedic medicine, vol I: diagnosis of soft tissue lesions, London, 1969, Baillière Tindall.

9 Cyriax J: Textbook of orthopedic medicine, vol II: treatment by manipulation, massage, and injection, Baltimore, 1974, Williams & Wilkins.

10 Grimsby O: Fundamentals of manual therapy: a course workbook, Vagsbygd, Norway, 1981, Sorlandets Fysikalske Institutt.

11 Harris F: Facilitation techniques and therapeutic exercise. In Basmajian J, editor: Therapeutic exercise, Baltimore, 1978, Williams & Wilkins.

12 Hollis M: Practical exercise, Oxford, 1981, Blackwell Scientific Publications Inc.

13 Kaltenborn F: Mobilization of the extremity joints: examination and basic treatment techniques, Norway, 1980, Olaf Norlis Bokhandel.

14 Knott M and Voss D: Proprioceptive neuromuscular facilitation: patterns and techniques, New York, 1968, Harper & Row, Publishers Inc.

15 Lloyd D: Facilitation and inhibition of spinal motorneurons, J Neurophysiol 9:421, 1946.

16 MacConaill M and Basmajian J: Muscles and movements: a basis for kinesiology, Baltimore, 1969, Williams & Wilkins.

17 Maitland G: Extremity manipulation, London, 1977, Butterworth Publishers.

18 Maitland G: Vertebral manipulation, London, 1978, Butterworth Publishers.

19 Mangine R: Orthopedic medicine, Springfield, Ill, 1976, Charles C Thomas, Publisher.

20 Markos P: Ipsilateral and contralateral effects of proprioceptive neuromuscular facilitation techniques on hip motion and electromyographic activity, Phys Ther 59(11): 1366–1373, 1979.

21 Mennell J: Joint pain and diagnosis using manipulative techniques, New York, 1964, Little, Brown & Co Inc.

22 Paris S: The spine: course notebook, Atlanta, 1979, Institute Press.

23 Paris S: Extremity dysfunction and mobilization, Atlanta, 1980, Prepublication Manual.

24 Prentice W: A comparison of static stretching and PNF stretching for improving hip joint flexibility, Athletic Training 18(1):56–59, 1983.

25 Prentice W: A manual resistance technique for strengthening tibial rotation, Athletic Training 23(3):230–233, 1988.

26 Prentice W: An electromyographic analysis of heat and cold and stretching for inducing muscular relaxation, J Orthop Sports Phys Ther 3:133–140, 1982.

27 Prentice W and Kooima E: The use of proprioceptive neuromuscular facilitation techniques in the rehabilitation of sport-related injuries, Athletic Training 21:26–31, 1986.

28 Rood M: Neurophysiologic reactions as a basis of physical therapy, Phys Ther Rev 34:444, 1954.

29 Schiotz E and Cyriax J: Manipulation past and present, London, 1978, William Heinemann Medical Books.

30 Sherrington C: The integrative action of the nervous sys-

tem, New Haven, 1947, Yale University Press.

31 Stoddard A: Manual of osteopathic practice, London, 1969, Hutchinson Ross Publishing Company.

32 Surberg P: Neuromuscular facilitation techniques in sportsmedicine, Phys Ther Rev 34:444, 1954.

33 Taniqawa M: Comparison of the hold-relax procedure and passive mobilization on increasing muscle length, Phys Ther 52(7):725–735, 1972.

34 Wadsworth C: Manual examination and treatment of the spine and extremities, Baltimore, 1988, Williams & Wilkins.

35 Zohn D and Mennell J: Musculoskeletal pain: diagnosis and physical treatment, Boston, 1976, Little, Brown & Co Inc.

36 Zusman M: Reappraisal of a proposed neurophysiological mechanism for the relief of joint pain with passive joint movements, Physiother Prac 1:61–70, 1985.

The Evaluation Process in Rehabilitation

5

David H. Perrin

OBJECTIVES

Following completion of this chapter, the student will be able to:

- Discuss the important components of a preparticipation physical examination.

- Understand the differences between on-field and off-field injury evaluations.

- Outline the protocol to be followed for an on-field injury evaluation.

- Understand the usefulness of upper- and lower-quarter screening in off-field evaluation.

- Describe the components and appropriate sequence for a comprehensive off-field evaluation.

- Appreciate and understand the importance and format for documentation of injury evaluation findings.

Evaluation of athletic injury typically occurs initially either on the field or court of competition or later in the athletic training room. In the first case, the sports therapist is at a distinct advantage over other health care providers. The sports therapist may have viewed the mechanism of injury, a component of injury evaluation that lends a great deal of insight into the anatomical structures involved. Moreover, the sports therapist is able to assess the nature of the injury prior to the onset of muscle spasm and swelling, factors that can confound the accurate assessment of severity. Either on or off the field, the examiner frequently has the advantage of knowing the athlete's personality, injury history, and pain threshold.

Effective injury evaluation includes a sequence of events that begins long before the occurrence of injury. The preparticipation examination is useful not only for preventing injury but also for establishing baseline information that may be helpful in determining the severity of an injury. Effective management of acute on-field injuries necessitates the establishment of an emergency plan that clarifies the roles and responsibilities of the personnel involved. Finally, effective off-field evaluation is accomplished only by a thorough and sequential injury evaluation format that includes documentation of significant findings.

PREPARTICIPATION EXAMINATION

Preparticipation examinations are an essential component of a comprehensive sports medicine health care plan. The National Collegiate Athletic Association (NCAA) lists it as the first component of a safe athletic program and recommends a thorough evaluation upon a student-athlete's initial entrance into an institution's intercollegiate athletic program.[16] A recent survey of the 50 states and the District of Columbia conducted to assess the requirements for scholastic preparticipation physical examinations showed that 35 states require a yearly examination of some type.[9]

The ideal preparticipation examination incorporates the expertise of medical doctors and sports therapists. The role of the physician is to assess the status of the cardiorespiratory and musculoskeletal systems and to review potential contraindications to participation. The team physician ultimately authorizes the athlete's participation in competitive sport. The nature and details of the medical evaluation are beyond the scope of this text.

The role of the sports therapist is to assess the strength, flexibility, and fitness of an athlete relative to the specific demands of the sport. The examination should be designed to screen for potential problem areas. A more definitive evaluation of problem areas should be conducted, and referral made to appropriate medical specialists if necessary.

History

The preparticipation examination should begin with a complete medical history that includes questions pertaining to prior illnesses, injuries, surgery, allergies, and immunizations, as well as any current medication therapy. An accurate family history should also be obtained, including any cardiovascular disease, diabetes, allergies, sudden death, or orthopedic problems experienced by members of the athlete's immediate family. Details of affirmative responses on the medical history form frequently need to be confirmed or explored through personal interview.

Flexibility

In making a determination of normal flexibility, the requirements of the sport in question must be considered. For example, inflexibility according to the standards of a gymnast is likely to be exceptional flexibility for an offensive lineman.

Assessment of flexibility should begin at the cervical region, include the trunk and all extremities, and focus especially on muscles frequently injured during athletic participation. Normal cervical motion should permit the athlete to place the chin on the chest, look at the ceiling, nearly align the chin with the shoulder on the right and left sides, and form a 45° angle while laterally

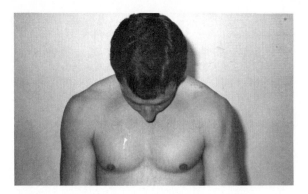

Fig. 5-1. Cervical flexion range of motion.

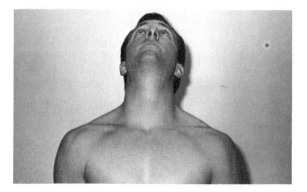

Fig. 5-2. Cervical extension range of motion.

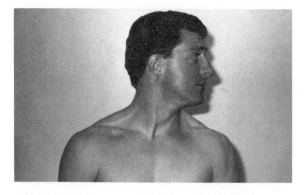

Fig. 5-3. Left cervical rotation range of motion.

flexing to the right and left (Figs. 5-1 to 5-4). Shoulder motion may be screened with Apley's range-of-motion tests, which assess abduction and external rotation (Fig. 5-5) and adduction and internal rotation (Fig. 5-6). Inability to per-

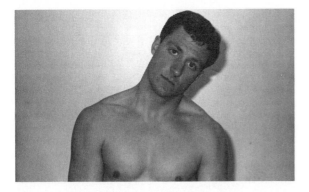

Fig. 5-4. Left lateral cervical flexion range of motion.

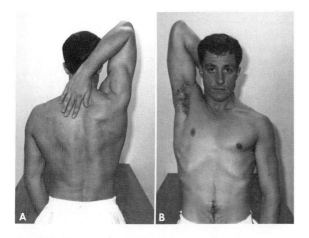

Fig. 5-5. Apley's range-of-motion test: abduction and external rotation.

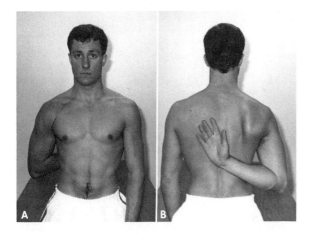

Fig. 5-6. Apley's range-of-motion test: adduction and internal rotation.

form these tests would necessitate careful evaluation of each motion inherent to the shoulder girdle-joint complex. Elbow, forearm, and wrist range of motion can quickly be assessed by having the athlete actively perform the motions inherent to these joints.

Evaluation of lower extremity flexibility should include motions about the hip, knee, and ankle joints. Figs. 5-7 and 5-8 illustrate simple tests for evaluating flexibility of the hip flexors and adductor muscle groups. Hamstring flexibility can be assessed from a supine position, and the hip stabilized at 90° (Fig. 5-9). Normal flexibility of the hamstring muscle group should permit the athlete to extend the knee completely. Low back and hamstring flexibility can be assessed by the sit-and-reach test (Fig. 5-10). Tautness of the iliotibial band, frequently a cause of disability, can be assessed through use of the Ober test, as illustrated in Fig. 5-11. Finally, flexibility of the triceps surae complex should be assessed with the knee first extended (gastrocnemius) and then flexed to 90° (soleus).

Any limitations in flexibility detected by the examiner should be confirmed and documented through the use of standard goniometry.[17] Only in this way can limitations in motion be confirmed and the usefulness of prescribed stretching programs be ascertained.

Strength

Manual muscle testing should be performed to assess strength of the cervical spine muscles and the major muscle groups of the extremities. Several resources describe the technique of manual muscle testing for all major muscle groups of the body.[7]

Athletes presenting with obvious deficiencies in strength or with histories of musculoskeletal injury should be evaluated by any one of several commercially available strength dynamometers. Isokinetic testing enables the accurate evaluation of single muscle group strength and its relationship to bilateral and reciprocal muscle groups. As with flexibility, the neuromuscular demands of a sport may dramatically influence the strength capacity of single muscle groups. This influence must be considered in the establishment of normal bilateral and reciprocal muscle group values for athletes in different sports.[18]

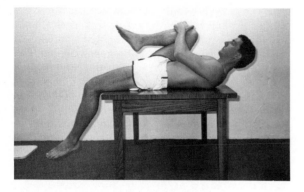

Fig. 5-7. Negative Thomas test for tightness of the left hip flexors.

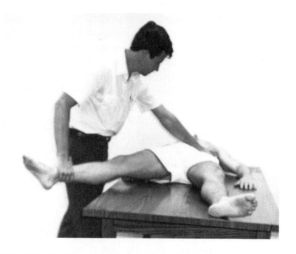

Fig. 5-8. Test for tightness of the adductors.

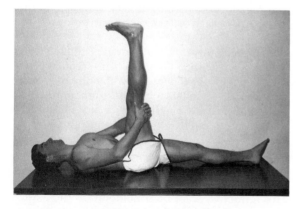

Fig. 5-9. Test for hamstring flexibility. Inability to completely extend the knee indicates a positive test.

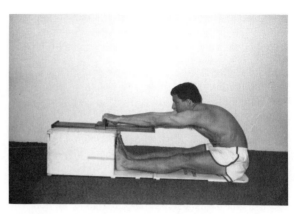

Fig. 5-10. Sit-and-reach test for low back and hamstring flexibility.

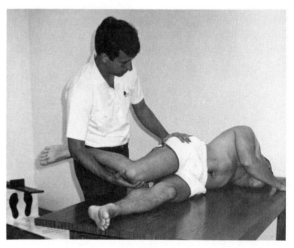

Fig. 5-11. Ober test for tightness of the iliotibial band.

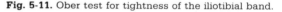

Body Composition

Assessment of body composition involves prediction of body density, from which the amount of body fat can be determined. The most accurate method for measuring body composition is hydrostatic weighing. Anthropometric techniques, which include height-weight indexes, skinfold fat, body circumference, and body diameters, are also available.[14]

When many athletes must be assessed during a physical examination, skinfold measurement of subcutaneous fat provides a rapid and reliable predictor of body density[14] (Fig. 5-12). Jackson

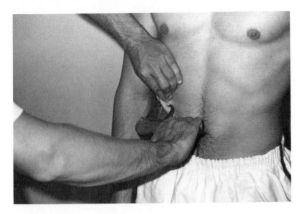

Fig. 5-12. Measurement of subcutaneous fat.

and Pollock[14] have recommended using the sum of three skinfolds to evaluate body composition in adults ranging in age from 18 to 61 years old. Subcutaneous fat is distributed differently in men and women, and so different sites are used for each group. For men, the sum of chest, abdomen, and thigh skinfolds are used; for women, the triceps, suprailium, and thigh skinfolds are recommended. Details of the technique for measuring skinfold fat have been presented in detail elsewhere.[14]

The generalized approach for determination of body composition proposed by Jackson and Pollock is appropriate for a large heterogeneous population (18 to 61 years old) but may not be appropriate for the high school athlete. Examiners dealing with prepubescent and pubescent athletes are encouraged to read the work of Slaughter and others.[21]

The purpose of determining body composition during the preparticipation examination is to provide the athlete with guidelines for desirable levels of body fatness. Optimal levels of body fatness vary considerably among sports. In general, highly trained athletes range from 4% to 10% for men and from 13% to 18% for women.[14]

Fitness

Fitness is most accurately determined through measurement of oxygen consumption during exhaustive work. However, this measurement also requires expensive laboratory equipment and is impractical for determining the fitness of many athletes during the preparticipation exam. Several techniques have been used that predict fitness from recovery heart rates following vigorous stepping or cycling exercises. Perhaps the most practical method for preparticipation screening of many athletes is the 12-minute run developed by Cooper.[5] This technique predicts maximal oxygen consumption from distance covered during a 12-minute run. From this information, athletes are categorized as having fitness levels falling somewhere between very poor and excellent. Based on test results and determined by the specific physiological demands of the sport, a conditioning program can be prescribed. A review of Wilmore's work [24] is helpful in designing conditioning programs appropriate for athletes in many different sports.

ON-FIELD EVALUATION

Although most on-field injuries in athletics are not life-threatening, the first responsibility of a sports therapist is to establish an emergency plan in the event that one does occur. The important components of such a plan include the acquisition of appropriate emergency care supplies and equipment such as airway devices, stretchers, spine boards, and splints.[20] Access to a telephone, whether competition is occurring indoors or outdoors, is essential. A mechanism for unlocking doors and gates along the path to the injured athlete is also a must. Finally, the lines of authority should be established early with regard to staff and student sports therapists, physicians, and coaches.

Prior knowledge of community rescue squad and hospital emergency room facilities and personnel can be very useful in assuring the appropriate disposition of the injured athlete. Voluntary in-service training on athletic injuries for the community emergency medical technicians (EMTs) and paramedics can be invaluable in establishing the expertise of the sports therapist. On-field management of a suspected cervical spine injury on Saturday afternoon is not the time to debate removal of a football helmet with an EMT.[10]

Another responsibility of the sports therapist is to be aware of the rules of each sport as they pertain to injury management. For example, intercollegiate wrestling permits only 2 minutes for evaluation of an athletic injury before the decision to continue wrestling or forfeit must be made. Stepping on a basketball court to evaluate an injured player necessitates either removing the player from the game or taking a team time-out. The implications of these rules to the sports therapist, especially in the final moments of a close contest, make injury evaluation an even greater challenge.

Evaluation Protocol for Life-Threatening Injury

The first responsibility during an on-field evaluation is to rule out serious and life-threatening injury via a primary survey. Such injuries on the athletic field are generally those in which the athlete is not breathing or has sustained trauma to the vital organs (e.g., central nervous system or internal organs). The components of a primary survey include the ABCs of emergency care: ensuring that there is an open *A*irway, *B*reathing is taking place, and *C*irculation is present. Once the ABCs have been established, injury to the cervical spine must be ruled out before the athlete is moved in any way. Should injury to the cervical spine be suspected, extreme care must be taken to avoid further injury from inappropriate movement. Several excellent sources have outlined the proper immobilization technique for the spinal cord-injured athlete.[8,23]

Injuries to the chest and abdomen may also pose a threat to the athlete's life. Signs of serious injury to the chest may include pain at the site, difficulty breathing, coughing up blood, cyanosis of the lips, a rapid, weak pulse, and low blood pressure.

Signs of injury to the abdomen may include tenderness when palpated, pain within the abdomen, difficulty in moving, low blood pressure, rapid pulse, and shallow respirations. Occasionally pain from injury to an internal structure may be referred elsewhere, as with pain in the left shoulder from injury to the spleen (Kehr's sign).

If injury to the chest or abdomen is suspected, the examiner should monitor the athlete's pulse, blood pressure, and respiration. Treatment should be directed toward the prevention of shock until emergency medical personnel arrive.

Evaluation Protocol for Non-Life-Threatening Injury

The first task of the sports therapist in the evaluation of an athlete on the field of play is to gain access to the athlete and establish control of the situation. Teams should be instructed never to touch or move an injured teammate; a nondisplaced cervical spine fracture could become crippling or fatal by the act of a well-intentioned teammate. Also, the sports therapist must never feel pressured by game officials or coaches to hasten the evaluation process.

The very early phase of acute injury evaluation may be simply to comfort the athlete and wait for the initial surge of pain to subside. Attempts to evaluate an injured athlete screaming and writhing in pain generally prove useless. Athletes usually gain control of their faculties within a few moments, at which time the evaluation may continue.

The next phase of the evaluation is to determine the mechanism of injury. Athletes can frequently describe the position of the body part or the point of contact by another player at the time of injury. Occasionally teammates, game officials, or coaches can provide useful information about the mechanism of injury.

The athlete should next be asked to identify the site of pain as precisely as possible. Occasionally the site of pain is quite diffuse immediately following injury but tends to become more circumscribed within a few minutes. Early in the on-field situation, the sports therapist should palpate the site of injury to rule out gross and obvious deformity and to determine the anatomical structures involved. The athlete's willingness to move the injured part can also be indicative of the severity of the injury.

Should the injury be determined to be ligamentous, stress tests should be employed immediately. Transporting an athlete even to the sideline can often lead to muscle spasm and guarding, which can confound the accurate assessment of joint laxity.

At this point in the evaluation, a determination should be made about transporting the athlete from the field of play. In most cases of upper extremity injury and with some lower extremity injuries, the athlete is capable of ambulating to the sideline. If any question exists, however, the athlete should be transported without bearing weight until a more definitive sideline evaluation can be conducted.

Once on the sideline, the injury evaluation should follow the guidelines described for the off-field evaluation. The sports therapist should note several important features of the injury that may be useful in determining severity. In particular, the degree and onset of swelling is noteworthy. For example, a knee joint that swells rapidly and substantially usually indicates significant ligamentous injury. Conversely, swelling that occurs slowly and overnight might suggest injury to a meniscal structure.

The amount of motion of the part following injury should also be noted. A knee injury possessing full range of motion following injury but lacking complete extension the following day is probably due to muscle spasm or joint effusion rather than to a displaced intraarticular structure.

Finally, the degree of laxity about a joint immediately following injury can be far more revealing than that observed the following day. Such information can be essential to the team physician's evaluation even several hours later and especially the next day.

Perhaps the most difficult questions the sports therapist must answer immediately following many injuries concern classifying the severity and predicting the length of disability. For the reasons stated earlier, the course an injury follows over a 24-hour period can be very revealing relative to its severity and to the period of time before full return to competition can be expected. Thus sports therapists should resist the attempts of others (coaches, press, and the like) to predict the period of disability associated with an injury immediately following its occurrence.

OFF-FIELD EVALUATION

Off-field evaluations are usually conducted in the athletic training room and allow the sports therapist the opportunity to perform a detailed and uninterrupted assessment of the injury. Two scenarios seem prevalent in athletics. The first is that of the injured athlete who knows exactly

what hurts and can vividly describe the mechanism of injury. The second situation is the athlete who reports pain of an insidious onset and has difficulty localizing the site of pain. In the first case, the evaluation may be more focused to the region where mechanism of injury and site of pain are known. In the latter situation, the injury evaluation protocol should begin with a series of range-of-motion, muscle, and neurological tests known as upper- or lower-quarter screening.

Quarter Screening

The purpose of upper- or lower-quarter screening is to isolate the site of pain and establish that the site of pain and location of injury are in fact the same. Embryology of the human body occurs in a longitudinal manner through development of dermatomes and myotomes. This formation is especially true in the extremities. The implication to the clinician is that pain from injury within a particular dermatome can be experienced at a point elsewhere than the actual site of injury. Also, injury to a nerve may manifest itself through sensory and/or motor deficit distally along the distribution of the nerve. This phenomenon of referred pain can confound the accurate assessment of injury to either an upper or lower extremity.

Upper-quarter screening involves the quick assessment of the neck, shoulder girdle region, and arm. Lower-quarter screening involves similar assessment of the low back, hip region, and leg.

UPPER-QUARTER SCREENING. Upper-quarter screening should begin with the athlete in a seated position. Visual inspection to assess posture of the head and shoulder girdle complex should precede the evaluation. The evaluation includes a series of range-of-motion (ROM) and manual muscle tests of the cervical region and proceeds distally along the upper extremity. Cervical spine motion is first assessed actively (Figs. 5-1 to 5-4) and then with slight overpressure, should active ROM produce no pain or limitation of motion (Fig. 5-13). (**Note:** In no instance should a suspected neck injury in the on-field situation include this assessment.) The muscles surrounding the cervical spine are then assessed with isometric resistance to examine for either neurological involvement or injury to a muscle (Figs. 5-14 to 5-17). During assessment of the cervical region, the sports therapist should observe not only for locally produced signs and symptoms but also for pain that may be emanating from the cervical region but referred distally elsewhere in the upper extremity.

Next the screening proceeds to the shoulder region and begins with range-of-motion tests (Figs. 5-5 and 5-6) for active motion of the shoulder girdle and glenohumeral joints. Resisted shoulder elevation (Fig. 5-18) and abduction (Fig. 5-19) are then tested to assess the C2 to C5 neurological levels. The screening continues along the upper extremity with testing in a similar manner at the elbow, wrist, and hand, as illustrated in Figs. 5-20 to 5-27.

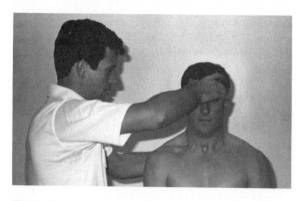

Fig. 5-15. Resisted cervical flexion.

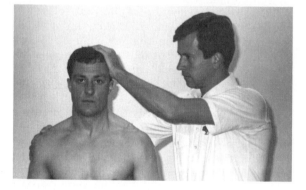

Fig. 5-16. Resisted left lateral flexion.

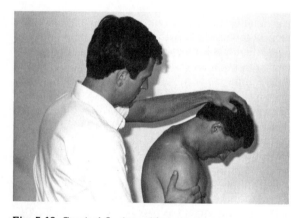

Fig. 5-13. Cervical flexion with overpressure.

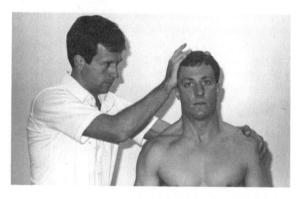

Fig. 5-17. Resisted right lateral flexion.

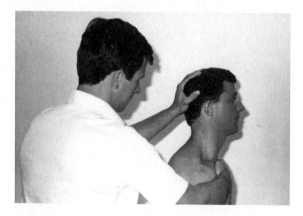

Fig. 5-14. Resisted cervical extension.

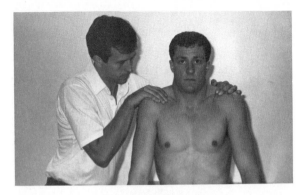

Fig. 5-18. Resisted shoulder elevation (C2, C3, C4).

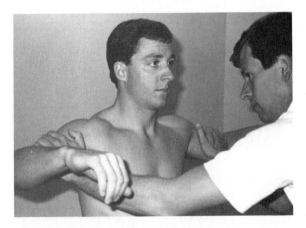

Fig. 5-19. Resisted shoulder abduction (C5).

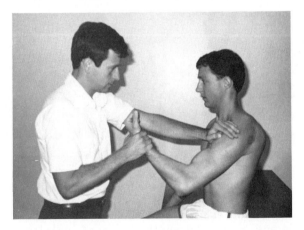

Fig. 5-20. Resisted elbow flexion (C6).

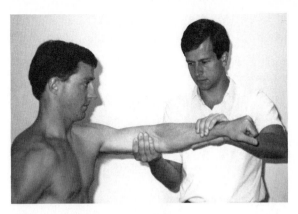

Fig. 5-21. Resisted elbow extension (C7).

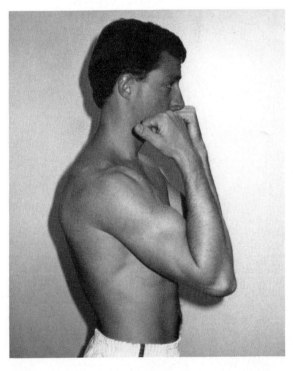

Fig. 5-22. Elbow flexion range of motion.

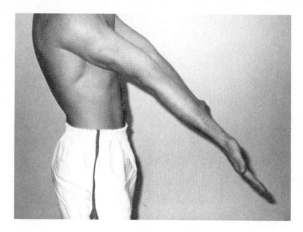

Fig. 5-23. Elbow extension range of motion.

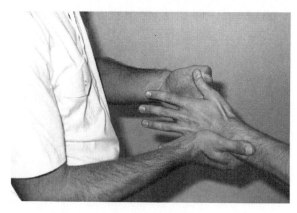

Fig. 5-26. Resisted thumb extension (C8).

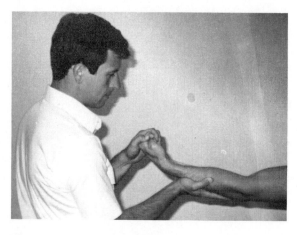

Fig. 5-24. Resisted wrist flexion (C7).

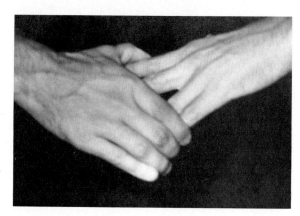

Fig. 5-27. Resisted finger abduction (T1).

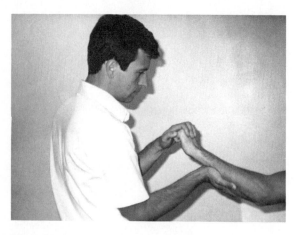

Fig. 5-25. Resisted wrist extension (C6).

As the upper-quarter screening proceeds distally from the cervical spine, the sports therapist should note pain or weakness. Should none be encountered, the site of injury is suspected to be elsewhere, and the procedure continues until the entire upper extremity has been examined. Should pain or weakness be found, a more detailed evaluation should be performed on the region of pain.

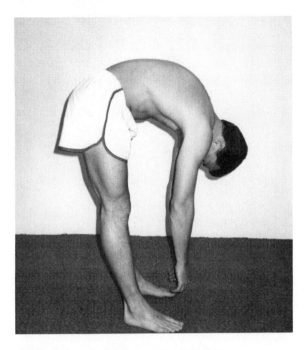

Fig. 5-28. Lumbar flexion range of motion.

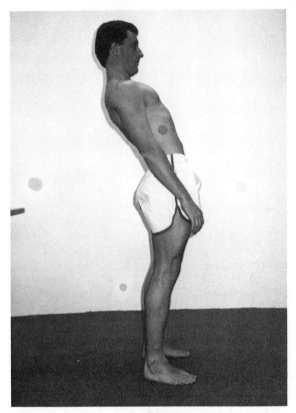

Fig. 5-29. Lumbar extension range of motion.

LOWER-QUARTER SCREENING. Lower-quarter screening involves a series of range-of-motion and manual muscle tests, beginning at the lumbar region and proceeding distally to include the entire lower extremity. As with the upper-quarter screening, the evaluation is preceded by a visual assessment of posture. The evaluation is conducted first while the athlete is standing and then in the sitting, supine, and prone positions.

While standing, the athlete is asked to perform active motion of the lumbar spine (Figs. 5-28 to 5-31). Locally or distally produced pain or limitation of lumbar motion should be noted.

Heel and toe walking should also be performed to assess neurological levels L4 and L5 (tibialis anterior and extensor hallucis longus; Fig. 5-32) and S1 (gastrocnemius and soleus; Fig. 5-33). Additional range-of-motion and manual muscle tests are performed as the athlete is sitting, supine, and prone (Figs. 5-34 to 5-42).

As with the upper-quarter screening, pain or weakness should be noted. A region free from pain or weakness is considered screened and thus not the site of injury. Should pain or weakness be found, a more detailed evaluation that focuses on the region of injury should follow.

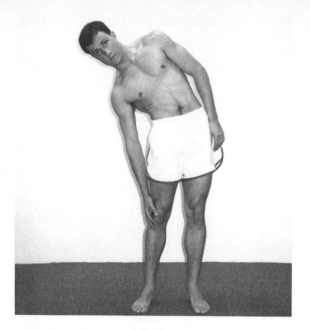

Fig. 5-30. Lumbar right lateral flexion.

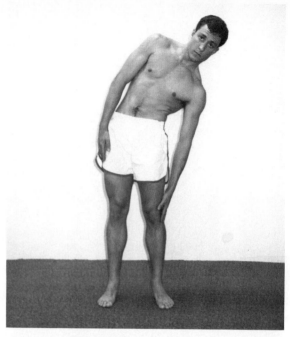

Fig. 5-31. Lumbar left lateral flexion.

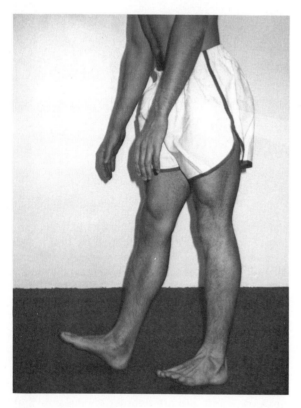

Fig. 5-32. Heel walking (L4, L5).

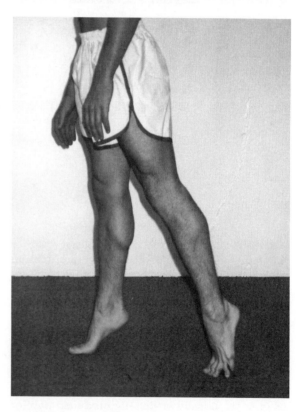

Fig. 5-33. Toe walking (S1).

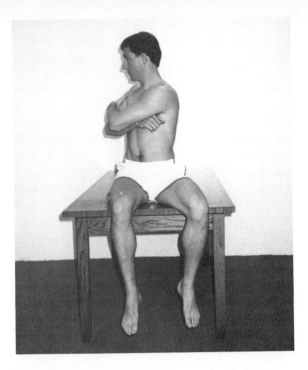

Fig. 5-34. Trunk right rotation.

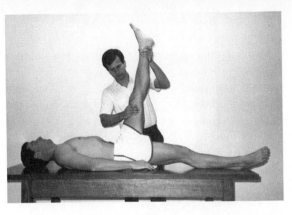

Fig. 5-36. Straight leg raise for sciatic nerve involvement.

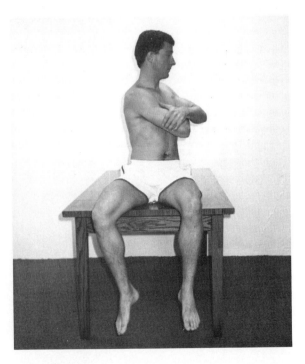

Fig. 5-35. Trunk left rotation.

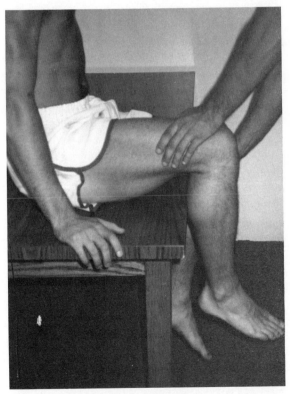

Fig. 5-37. Resisted hip flexion (L1, L2).

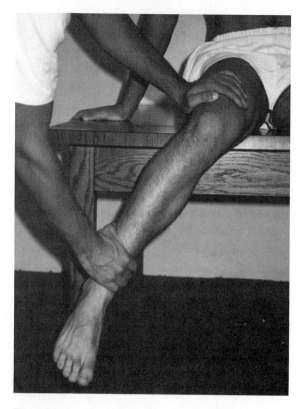

Fig. 5-38. Hip internal rotation range of motion.

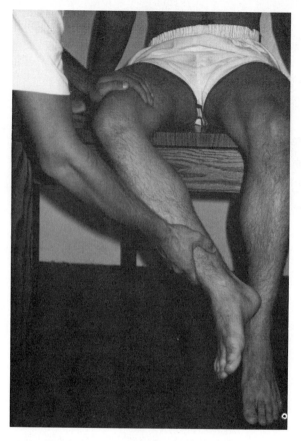

Fig. 5-39. Hip external rotation range of motion.

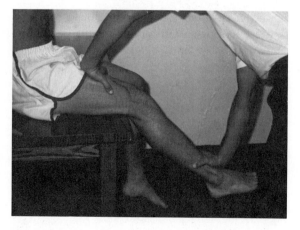

Fig. 5-40. Resisted knee extension (L3, L4).

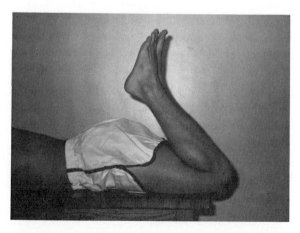

Fig. 5-41. Knee flexion range of motion.

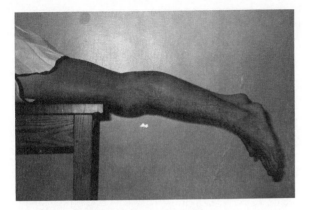

Fig. 5-42. Knee extension range of motion.

Off-Field Evaluation Protocol

The key to successful injury evaluation is to establish a sequential and systematic approach that is followed in every case. Only through a systematic approach can the sports therapist be confident that an important component of the evaluation will not be forgotten. Every injury is different and may present with unique signs and symptoms. Thus, although a systematic approach is important, the athletic trainer must take care not to become robotized during the evaluation process. With this in mind, the box on p. 102 is an example injury evaluation format to assist the beginning athletic trainer in establishing a sequential injury evaluation plan.

HISTORY. Perhaps the single most revealing component of injury evaluation is the history. The primary goals of the history are to determine the mechanism and site of injury. History taking includes not only a recounting of recent events leading to the injury but also an accounting of previous injuries to the body part in question. The sports therapist should also refer to the injury profile obtained from the athlete during the preparticipation examination.

The role of the sports therapist in obtaining an accurate and pertinent history is to ask the right questions and listen carefully. Questions must be asked in a nonleading manner. For example, "What activities cause your knee to hurt?" is more likely to elicit an unbiased response than "Your knee probably hurts when you sit at the movies, right?"

From the athlete's responses, the evaluator must note the pertinent and disregard the irrel-

evant. Each response provides a key to the nature of the next question.

From the history, the sports therapist should determine whether the injury episode is acute or recurrent. If acute, knowledge of the athlete's posture at the moment of injury is important in determining the mechanism. If swelling is present, the sports therapist should determine if the onset was immediate or slow. The athlete's ability to continue playing or need to stop immediately following the injury can be indicative of severity.

If chronic, the course of the injury should be ascertained relative to an increase or decrease of symptoms and the efficacy of previous treatment regimens. Asking whether it is getting better, getting worse, or staying the same provides the evaluator with information relative to the anatomical structures involved and the usefulness of previous or current treatments.

From the history, the evaluator should have a visual image of the injury mechanism and a general impression of the injury. With this information the evaluator is ready to proceed with a specific injury evaluation plan.

INSPECTION. Visual inspection of the injury begins as the athlete enters the training room. Of special interest is the athlete's gait in the case of lower-extremity injury. If an upper extremity is involved, the carrying position of the part should be noted.

A bilateral comparison of the anatomical region in question must be made. This will necessitate removal of clothing in many cases. In all instances, the modesty of the athlete must be protected. Shorts alone may be worn by the male athlete; female athletes should wear sleeveless shirts or halter tops for evaluation of upper-extremity injury. As the athlete removes clothing, limitations in motion and weight bearing should be observed.

The primary purpose of the visual inspection is to rule out the presence of gross or obvious deformity. Articular dislocations, such as those of the finger or shoulder, are easily visualized with careful inspection. Fractures of superficially located bones may also be noted in some cases, although nondisplaced fractures of a bone such as the clavicle may be impossible to ascertain from physical examination. The presence of swelling at the injury site should be noted, as should the nature of its onset, that is, rapid and

KNEE INJURY EVALUATION CHECKSHEET

I. HISTORY

    1. Ask what happened   _____
    2. Ask for description of mechanism   _____
    3. Ask for site of pain   _____
    4. Ask if any previous history   _____

II. INSPECTION

    1. Look for obvious deformity   _____
    2. Look for swelling and effusion   _____
    3. Compare bilaterally   _____

III. PALPATION

  A. Medial aspect

    1. MCL—femoral attachment   _____
    2. MCL—tibial attachment   _____
    3. Joint line   _____

  B. Lateral aspect

    1. LCL—femoral attachment   _____
    2. LCL—fibular attachment   _____
    3. Joint line   _____
    4. Fibular head   _____

  C. Anterior aspect

    1. Suprapatellar pouch (for swelling   _____
    2. Quadriceps tendon   _____
    3. Patella (superior pole)   _____
    4. Patella (inferior pole)   _____
    5. Patellar tendon   _____
    6. Tibial tuberosity   _____

  D. Posterior Aspect

    1. Popliteal fossa   _____
    2. Hamstring tendons   _____

IV. ACTIVE RANGE OF MOTION

    1. Knee flexion   _____
    2. Knee extension   _____
    3. Compare bilaterally   _____

V. PASSIVE RANGE OF MOTION

    1. Knee flexion   _____
    2. Knee extension   _____
    3. Compares bilaterally   _____

VI. RESISTIVE RANGE OF MOTION

    1. Knee extension   _____
    2. Knee flexion   _____
    3. Ankle plantar flexion   _____

VII. SPECIAL TESTS

  A. Menisci

    1. Check for terminal extension   _____
    2. McMurray test   _____

  B. MCL valgus stress test

    1. Correct hand placement   _____
    2. Ensure muscular relaxation   _____
    3. Stressed with terminal extension   _____
    4. Stressed with slight flexion   _____
    5. Compare bilaterally   _____

  C. LCL varus stress test

    1. Correct hand placement   _____
    2. Ensure muscular relaxation   _____
    3. Stressed with slight flexion   _____
    4. Compare bilaterally   _____

  D. ACL anterior drawer stress test

    1. Correct hand placement   _____
    2. Ensure hamstring relaxation   _____
    3. Stressed at 90° flexion   _____
    4. Compares bilaterally   _____

  E. ACL Lachman stress test

    1. Correct hand placement   _____
    2. Ensure muscular relaxation   _____
    3. Stressed at 20° flexion   _____
    4. Compare bilaterally   _____

immediate or gradual and slow. Finally, in the case of chronic injury, the presence of atrophy of muscles surrounding the region should be noted. For example, an athlete experiencing patellofemoral pain over an extended period of time may present with a substantial deficit in thigh girth.

PALPATION. Palpation of the injury site should occur early in the on-field evaluation for reasons previously described. During the more detailed off-field evaluation, palpating later in the injury evaluation process may be better. The disadvantage of palpating the injury site early is that such manual probing may elicit a pain response that will detract from the findings of the active, passive, and resistive motions that follow. Furthermore, the phenomenon of referred pain may make localization of the injury site difficult until other components of the evaluation have been performed. In any event, palpation of the injury will be discussed here, with its place in the injury evaluation protocol left to the individual examiner.

The purpose of palpation is to identify as closely as possible the exact anatomical structures involved in the injury. Palpation may be quite revealing at some regions (ankle, knee, elbow) but far less helpful at others (shoulder, hip). From palpation the presence of excessive heat from infection or inflammation should be noted. The volume and consistency of swelling may indicate effusion or hemarthrosis at a joint, and calcification may be identified in the residual hematoma from a soft tissue contusion. Rupture of a muscle or tendon may present as a gap at the point of separation. Some believe malalignment of a skeletal structure such as a vertebra can be ascertained through careful palpation.

ASSESSMENT OF MOTION. The goal of testing the motion of the injured part is to determine the nature of the anatomical structures involved. Injuries to the athlete are generally either those involving the muscle-tendon unit (contractile structures) or those having no capacity to generate tension (inert or noncontractile structures). Contractile structures include the muscle belly, muscle-tendon junction, and tendon attachment to bone. Inert structures commonly implicated in athletic injury include ligament, joint capsule, nerve, and bone. Through evaluating a series of active, passive, and resistive movements the sports therapist can usually identify the injured structure as falling into one of these two categories.

Active motion. Active motion is movement performed by the athlete without the assistance or resistance of the examiner. The goals of active motion are to assess the athlete's willingness to move the injured part and to localize generally the site of injury. Active motion by itself tells little of the nature of the involved structure because contractile structures move the part, and inert structures are stretched at the extremes of motion. Thus pain arising during active motion may originate from either the muscle-tendon unit or any one of several inert structures.

Assessment of active motion should include all movements normally found at the joint. Moreover, assessment of the joints both proximal and distal to the injury site is frequently indicated.

Passive motion. Passive motion is movement performed by the examiner with no active participation by the injured athlete. The challenge for the examiner is to obtain the athlete's complete muscular relaxation. The purpose of passive motion is to assess the state of the inert structures because movement is being imparted by the examiner rather than by the athlete's volitional muscular contraction. Thus injury to an inert structure is suspected if pain arises during passive motion. Because contractile structures will also be stretched at the extreme of motion, however, only in combination with resistive movement can this suspicion be confirmed.

Also of significance during the performance of passive motion is the presence of crepitus or clicking. Crepitus may indicate roughening of one or more articular surfaces such as found in advanced patellofemoral disease. Clicking may result from a subluxing tendon or displaced intraarticular cartilage. A biceps tendon subluxing from the intertubercular groove of the humerus and a torn meniscus catching between tibia and femur during knee motion are two forms of clicking.

Also of significance during the assessment of passive motion is the sensation experienced by the examiner at the extreme of motion and known as **end-feel.** Figs. 5-43 to 5-45 illustrate normal end-feels typically encountered during assessment of passive motion at the elbow. Common abnormal end-feels experienced during passive motion are the resistance caused by a muscle in spasm or the springy block sensation resulting from a displaced intraarticular cartilage.

Occasionally the examiner may encounter a phenomenon during passive motion known as **painful arc.** Painful arc is present when the athlete experiences pain at a particular point in the range of motion, with the discomfort subsiding as the point is passed in either direction. Painful arc is usually indicative of an impingement syndrome; that is, a soft tissue structure is being pinched between two bony structures. A painful arc is frequently found at the shoulder region as the subacromial bursa or supraspinatus tendon is pinched during movements inherent to activities such as swimming and throwing.

Resistive motion. Resistive motion is movement performed by the athlete but against the opposite and equal resistance of the examiner. The goal of resistive motion is to assess the state of the contractile unit. Injury to any component of the muscle-tendon unit can result in pain or weakness during resistive motion. Also, injury to a component of the nervous system can manifest itself through muscular weakness, a situation

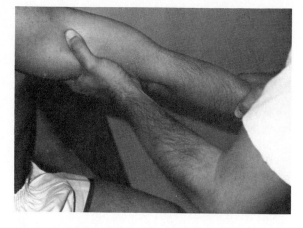

Fig. 5-43. Passive elbow extension illustrating bone-to-bone end-feel.

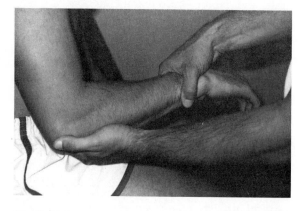

Fig. 5-44. Passive elbow pronation illustrating capsular end-feel.

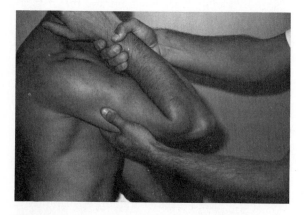

Fig. 5-45. Passive elbow flexion illustrating tissue approximation end-feel.

RESULTS OF RESISTIVE MOTION	
INTERPRETATION	**POSSIBLE PATHOLOGY**
Strong and painful	Muscle-tendon unit
Strong and painless	Healthy muscle-tendon unit
Weak and painful	Fracture or tendon avulsion
Weak and painless	Muscle rupture or nerve palsy

that can confound the injury evaluation. Only through an integration of findings during active, passive, and resistive motion can the injured structure accurately be identified. The accompanying box describes the potential findings of resistive motion.

Resistive motion must be performed from a stationary joint position and while in the midrange of motion. Resistive motion assessed dynamically and allowed to progress to an extreme in the range of motion not only tests contractile capacity of the muscle in question but also stretches the antagonist muscle as well as inert tissue. Several excellent resources illustrate manual muscle examination.[7] Figs. 5-20 and 5-40 illustrate the resistance, counterpressure, and joint positions for an upper- and lower-extremity muscle group.

SPECIAL TESTS. At this point in the evaluation, the examiner should have identified the structures involved in the injury. Depending on the examiner's findings, special tests are employed to confirm suspicions or to assess severity of injury. For example, suspicion of recurrent anterior shoulder dislocation may be confirmed through use of an apprehension test designed to reproduce the typical mechanism of injury (Fig. 5-46). Stress testing of knee ligaments is performed not only to confirm the structures involved but also to determine the degree of laxity and thus the severity of injury (Fig. 5-47). Special tests are described in detail in the chapters discussing each body region.

ARRIVING AT AN IMPRESSION. Only through a complete and systematic evaluation can a valid impression of an injury be made. One component of the evaluation alone usually provides insufficient information. Only through an integration of findings from the history and physical examination can the examiner arrive at a reasonable impression of injury. With this information an appropriate treatment and rehabilitation plan can be implemented.

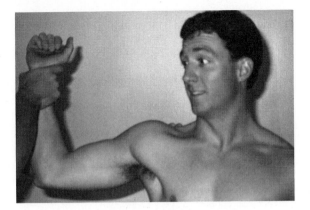

Fig. 5-46. Apley's apprehension test for anterior shoulder dislocation.

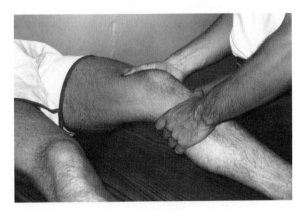

Fig. 5-47. Lachman's test for anterior cruciate ligament insufficiency.

DOCUMENTATION OF FINDINGS

The final phase of the injury evaluation format is the documentation of findings. The medicolegal climate of sport necessitates careful and systematic documentation of injuries. Of no less importance is the role documentation of injury plays in the establishment of a bona fide profession. An effective system of documentation should gather and record specific information about an injury with respect to subjective and objective information, clinician assessment, and plan of treatment (SOAP notes).

SOAP Notes

Documentation of acute athletic injury can be effectively accomplished through a system de-

---

INJURY REPORT FORM

ATHLETE NAME _____   DATE OF INJURY _____

INJURY SITE: R L _____   TODAY'S DATE _____
                                          (CIRCLE ONE)

                                          SPORT _____

Subjective findings (history):

Objective findings (inspection, palpation, mobility, and special tests):

Assessment (impression):

Plan (treatment administered and disposition):

Follow-up notes: Date _____

EVALUATED BY _____

RECORDED BY _____

---

signed to record both subjective and objective findings and to document the immediate and future treatment plan for the athlete. This method combines information provided by the athlete and the observations of the examiner.

The accompanying box presents a recommended injury report form that includes the components of documentation discussed above. This form also includes a provision to document findings arising from more definitive evaluation or from the examiner's subsequent day evaluation.

S (SUBJECTIVE). This component includes the subjective statements provided by the injured athlete. History taking is designed to elicit the athlete's subjective impressions relative to time, mechanism, and site of injury. The type and course of the pain and the degree of disability experienced by the athlete are also noteworthy.

O (OBJECTIVE). Objective findings result from the sports therapist's visual inspection, palpation, and assessment of active, passive, and resistive motion. Findings of special testing should also be noted here. Thus the objective report would include assessment of posture, presence of deformity or swelling, and location of point tenderness. Also, limitations of active motion and pain arising or disappearing during passive and resistive motion should be noted. Finally, the results of special tests relative to joint stability or apprehension or others are also included.

A (ASSESSMENT). Assessment of the injury is the sports therapist's professional judgment with regard to impression and nature of injury. Although the exact nature of the injury will not always be known initially, information pertaining to suspected site and anatomical structures involved is appropriate. A judgment of severity may be included but is not essential at the time of acute injury evaluation.

P (PLAN). The plan should include the first aid treatment rendered to the athlete and the sports trainer's intentions relative to disposition. Disposition may include referral for more definitive evaluation or simply the application of splint, wrap, or crutches and a request to report for reevaluation the following day. If the injury is of a more chronic nature, the examiner's plan for treatment and therapeutic exercise would be appropriate.

SUMMARY

1. The components of the preparticipation exam include a medical history and evaluation of flexibility, strength, body composition, and fitness.
2. On-field evaluation requires the establishment of an emergency plan and early recognition of life-threatening injury.
3. Off-field evaluation permits a more detailed assessment of injury and may begin with upper- or lower-quarter screening.
4. The important components of off-field evaluation include history, inspection, palpation, assessment of active, passive, and resistive motion, and special tests.
5. The final phase of injury evaluation is effective record keeping, which includes documentation of subjective and objective findings, the evaluator's assessment, and the plan for injury management and treatment.

REFERENCES

1 Cooper KH: A means of assessing maximal oxygen intake, JAMA 203:135–138, 1968.
2 Daniels L and Worthingham C: Muscle testing: techniques of manual examination, Philadelphia, 1980, WB Saunders Co.
3 Denegar CR and Saliba EN: On the field management of the potentially cervical spine injured football player, Athletic Training (in press).
4 Feinstein RA, Soileau EJ, and Daniel WA: A national survey of preparticipation requirements, Physician Sports Med 16:51–59, 1988.
5 Feld F and Blanc R: Immobilizing the spine-injured football player, J Emerg Med Serv 12:38–40, 1988.
6 Jackson AS and Pollock ML: Practical assessment of body composition, Physician Sports Med 13:76–90, 1985.
7 National Collegiate Athletic Association: NCAA sports medicine handbook, Mission, Kans, 1987, NCAA.
8 Nockin CC and White JD: Measurement of joint motion: a guide to goniometry, Philadelphia, 1985, FA Davis Co.
9 Perrin DH, Robertson RJ, and Ray RL: Bilateral isokinetic peak torque, torque acceleration energy, power, and work relationships in athletes and nonathletes, J Ortho Sports Phys Ther 9:184–189, 1987.
10 Powell J: 635,000 injuries annually in high school football, Athletic Training 22:19–22, 1987.
11 Ray RL and Feld FX: The team physician's medical bag. In Emergency Treatment of the Injured Athlete, Clin Sports Med 8:139–146, 1989.
12 Slaughter MH and others: Skinfold equations for estimation of body fatness in children and youth, Human Biol 60:709–723, 1988.
13 Vegso JJ, Bryant MH, and Torg JS: Field evaluation of head and neck injuries. In Torg JS, editor: Injuries to the head, neck, and face, Philadelphia, 1982, Lea & Febiger.
14 Wilmore JH: Training for sport and activity: the physiological basis of the conditioning process, ed 2, Boston, 1982, Allyn & Bacon Inc.

SUGGESTED READINGS

American Academy of Orthopaedic Surgeons: Emergency care and transportation of the sick and injured, Menasha, Wisc, 1981, George Banta Co, Inc.
American Academy of Pediatrics Committee on Sports Medicine: Sports medicine: health care for young athletes, Evanston, Ill, 1983, AAP.
Booher JM and Thibodeau GA: Athletic injury assessment, St Louis, 1985, The CV Mosby Co.
Brody DM: Running injuries. Ciba Clin Symp 32:1–36, 1980.
Cyriax J: Textbook of orthopaedic medicine, vol 1, diagnosis of soft tissue lesions, London, 1982, Baillière Tindall.
Gould JA and Davies GJ, editors: Orthopaedic and sports physical therapy, St Louis, 1985, The CV Mosby Co.
Hoppenfeld S: Physical examination of the spine and extremities, New York, 1976, Appleton-Century-Crofts.
Hoppenfeld S: Orthopaedic neurology, Philadelphia, 1977, JB Lippincott Co.
Magee DJ: Orthopedic physical assessment, Philadelphia, 1987, WB Saunders Co.
Saunders DH: Evaluation, treatment and prevention of musculoskeletal disorders, Minneapolis, 1985, Viking Press, Inc.

Psychological Considerations of Rehabilitation

6

Joe Gieck

OBJECTIVES

Following completion of this chapter, the student will be able to:

- Understand how different athletes deal with similar injuries.

- Understand the injury-prone athlete.

- Be able to identify stressors in the athlete's life and effective methods with which to deal with them.

- Identify the four phases of injury in the athlete's perception of it.

- Understand the importance of athletes taking responsibility for their actions in regard to injury.

- Recognize irrational thinking and its resolution.

- Understand the importance, physically and mentally, of short-term goals in rehabilitation.

- Understand the strategies the athlete can use for gaining control of the injury situation.

- Understand the importance of the relationship between the sports therapist and the athlete.

- Appreciate the importance of rehabilitation adherence and its deviations.

- Understand the coping skills necessary for successful rehabilitation.

- Appreciate the problems associated with long-term rehabilitation.

Sports medicine and athletic training are still inexact sciences, and nowhere within this area is this more evident than in the psychological phase of recovery from injury. Plato mentioned never attempting to cure the body without curing the soul. Current clinicians have found that people with negative self-concepts suffer more injuries.

Most athletes have the self-confidence to adapt to a mild or moderate injury, and most have the support, understanding, and proper encouragement to adapt to more severe injury, but even the most self-confident have their doubts. One athlete put it this way: "The best competitors like to compete and to me this is just a game—an inner game. It's an inner soul game.

Can I beat my knee back?" But he also expressed doubts about the real test when a tackler "takes a whack at the knee" and "how I haven't thought about it, but I've had nightmares about it. My buddy told me he broke his ankle. He said once you get that real good hit and you pop up and it pops up with you, then everything is going to fall into place and you're going to be rolling. You're going to go out there like it's never been hurt and just play." This quote expresses the positive aspects of return to competition but also some of the doubts involved.

With the emergence of sports psychology, more attention is paid to getting the mind ready to return to competition to match the adjustment of the body. Athletes have begun to describe the nightmares, fears, and anxiety of returning to competition. Also, in the current trend of high-salaried athletes, some describe their knee or other injuries and surgery as the most important things in their lives as they will either going to make or break them. These operations can allow the athletes to make either millions of dollars in a sports career or only thousands in a regular job if their careers end.

Athletes don't all deal with injury in the same manner. Rotella[8] describes how one may view the injury as disastrous, another may view it as an opportunity to show courage, and another athlete may relish the injury as it prevents his embarrassment over poor physical performance, provides an escape from a losing team, or discourages a pushy parent. If the injury is career-threatening, the athlete whose whole life has evolved around a sport may have an identity crisis.

Fig. 6-1 demonstrates the physical and emotional aspects of return to performance. The return performance is either enhanced or negated by the physiological and psychological results of both.

THE INJURY-PRONE ATHLETE

Some athletes seem to have a pattern of injury, whereas others in exactly the same position with the same physical makeup are injury-free. Certain researchers suggest that some psychological traits may predispose the athlete to a repeated injury cycle. No one particular personality type has been recognized as injury-prone. However, the individual who likes to take risks seems to represent the injury-prone athlete. This individual usually also lacks the ability to cope with the stresses associated with these risks and their consequences.

Much has been written about life's stress events and the likelihood of illness. These events are changes that require a readjustment, such as death of family members, divorce, school change, and job change. Sports researchers are suggesting that the inner thoughts and anxieties of the athlete create stresses within the athlete, and these stresses make the likelihood of injury and reinjury more likely, especially for the athlete who is inflexible and resistant to change.

Stressors are both positive, such as making All-American, and negative, such as being arrested. Each requires a life-style readjustment.

Examples of life's stress events, including some related to football, are listed in the box on page 109. The scale is based on a 0 to 100 rating, with 100 being the most stressful events.

Obviously the staff of a smaller team is more familiar with the athletes and their problems and can more effectively deal with them, but larger teams' staffs should attempt to deal with the individual through the position coach, with the individual problems being solved in the smaller unit. Unfortunately, many coaches do not have the interest or ability to work with athletes needing help. Some sort of a screening device should be used to identify those individuals who are

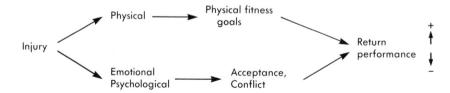

Fig. 6-1. Physical and emotional aspects of return to performance.

experiencing some of life's situations that they are unprepared to handle.

These individuals need someone to interact with to reduce the stress in their lives. In this way they can reduce the stress by talking about their feelings rather than holding them to themselves. Programs such as relaxation training, thought reorganization, simple support and empathy, or, in extreme stress situations, psychiatric intervention are necessary. In many instances the sport is the one positive thing in life that helps the athlete get through times of extreme stress (Fig. 6-2). Areas outside sports are often stressful; intervention has to be within their comfortable emotional framework.

This life stress information on the athlete is important for the athletic sports therapist in rehabilitation work. Early detection of stresses and their relief are the avenues of choice for a more speedy rehabilitation after injury.

Each athlete copes with life stress differently. One athlete may adjust to a new coach with ease, especially if the coach is one in a long series, whereas another, who may have had only one or two coaches, may have a more difficult time with the adjustment, especially if the athlete goes from an easygoing coach to a strict disciplinarian. However, the individual with multiple coaches may have had difficulty adjusting to each new coach. Experience in the situation benefits the adjustment if the athlete has successfully handled the experience before.

Those with good support and, most important, perception of support from their friends, family, and athletic staff also have an easier time with life's stress events. Often those with poor coping mechanisms and those who are inflexible are injury-prone.

Few athletes react to stress events by verbalizing them, yet most handle them very well by themselves. James Michener[6] makes the following point:

> For many athletes physical activity, rather than talking things out, appears to offer a means of expressing feelings and aggressions. Perhaps this substitution of actions for words contributes to the seeming reluctance of athletes to come to a service that requires that they articulate their feelings.

ATTITUDES SETTING UP INJURY

Certain attitudes toward sports have fostered injury and more important reinjury. The phrase "you have to play with pain" has been interpreted more literally to mean that the athlete has to play through an injury. The difference is that

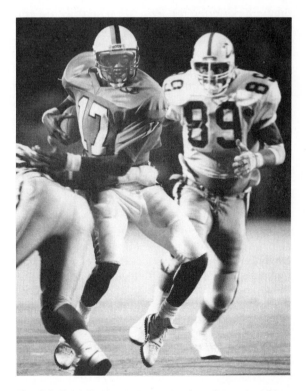

Fig. 6-2. Participation in sports is often the one positive aspect of life that helps the athlete get through times of extreme stress.

LIFE STRESS EVENTS

Death of family member—100
Detention in jail—63
Injury—46
Death of close friend—37
Playing for new coach—35
Playing on new team—31
Outstanding personal achievement—28
Major change in living habits—25
Social readjustment—24
Change to new school—20
Major change in social activities—18
Sleep habit change—16

some injuries may be mild and only somewhat painful, resulting in no reinjury in competition, whereas a more severe injury is made worse by continuing to compete. The importance of a certified sports trainer to make this decision is obvious.

Unfortunately, untrained personnel such as coaches are assuming this responsibility when no certified sports trainer is present or when the certified sports trainer is easily intimidated by the coach and not backed up by the athletic director. Either situation results in poor medical care and leaves the management vulnerable to legal action as a result of negligence. Courts expect competent medical care to be provided to the athletes. That care can be provided only by a certified sports trainer or a physician (Fig. 6-3). Players who feel that a missed practice or game will relegate them to the bench for the year or those who have been encouraged to play no matter what are candidates for injury and reinjury. Usually what happens, however, is that they are performing poorly because they are not at full strength and thus they only reinforce the decision of the coach to play someone else. The role of the certified sports trainer is to determine when the player is functioning at top potential without risk of injury or reinjury and to keep the coach abreast of the player's status. A clear perception of the injury and its limitations by the athlete is important. An important role of the sports therapist is to inform the athlete of the difference between pain and injury.

The athlete who continues to play with an unhealed injury or repeated reinjury is constantly reducing the chances of a healthy life of activity. The athlete has to live past the few years of competition. Most, however, have difficulty seeing past the present season, or at best have the goal of participating in their sport until they can no longer compete, regardless of the consequences. The rewards of competition and the admiration of others take sports out of perspective and retard a healthy attitude toward sports. The attitude of the athlete is "Sacrifice everything for the sport; besides, I'm bulletproof." Lack of this attitude is viewed by some as weakness. These athletes have difficulty adjusting to injury, especially a career-ending one.

The attitude of neglecting the injured athletes or giving them the perception that they are lep-

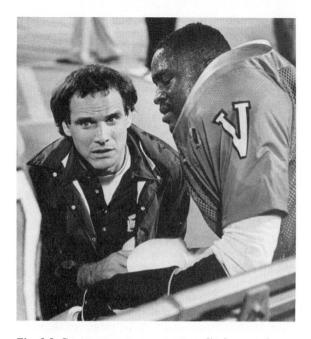

Fig. 6-3. Courts expect competent medical care to be provided to athletes by a certified athletic trainer or physician.

ers also can contribute to injury and reinjury. Coaches who foster this attitude are saying to the players that they have no self-worth if they are injured. Some coaches go so far as to prevent team contact until injured players are ready to return or to belittle them in front of their peers, believing that this will make the athlete want to get back to competition quicker. This tactic may work with some players with minor injuries, but only causes major adjustment difficulties for athletes who suffer severe injury.

Some coaches refuse to talk to the athlete or tell others the athlete really doesn't want to play or isn't tough enough. The coach is experiencing frustration with the fact that the athlete is injured and is unable to come to grips with the injury. Counseling with the coach in this situation to point out the effects of such attitudes may be helpful. Fortunately, these coaches are in the minority.

During this period either the athletic staff is showing its concern for the athlete and in return winning the athlete's loyalty and dedication to them down the road, or they are undermining the athlete's trust and setting up a future situation for the athlete to let them down when the athlete gets in the position of controlling the outcome of a contest and may just underperform in spite. Commitment is a two-way street. The athletic staff has to show its commitment to the athlete to receive the athlete's commitment.

PHASES OF INJURY

The athlete has to deal with four phases of injury: denial, anger, depression, and acceptance. These closely follow Elisabeth Kübler-Ross's model of the stages of death and dying. Following injury, the athlete faces three possible situations. The injury may be minimal and allow a speedy return, the athlete may have a prolonged period of rehabilitation, or the playing career may be at an end. The athlete must be encouraged along positive avenues to have the best opportunity to achieve complete rehabilitation, both emotionally and physically.

Early denial of the injury is commonplace, as the athlete attempts to rationalize that everything will be all right. The athlete feels that the injury will be fine the next day and that the early diagnosis is wrong. However, when the next day arrives and the injury is not better, the athlete begins to have difficulty dealing with the fact that recovery is not imminent. As a consequence, the athlete often feels anxious, isolated, and lonely.

Anger may soon replace this feeling of disbelief as the injured player vents feelings. Whoever happens to be around the athlete often bears the brunt of the anger. Anger cannot be reasoned with, and the athletic health care personnel must understand and not react to the anger of the athlete. This response is merely emotional, a release of frustration. The sports therapist must act as an emotional blotter and, if possible, not further aggravate the situation by attempting to exert power to calm down the athlete. Listen to what the athlete is feeling rather than to what is said. This active listening requires time and effort on the part of the sports therapist. The athlete has lost control of the situation and is seeking to regain it (Fig. 6-4).

Next, moods of anger, bargaining, and depression often are interrelated, with the athlete swinging from one to the other and back. Bargaining may also begin after the initial phase of

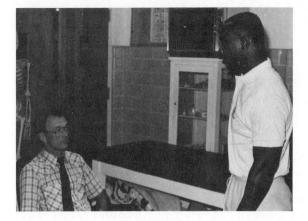

Fig. 6-4. Listen to what the athlete is feeling rather than to what he or she is saying.

denial, as the athlete is saying the injury isn't real. The athlete may put a concentrated effort into treatment and rehabilitation for a brief period to get back into competition for the game. When this fails, the athlete often drops into depression and slacks off on rehabilitation effort.

In this phase the athlete has lost control of the physical situation and often the emotional control that goes with it. Team and individual identity are gone, and the athlete is an outsider watching from the sidelines or often from the stands. Being in the stands often further isolates the athlete. This action alone often solidifies the phase of depression and should be avoided wherever possible.

Success or failure of the team may produce anxiety within the injured athlete. If the team wins, the athlete wonders what role is left; if the team loses, the anxiety is great for the athlete to return to help the team.

Acceptance is a phase many well-managed athletes move into with ease. Fortunately, this group comprises most of the athletes with whom the competent sports therapist will work. The positive interest, energy, and empathy shown by the sports therapist make the transition from initial injury and denial to the acceptance phase a quicker recovery for the athlete. This explains why some rehabilitation personnel who rapidly get their athletes to acceptance rarely see the athlete who is not psychologically adjusting to injury, whereas some who poorly manage their athletes continually see a great number of these individuals.

IT IS THE ATHLETE'S INJURY

The athlete who has reached the acceptance phase should have taken the responsibility for the injury. It is not the sports therapist's injury. The athlete has to accept the responsibility for the pain and the condition and deal with it. At this time the athlete is encouraged to transfer the time and energy given to the sport into the rehabilitation process. The athlete has to become an active and not a passive participant. The knee injury is now the competitor rather than the next week's opponent.

Care should be taken so the athlete does not become a dependent patient. Some want the sports therapist to be responsible for their welfare and want the sports therapist to meet their every need at their whim and command. They demand more time be spent on them. Failure of one staff member to meet their demands results in their selecting a staff member who will meet their demands. Staff members with the greatest need to help others will be easily taken advantage of at the sacrifice of time needed for other athletes.

When these dependent patients no longer receive the special attention they feel they deserve, they often lash out in anger or frustration. The sports therapist needs to head off this response by firmly yet emphatically explaining the restrictions on time and what is required of the athlete in terms of rehabilitation. This response should be pointed out to the athlete as inappropriate and needs examination on the part of the sports therapist and the athlete if it becomes a continual problem, as it is only a detriment to recovery.

The athlete is guided in rehabilitation but must push within these guidelines. The athlete has to be encouraged and believe in future success. All efforts should point toward a positive result with the athlete working with what is available and not with wishful thinking.

IRRATIONAL THINKING

With injury a very real stressor in the life of the athlete, irrational thinking often sets in. Percep-

tions of situations that before have been rational now become irrational as self-destructive emotion colors the thought process. Emotional reaction is exacerbated, as the athlete fails to return to normal in a few days. The athlete's common sense and judgment have become altered. This may occur with a daily mood change, so continual interaction with the athlete is necessary to restore rationality. The technique of cognitive restructuring helps the athlete become aware of these destructive, self-defeating behaviors. The athlete has often put in years of training and imposes pressures to return quickly. Fortunately, the certified sports trainer will prevent premature return and consequent reinjury by setting short-term goals and functional criteria prior to return.

The athlete, however, may fall into the mode of "I can't do it, I'll never get well." This irrational thinking produces anxiety, fear, and possibly depression that are detrimental to progress in rehabilitation. The athlete may be illogical, distort perceptions of events, or reach unrealistic decisions and conclusions. The athlete has replaced the old set of worries about simply playing well and helping the team win with the set of "Woe is me," with its resultant anxiety. Obviously, these thought patterns are detrimental to the positive attitude necessary in the rehabilitation process. Some examples of irrational thinking are shown in the box.

The sports therapist must recognize and intervene in this irrational thinking and challenge these thoughts with the athlete. Examination of these thoughts with athletes reassures them that it is "normal" to feel unhappy, frustrated,

---

EXAMPLES OF IRRATIONAL THINKING TOWARD INJURY

Exaggeration: athletes exaggerate the severity of the injury.

Disregard: athletes pay no attention to the aspects of the injury that are important for the healing and rehabilitation to occur.

Oversimplification: athletes think of the injury as good, bad, right, or wrong.

Overgeneralization: athletes tend to complicate the simple facts of the injury.

Unwarranted conclusions: athletes draw conclusions about the injury based on unsound or erroneous facts.

angry, insecure, or depressed, but the injury is not hopeless, they do not lack courage, and all is not lost and life is not over. The athlete should be challenged to replace irrational thoughts with positive and rational ones. In short, the injury is aggravating and unfortunate, but it can be handled and overcome. The injury is placed in perspective and viewed the same as the athlete would consider preparation for the next contest.

The athlete has to identify faulty thinking, gain understanding of it, and actively work for its change. Research indicates that the self-thoughts, images, and attitudes during the recovery period determine the length and quality of the rehabilitation.

The many concerns on the mind of the athlete prevent listening to the sports therapist until the acceptance phase of injury. Thus the sports therapist spends a lot of time repeating and reinforcing goals and exercise regimens (Fig. 6-5).

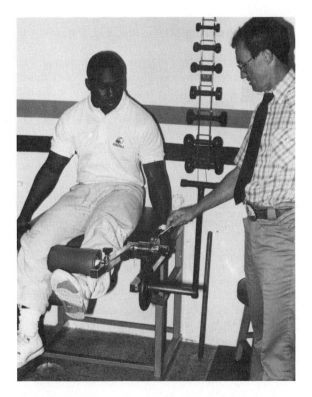

Fig. 6-5. The athlete may not be listening to the sports therapist until the acceptance phase of injury; thus the sports therapist may have to repeat and reinforce goals and exercise regimens.

This process is important but often frustrating to the sports therapist, especially for those with no insight into the personality of the athlete. During this phase, close observation of the exercise routines is necessary to make sure the athlete is following instructions and performing the exercises correctly. Athletes in the adjustment phase do not have this problem and thus do not need the close supervision.

Obviously, the sports therapist must note any deviation in mood or personality from the normal and counsel the athlete as to its cause. Often the athlete simply has become discouraged because the rehabilitation is taking too long, even though the athlete has been advised that the whole process requires even more weeks or months of rehabilitation.

During this time the athlete is often experiencing peaks and valleys in the recovery process. The athlete is used to two speeds: nothing and full speed. The athlete is frustrated to have to spend time in the crutch phase, then the walking phase, then the fast walk phase, then the walk-jog phase, then the jog phase, then the jog-run phase, then the run phase, and then finally the full-speed activity phase.

The athlete ends up with two problems: the physical injury and, what is often worse, the emotional frustration of the injury. The frustration often overshadows the injury as the athlete cannot adjust to restrictions. Adaptation to the frustration is hard work in the rehabilitative process. The work the athlete is doing is not producing the same rewards as participation in the sport, plus the athlete is becoming anxious about becoming further behind in the sport. Mind and body are out of sync, with the mind going ahead at a rapid pace while the body falls behind expectations.

At this point reinjury often occurs. The athlete skips the intermediate goals because of frustration and thus ends up with a setback because of reinjury. The athlete desperately wants to return to previous form. The sports therapist often has to explain over and over the purpose of the intermediate goals and the setbacks that occur without their attainment. The athlete must understand that this phase has to be gone through and that frustration, hopelessness, and self-pity are part of the adjustment process. Athletes often describe this inactivity during injury as harder than playing. When they are playing, all their energy is directed toward the one goal of simply running plays and completing their assignments.

In the early phases of rehabilitation, athletes are not listening to the sports therapist, so they must be observed in their daily routines to make sure that they are doing what has been prescribed. Close supervision may be necessary for several sessions; they are listening but not hearing. Injury is a major stressor, and the trainer-therapist needs patience. Texts such as Gordon's *Teacher Effectiveness Training*[3] can help the sports therapist understand this problem in the life of the athlete.

With an injury that requires weeks or months of rehabilitation before returning to competition, the athlete often feels that the coaches have ceased to care, which reinforces the depression. The athlete must understand that the coach cares but has to spend time to get a replacement ready for competition.

STRATEGIES FOR GAINING CONTROL

The athlete will be unable to return and play successfully without gaining the emotional self-control to think rationally about the injury and cope successfully with it. Several strategies used by sports psychologists to aid with those who need this help are:

> Relaxation training
> Thought stoppage
> Imagery
>> Visual rehearsal
>> Emotive rehearsal
>> Body rehearsal

A strategy suggested for getting the athlete over the passive phase of injury is a model of regaining an active role in the injury. The model outlines four tasks in the strategy:

1. Accept the reality of the loss.
2. Experience the pain of grief.
3. Adjust to the new environment that is void of the loss.
4. Withdraw emotional energy and refocus it into another direction or activity.

Questions such as "How are you coping with your knee injury and the time you now have on your hands?" and "How do you perceive your rehabilitation is coming?" give the sports therapist a guide to the athlete's phase. Athletes should be encouraged to express their feelings.

Athletes who are successfully coping with their injuries are rational in their assessments and thoughts. Fortunately, these athletes make up the great majority of people encountered if they are managed properly.

Relaxation Training

Pain, lack of confidence, and anxiety may prevent athletes from achieving their potential in the rehabilitation setting. Relaxation training allows athletes to control these feelings with a series of deep breathing, voluntary muscular contractions, and relaxation exercises, in combination with thought control. In this manner athletes may concentrate more on the tasks at hand.

Negative Thought Stoppers

One of the most difficult aspects of adjusting to injury is the stoppage of negative thoughts. They become detrimental to the return. These have to be recognized by the athlete and controlled. Teaching athletes to control their inner thoughts helps to determine their future behavior. This technique is an ongoing process of awareness, education for removing negative thoughts, and encouragement for ultimate change.

Early education stresses the aspect that negative thoughts have a detrimental effect on both mental and physical performance. Keeping a daily record of when these thoughts take place and the circumstances in which they occur is helpful. Then athletes are helped to stop these negative thoughts and instill a positive regimen. This step is followed by an evaluation of the whole negative thought-stopping program on a regular basis. In this manner, athletes have the practice and feedback to begin their own positive outlook in terms of constructive thoughts, concentration, cues, images, and calming responses to change inappropriate attitudes. This positive outlook can assist athletes in returning more quickly to competition with better abilities to perform.

The reinforcement of phrases such as "You will get better" and "This too will pass" aid in the blockage of the negative thoughts that often occur. Negative thoughts block the athlete's road to recovery by increasing pain, anxiety, and anger. Athletes should be encouraged to put their efforts into recovery rather than into the downward spiral of self-pity. Thoughts create emotions; therefore, these negative thoughts have to be recognized and dealt with for a more rapid recovery.

Imagery

Imagery is used by athletes to reduce the anxieties associated with the return procedure. Visual images used in the process include visual rehearsal, emotive imagery rehearsal, and body rehearsal.

Visual rehearsal uses both coping and mastery rehearsal. Coping rehearsal has athletes visually rehearsing problems they feel may stand in their way to return. They then rehearse how they will overcome these problems.

Mastery rehearsal aids in gaining the confidence and motivational skills necessary. Athletes visualize their successful return to competition from the early drills of the sport to practice to the game situation.

Emotive rehearsal aids the athlete in gaining confidence and security by visualizing scenes relating to positive feelings of enthusiasm, confidence, and pride, in other words, the emotional rewards of praise and success from participating well in competition.

Body rehearsal empirically helps athletes in the healing process. Athletes visualize their bodies healing internally both during the rehabilitation process and during the day. To do this, they have to have a good understanding of the injury and of the type of healing occurring in relation to the rehabilitation procedures.

Care should be taken to explain the healing and rehabilitative process clearly, but not to overwhelm athletes with so much information that they become intimidated and fearful. This mistake is often made by the inexperienced counselor who wants to impress the athletes. Educate athletes only to the amount of knowledge required. By the same token, don't hold back information athletes require for this imagery.

INTERPERSONAL RELATIONSHIPS OF THE ATHLETE AND THE SPORTS THERAPIST

The sports therapist is often the first person athletes interact with after injury and the one who will direct the recovery. As a result, the sports therapist has to deal with the athlete as a person and not as just as a patient. When athletes enter the treatment setting, they should get the perception that the sports therapist cares for the athlete as a person and not just as part of the job. Their perception of the sports therapist makes a difference in terms of recovery time and effort. First they have to respect the sports therapist as a person before they can trust the therapist-trainer in the rehabilitative setting. Successful communication between the sports therapist and the athlete is essential for effective rehabilitation. Taking an interest in the athletes before injuries have occurred enables the sports therapist to know the personalities of the athletes and be able to work with them in helping to build their confidence.

With injury athletes lose control over their physical efforts. They have gone from 4 to 5 hours a day of practice or competition to no activity. They are in a temporary life-style change. Their feelings are going to affect the success or failure of the rehabilitation process. The sports therapist must establish rapport and a sense of genuine concern and caring for the athlete, who is not fooled by the superficial concerns of the sports therapist.

The sports therapist is often the person who effectively explains the injury to the athlete. Care should be taken to explain the situation to the athlete in understandable terms. In most cases the simplest explanation acceptable to the athlete is the best. With mild and moderate injuries, the use of *sprain, strain,* or *bruise* suffices. The example of a sprained knee and torn ligaments of the knee can be descriptions of the same grade-two injury, but the athlete may interpret the two terms altogether differently.

With the more severe grade-three injuries, care should be taken to inform athletes accurately, while at the same time not frightening them. Knowledge of the injury, its healing mechanism, and the rehabilitation process and progression give athletes an orderly timetable within which to proceed. If information is broken down this way, athletes do not become overwhelmed by the whole process. In this manner the anxiety and uncertainty manifested in the early denial and anger phases may be lessened. Athletes thus can put all their efforts into the rehabilitation process, with actions replacing anxiety.

Athletes must have injuries explained to them to their satisfaction. Disseminating injury information appropriate to athletes' emotional and intellectual level can be a real challenge. The rate and degree of acceptance is not the same with all athletes. Severity of injury is certainly important, but the athlete's perception of that severity is what matters in the rehabilitation process. Thus the physiological must be interrelated with the psychological. In working with athletes, the sports therapist should be not only empathetic but also nonjudgmental (Fig. 6-6).

Athletes are expected to report for rehabilitation, but the coach is the disciplinarian, not the sports therapist, and the coach institutes punishment for lack of participation in the rehabilitation process. The coach must support the rehabilitation concept or athletes soon know that this is not a priority with the coach and begin to lose interest if they are not highly motivated to return.

The real challenge of rehabilitation is how to motivate athletes to do their best in the rehabilitation process. Athletes who are not reporting for rehabilitation have a reason.

Everything is done for some need. The rehabilitation program must be established within these needs. If athletes are not reporting, either something is more important to them than a hastened recovery, or they have not had the importance of the process adequately explained to them. Reexamine the program and the athlete's goals. If the program has not been well explained and they are not committed to the program, the program either is doomed to failure or will be less than successful. Motivation must come from within, but the sports therapist can provide the encouragement and positive reinforcement necessary for the athlete to make a commitment.

Lack of commitment may indicate frustration, boredom, of feelings of a lack of progress. In this case, further explanations or changes in routine are necessary. The athlete may need the oppor-

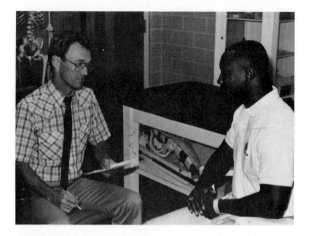

Fig. 6-6. In working with the athlete, the sports therapist has to be not only empathetic but also nonjudgmental.

tunity to comment on the program and make a commitment to the rehabilitation before being structured into a strict regimen of rehabilitative procedures.

An angry, hostile, or surly attitude toward the personnel or program should not offend the sports therapist. In anger the athlete is usually reacting to the situation and not necessarily to the individual. Whenever possible, anger should not be challenged, as no one can reason with anger. Instead, wait until the individual is in control to discuss inappropriate behavior that cannot be tolerated in the rehabilitation setting. Then the sports therapist and the athlete can work out the cause of the anger and its solution.

As stressed before, knowing the personality of the athlete enables the sports therapist to have a better understanding of what the athlete is going through. This insight can make all the difference in getting the athlete into a proper frame of mind for successful completion of the rehabilitation process.

ADHERENCE TO THE REHABILITATION PROCESS

Shank[11] found that athletes who are committed to the rehabilitation program work harder and thus return more quickly with better results than those who are nonadherents. Their pain tolerance is greater and of less concern, and they are more self-motivated, as opposed to the apathy of the nonadherents.

Also support from peers, coaches, and rehabilitation staff is important in influencing adherence. Those with support show a greater effort to fit the rehabilitation effort into their schedules. They are more likely to keep commitments to those who support them than they are to themselves. Those who are nonadherents respond better to support and motivation from their support group than do the adherents. Thus, extra encouragement from this support group for the nonadherents can really pay dividends in getting them motivated for successful completion of their rehabilitation.

Keep in mind that athletes may have many activities in their daily schedules, and fitting the rehabilitation to their schedules rather than the reverse can also encourage compliance. The more the athlete is allowed input and flexibility, the more successful the compliance will be.

As mentioned, pain is better tolerated by the compliant athlete. Rehabilitation programs should be examined to determine the aspects that may be painful. Almost all rehabilitation should be pain-free, and what is not is usually detrimental to the return of the athlete. Painful exercise, therefore, is not only harmful but also reduces compliance, especially in the nonadherent.

Another aspect of compliance has to do with athletes' perception of their ability. Athletes who perceive themselves ready to continue to a more advanced level of competition tend to shirk rehabilitation. They usually are the better athletes who do not have to work as hard as but perform better than their peers, so they assume the same attitude about rehabilitation. With this attitude, these good athletes never become truly great athletes because of their lack of commitment to their sport. Once they have risen to the top level where most have the same skills, the work habit is not there to put them in the top of the elite athlete group.

Other factors of compliance for student athletes are the length of time at a particular school, semester grade-point average, perception of class load, career goals, amount of participation time in contests, perception of time available for treatments, and previous experience with rehabilitation programs.

The more formal education a person has, the higher the level of compliance to treatments; the higher the semester grade-point average, the higher the treatment compliance. Interestingly enough, an inverse relationship exists between athletes' perception of difficulty of their class load and compliance. Often athletes do better academically during the season than at other times, possibly because they budget their time with better discipline during the season, and this approach carries over into the rehabilitation setting.

Those who have better-defined career goals and those who have the greatest amount of participation time have higher levels of compliance, as do those who perceive they have a greater amount of time available for treatments and those who have previous experience with rehabilitation programs.

COPING WITH INJURY

The sports therapist has to remember that a big part of rehabilitation is to help the athlete cope with the injury. A mild physical injury can be a severe emotional one. At this time the athlete's abilities to cope with the situation are impaired or overwhelmed. The sports therapist must assist the athlete in getting through this time of crisis until the athlete becomes more in control of the situation. This situation may last from several hours to several days.

Athletes feel helpless because their whole lives may revolve around sports and now they have lost the ability to perform. After this period, injured athletes take either the positive and recovering attitude or one of self-defeat and negativism. This period of limbo should be managed positively to benefit the athlete both on and off the field. Athletes often cope more successfully than the average person because they have self-discipline, emotional control, and better coping skills as a result of their years of competing and adjusting to these demands.

Moos and Tsu[4] talk about major adaptive tasks for the athlete and divide them into eight areas. The first adaptive task has the athlete responding to pain and loss of function and control. Second, the athlete copes with the stresses of the foreign situation of emergency rooms, surgical conditions, casts, braces, or crutches. Also with this coping is the unfamiliar situation of the tremendous amount of effort required of the rehabilitative process, in terms of both time and energy, all without the satisfaction of performing in a competitive setting. Stress is further added as athletes are no longer in the inner circle of their sport with their friends.

The third area has athletes reaching out to establish relationships with the rehabilitative staff. This step is often difficult for athletes who have been catered to when healthy and are now in a reversed role. At this time athletes question many of the aspects of the rehabilitation procedure. They question the doctor's diagnosis, the trainer for working them possibly too much, and the coach for not paying attention to them. They question whether they themselves are malingerers and the rehabilitation personnel as to whether they know how important competition is to them.

The fourth stage requires athletes to acquire emotional balance. Before, they may have had many emotional outbursts to coaches, doctors, sports therapists, and friends as part of the anger mentioned earlier. This frustration is often the result of having been dedicated to a single sport or activity. Many top athletes are emotionally immature, which is one of the disadvantages of sports. Olympic and other top-caliber athletes are often emotionally and socially years behind their chronological peers because they have spent so much time in their sport that their social interactions have suffered. Therefore, many top or single-minded athletes have difficulty with emotional control when they sustain a serious injury.

Next, athletes enter the fifth stage, that of maintaining a healthy self-image. This phase has athletes sustaining a sense of competence and mastery. Athletes have had to undergo a change in identity that is often difficult. They have had to remain upbeat and positive while at the same time revising their expectations. This phase is difficult for athletes who have had high expectations and lack the ability to attain these goals.

Athletes who are injured and do not regain their previous form are faced with the same problem. Athletics now takes on a different perspective, and a healthy self-image is required for successful adaptation. At this time athletes have to adjust to dependence on others for their reha-

bilitation needs, as their independence and self-control have been compromised.

The sixth phase is that of injured athletes maintaining or regaining normal relationships with peers, family, coaches, and rehabilitation personnel. They may have had little support from this group, as everyone is concerned with the results of the team. Injured athletes feel neglected because their communication lines revolve around the sport, and they are no longer part of the sport. When athletes are involved around the team, however, they feel less isolated and guilty.

The seventh area requires athletes to get ready for future competition. This phase is often difficult for athletes, as the time necessary is constantly being reduced by surgical and rehabilitation philosophies and techniques. This reduced time may not allow the athletes adequate mental preparation for the return. Prospective return dates should be discussed with athletes so they may begin to anticipate their return.

Accepting the limitations of injury and fitting into the athletic life-style's restrictions and limitations is the eighth and final task area of adaptation. It can range from the athlete who continues a normal life-style with the exception of sports competition to the athlete who is a quadriplegic.

In the area of coping, the sports therapist needs to help athletes with short-term problems rather than with what may happen in the future. Trying to see the total picture right away may be too overwhelming for athletes. This emphasis is important from the time the injury is first assessed on the sidelines. In most cases this situation is foreign and hostile for athletes and care should be taken to make them as much at ease as possible. How this situation is handled can determine their future attitude toward recovery. Accept their present conceptions but direct them toward a more positive outlook of the situation.

After injury, athletes need the support of those who have been important and around them. To prevent possible feelings of negative self-worth and problems of loss of identity for athletes, their support groups need to stress the fact that they are interested in the athlete as a person rather than as a team member. Friendships based on athletic identification are now compromised, as the athletic identification is gone, and they can be related to in athletic terms only by what they did yesterday or as injured teammates and not as individuals. If the rehabilitation personnel have established prior personal contact with the athlete as a worthwhile person, this transition can be easier.

GOALS

Goal setting is an important aspect of the rehabilitation of the athlete. First, the goal must be mutually acceptable to both athlete and sports therapist. If the goal is not acceptable to the athlete, the rehabilitation will fail. A goal of return to competitive athletics requires a different program than the goal of leisure athletics or one of just casual exercise.

The time in the season determines certain goals. The individual injured early in the season may be held out for the year as a red shirt or may have an accelerated rehabilitation program for return as soon as possible. The Little League player will have different goals than the high school participant, who will have different goals than the professional player. Remember, the injury belongs to the athlete, who has to accept the goals and be responsible for them if the program is to be a success.

Short-term goals emphasize progress and help to maintain motivation better than a long-term goal that will often seem unobtainable. The completion of short-term goals gives the athlete experience with success and helps to maintain a positive attitude. An increase in range of motion, lifting another set of weights, and walking without crutches are such short-term goals. Progress is easier to see when the goal is to walk without crutches than when the goal is playing competitive basketball.

Attainment of short-term goals emphasizes to athletes that they are regaining physical control of the situation once more and that they are getting better (Fig. 6-7). Athletes should be kept busy working toward the attainment of these goals to help prevent negative thinking about the negative aspects of the injury.

At this time, the trainer-therapist should reassess the strengths and weaknesses of the athlete who will be disabled for several weeks or more. Strength, power, endurance, speed, agility, and flexibility indexes should be evaluated,

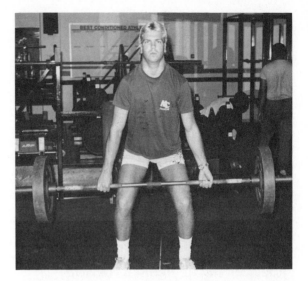

Fig. 6-7. Attainment of short-term goals emphasizes to athletes that they are regaining physical control of their situations and that they are getting better.

as well as the percentage of body fat. Past physical fitness tests should be evaluated and their results integrated into the "new" program. Dietary habits should be investigated and corrected if necessary. With this positive approach toward the rehabilitation program, athletes may return to active status in better condition than before they were injured.

The sports therapist must clarify what is expected from the athlete in terms that are within the athlete's ability. The athlete must make a commitment to the rehabilitation process and comply with its demands. However, the goal must be important enough to the athlete to make the commitment. Here often lies the challenge for the sports therapist: making the goals of the athlete compatible with those of complete recovery.

Care must be taken not to promise more than is possible. A promise that "your knee will be as good as new after surgery" is not possible, but "we have a goal of 90 to 100% result for your knee after surgery" says much of the same without overstating the result.

Mastery of short-term goals allows athletes to feel they are regaining control of the situation. Written short-term goals are desirable because athletes can see their progress. For the same reason, athletes should be encouraged to keep workout journals that give them a more orderly sense of progression about the recuperation.

Return criteria must be explained to the athlete. All concerned—sports therapist, physician, coach, and, most of all, the athlete—must be in agreement about the readiness to return to competition. Positive reinforcement and successful completion of functional short-term goals should have reduced any fears, and the athlete should have relaxed and gained the confidence needed to put all the external factors out of mind. With successful rehabilitation the athlete's instincts return to replace the hesitation the athlete previously had in earlier phases of recovery after the injury.

PROBLEMS IN THE REHABILITATION PROCESS

Some athletes are problems who tax even the most empathetic and understanding of personnel. The better the athlete is dealt with prior to injury in terms of positive personal interaction, the more successful will be the result. The sports therapist spends 95% of the time with 5% of the athletes. Within this group are the athletes who do not seem to be getting better.

With treatment and rehabilitation, athletes are expected to improve. When they do not, the athlete, physician, sports therapist, and coach become anxious. The self-esteem of the rehabilitation team is based on their ability to cure the athlete and the athlete is denying them of that achievement.

Anxiety turns to frustration, antagonism, and hostility on the part of all involved. Often the athlete is described as crazy or unmotivated to explain the lack of improvement. "It certainly can't be the fault of the medical staff or coach."

This indirect communication to players tells them they are not worthwhile in the eyes of the staff. Lack of improvement may be a way that athletes, especially those with low self-esteem, get back at the coach or the system. Athletes may feel that they are not cared for and therefore not getting the attention they deserve. This is the environment for a lawsuit. Often the *perception* of poor care rather than actual poor care fosters most of these hostile feelings toward the athletic and rehabilitation staff.

During this time athletes may often be able to give some insight to the staff as to the reason why they are not improving. Maybe a change in routine, a missed diagnosis, or improper treatment is the cause. The more athletes are involved in their rehabilitation, the more they will move toward a speedy recovery. Athletes may be afraid to return or have other hidden reasons for not returning.

The hypochondriac and the malingerer present two types of returning problems. The hypochondriac is often nervous and irritable and seems to be eccentric but often competes with a high tolerance to pain upon returning to the sport. These athletes perceive their lives to be extremely complicated, and they feel they have lost control of their lives both athletically and emotionally.

Many people are taught that all things can be overcome, which is not true. Athletes must be helped to perform within the limits of what they can control. Often hypochondriacs are used to a great deal of support that is suddenly gone. They face a new coach, new environment, new peers, a new athletic philosophy—all situations of change. Their only support is their self-confidence and coping skills, both of which are infantile.

Malingerers, however, claim nothing works in relieving their pain and symptoms. Everything is directed to a constant emphasis of symptoms. "Good morning" may be met with the response, "My ankle still hurts today; yesterday's treatment didn't help a bit." Bizarre symptoms, glove paresthesia, and the like are often tips. Malingerers often have reasons, whether it's saving face because they lack the athletic ability or hostility toward someone involved in the sport. They may fear loss of scholarship aid but not want to do the work required to maintain it, or they may be concerned with litigation at some future time because of some perceived injustice imposed by someone in the system.

Attacks on these individuals result in lowering their self-esteem and further exaggerating their problems. Only by active support and empathy can these individuals be helped, and professional counseling or psychiatric attention may be necessary.

The rehabilitation staff may be partially responsible for some of the problems experienced in the rehabilitation setting. The sports therapist that becomes more sympathetic than empathetic

TABLE 6-1
Effectiveness of the Sports Therapist

Type of Therapist	Knowledgeable	Convincing	Sincerely Concerned
Great sports therapist	x	x	x
Good sports therapist	x	x	o
Fair sports therapist	x	o	o
Quack	o	x	o
Bad sports therapist	o	o	o

may be reinforcing behavior that is detrimental to the athlete. Chronic pain behaviors, complaining, dependence on the sports therapist, focusing only on the injury, and lack of desire to compete are examples of situations when the attention of the staff may reinforce this aberrant behavior. In this period, the athlete may be in a mood of self-pity just prior to entering the acceptance phase of the injury.

Hard work in the rehabilitation process should be praised so the athlete is rewarded for positive responses as opposed to overconcern for the athlete's condition, which results in reinforcement of negative responses.

REHABILITATION PERSONNEL

Sports therapists should examine their motives for being in the field, especially when problems are continually cropping up in day-to-day operations. Are they in it for the power or to help people? Some thrive on the following they get from the athletes and thus boost their egos.

Techniques and philosophies should be continually examined to judge their effectiveness. Outdated or invalid theories need to be eliminated to maintain a current rehabilitation program. But remember that many of the athletes will get well anyway if the sports therapist does not mess them up. Table 6-1 explains the effectiveness of the sports therapist. Without rapport or perceived concern, programs often fail as the athlete loses confidence in the sports therapist.

CONCLUSION

Injury is a foreign, emotional, and unpleasant experience for the athlete. Tradition says that injuries are to be shrugged off and the battle con-

tinued. When injuries cannot be ignored, the athlete can become psychologically upset. For this reason all teams should have access to the skills of a sports psychologist, when and if needs arise above the abilities of the coach, team physician, or sports therapist. Rehabilitation is a physical and mental process. No two injuries are alike, and no two individuals necessarily react alike. Often attitudes and strategies for a rehabilitation process must be addressed for the troubled athlete. Only the sports therapist, with the necessary commitment, skills, and empathy, will be able to guide the athlete to a successful resolution of the symptoms and to a successful return to active status.

SUMMARY

1. Athletes do not deal with injuries in the same way. The sports therapist has to understand their views of injury. The manner in which the sports therapist manages these athletes often determines their time away from the sport.
2. Life's stress events play an important role in the adjustment to a certain system or coach. The successful program takes this factor into consideration and adjusts to the individual player whenever possible.
3. Attitudes on the part of coaches and staff have a direct bearing on the performance of the athlete. These personnel direct the athlete in the right direction for successful maturation and athletic competition.
4. After injury the athlete must adjust to denial, anger, depression, and acceptance. Each phase requires empathy on the part of all rehabilitation personnel.
5. The athlete must take responsibility for the

injury and deal with it as such. Guiding the athlete toward this goal is an integral part in injury management.

6. Irrational thinking on the part of the athlete is natural after injury. The role of rehabilitation personnel is to change this thinking through such strategies as relaxation training, thought stoppage, visual rehearsal, emotive rehearsal, and body rehearsal.

7. The interpersonal relationships of the athlete and sports therapist are most important and often the key to the return for the athlete.

8. Coping with the injury and adherence to the rehabilitation program are most important, as is the establishment of short- and long-term realistic goals.

REFERENCES

1 Fisher AC and others: Adherence to sports injury rehabilitation programs, Physician Sports Med 16(7):47–53, 1988.

2 Gieck J: Stress management and the athletic trainer, Athletic Training 19(2):115–119, 1984.

3 Gordon T: Teacher effectiveness training, New York, 1974, David McKay Co Inc.

4 Journal of Physical Education and Physical Fitness 48(4):66–69, 1987.

5 Journal of Sports Medicine and Physical Fitness: A Quarterly Review, 279–284, 1987.

6 Michener J: Sports in America, New York, 1976, Random House Inc.

7 Moos RH, Tsu VD: Coping with physical illness, New York, Plenum Medical Books Company, 1984.

8 Rotella RJ: The psychological care of the injured athlete. In Bunker L, Rotella RJ, and Reilly A, editors: Sport psychology: psychological considerations in maximizing sport performance, Michigan, 1985, Movement Publications.

9 Rotella RJ: Psychological care of the injured athlete. In Kulund D, editor: The injured athlete, Philadelphia, 1988, JB Lippincott Co.

10 Rotella RJ and Heyman S: Stress, injury and the psychological rehabilitation of athletes. In Williams J, editor: Applied Sport Psychology: Personal Growth to Peak Performance, Palo Alto, Calif., 1986, Mayfield.

11 Shank R: Academic and athletic factors related to predicting compliance by athletes to treatments, dissertation, Charlottesville, 1987, University of Virginia.

Therapeutic Modalities in Rehabilitation

7

William E. Prentice and Charles L. Henry

OBJECTIVES

Following completion of this chapter, the student will be able to:

- Describe the approach of the sports therapist in using therapeutic modalities.

- Discuss the potential physiological responses of biological tissue to electrical stimulating currents.

- Discuss the use of diathermy in rehabilitation.

- Compare ultrasound with diathermy as a deep-heating modality.

- Discuss the physiological effect of thermotherapy and cryotherapy techniques.

- Describe the possible uses for the low-power laser in sports medicine.

- Discuss the progression of modality use following acute injury.

- Discuss how various modalities can best be used in treating chronic injury.

- List indications and contraindications for use of the various modalities.

- Discuss the physiological effects associated with the use of the different modalities.

Therapeutic modalities, when used appropriately, can be extremely useful tools in the rehabilitation of the injured athlete. Like any other tool, their effectiveness is limited by the knowledge, skill, and experience of the person using them. For the sports therapist, decisions regarding how and when a modality may best be employed should be based on a combination of theoretical knowledge and practical experience. Modalities should not be used at random, nor should their use be based on what has always been done before. Instead, consideration must always be given to what should work best in a specific clinical situation.

In any program of rehabilitation, modalities should be used primarily as adjuncts to therapeutic exercise and certainly not at the exclusion of range-of-motion and strengthening exercises.

There are many different approaches and ideas regarding the use of modalities in injury rehabilitation. Therefore, no "cookbook" exists for modality use. Instead, sports therapists should make their own decisions from the options in a given clinical situation about which modality will be most effective.

ELECTRICAL STIMULATING CURRENTS

Electrical stimulating currents are among the therapeutic modalities most often used by the sports therapist. The effects of electrical current passing through biological tissues may be physiological, chemical, or thermal. All biological tissue has some response to this current flow. The type and extent of the response depends on (1) the type of tissue and its physiological response characteristics and (2) the parameters of the electrical current applied, that is, its intensity, duration, waveform, modulation, and polarity. Biological tissue responds to electrical energy in a manner similar to that manner in which it normally functions and grows.

Clinically, the sports therapist uses electrical currents for several purposes: (1) producing muscle contraction through stimulation of nerve and muscle; (2) stimulation of sensory nerves to help in the treatment of pain; (3) creating an electrical field on the skin surface to drive ions into the tissues (iontophoresis); and (4) creating an electrical field within the tissues to stimulate or alter the healing process (medical galvanism). In a sports medicine environment, the major therapeutic uses of electricity center on muscle contraction, sensory stimulation, or both.[13]

To produce any physiological response in the nerve and muscle fibers, an electrical current must be of sufficient intensity and last long enough to equal or exceed the nerve membrane's basic threshold for excitation. When this occurs, depolarization of the nerve fiber results in an action potential.[13]

Different types (sizes) of nerves have different thresholds for depolarization. The strength-duration curves in Fig. 7-1 represent graphically the thresholds for depolarization of sensory, motor, and pain nerve fibers. If current intensity and/or current duration are increased to a level great enough to reach the minimal threshold for depolarization of sensory fibers, the electrical current can be felt. If current intensity and/or duration are increased further, a muscle contraction may be elicited by reaching the threshold for depolarization of the motor fibers. If the intensity/duration continues to increase, eventually a level is reached that causes depolarization of the smaller fibers and pain. By simply changing current intensity, current duration, or some combination of the two, very different physiological responses can be achieved.[2]

Traditionally, various types of electric currents have been classified by attaching specific names, such as high volt, low volt, alternating, direct, interferential, Russian, and microamperage (MENS). Electrical stimulators that output any of these varieties of current (with the possible exception of some new MENS units in which the intensity is not great enough) have the capability of producing any of these physiological responses if the current parameters are adjusted appropriately. Thus a discussion of the physiological effects of electrical current on the stimulation of sensory nerves and motor nerves is appropriate.[1]

Stimulation of Sensory Nerves

Transcutaneous electrical nerve stimulation (TENS) has been traditionally defined as a technique used for the purpose of stimulating large-diameter sensory nerve fibers with electrodes placed on the skin specifically for the purpose of relieving either chronic or acute pain. This modality is an effective, noninvasive, nonpharmacological method of pain modulation.[20]

Electrodes are placed on the skin surface generally in or over the area of pain. Electrodes placed at the painful region may be within the dermatome, on a specific point, or over a peripheral nerve supplying the painful region. Spinal cord segments that give rise to a specific nerve root conveying nociceptive input provide another choice for electrode placement. Electrodes are often placed along vertebrae or between spinous processes in conjunction with electrodes placed over specific dermatomal regions.[15] These stimulators are designed to deliver pulses with a waveform that generally differs depending on the manufacturer. Electrical currents are either monophasic (DC) or biphasic (AC) and may take on sine, square, or triangular waveforms.[1] Various claims concerning the effectiveness of specific waveforms have been made by manufacturers and, although one type of waveform may be more effective for a particular patient, generalizations are difficult to make. These waveforms refer to the waveform produced by the stimulator and delivered to the patient and not the waveform of the current used to drive the generator.

The mechanism by which TENS produces relief of pain is a matter for debate. Certainly, the first units were designed and tried clinically on

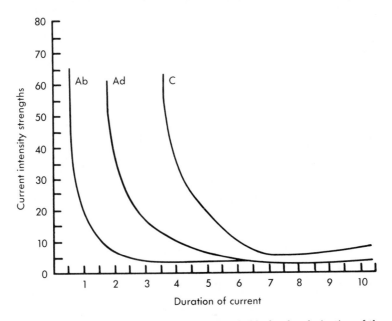

Fig. 7-1. Strength-duration curves represent the thresholds for depolarization of the various types of nerve fibers. *Ab*, sensory fibers; *Ad*, motor fibers; *C*, pain fibers.

the basis of Melzak and Wall's gate control theory of pain, originally proposed in 1965 with several later modifications.[21] To summarize this theory, nociceptive information is conveyed from the periphery to the spinal cord by small unmyelinated C fibers and small myelinated A fibers. These fibers directly or indirectly excite T cells in lamina V of the dorsal horn, which transmit nociceptive information to higher conscious pain centers in the thalamus and somatosensory cortex. By exciting large-diameter A fibers (which innervate cutaneous receptors), synaptic transmission between the pain fibers and the T cells is presynaptically inhibited and thus pain is not consciously perceived.

Most recent theories concerning the mechanism of TENS in the relief of pain involve endogenously produced opiatelike substances called **enkephalins.** Enkephalins have been implicated in a pain-relief mechanism in the dorsal horn of the spinal cord. Stimulation of large-diameter afferent fibers may locally release enkephalins from small enkephalin interneurons that presynaptically inhibit synaptic transmission of nociceptive input to the thalamus and somatosensory cortex and thereby eliminate conscious appreciation of pain.[13]

Conventional TENS involves stimulation of large-diameter afferent fibers. How is this accomplished with commercially available TENS units? Peripheral nerves are actually bundles of a large number of large and small sensory and motor nerve fibers, innervating skin, muscle, and visceral structures. Because the electrodes connected to the TENS stimulator are placed on the skin (and thus in proximity to cutaneous sensory receptors), sensory fibers are preferentially stimulated. In addition, as stimulus intensity (or duration) is increased, large-diameter afferent fibers are excited (or recruited) before small ones. Of course, if the intensity or duration of the stimulus is increased sufficiently, motor and small-diameter sensory fibers (pain fibers) are excited. With TENS, the objective is to stimulate maximally the large-diameter afferent fibers without concomitant motor responses or pain.

Nerve and muscle tissue have characteristic strength-duration (S-D) curves. If S-D curves for single nerve fibers are constructed, that different-sized nerve fibers have characteristic curves becomes apparent. Large fibers are more easily excited by an electrical stimulus than small fibers.[13]

At very short pulse durations (on an order of

10 microseconds), the difference between the stimulus intensity necessary to excite large-diameter type A sensory fibers and that necessary to excite very-small-diameter type C pain fibers is maximized. Many commercial TENS units have variable adjustments for pulse duration, amplitude or intensity, and frequency. Optimal stimulation of large-diameter fibers (and, therefore, maximal pain relief) is obtained if a short-duration pulse is chosen and the intensity is gradually increased until a tingling sensation is perceived. Although optimal frequency of stimulation has not been determined, frequencies greater than 100 cycles per second are rarely used because subjective increases in pain relief do not seem to occur at these frequencies.

A second pain-control system is located in the brainstem and has been shown to exert a powerful inhibitory influence on transmission of impulses conveying nociceptive information. These areas are located primarily in the periaqueductal gray matter as well as in the Raphe nucleus and are preferentially activated by small fibers (C fibers and A fibers). Intense electrical stimulation of peripheral pain fibers by either low-frequency, high-intensity TENS or electroacupuncture techniques results in what may be called **hyperstimulation analgesia.** Whereas in conventional TENS the duration of relief is generally short due to the relatively short half-life of enkephalins, the duration of relief following hyperstimulation using high-intensity electrical stimulation is generally days or weeks, and in some cases the relief may be permanent.[13]

The Raphe nucleus appears to be a source of descending pain control. Descending sertonergic neurons originating in the Raphe nucleus and descending in the dorsolateral tract to various levels of the spinal cord are activated by intense electrical stimulation. This descending inhibitory system acts at various levels of the spinal cord through stimulation of the enkephalin interneurons discussed earlier. The resulting presynaptic inhibition of primary afferent pain fibers results in a reduction of pain sensation.

Hyperstimulation analgesia may result from intense electrical stimulation of acupuncture points as well as trigger points. The most effective type of stimulus is a long-duration, monophasic pulse, which results in intense stimulation of pain fibers.

Another effect of such intense electrical stimulation is the release of another opiatelike polypeptide called **endorphin,** from the anterior pituitary gland. A large molecular complex known as ACTH/β-lipotropin is broken down to produce β-endorphin, certain types of enkephalins, and ACTH. This process is stimulated through low-frequency, high-intensity stimulation of peripheral pain fibers. The release of ACTH results in corticosteroid release from the adrenal glands. These antiinflammatory substances may play a part in the pain reduction seen following high-intensity stimulation. The released endorphins may serve to reduce pain locally by increasing the rate of degradation of prostaglandins and bradykinin. However, their most important function in the reduction of chronic and acute pain is through their direct stimulation of cells in the Raphe nucleus. This stimulation results in the increase of the activity of the descending pain-control mechanisms discussed earlier. One hypothesis is that β-endorphin is released in response to intense, low-frequency (1–5 Hz) stimulation of specific acupuncture or trigger points. This technique has been referred to as **acustim** or **electroacutherapy.**[13]

Stimulation of Motor Nerves

Electrical stimulation of motor nerve fibers at sufficient intensity and duration to produce depolarization results in muscular contraction. Once a stimulus reaches the depolarizing threshold, an increase in the intensity of the stimulus does not alter the quality of the contraction. However, if the frequency of stimulation is increased, the time for repolarization of the muscle fiber is decreased, and thus the contractions tend to summate. When the stimulation frequency reaches 50 Hz or greater, the muscle exhibits a tetanic contraction.

Several therapeutic gains can be accomplished by electrically stimulating a muscle contraction. Electrically induced contractions can be used to facilitate circulation by pumping fluid and blood through the venous and lymphatic channels away from an area of swelling.[13]

Muscular inhibition following periods of immobilization or surgery is an indication for muscle reeducation. Electrically stimulating the muscle to contract produces an increase in the sensory input from the muscle and assists the patient in relearning a muscular response or pattern.[13]

Muscular strengthening may be accomplished using high-frequency AC current in conjunction with voluntary muscle contractions. The exclusive use of electrical current does not appear to increase muscle strength.[8] Electrically stimulating the muscle to contract during periods of immobilization retards muscle atrophy and may potentially reduce the time required for rehabilitation following immobilization.

Electrical currents may also assist in increasing range of motion about a joint where contractures are limiting motion. Repeated contraction over an extended time appears to make the contracted joint structures and muscle modify and lengthen.[13]

Iontophoresis

Electrical stimulating currents may also be used to produce chemical changes. Electricity is used in the clinic to cause chemical change in two important ways. The first is called **iontophoresis** or **ion transfer,** defined as the introduction of chemical ions into superficial body tissues for medicinal purposes with the use of direct current. For iontophoresis to work, the chemical substance must be in an ionic form. Because like charges repel, chemical substances with a positive charge are introduced through the skin with the positive electrode or anode, and substances with a negative charge must be introduced with the negative electrode or cathode.[13]

If the drug is in solution form, it is generally applied to a gauze pad that is placed directly over the area to be treated. The active electrode of the same polarity as the charge of the ion is then placed on top of the drug-soaked gauze and secured firmly in place. The dispersive or indifferent electrode is generally placed at a remote area of the same extremity. Drugs in paste form are usually rubbed onto the skin surface, and a moist electrode with the proper polarity is then secured. In general, intensity is adjusted to tolerance. Treatment time is generally indicated by the physician, but 10 to 15 minutes is a typical treatment time.

Some care must be taken with very potent drugs that could potentially have deleterious systemic effects. However, iontophoretically applied medicinal ions generally do not migrate far below the surface of the skin or mucous membranes.

Some of the more common substances that may be iontophoretically applied are:
1. Heavy metal ions such as zinc and copper to fight certain types of skin infections
2. Chloride ions to loosen superficial scars
3. Local anesthetics
4. Vasodilating drugs
5. Magnesium ions for plantar warts

Medical Galvanism

The other major use of direct current that may be included under the general category of chemical effects has been termed **medical galvanism,** defined as the use of low-voltage galvanic or direct current for therapeutic purposes without the introduction of pharmacological substances. The therapeutic benefit is thought to result largely from local ionic changes that result in increased circulation to body parts between the electrodes. Presumably the improved circulation speeds up absorption of inflammatory products such as accumulated metabolites with subsequent pain relief. Low-volt electrical currents may speed wound healing, decrease edema, and help fight localized infection. Some conditions for which galvanic current has been used effectively include contusions, sprains, myositis, acute edema, certain forms of arthritis, tenosynovitis, and neuritis.

Some other effects of long-duration, low-volt current, which seem to be polarity specific and a result of local ionic and electrical changes, are:

Positive pole (anode)	hardening of tissues	decreases nerve excitability
Negative pole (cathode)	softening of tissues	increases nerve excitability

Diathermy

Direct currents and low-frequency alternating currents are not used to generate thermal effects clinically. The reason is not that such currents are incapable of generating thermal effects, but that the intensities necessary would be prohibitively high and result in severe pain and cutaneous or subcutaneous tissue burns. Slight thermal effects, however, occur as a result of local circulation increases.

High-frequency currents may be used to produce a tissue temperature increase. Electrical current flowing through a conductor results in the development of a magnetic field around the conductor. The strength of this field varies with the strength of the current carried by the conductor. Electronic instruments have been devised that are capable of generating extremely high frequency (alternating) magnetic fields, which in turn are capable of generating extremely high frequency alternating "currents" within human tissues.

If a long length of very fine wire (conductor) is tightly coiled and a bar magnet (magnetic field) is passed through the coil, an electrical current is induced in the coiled wire. In other words, a changing or alternating magnetic field can induce an electrical current in a nearby conductor.

In the clinic, diathermies are used to generate rapidly alternating magnetic fields and in some cases electrical fields. These high-frequency magnetic fields (analogous to the bar magnet moving back and forth) generate induced high-frequency alternating currents (sometimes called **eddy currents**) in body tissues (analogous to the coiled wire). Everyday experience demonstrates that substances conducting electricity heat up (e.g., filament of a light bulb). Thus, the end result of these high-frequency alternating currents is the heating of body tissues.[6]

Electrical currents induced in highly conductive materials are more intense, and, therefore, the generation of heat per unit of time is greater than in less conductive substances. The human body is composed of materials of different electrical resistances, and consequently the rate of heat generation is different in different tissues and organs. The conductivity of various body tissues is generally a function of their fluid (water and electrolyte) content. Thus, muscle is heated by the diathermies much more readily than skin, bone, and fat. In general, diathermy is most effective in heating highly vascularized tissues. One of the most important precautions to take when treating a patient with diathermy is to find out whether the patient has any type of metal implant such as a pin, plate, or joint prosthesis.

Metal is an excellent conductor of electricity and may heat to the point of causing a severe burn. Other precautions are discussed later.

Primarily two forms of diathermy are used clinically today. The first has been called **shortwave diathermy** (Fig. 7-2). The operating frequency of these devices is about 27 million cycles per second. Calculations based on the frequency-wavelength relationship of electromagnetic energy (which is the output of these devices) yield a wavelength of approximately 11 meters. Several types of electrodes are used to transmit this shortwave energy to a patient, including pads, cuffs, air-spaced plates, drums, and induction field cables.[10]

Owing to electrode configurations, some shortwave diathermies generate rapidly alternating electrical fields as well as magnetic fields. An example is air-spaced plate electrodes, which function much like a capacitor. The result of the high-frequency oscillating electric field is much the same as the oscillating magnetic field; that is, tissue temperature rises. Claims have been made that diathermy units utilizing electrical field energy (so-called electrostatic devices) heat adipose tissue more than units utilizing magnetic field energy (electromagnetic devices). Fat seems to be more resistant to the passage of an electrical field than a magnetic field and therefore is heated more. In the case of shortwave diathermy units utilizing air-spaced plates, the body part to be treated is placed directly between the plates. Energy passing from plate to plate must therefore pass directly through the patient, who actually becomes part of the circuit. With a drum or induction field cable, the patient does not actually become a part of the circuit but rather is within the magnetic field resulting from current flow within the circuit.

The other type of diathermy unit used in the clinic is the microwave diathermy, which has certain advantages over shortwave diathermy. The operating frequency of microwave diathermy is on the order of 2450 million cycles per second yielding a wavelength of approximately 12 cm (as contrasted to a wavelength of over 10 meters for shortwave diathermy). With microwave diathermy, the wavelength is short enough to have some of the properties of visible light, and therefore the energy can be focused toward the body part to be treated. This allows for greater pen-

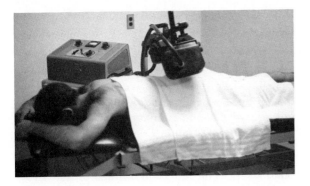

Fig. 7-2. Short wave diathermy using drum electrodes applied to the back.

duction of heat deep within the tissues.[19]

Neither type of diathermy is in as widespread use today as in past years. One major problem is that with significant subcutaneous fat the temperature of the fat may rise to dangerous levels, especially when the diathermy device produces its effects primarily with electrical fields. Furthermore, electrode choice and placement takes a significant amount of time, and body areas needing treatment may not always be optimally accessible to available electrode types. Perhaps the main reason for the decline in the use of diathermy has been the development of ultrasound, which is cheaper, provides deep-tissue temperature rise, is safer, and requires a much shorter treatment time.

ULTRASOUND

By definition, **ultrasonic energy** is vibrational energy with a frequency above 20,000 Hz. Unlike sound energy in the audible range, ultrasonic energy is for the most part absorbed by gases. For this reason, a liquid or ointment must be used as a coupling agent to ensure significant transfer of energy from the source of ultrasound to the patient.[9]

Ultrasonic energy is generally produced in the clinic by a device that generates a high-frequency alternating current. This high-frequency current then sets a crystal (usually quartz or a synthetic crystal), which is housed in a handheld transducer, into vibration (Fig. 7-3). The most common clinical ultrasonic generators operate at a frequency of 1 million Hz.

As used in the clinic, ultrasound is usually delivered at an intensity of about 1.5 watts per square cm of transducer surface. At this intensity, significant deep-heating effects occur, due primarily to the absorption of high-frequency sound energy and the transduction of this energy into heat. Because of the considerable reflection of ultrasonic energy at tissue interfaces (e.g., tendon-bone), sharply localized tissue temperature increases can occur at these junctions, particularly those junctions having limited vascularization. Such a temperature increase sometimes occurs at the junction of bone and periosteum. Because the periosteum is rich in sensory endings, a deep, dull ache of very sudden onset may occur.[26]

etration because more of the energy strikes the skin perpendicularly. Scatter of the energy is minimized, and absorption is maximized. Because of its longer wavelength, shortwave energy cannot be focused with equipment available to clinical settings, and consequently much energy is lost due to scatter.

For the forms of electromagnetic energy used by sports therapists, as the wavelength of electromagnetic energy decreases (frequency increases), the depth of penetration into body tissues also decreases, all other things being equal. From this alone, one might conclude that microwave energy might not penetrate as deeply as shortwave energy because of its short wavelength. Given the extremes of the electromagnetic spectrum, however, the difference between the wavelengths of microwave and shortwave diathermy is relatively very small. In addition, because microwave energy can be focused, therapeutic tissue temperature rise can occur up to a depth of 5 cm, and microwave diathermy is probably as effective as shortwave diathermy in producing deep-tissue temperature rise.

Energy of clinical shortwave diathermy wavelengths is thought to cause a deep-heating effect largely through the oscillation of polar molecules, such as water. High-frequency microwaves result in intraatomic vibrations or disturbances but probably have too high a frequency to result in molecular oscillation or spin. However, the increase in intramolecular vibration has the same effect as molecular oscillation, that is, the pro-

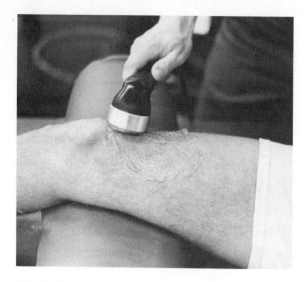

Fig. 7-3. Technique for applying ultrasound.

In addition to thermal effects, other physiological effects of ultrasound have been reported. Ultrasonic energy has been shown to be largely absorbed by proteins and to cause changes in cell permeability to sodium and potassium. Ultrasound has also been shown to be effective in decreasing pain due to neuromas, increasing range of motion limited by scar formation, and relieving pain resulting from tendonitis, bursitis, or fibrosis with or without evidence of mineral deposition. Whether ultrasound exerts these effects via thermal or nonthermal changes cannot yet be clearly determined.

Ultrasonic energy is not transmitted efficiently through gas or, for that matter, through fluids containing high concentrations of gases because most of the energy is absorbed by the gas. Therefore, an appropriate ultrasonic conducting medium or coupling agent must be placed between the transducer or sonator and the patient. For fairly large and smooth body surfaces, a coating of commercial gel or mineral oil may be placed directly on the surface. The transducer is placed directly in contact with this and is either continually moved in a circular or longitudinal motion or remains stationary with the unit set in either a pulsed mode or at a duty cycle of 50% or less. For very irregular body surfaces or areas with bony prominences, immersion techniques are often preferred. The body part is immersed in a container of fluid such as distilled water (previously boiled so as to remove gas bubbles). The transducer is then held 1 inch from the part to be treated and usually moved continuously.

Ultrasound is sometimes also used to introduce pharmacological agents subcutaneously, possibly by causing changes in the permeability of the cell membrane. This technique is called **phonophoresis.** The medicinal agent is mixed with an ointment or liquid that serves as a coupling agent. The radiating surface of the transducer is placed into the coupling agent containing the pharmacological agent and energized using either the moving or stationary technique.[23]

Phonophoresis may be superior to iontophoresis as a method of introducing topically applied medication deep into underlying tissue. It has no danger of skin damage and no tendency to dissociate the introduced compound into ionized fragments. In addition, pharmacological agents may be introduced more deeply into subcutaneous tissues with phonophoresis than with iontophoresis without concern for the pH of the coupling agent. Treatment time may also be cut by as much as one half.

Ultrasound has many advantages over the use of diathermy. In general, ultrasound can provide the deep-heating effects of diathermy and possibly useful nonthermal effects. Ultrasound units are generally much less expensive than diathermy units and usually much more portable. Another important clinical advantage is that ultrasound is poorly absorbed by homogeneous tissues such as fat, and therefore excessive heating of fat (which is superficial to tissues where deep heating is desired) is not a problem. Another advantage is that ultrasound can usually be used in the area of metal implants if they are deep enough. Metal, which is extremely homogeneous, does not absorb energy to as high a degree with ultrasound as with shortwave or microwave energy. Some reflection of ultrasound does occur, and some increase in temperature can occur at tissue-implant interfaces.

INFRARED MODALITIES

The superficial heating and cooling modalities used in a sports medicine setting are all classified as infrared modalities. Heat modalities are referred to as **thermotherapy.** Thermotherapy is used when a rise in tissue temperature is the goal of treatment. The use of cold, or **cryotherapy,** is most effective in the acute stages of the healing process immediately following injury when tissue temperature loss is the goal of therapy (Fig. 7-4). Cold applications can be continued into the reconditioning stage of athletic injury management. The term **hydrotherapy** can be applied to any cryotherapy or thermotherapy technique that uses water as the medium for heat transfer.[3]

Clinical Use of Heat and Cold

The physiological effects of heat and cold are rarely the result of direct absorption of infrared energy. There is general agreement that no form of infrared energy can have a depth of penetration greater than 1 cm. Thus the effects of the infrared modalities are primarily superficial and directly affect the cutaneous blood vessels and the cutaneous nerve receptors.[3]

Absorption of infrared energy cutaneously increases and decreases circulation subcutaneously in both the muscle and fat layers. If the energy is absorbed cutaneously over a long enough period of time to raise the temperature of the circulating blood, the hypothalamus will reflexly increase blood flow to the underlying tissue. Likewise, absorption of cold cutaneously can decrease blood flow via a similar mechanism in the area of treatment.

Thus if the primary treatment goal is a tissue temperature increase with a corresponding increase in blood flow to the deeper tissues, a wiser choice is perhaps a modality, such as diathermy or ultrasound, that produces energy that can penetrate the cutaneous tissues and be directly absorbed by the deep tissues.

If the primary treatment goal is to reduce tissue temperature and decrease blood flow to an injured area, the superficial application of ice or cold is the only modality capable of producing such a response.

Perhaps the most effective use of the infrared modalities is for the purpose of **analgesia**, that is, reducing the sensation of pain associated with injury. The infrared modalities stimulate primarily the cutaneous nerve receptors. Through one of the mechanisms of pain modulation, most

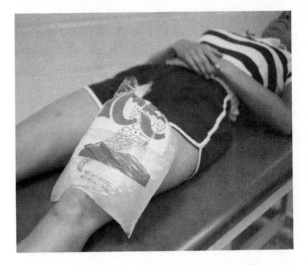

Fig. 7-4. Cryotherapy is an important technique used in the acute phase of injury.

likely the gate control theory, hyperstimulation of these nerve receptors by heating or cooling reduces pain. Within the philosophy of an aggressive program of rehabilitation, as is standard in most sports medicine settings, the reduction of pain as a means of facilitating therapeutic exercise is a common practice. As emphasized earlier, therapeutic modalities are perhaps best used as an adjunct to therapeutic exercise. Certainly, this should be a prime consideration when selecting an infrared modality for use in any treatment program.[3]

Continued investigation and research into the use of heat and cold is warranted to provide useful data for the sports medicine professional. Heat and cold applications, when used properly and efficiently, provide the sports therapist with tools to enhance recovery and provide the athlete with optimal health care management. Thermotherapy and cryotherapy are only two of the tools available to assist in the well-being and reconditioning of the injured athlete.

Cryotherapy

Cryotherapy is the use of cold in the treatment of acute trauma and subacute injury and for the decrease of discomfort following athletic reconditioning and rehabilitation. Tools of cryotherapy include ice packs, cold whirlpool, ice whirlpool, ice massage, commercial chemical cold spray, and contrast baths. Application of cryotherapy produces a three- to four-stage sensation. The first sensation of cold is followed by a stinging, then a burning or aching feeling, and finally numbness. Each stage is related to the nerve endings as they temporarily cease to function as a result of decreased blood flow. The time required for this sequence varies from 5 to 15 minutes. After 12 to 15 minutes, a reflex deep-tissue vasodilation called the **hunting response** is sometimes demonstrable with intense cold (10° C or 50° F).[16] Thus a minimum of 15 minutes is necessary to achieve extreme analgesic effects.

Application of ice is safe, simple, and inexpensive. Cryotherapy is contraindicated in patients with cold allergies (hives, joint pain, nausea), Raynaud's phenomenon (arterial spasm), and some rheumatoid conditions.[12]

Depth of penetration depends on the amount of cold and the length of the treatment time. The body is well equipped to maintain skin and subcutaneous tissue viability through the capillary bed by reflex vasodilation of up to 4 times normal blood flow. The body has the ability to decrease blood flow to the body segment that is supposedly losing too much body heat by shunting the blood flow. Depth of penetration is also related to intensity and duration of cold application and the circulatory response to the body segment exposed. If the person has normal circulatory responses, frostbite should not be a concern. Even so, caution should be exercised when applying intense cold directly to the skin. If deeper penetration is desired, ice therapy is most effective with ice towels, ice packs, ice massage, and ice whirlpools.[17] Patients should be advised of the four stages of cryotherapy and the discomfort they will experience. The sports therapist should explain this sequence and advise the athlete of the expected outcome, which may include a rapid decrease in pain.[3]

Thermotherapy

Heat is still used as a universal treatment for pain and discomfort. Much of the benefit is derived because the treatment simply feels good. In the early stages following injury, however, heat causes increased capillary blood pressure and increased cellular permeability, which results in additional swelling or edema accumulation.[3] No athlete with edema should be treated with any heat modality until the reasons for edema are determined. The best interest of the sports therapist is to use cryotherapy techniques or contrast baths to reduce the edema prior to heat applications. Superficial heat applications seem to feel more comfortable for complaints of the neck, back, low back, and pelvic areas and may be most appropriate for the athlete who exhibits some allergic response to cold applications. However, the tissues in these areas are absolutely no different from those in the extremities. Thus, the same physiological responses to the use of heat or cold are elicited in all areas of the body.

Primary goals of thermotherapy include increased blood flow and increased muscle temperature to stimulate analgesia, increased nutrition to the cellular level, reduction of edema, and removal of metabolites and other products of the inflammatory process.[3]

INTERMITTENT COMPRESSION

Intermittent compression units are used to control or reduce swelling following acute injury or pitting edema, which tends to develop in the injured area several hours after injury.

Intermittent compression makes use of a nylon pneumatic inflatable sleeve applied around the injured extremity (Fig. 7-5). The sleeve can be inflated to a specific pressure that forces excessive fluid accumulated in the interstitial spaces into vascular and lymphatic channels, through which it is removed from the area of injury. Compression facilitates the movement of lymphatic fluid, which helps to eliminate the byproducts of the injury process.[24]

Intermittent compression devices have essentially three parameters that may be adjusted: on-off time, inflation pressures, and treatment time. Recommended treatment protocols have been established through clinical trial and error with little experimental data currently available to support any protocol.[14]

On-off times include 1 minute on and 2 minutes off, 2 minutes on and 1 minute off, and 4 minutes on and 1 minute off. These recommendations are not based on research. Thus, patient comfort should be the primary guide.

Recommended inflation pressures have been

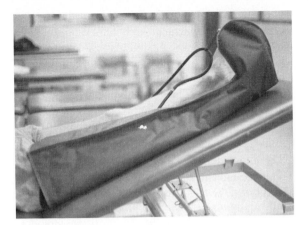

Fig. 7-5. A Jobst full leg sleeve used for facilitating lymphatic flow.

loosely correlated with blood pressures. The Jobst Institute recommends that pressure be set at 30 to 50 mm Hg for the upper extremity and at 30 to 60 mm Hg for the lower extremity. Because arterial capillary pressures are approximately 30 mm Hg, any pressure that exceeds this should encourage the absorption of edema and the flow of lymphatic fluid.[14]

Clinical studies have demonstrated a significant reduction in limb volume after 30 minutes of compression.[14] Thus, a 30-minute treatment time seems to be efficient in reducing edema.

Some intermittent compression units have the capability of combining cold along with compression. Electrical stimulating currents are not uncommonly used to produce muscle pumping and thus facilitating lymphatic flow.

LOW-POWER LASER

Laser is an acronym that stands for light amplification of stimulated emissions of radiation. Lasers are relatively new to the medical community and are certainly the newest of the modalities used by sports therapists.

The principles of physics under which laser energy is produced are complex. Basically, an atom is excited when energy is applied and raises an orbiting electron to a higher orbit. When the electron returns to its original orbit, it releases energy (photons) through a process called **spontaneous emission**. Stimulated emission occurs when the photon is released from an excited atom and it promotes the release of an identical photon to be released from a similarly excited atom. For lasers to operate, a medium of excited atoms must be generated. This is termed **population inversion** and results when an external energy source or pumping device is applied to the medium.[25]

Laser light differs from conventional light in that laser light is monochromic (single color or wavelength), coherent (in phase), and collimated (minimal divergence). Laser can be thermal (hot) or non-thermal (low power, soft, cold). The categories include solid-state (glass or crystal), gas, semiconductor, dye, and chemical lasers.[22]

Helium-neon (HeNe gas) and gallium arsenide (GaAs semiconductor) lasers are two low-power lasers currently being investigated by the FDA for potential application in physical medicine. The HeNe lasers deliver a characteristic red beam with a wavelength of 632.8 nanometers. They are delivered in a continuous wave and have a direct penetration of 2 to 5 mm and an indirect penetration of 10 to 15 mm. The GaAs laser is invisible, with a wavelength of 904 nanometers. It is delivered in a pulse mode at a very low power output. They have a direct penetration of 1 to 2 cm and an indirect penetration of 5 cm.[25]

The proposed therapeutic applications of lasers in physical medicine include acceleration of collagen synthesis, decrease in microorganisms, increase in vascularization, and reduction of pain and inflammation.[5,7]

The technique of laser application is ideally done with light contact to the surface and should be perpendicular to the target surface. Dosage appears to be the critical factor in eliciting a response, but exact dosages have not been determined. Dosage is altered by varying the pulse frequency and the treatment times. The treatment is applied by developing an imaginary grid over the target area. The grid comprises 1-cm squares, and the laser is applied to each square for a predetermined time. Trigger or acupuncture points are also treated for painful conditions.

The FDA considers low-power lasers as low-risk devices. Although no deleterious effects have been reported, certain precautions and contraindications do exist, including lasing over cancerous tissue, directly into the eyes, and during the first trimester of pregnancy. Initial pain increases and episodes of syncope have been reported but do not warrant treatment cessation.

Future research for determining the efficacy and treatment parameters is needed to substantiate the application of low-power laser in a sports medicine setting.

TREATMENT OF ACUTE INJURY

In a sports medicine environment, injuries may be classified as either acute or chronic. Acute injuries result from trauma, and chronic injuries result primarily from overuse. The rehabilitation progression in acute injuries may be loosely classified in four stages: acute, inflammatory, fibroplastic, and maturation. These stages overlap, and the estimated time frames show extreme variability between patients. Table 7-1 summa-

rizes the various modalities that may be used in each of the four stages.

Initial Acute Injury Stage

Modality use in the initial treatment phase should be directed toward limiting the amount of swelling and reducing pain that occurs acutely. The acute phase is marked by swelling, pain when touched, and pain on both active and passive motion. In general, the less initial swelling, the less the time required for rehabilitation. Traditionally, the modality of choice has been and still is **ice**.

Cryotherapy is known to produce vasoconstriction, at least superficially and perhaps indirectly in the deeper tissues, and thus limits the bleeding that always occurs with injury. Ice

TABLE 7-1

Clinical Decision Making on the Use of Various Therapeutic Modalities in Treatment of Acute Injury

Stage	Time Frame	Clinical Picture	Possible Modalities Used	Rationale for Use
Acute	Injury–day 3	Swelling Pain to touch Pain on motion	CRYO ESC IC LPL Rest	↓ Swelling, ↓ pain ↓ Pain ↓ Swelling ↓ Pain
Postacute	Day 2–day 6	Swelling subsides Warm to touch Discoloration Pain to touch Pain on motion	CRYO ESC IC LPL Range of motion	↓ Swelling, ↓ pain ↓ Pain ↓ Swelling ↓ Pain
Regeneration	Day 4–day 10	Pain to touch Pain on motion Swollen	THERMO ESC LPL IC Range of motion Strengthening	Mildly ↑ circulation ↓ Pain—muscle pumping ↓ Pain Facilitate lymphatic flow
Repair	Day 7–recovery	Swollen No more pain to touch Decreasing pain on motion	ULTRA ESC LPL SWD MWD Range of motion Strengthening Functional activities	Deep heating to ↑ circulation ↑ Range of motion, ↑ strength, ↓ pain ↓ Pain Deep heating to ↑ circulation Deep heating to ↑ circulation

CRYO, cryotherapy; ESC, electrical stimulating currents; IC, intermittent compression; LPL, low-power laser; MWD, microwave diathermy; SWD, shortwave diathermy; THERMO, thermotherapy; ULTRA, ultrasound; ↓, decrease; ↑, increase.

bags, cold packs, and ice massage may all be used effectively. Cold baths should be avoided because the foot is placed in the gravity-dependent position. Cold whirlpools also place the foot in the gravity-dependent position and produce a massaging action that is likely to retard clotting. The importance of cryotherapy techniques for reducing acute swelling has probably been exaggerated. Cryotherapy is perhaps best used for producing analgesia, which most likely results from stimulation of sensory cutaneous nerves that, via the gating mechanism, blocks or reduces pain.

Compression is perhaps the most critical element in controlling swelling acutely. An intermittent compression device may be used to provide even pressure around an injured extremity. The pressurized sleeve mechanically reduces the amount of space available for swelling to accumulate. Units that combine both compression and cold are extremely useful in this phase.

Regardless of the specific techniques selected, cold and compression should always be combined with elevation to avoid any additional pooling of blood in the injured area due to the effects of gravity.

Electrical stimulating currents may also be used in the acute phase for pain reduction. Parameters should be adjusted to maximally stimulate sensory cutaneous nerve fibers, again to take advantage of the gate control mechanism of pain modulation. Intensities that produce muscle contractions should be avoided because they may increase clotting time.

The low-power laser has also been demonstrated to be effective in pain modulation through the stimulation of trigger points and may be used acutely.

The injured part should be rested and protected for at least the first 48 to 72 hours to allow the inflammatory phase of the healing process to do what it is supposed to.

Inflammatory Stage

The inflammatory stage begins as early as day 1 and may last as long as day 6 following injury. Clinically, swelling begins to subside and eventually stops altogether. The injured area may feel warm to the touch, and some discoloration is usually apparent. The injury is still painful to the touch, and pain is elicited on movement of the injured part.

As in the acute stage, modalities should be used to control pain and reduce swelling. Cryotherapy should still be used early in the postacute phase. Ice bags, cold packs, or ice massages provide analgesic effects. The use of cold also reduces the likelihood of swelling, which may continue during this stage. Swelling does subside completely by the end of this phase. Once swelling has stopped, the sports therapist may elect to begin contrast baths with a longer cold-to-hot ratio. Many sports therapists elect to stay with cryotherapy for weeks following injury; in fact, some never switch to the superficial heating techniques. This procedure is simply a matter of personal preference that should be dictated by experience.

An intermittent compression device may be used to decrease swelling by facilitating resorption of the by-products of injury by the lymphatic system. Electrical stimulating currents and low-power laser can be used to help reduce pain.

After the acute stage, the athlete should begin to work on active and passive range of motion. Decisions regarding how rapidly to progress exercise should be determined by the response of the injury to that exercise. If exercise produces additional swelling and markedly exacerbates pain, then the level or intensity of the exercise is too great and should be reduced. Sports therapists should be aggressive in their approach to rehabilitation, but the approach will always be limited by the healing process.

Fibroplastic Stage

During the fibroplastic stage, fibroblastic cells are laying down a matrix of collagen fibers and forming scar tissue. This stage may begin as early as 4 days after the injury and may last for a week. At this point, swelling has stopped completely. The injury is still tender to the touch but is not as painful as during the last stage. Pain is also less on active and passive motion.

Treatments may change during this stage from cold to heat, once again using increased swelling as a precautionary indicator. Thermotherapy techniques including hydrocollator packs, paraffin, or eventually warm whirlpool may be safely employed. The purpose of ther-

TABLE 7-2

Clinical Decision Making on the Use of Various Therapeutic Modalities in Treatment of Chronic Injury

Clinical Picture	Possible Modalities	Rationale for Use
Pain on motion	Ultrasound	Deep heating to ↑ circulation
Pain to touch	Shortwave and microwave diathermy	Deep heating to ↑ circulation
Swelling	Cryotherapy	↓ Pain
Warm to touch	Electrical stimulating currents	↓ Pain, ↑ strength, ↑ range of motion
Possible crepitus	Low-power laser	↓ Pain
	Antiinflammatory medication	↓ Pain
	(Range of motion Strengthening)	

↑, increase; ↓, decrease.

motherapy is to increase circulation to the injured area to promote healing. These modalities can also produce some degree of analgesia.

Intermittent compression can once again be used to facilitate removal of injury by-products from the area. Electrical stimulating currents can be used to assist this process by eliciting a muscle contraction and thus inducing a muscle pumping action. This aids in facilitating lymphatic flow. Electrical currents can once again be used for modulation of pain, as can stimulation of trigger points with the low-powered laser.

The sports therapist must continue to stress the importance of range-of-motion and strengthening exercises and progress them appropriately during this phase.

Maturation Stage

The maturation stage is the longest of the four stages and may last for several years, depending on the severity of the injury. The ultimate goal during this phase is return to activity. The injury is no longer painful to the touch, although some progressively decreasing pain may still be felt on motion. The collagen fibers must be realigned according to tensile stresses and strains placed upon them. Virtually all modalities may be safely used during this stage; thus decisions should be based on what seems to work most effectively in a given situation.

At this point some type of heating modality is beneficial to the healing process. The deep-heating modalities, ultrasound, or shortwave and mi-

crowave diathermy should be used to increase circulation to the deeper tissues. Increased blood flow delivers the essential nutrients to the injured area to promote healing, and increased lymphatic flow assists in breakdown and removal of waste products. The superficial heating modalities are certainly less effective at this point.

Electrical stimulating currents can be used for a number of purposes. As before, they may be used in pain modulation. They may also be used to assist in increasing range of motion or muscular strength.

Low-power laser can also assist in modulating pain. If pain is reduced, therapeutic exercises may be progressed more quickly.

Range-of-motion and strengthening exercises can be increased relatively quickly and progress toward a full, pain-free return to levels required for successful participation in sport activities.

Other Considerations in Treating Acute Injury

Generally some type of cold treatment is used following activity. Most often either ice packs or cold whirlpools are recommended. The rationale for use of these cryotherapy tools is to limit swelling in the injured area. Because the primary effects of ice on circulation are superficial, a more effective treatment may rely on compression in the form of either an intermittent compression unit that also uses cold or an elastic wrap along with elevation. Cold whirlpools should be avoided following activity because they place the injured extremity in the gravity-dependent position.

During the rehabilitation period following injury, athletes must alter their training and conditioning habits to allow the injury to heal sufficiently. The sports therapist must not neglect fitness training in designing a rehabilitation program. Consideration must be given to maintaining strength, flexibility, and cardiorespiratory endurance.

TREATMENT OF CHRONIC INJURY

The treatment of chronic injury can be frustrating for the sports therapist. Chronic injuries generally result from overuse of a particular part and tend to persist without intervention into the cause of the injury. Chronic injuries usually involve some degree of inflammation, some swelling, and possible crepitus on motion. They are often warm to the touch, with pain on motion and some tenderness to touch. Modalities should generally be used in chronic injuries to reduce inflammation and pain and thus facilitate return to normal activity levels.

Deep-heating modalities such as ultrasound, shortwave diathermy, and microwave diathermy are most effective in increasing circulation to the deep inflamed tissues. Techniques of thermotherapy and cryotherapy have only superficial effects on circulation; however, they can be useful in producing analgesia. Low-power laser can also be used for the purpose of pain modulation.

Electrical stimulating currents can also be used to reduce pain but may in addition be used to facilitate increases in both strength and range of motion as well.

Modality use should be combined with antiinflammatory medication and exercise to maintain strength, flexibility, and cardiorespiratory endurance.

Table 7-2 summarizes the clinical decision-making process with regard to selection of various modalities during treatment of chronic injury.

INDICATIONS AND CONTRAINDICATIONS

Table 7-3 is a summary list of indications for use, contraindications, and precautions in using the various modalities. This list should aid the sports therapist in making decisions regarding the appropriate use of a therapeutic modality in a given clinical situation.

SUMMARY

1. Modalities are best used by the sports therapist as adjuncts to other forms of therapeutic exercise. Decisions on how a particular modality may best be employed should be based on both theoretical knowledge and practical experience.
2. Electrical stimulating currents may be used for the purpose of stimulating sensory nerves to modulate pain, stimulating motor nerves to elicit a muscle contraction, introducing chemical ions into superficial tissues for medicinal purposes, and creating an electrical field in the tissues to stimulate or alter the healing process.
3. The physiological response of the biological tissues to electrical stimulating currents is to a great extent determined by the treatment parameters of the current selected by the sports therapist.
4. Shortwave and microwave diathermy units utilize extremely high frequency electrical currents to produce a tissue temperature increase in the deeper tissues.
5. Ultrasound is vibrational acoustic energy that causes a tissue temperature increase in addition to other physiological effects that aid healing.
6. Ultrasound has a number of advantages over diathermy including deeper penetration and more portable and less expensive equipment.
7. The effects of thermotherapy and cryotherapy are primarily superficial. These modalities are perhaps most effectively used for the purpose of producing analgesia. They also have an indirect effect on circulation in the deeper tissues.
8. Low-powered lasers are the newest modality used in sports medicine settings, primarily for the purpose of promoting wound healing and also for pain modulation through stimulation of acupuncture and trigger points.
9. Modality use in the initial or acute stages

TABLE 7-3

Indications and Contraindications for Therapeutic Modalities

Therapeutic Modality	Indications for Use	Contraindications and Precautions
Electrical stimulating currents—high voltage	Pain modulation Muscle reeducation Muscle pumping contractions Retard atrophy Muscle strengthening Increase ROM Fracture healing Acute injury	Pacemakers Thrombophlebitis Superficial skin lesions
Electrical stimulating currents—low voltage	Wound healing Fracture healing Iontophoresis	Malignancy Skin hypersensitivities Allergies to certain drugs
Shortwave diathermy and microwave diathermy	Increase deep circulation Increase metabolic activity Reduce muscle guarding/spasm Reduce inflammation Facilitate wound healing Analgesia	Metal implants Pacemakers Malignancy Wet dressings Anesthetized areas Pregnancy Acute injury and inflammation Eyes Areas of reduced blood flow Anesthetized areas
Cryotherapy—cold packs, ice massage	Acute injury Vasoconstriction—decreased blood flow Analgesia Reduce inflammation Reduce muscle guarding/spasm	Allergy to cold Circulatory impairments Wound healing Hypertension
Thermotherapy—hot whirlpool, paraffin, hydrocollator, infrared lamps	Vasodilation—increased blood flow Analgesia Reduce muscle guarding/spasm Reduce inflammation Increase metabolic activity Facilitate tissue healing	Acute and postacute trauma Poor circulation Circulatory impairments Malignancy
Low-power laser	Pain modulation (trigger points) Facilitate wound healing	Pregnancy Eyes
Ultraviolet	Acne Aseptic wounds Folliculitis Pityriasis rosea Tinea Septic wounds Sinusitis Increase calcium metabolism	Psoriasis Eczema Herpes Diabetes Pellagra Lupus erythematosus Hyperthyroidism Renal and hepatic insufficiency Generalized dermatitis Advanced atherosclerosis
Ultrasound	Increase connective tissue extensibility Deep heat Increased circulation Treatment of most soft tissue injuries Reduce inflammation Reduce muscle spasm	Infection Acute and postacute injury Epiphyseal areas Pregnancy Thrombophlebitis Impaired sensation Eyes
Intermittent compression	Decrease acute bleeding Decrease edema	Circulatory impairment

following injury should be directed toward one goal, that being to reduce the amount of swelling that occurs. The less the amount of initial swelling, the less time will be required for rehabilitation.

10. During the inflammatory stage of healing, modalities should be used to reduce pain and limit the amount of swelling. The injured part should be rested to allow the healing process to work.

11. During the fibroplastic stage, thermotherapy may be used to help increase blood flow to the injured area. Also during this time, strengthening and range-of-motion exercises should begin.

12. Maturation is a long-term process during which the athlete returns to activity. Deepheating modalities that increase blood flow and assist in the breakdown and removal of the by-products of the healing process should be used. The quantity and intensity of therapeutic exercise should be progressively increased during this phase of healing.

13. In chronic injuries, modalities should be used along with appropriate antiinflammatory medication for the purpose of reducing or controlling inflammation.

REFERENCES

1 Alon G: High voltage stimulation: a monograph, Chattanooga Corporation, 1984.

2 Barr J: Transcutaneous electrical nerve stimulation characteristics for altering pain perception, Phys Ther 66(10):1037–1048, 1987.

3 Bell G: Infrared modalities. In Prentice W, editor: Therapeutic modalities in sports medicine, St Louis 1990, Times Mirror/Mosby College Publishing.

4 Benton L and others: Functional electrical stimulation: a practical clinical guide, Downet, Calif, 1980, Rancho Los Amigos Hospital.

5 Castel M: A clinical guide to low-power laser therapy, Downsview, Ont, 1985, Physiotechnology, Ltd.

6 Donley P: Shortwave and microwave diathermy. In Prentice W, editor: Therapeutic modalities in sports medicine, St Louis, 1990, Times Mirror/Mosby College Publishing.

7 Enwemeka C: Laser biostimulation of healing wounds: specific effects and mechanisms of action, J Ortho Sports Phys Ther 9:333–338, 1988.

8 Eriksson E and Haggmark T: Comparison of isometric muscle training and electrical stimulation supplement, isometric training in recovery after major knee ligament surgery, Am J Sports Med 7:169–171, 1979.

9 Geick J and others: Therapeutic ultrasound: technology, performance standards, biological effect, and clinical application, HSH Publication, FOA 84-XXXX, August, 1984.

10 Griffin J and Karselis T: The diathermies. In Griffin J and Karselis T, editors: Physical agents for physical therapists, Springfield, Ill, 1982, Charles C Thomas, Publisher.

11 Haar G: Basic physics of therapeutic ultrasound, Physiotherapy 64(4):100–102, 1978.

12 Hocutt J and others: Cryotherapy in ankle sprains, Am J Sports Med 10(5):316–319, 1982.

13 Hooker D: Electrical stimulating currents. In Prentice W, editor: Therapeutic modalities in sports medicine, St Louis, 1990, Times Mirror/Mosby College Publishing.

14 Hooker D: Intermittent compression devices. In Prentice W, editor: Therapeutic modalities in sports medicine, St Louis, 1990, Times Mirror/Mosby College Publishing.

15 Howson D: Peripheral neural excitability, Phys Ther 58:1467–1473, 1978.

16 Knight K and others: A reexamination of Lewis cold induced vasodilation in the finger and ankle, Ath Train 15:248–250, 1980.

17 Knight K and Londeree B: Comparison of blood flow in the ankle of uninjured subjects during therapeutic applications of heat, cold, and exercise, Med Sci Sport Exer 12(1):76–80, 1980.

18 Laughman RK and others: Strength changes in the normal quadriceps femoris muscle as a result of electrical stimulation, Phys Ther 63:494–499, 1983.

19 Lehmann J and Delauter B: Diathermy and superficial heat and cold. In Krusen F, editor: Handbook of physical medicine and rehabilitation, Philadelphia, 1982, WB Saunders Co.

20 Mannheimer J and Lampe G: Clinical transcutaneous electrical nerve stimulation, Philadelphia, 1984, FA Davis Co.

21 Melzack R: Prolonged relief of pain by brief intense transcutaneous electrical stimulation, Pain 1(4):357–373, 1975.

22 Mester E, Mester A and Mester A: Biomedical effects of laser application, Laser Surg Med 5:31–39, 1985.

23 Quillen S: Phonophoresis: a review of the literature and technique, Ath Train 15(2):109–110, 1980.

24 Quillen W and Rouiller L: Initial management of acute ankle sprains with rapid pulsed pneumatic compression and cold, J Ortho Sports Phys Ther 4(1):39–43, 1982.

25 Saliba E: Low-power laser. In Prentice W, editor: Therapeutic modalities in sports medicine, St Louis, 1990, Times Mirror/Mosby College Publishing.

26 Spiker J: Ultrasound. In Prentice W, editor: Therapeutic modalities in sports medicine, St Louis, 1990, Times Mirror/Mosby College Publishing.

Pharmacological Considerations in a Rehabilitation Program

8

William E. Prentice

OBJECTIVES

Following completion of this chapter, the student will be able to:

- Discuss the reasons for use of various analgesics, antiinflammatories, and antipyretics as an adjunct form of treatment in a rehabilitation program.

- Identify the potential side effects and reactions of medications that act on the respiratory tract, medications that affect the gastrointestinal tract, and antibiotics.

- Discuss the importance of record keeping when administering medications in a sports medicine environment.

- Be aware of the legalities of dispensing versus administering medications by sports medicine personnel.

- Discuss the impact of drug testing programs on the use of various medications in a rehabilitation setting.

The use of medications prescribed for various medical conditions by qualified physicians may be of great value to the athlete as it may with any other individual in the population. Under normal circumstances an athlete would be expected to respond to medication just as anyone else would. However, due to the nature of physical activity, the athlete's situation is not normal; with intense physical activity, special consideration should be given to the effects of certain types of medication.

For the sports therapist supervising a program of rehabilitation, some knowledge of the potential effects of certain types of drugs on performance during the rehabilitation program is essential.

The sports therapist working under the direction of a team physician is responsible for keeping the athlete healthy and ready to train and compete under physically, mentally, and emotionally demanding circumstances. The sports therapist should be concerned not only with rehabilitation but also with prevention, acute management, and evaluation of sports-related injuries. On occasion, the sports therapist must make decisions regarding the appropriate use of medications based on knowledge of the indications for use and the possible side effects in athletes who are involved in programs of rehabilitation.

The sports therapist must be cognizant of the potential effects and side effects of both over-the-counter and prescription medications on the athlete during rehabilitation as well as during competition.

This chapter concentrates on the special considerations that must be given regarding those medications most commonly used in a sports medicine environment.

COMMON MEDICATIONS

This section provides the sports therapist with some special considerations regarding those medications most commonly prescribed for and used by individuals involved in some sports-related activity. The classifications of medication discussed include (1) analgesics, antipyretics, and antiinflammatories; (2) drugs that affect the respiratory tract; (3) drugs that affect the gastrointestinal tract; and (4) use of antibiotic medications. (See also Table 8-1.)

Analgesics, Antipyretics, and Antiinflammatories

Perhaps medications are most commonly used in a sports medicine environment for pain relief. The athlete is continuously in situations where injuries are very likely. Fortunately, most of the injuries that occur are not serious and lend themselves to rapid rehabilitation. However, pain is associated with even minor injury.

The three nonnarcotic analgesics most often used are aspirin (salicylate), acetaminophen, and ibuprofen. Aspirin is the most commonly used drug in the world.[25] Because of its easy availability, it is also likely the most misused drug as well. Aspirin is a derivative of salicylic acid and is used for its analgesic, antiinflammatory, and antipyretic capabilities.

Analgesia may result from several mechanisms; aspirin may interfere with the transmission of painful impulses in the thalamus; sensitivity of pain receptors may increase due to interference with synthesis of prostaglandins that cause redness, swelling, and pain; and it may facilitate fluid resorption from injured tissues by blocking the release of lysosomal enzymes, thus reducing capillary permeability and the fluid loss that produces swelling.[19] Aspirin also is capable of reducing fever by altering sympathetic outflow from the hypothalamus, which produces increased vasodilation and heat loss through sweating.[19] Among the side effects of aspirin usage are gastric distress, heartburn, some nausea, tinnitus, headache, and diarrhea. More serious consequences can develop with prolonged use or high dosages.[1]

An athlete should be very cautious about selecting aspirin as a pain reliever for a number of reasons. Most important is the fact that aspirin decreases aggregation of platelets and thus impairs the clotting mechanism, should injury occur.[21] Prolonged bleeding at an injured site will increase the amount of swelling, which has a direct effect on the time required for rehabilitation.

Use of aspirin as an antiinflammatory should be recommended with caution. Other prescription antiinflammatory medications do not produce many of the undesirable side effects of aspirin. Generally, prescription antiinflammatories are considered to be more effective.

Aspirin sometimes produces gastric discomfort. In the case of an athlete, intense physical activity may exacerbate this side effect. Buffered aspirin is no less irritating to the stomach than is regular aspirin, but enteric-coated tablets do resist aspirin breakdown in the stomach and may minimize gastric discomfort. Regardless of the form of aspirin ingested, it should be taken with meals and/or with large quantities of water (8 to 10 oz/tablet) to reduce the likelihood of gastric irritation.

Ibuprofen is classified as a non-steroidal antiinflammatory drug (NSAID); however, it also has both analgesic and antipyretic effects. Ibuprofen, like aspirin, has a number of side effects, including the potential for gastric irritation. It is not as likely to affect platelet aggregation as is aspirin. Ibuprofen administered at a dose of 200 mg does not require a prescription and at that dosage may be used for analgesia. At a dose of 400 mg, the effects are both analgesic and antiinflammatory. At this dosage, a prescription is required for administration.

Acetaminophen, like aspirin, has both analgesic and antipyretic effects, but it does not have significant antiinflammatory capabilities. Acetaminophen is indicated for relief of mild somatic pain and fever reduction through mechanisms similar to those of aspirin.[14]

The primary advantage of acetaminophen for the athlete is that it does not produce gastritis, irritation, or gastrointestinal bleeding. Likewise, it does not affect platelet aggregation and thus does not increase clotting time following an injury.

For the athlete who is not in need of some antiinflammatory medication but who requires some pain-relieving medication, acetaminophen

TABLE 8-1

Sports Therapists' Guide to Commonly Used Medications

Generic Name	Trade Name	Primary Use of Drug	Sport Medicine Consideration
ANALGESICS, ANTIPYRETICS, AND ANTIINFLAMMATORIES			
Aspirin	Many trade names	Analgesic, antipyretic, antiinflammatory	Gastric irritation, nausea, tinnitus
Acetaminophen	Tylenol, Datril, others	Analgesia, antipyretic	None
Nonsteroidal antiinflammatories		All are analgesic, antipyretic, antiinflammatory	Gastric irritation less common than with aspirin except for indomethacin These should be used on a long-term basis for reducing inflammation; should not be substituted for aspirin or acetaminophen in cases of mild headache or low fever
Indomethacin	Indocin		
Ibuprofen	Advil, Motrin, Nuprin		
Naproxen	Naprosyn, Anaprox		
Piroxicam	Feldene		
Zomepirac	Zomax		
Tolmetin	Tolectin		
Fenoprofen	Nalfon		
Meclofenamate	Meclomen		
DRUGS THAT AFFECT THE RESPIRATORY TRACT			
Chlorpheniramine	Chlor-Trimeton	Antihistamine for allergies	Used primarily for treatment of allergic reaction Causes drowsiness, decreased coordination
Dimenhydrinite	Dramamine	Antihistamine used for treatment of motion sickness, nausea, vomiting	Should be administered before travel begins, produces drowsiness
Oxymetazoline	Afrin, Dristan Long Lasting, Neo-synephrine 12 Hour, Nostrilla, Sinex Long Lasting	Adrenergic decongestant applied topically as spray	Do not exceed recommended dosage because of rebound congestion; may cause sneezing, dryness of nasal mucosa, and headache
Pseudo-ephedrine	Sudafed, Sudrin, Afrinol, Cenafed, Neofed, others	Adrenergic decongestant used orally	Produces stimulation of the central nervous system; topically applied decongestants work faster but oral decongestants are preferred in long-term use
Diphenhydramine	Benylin cough syrup, Benydryl	Antihistamine used primarily for its drying effect in reducing coughing; also used for motion sickness and preventing nausea and vomiting	Produces drowsiness and dry mouth found in over-the-counter sleeping medication
Dextromethorphan	Benylin DM, Romilar CF, Coughettes, Sucrets Lozenge	Nonnarcotic antitussive used for suppression of cough	Very effective in case of unproductive cough; doesn't produce drowsiness and other side effects as commonly

TABLE 8-1
Sports Therapists' Guide to Commonly Used Medications

Generic Name	Trade Name	Primary Use of Drug	Sport Medicine Consideration
Benzonatate	Tessalon	Peripherally acting anti-tussive that acts as an anesthetic	May produce drowsiness and a chilled sensation
Codeine or hydrocodone		Narcotic antitussive that depresses the central cough mechanism	Used in combination with decongestant, an antihista-mine, or expectorant, can produce sedation, dizzi-ness, constipation, nausea
Guaifenesin	Robitussin, Glycotus, Anti-tuss	Expectorant used for symptomatic relief of un-productive cough	Used for treating a dry or sore throat; may cause drowsiness and nausea

DRUGS THAT AFFECT THE GASTROINTESTINAL TRACT

Generic Name	Trade Name	Primary Use of Drug	Sport Medicine Consideration
Sodium bicarbonate	Soda Mint, Bell/ans	Antacid used for quick relief of upset stomach	Produces gas belching and tension; may cause sys-temic alkalinity
Aluminum hydroxide	Amphagel, Dialume, Alterrabel	Antacid used for upset stomach	May produce constipation; moderate acid neutralizer
Calcium carbonate	Mallamint, Alka-2, Amitone, Chooz, Ti-tralac	Antiacid used for stom-ach upset	May produce constipation and acid rebound; high acid-neutralizing capability
Dihydroxyaluminum sodium carbonate	Rolaids	Antacid used for upset stomach	May cause constipation; rapid neutralizing capabili-ties, but transient
Magnesium hydroxide, car-bonate oxide, or phosphate	Milk of Magnesia	Antacid used for upset stomach	May cause diarrhea and lasting neutralization of acid without rebound
Cimetidine	Tagamet	Antihistamine used for relief of upset stomach	May produce drowsiness and either constipation or diarrhea
Common combination antacids and antiemetics	Alka-Seltzer, Di-Gel, Gaviscon, Gelusil, Maalox, Mylanta, Tempo, Titralac, Wingel, others	Over-the-counter combi-nation drugs used for controlling nausea and vomiting	May produce either diar-rhea or constipation
Promethazine hydrochloride	Phenergan	Antiemetic used for pre-venting motion sickness, nausea, and vomiting	Causes sedation and drowsiness
Diphenoxylate HCl	Lomotil, Enoxa, Co-lonil	Narcotic antidiarrheal	Causes dry mouth, nausea, drowsiness
Loperamide	Imodium	Systemic antidiarrheal	Abdominal discomfort and drowsiness
Common over-the-counter an-tidiarrheals	Donnagel, Kaopec-tate, Pepto-Bismol, Amogel, Devrom	Relief of diarrhea	All are relatively safe with few side effects, although their effectiveness is ques-tionable

should be the drug of choice. If inflammation is a consideration, the team physician may elect to use either aspirin or a type of NSAID. These NSAIDs are prescription medications that, like aspirin, have not only antiinflammatory but also analgesic and antipyretic effects. They are effective for patients who cannot tolerate aspirin and who tend to experience GI distress associated with aspirin use. Their antiinflammatory capabilities are thought to be equal to those of aspirin, their advantages being that NSAIDs have fewer side effects and relatively longer duration of action. Perhaps the biggest disadvantage of the NSAIDs is that they tend to be expensive.[17] Even though NSAIDs have analgesic and antipyretic capabilities, they should not be used in cases of mild headache or increased body temperature in place of aspirin or acetaminophen. However, they can be used to relieve many other mild to moderately painful somatic conditions like menstrual cramps and soft tissue injury.[17]

The NSAIDs are used primarily for reducing the pain, stiffness, swelling, redness, and fever associated with localized inflammation, most likely by inhibiting the synthesis of prostaglandins. The sports therapist must be aware that inflammation is simply a response to some underlying trauma or condition and that the source of irritation must be corrected and/or eliminated for these antiinflammatory medications to be effective.

Muscle spasm and guarding accompanies many musculoskeletal injuries. Elimination of this spasm and guarding should facilitate programs of rehabilitation. In many situations, centrally acting oral muscle relaxants are used to reduce spasm and guarding. However, to date the efficacy of using muscle relaxants has not been substantiated, and they do not appear to be superior to analgesics or sedatives in either acute or chronic conditions.[12]

Drugs that Affect the Respiratory Tract

ANTIHISTAMINES. Antihistamines reduce the effects of the chemical histamine on various tissues by selectively blocking receptor sites to which histamines attach. Histamine is abundant in the mast cells of the skin and lungs and in the basophils of blood. It is also found in the gastro-

intestinal tract and in the brain, where it acts as a neurotransmitter.[6] Histamine is released in response to some toxin, physical or chemical agent, drug, or antigen that has been introduced into the system. Thus it has a major function in many allergic or hypersensitivity reactions.[20]

Antihistamines are most typically used in the treatment of allergic reactions but may also be used as an antiemetic in the prevention of nausea and vomiting.[15] Histamine produces a number of systemic responses: (1) swelling and inflammation in the skin or mucous membranes (angioedema), (2) spasm of smooth bronchial muscle (asthma), (3) inflammation of nasal membranes (rhinitis), and (4) the possibility of anaphylaxis. These responses in varying degrees are typical of allergic reactions to insect stings, food reactions, drug hypersensitivities, and anything else that may facilitate the release of histamine.

Histamine produces these reactions by binding with the cells that compose the various tissues at specific receptor sites. An antihistamine medication has the capability of competitively blocking these receptor sites and thus preventing the typical histamine response. Antihistamines are classified as either H1 or H2 receptor blockers. The so-called true antihistamines affect the H1 receptors only; H2 blockers affect cells in the stomach that secrete hydrochloric acid. Antihistamines do not reverse the effects of histamine; they simply block the receptor sites. An athlete would benefit from different types of antihistamine medications for (1) relief from various types of allergic reactions, (2) prevention of motion sickness, or (3) relief of coughing due to colds or throat irritations.

Athletes, particularly those involved with fall and spring sports, practice outdoors where they are exposed to a number of allergens (e.g., pollen, insects) that potentially can produce a histamine response. Most cases are mild allergic reactions that may be treated by the sports therapist with an over-the-counter antihistamine. These medications are most effective in reducing the effects of histamine on the vascular system, which symptomatically include urticaria, rhinitis, and angioedema. These medications are effective in approximately 70% of the patients treated.[6] Chlorpheniramine is the antihistamine most commonly used for the treatment of these mild allergic reactions.

A competitive schedule may require the athlete to do a great deal of traveling. People riding in a bus, car, or airplane often develop nausea and discomfort in response to motion. This motion sickness may be treated with a number of antihistamine medications. Dimenhydrinate and meclizine are the most commonly used drugs for the prevention of motion sickness. They are best used prophylactically before motion sickness occurs. Like other antihistamines, the major side effect is drowsiness and sedation.[4]

In the case of the athlete, antihistamines should be used with caution. The most common side effects of antihistamines are drowsiness and in some cases decreased coordination. Both of these side effects may adversely affect athletic performance and potentially predispose the athlete to unnecessary injury. Thus, use of antihistamine medication immediately prior to athletic competition is not recommended. The athlete should also be reminded that use of any antihistamine along with consumption of alcohol will markedly increase drowsiness.

DECONGESTANTS. Nasal congestion may be associated with a number of causes including pollinosis or hay fever; perennial rhinitis, a chronic inflammatory condition that occurs with constant exposure to an allergen; and infectious rhinitis, which is symptomatic of the common cold.[25] Antihistamines also have anticholinergic effects and can often help to dry up a runny nose. In addition, nasal congestion may be treated with sympathomimetic or decongestant medications that may be used topically or orally. Oxymetazoline is an adrenergic topical nasal decongestant that, when sprayed on the nasal mucosa, produces prolonged vasoconstriction and reduces edema and fluid exudation. Pseudoephedrine is also an adrenergic decongestant taken orally. Nose drops act more rapidly than do the oral decongestants, and oral medications cause more side effects such as stimulation of the CNS. However, oral medications are preferred in long-term use.[17]

Some medications combine both antihistamines and nasal decongestants into a single tablet taken orally, which produces relatively lower degrees of drowsiness and other side effects.

ANTITUSSIVES AND EXPECTORANTS. Drugs that suppress coughing are called **antitussives.** Coughing is a reflex response to some irritation of the throat or airway. A cough is productive if some material is brought up. This type of cough is beneficial in clearing excessive mucus or sputum. An unproductive cough may be caused by post-nasal drip, dry air, a sore throat, or anything else that may irritate the throat. An unproductive cough is of no benefit and should be treated with medication. If the cause of the cough is a dry throat or a sore throat, an expectorant medication may be used to increase production of fluid in the respiratory system to coat the dry and irritated mucosal linings.[17]

Antitussive drugs are divided into those that depress the central cough center in the medulla and may be either narcotic or nonnarcotic drugs, and those that act peripherally to reduce irritation in the throat or trachea. Codeine and hydrocodone are two of the more common narcotic antitussives that also have analgesic effects. They are relatively weak narcotics that are considered safe. Codeine is found primarily in liquid form and is often combined with a decongestant, an analgesic, an expectorant, and/or an antihistamine. Any liquid preparation that contains codeine is a prescription medication. The side effects of codeine include sedation, dizziness, constipation, and nausea.[6]

The most common nonnarcotic antitussives are diphenhydramine, dextromethorphan, and benzonatate. Perhaps their biggest advantage is that they have no analgesic effects and do not produce dependence. Diphenhydramine is an antihistamine-antitussive that produces both drowsiness and a drying effect. Dextromethorphan is the most widely used antitussive. It has been shown to be as effective as codeine in medicating an unproductive cough but does not cause side effects as severe as those of codeine. Benzonatate causes a local anesthetic action on the stretch receptors in the throat and thus dampens the cough reflex. Its side effects include drowsiness and a chilled sensation.[6]

The peripherally acting antitussives are primarily expectorants. Although expectorants are thought to increase production of fluid in the throat, little experimental evidence suggests that the use of an expectorant is any more effective than drinking water or sucking a piece of hard candy. In many cases an expectorant is combined with some other medication such as an antihistamine or a decongestant.[5]

The athlete who is in need of antitussive or expectorant medication may benefit greatly from it. Physical activity tends to exacerbate the problem of a dry sore throat that may be responsible for an unproductive cough. The biggest consideration for the sports therapist would be the effects of other medications (e.g., antihistamines or decongestants) that may also be contained in these fluids or lozenges. The drowsiness, gastric irritability, and lack of coordination that may occur will detract from athletic performance.

DRUGS FOR ASTHMA. Asthma, also known as exercise-induced bronchial obstruction, is one of the more common respiratory diseases. The problem may result from a number of respiratory stressors but is always characterized by spasm of smooth muscle, inflammation of mucous linings, and edema, each of which leads to shortness of breath. The medications used for the treatment of asthma are classified as sympathomimetic drugs administered most often as aerosols. Sympathomimetics are bronchodilators that generally reverse the symptoms. Perhaps the greatest side effect of the sympathomimetics is that they may cause some problems in hot environments.

Drugs That Affect the Gastrointestinal Tract

The gastrointestinal tract is subject to numerous disturbances and disorders that are probably among the most common human ailments. The ailments include indigestion, nausea, diarrhea, and constipation problems that virtually everyone has experienced at one time or another. Because of factors such as the stress associated with competition, inconsistent travel schedules, eating patterns on road trips, and even motion sickness during travel, the athlete is even more likely to experience gastric upset.

ANTACIDS. The primary function of an antacid is to neutralize acidity in the upper GI by raising the pH, inhibiting the activity of the digestive enzyme pepsin, and thus reducing its action on the gastric mucosal nerve endings. Antacids are effective not only for relief of acid indigestion and heart burn but also in the treatment of peptic ulcer. Antacids available in the market possess a wide range of acid-neutralizing capabilities and side effects. The sports therapist has to be aware of these side effects when selecting a specific antacid preparation.

One of the most commonly used antacid preparations is sodium bicarbonate or baking soda, which quickly neutralizes hydrochloric acid and yields carbon dioxide gas and water. Sodium bicarbonate is rapidly absorbed by the blood to produce systemic alkalinity. Belching is usually associated with sodium bicarbonate ingestion, and ingestion of excess sodium bicarbonate often produces a rebound effect in which gastric acid secretion increases in response to an alkaline environment.[18]

Other antacids include alkaline salts, which again neutralize hyperacidity but are not easily absorbed in the blood. They also produce disturbances in the lower GI. Many of these nonsystemic antacids slow absorption of other medications from the GI tract. Ingestion of antacids containing magnesium tends to have a laxative effect; those containing aluminum and/or calcium seem to cause constipation. Consequently, many antacid liquids or tablets are combinations of magnesium and either aluminum or calcium hydroxides.[6] If use of a specific antacid produces diarrhea, for example, it may be replaced by another antacid that is higher in aluminum or calcium content to counteract the effects of the magnesium. Conversely, an antacid high in magnesium content may reduce constipation. Simethicone is a silicone added to many of these preparations to reduce gas trapped in the upper GI through its antifoaming action.[25]

Sodium bicarbonate is best used on a short-term basis for rapid relief of heartburn or acid indigestion because of the subsequent rebound effect, but the hydroxide salt preparations may be used on a long-term basis.

Selection of specific antacids should be based on consideration of their potential side effects, such as tendency to produce diarrhea or constipation, and on how well the patient tolerates their use in terms of taste, side effects, and finally cost.[17]

Calcium supplementation for the purpose of increasing calcium uptake by bone and hence increasing bone density as a means of reducing the incidence of fractures is being recommended by some sports medicine specialists. Caution should be exercised in ingesting large amounts of calcium carbonate from antacids because of the potential constipation that may accompany prolonged use.

Another medication used for relief of gastric

discomfort is an antihistamine that is an H2 receptor blocker. Cimetidine inhibits the action of histamine on cells in the stomach that secrete hydrochloric acid and is most typically used to treat ulcers. However, its use in the treatment of indigestion is thought to be no more effective than other antacid preparations.[23]

ANTIEMETICS. This group of drugs is used to treat the nausea and vomiting that may result from a variety of causes. Vomiting serves as a means of eliminating irritants from the stomach before they can be absorbed. Most of the time, however, purging the stomach is not necessary, and vomiting serves only to make the athlete uncomfortable. Frequently, nausea may be treated by giving the individual carbonated soda, tea, or ice to suck. If nausea and vomiting persists, some medication may be beneficial.

Antiemetics are classified as acting either locally or centrally. The locally acting drugs such as most over-the-counter medications (e.g., Pepto-Bismol, Alka-Seltzer) are topical anesthetics that reportedly affect the mucosal lining of the stomach. However, the effects of soothing an upset stomach may be more of a placebo effect.[25] The centrally acting drugs affect the chemoreceptor trigger zone in the medulla by making it less sensitive to irritating nerve impulses from the inner ear or stomach.

A variety of prescription antiemetics can be used for controlling nausea and vomiting, including phenothiazines, antihistamines, anticholinergic drugs for preventing motion sickness, and sedative drugs. The primary side effect of these medications is again extreme drowsiness.

The sports therapist should deal with nausea and vomiting first by using fluids, which have a calming effect on the stomach, followed by the administration of one of the locally acting medications. If vomiting persists, the athlete will become drowsy and thus may be unable to perform at competitive levels, and dehydration and the problems that accompany it are important considerations for an athlete who has been nauseated and vomiting. Antiemetics may also potentiate central nervous system depressants.

ANTIDIARRHEALS. Diarrhea may result from many causes, but it is generally considered to be a symptom rather than a disease. It can occur as a result of emotional stress, allergies to food or drugs, or many different types of intestinal problems. Diarrhea may be acute or chronic. Acute

diarrhea, the most common, comes on suddenly and may be accompanied by nausea, vomiting, chills, and intense abdominal pain. It typically runs its course very rapidly, and symptoms subside once the irritating agent is removed from the system. Chronic diarrhea, which may last for weeks, may result from more serious disease states.

The athlete suffering from acute diarrhea may be totally incapacitated in terms of athletical performance. The major problem of diarrhea is potential dehydration. An athlete, particularly when exercising in a hot environment, depends on body fluids to maintain normal temperature. An individual who becomes dehydrated has difficulty with regulation of temperature and may experience some heat-related problem. The sports therapist's primary concern should be replacing lost body fluids and electrolytes. Medication may be used on a short-term basis for relief of the symptoms, but identifying and treating the cause of the problem are important as well.

Medications used for control of diarrhea are either locally acting or systemic. The locally acting medications most typically contain kaolin, which absorbs other chemicals, and pectin, which sooths irritated bowel. Some contain substances that add bulk to the stool. The effectiveness of locally acting medications is questionable, but they are considered safe and inexpensive.[9]

The systemic agents, which are generally antiperistaltic or antispasmodic medications, are considered to be much more effective in relieving symptoms of diarrhea, but most are prescription drugs. The systemic medications are either opiate derivatives or anticholinergic agents, both of which reduce peristalsis. Common side effects of the systemic antidiarrheals include drowsiness, nausea, dry mouth, and constipation. Long-term use of the opiate drugs may lead to dependence.[3]

If the cause of diarrhea is a noninvasive bacteria, a physician may choose to administer multispectrum antibiotics along with an antiperistaltic agent.

CATHARTICS. Laxatives may be used to empty the GI tract and eliminate constipation. In most cases, constipation may be relieved by proper diet, sufficient fluid intake, and exercise.[17] A cathartic medication is generally not necessary.

An athlete who complains of constipation should first be advised to consume those foods and juices that cause bulk in the feces and stimulate gastrointestinal peristalsis such as bran cereals, fresh fruits, coffee, and chocolate. Increased fluid intake also facilitates peristalsis in the bowel.

Generally speaking, athletes seem to suffer less from constipation than from diarrhea. This tendency may be attributed as much to activity levels as to any other single factor.

If a laxative medication is necessary, the bulk-forming laxatives are among the safest but should be utilized only for short periods, and dietary modifications should also be encouraged.

Antibiotic Medications

Many of the medications discussed have been over-the-counter medications that may be selected and administered by the sports therapist following strict guidelines and protocols for administration established by the team physician. In the case of infectious diseases, the team physician must be directly involved in the selection of specific antimicrobial agents. The sports therapist is often the individual who first recognizes an athlete's signs of developing infection, such as fever, redness, swelling, tenderness, purulent drainage, and swollen lymph nodes. The sports therapist should have the responsibility of referring the athlete with a suspected infection to the physician for a total assessment, including physical examination and laboratory tests. The team physician will then prescribe for the athlete an appropriate antibiotic medication that is selectively capable of destroying the invading microorganism without affecting the patient.[24] The sports therapist may be asked to provide adjunctive therapy such as applying hot compresses or soaks in antiseptic solutions in open infections.

In the case of an athlete who is using an antibiotic medication, the sports therapist's role should be to monitor the patient for signs and symptoms of allergic response or drug-induced toxicity. Many individuals exhibit hypersensitivity reactions to antimicrobial agents. Perhaps the most common reaction occurs with the use of penicillin. Antibiotics are also capable of damaging the tissues they contact. They may damage the mucosa of the stomach and cause diarrhea, nausea, and vomiting. They can also affect kidney function and may interfere with nervous system function. Should these reactions occur, the athlete should be sent back to the physician, who may elect to change to another type of antibiotic medication.[31]

An athlete who has an infection, be it localized or systemic, that requires use of an antibiotic will usually be advised not to train or compete until the infection is under control. The sports therapist should be certain that the athlete adheres to this recommendation both to benefit the infected athlete and to limit the possibility of the infection spreading or being transmitted to other athletes.

ADMINISTERING VERSUS DISPENSING OF MEDICATION

The methods by which drugs may be administered and dispensed vary according to individual state laws. Sports medicine settings are subject to those laws. Administration of a drug is giving the athlete a single dose of a particular medication. Dispensing of medication is giving the athlete a drug in a quantity greater than would be used in a single dose. In most cases, the team physician is the individual ultimately responsible for prescribing medications. These prescription medications are then dispensed by either the physician, a pharmacist, or a nurse. The sports therapist may not dispense medication. However, in most states they may legally administer a single dose of a nonprescription medication. The sports therapist typically does not possess the background or the experience to make decisions about the appropriate use of medication and should be subject to strict protocols if and when administering medication.

On occasion over-the-counter medications are placed on a countertop in the sports medicine clinic for use as the athlete sees fit. Although this method of administering medication saves time for the clinician, this somewhat indiscriminate use of even the over-the-counter drugs by an athlete should be discouraged. The sports therapist who is administering over-the-counter medication of any variety should be knowledgeable about the possible effects of various drugs during exercise. Likewise, sports therapists should be subject to strict protocols established by the team physician for administering medication. Failure to follow these guidelines or protocols may make the sports therapist legally liable should something happen to the athlete that can be attributed to use or misuse of a particular drug.

Record Keeping

Those involved in any health care profession are acutely aware of the necessity of maintaining complete up-to-date medical records. Again the sports medicine setting is no exception. If medications are administered by a sports therapist, maintaining accurate records of the types of medications administered is just as important as recording progress notes, treatments given, and rehabilitation plans. The sports therapist may be dealing with a number of different patients simultaneously while trying to get a team ready for practice or competition. At times things become hectic, and stopping to record each time a medication is administered is difficult. Nevertheless, the sports therapist should include the following information on a type of medication administration log: (1) name of the athlete, (2) complaint and/or symptoms, (3) type of medication given, (4) quantity of medication given, and (5) time of administration.

DRUG TESTING

Perhaps no other topic related to pharmacology has received more attention from the media during recent years than the use and abuse of drugs by athletes. Much has been written and discussed regarding the use of performance-enhancing drugs among Olympic athletes, the widespread use of "street drugs" by professional athletes, and the use of pain-relieving drugs by athletes at all levels.[7,11]

Although much of the information being disseminated to the public by the media may be based on hearsay and innuendo, the use and abuse of many different types of drugs can have a profound impact on athletic performance.

To say many experts in the field of sports medicine regard drug abuse among athletes with growing concern is a gross understatement. Drug testing of athletes at all levels for the pur-

pose of identifying individuals who may have some problems with drug abuse is becoming commonplace. Both the NCAA and the International Olympic Committee have established lists of substances that are banned from use by athletes. The lists include performance-enhancing drugs and "street" or "recreational" drugs, as well as many over-the-counter and prescription drugs. The legality and ethics of testing only those individuals involved with sports are still open to debate. The pattern of drug usage among athletes may simply reflect that of our society in general.

The sports therapist who is working with an athlete who may be tested for drugs at the NCAA level or with world-class or Olympic athletes should be very familiar with the list of banned drugs. Having an athlete disqualified because of the indiscriminate use of some over-the-counter drug during a rehabilitation program would be most unfortunate.

SUMMARY

1. An athlete who requires an analgesic for the purpose of pain relief should be given acetaminophen because aspirin may produce gastric upset and slow clotting time.
2. For treating inflammation, NSAIDs are recommended because they do not produce many of the side effects associated with aspirin use.
3. Antihistamines are used primarily in the treatment of allergic reactions and may produce drowsiness and sedation.
4. Decongestants are used to reduce nasal congestion and may be used orally or topically.
5. Antitussives and expectorants are used to suppress coughing and keep the throat moist. They generally produce drowsiness, gastric irritability, and some lack of coordination.
6. Antacids neutralize acidity in the upper GI tract and may produce diarrhea or constipation.
7. Antiemetics are used to treat nausea and vomiting and should be used with large quantities of fluid to prevent dehydration.
8. Antidiarrheals act to reduce peristaltic action in the lower GI tract and may produce

drowsiness, nausea, dry mouth, and constipation.

9. Cathartics are used to empty the GI tract and reduce constipation.

10. Antibiotics are used to treat various infections and may produce hypersensitivity reactions in the athlete. Generally an athlete who is using an antibiotic should avoid training and competition until the infection subsides.

11. The use of medication in a sports medicine setting should be subject to strict preestablished guidelines and protocols and monitored closely by the sports therapist supervising a rehabilitation program.

12. The sports therapist should maintain a log that documents all medications being administered during a rehabilitation program.

13. The sports therapist must be aware of medications commonly used in treatment of various disorders that may be detected in a drug test as banned substances.

REFERENCES

1 Beaver W, Kantor T, and Levy G: On guard for aspirin's harmful side effects, Patient Care 13:48, 1975.
2 Beaver WT: Aspirin and acetaminophen as constituents of analgesic combinations, Arch Intern Med 141:293–300, 1981.
3 Bertholf C: Protocol, acute diarrhea, Nurse Pract 3:8, 1980.
4 Black F, Correia M, and Stucker F: Easing proneness to motion sickness, Patient Care 14(6):114, 1980.
5 Boyd E: A review of expectorants and inhalents, Int J Clin Pharmacol Ther Toxicol 3:55, 1970.
6 Clark J, Queener S, and Karb V: Pharmacology basis of nursing practice, St Louis, 1982, The CV Mosby Co.
7 Clarke KS: Sports medicine and drug control programs of the US Olympic Committee, J Allergy Clin Immunol 73:740–744, 1984.
8 Clyman B: Role of the non-steroidal anti-inflammatory drugs in sports medicine, Sports Med 3:212–246, 1986.
9 Dahr G and Soergel K: Principles of diarrhea therapy, Am

Fam Phy 19(1):165, 1979.
10 Dretchen K, Hollander D, and Kirsner J: Roundup on antiacids and anticholinergics, Patient Care 9(6):94, 1975.
11 Drugs in the Olympics, Med Lett Drugs Ther 26:66, 1984.
12 Elenbaas JK: Centrally acting skeletal muscle relaxants, Am J Hosp Pharm 37:1313–1323, 1980.
13 Hill J and others: The athletic polydrug abuse phenomenon, Am J Sports Med 11:269–271, 1983.
14 Koch-Weser J: Acetaminophen, N Eng J Med 255:1297, 1976.
15 Krausen A: Antihistamines guidelines and implications, Ann Otol Rhinol Laryngol 85:686, 1979.
16 Levy G: Comparative pharmacokinetics of aspirin and acetaminophen, Arch Intern Med 141:279–281, 1981.
17 Malseed R: Pharmacology: Drug therapy and nursing considerations, Philadelphia, 1985, JB Lippincott Co.
18 Mehlisch DR: Review of the comparative analgesic efficacy of salicylates, acetaminophen and pyrazolones, Am J Med 75(A):47–52, 1983.
19 Moncada S and Vane J: Mode of action of aspirin-like drugs, Adv Int Med 24:1, 1979.
20 Pearlman D: Antihistamines: pharmacology and clinical use, Drugs 12:258, 1976.
21 Quick A: Salicylates and bleeding: the aspirin tolerance test, Am J Med Sci 252:265–269, 1966.
22 Reynolds RC, Floetz P, and Thielke TS: Comparative analysis of drug distribution costs for controlled versus noncontrolled oral analgesics, Am J Hosp Pharm 41:1558–1563, 1984.
23 Rodman M: A fresh look at OTC drug interactions: antiacid preparations, RN 46:84, 1981.
24 Rodman M: Antiinfectives you administer: choosing the right drug for every job, RN 40:73, 1977.
25 Rodman M and Smith D: Clinical pharmacology in nursing, Philadelphia, 1984, JB Lippincott Co.
26 Settipane GA: Adverse reactions to aspirin and related drugs, Arch Intern Med 141:328–332, 1981.
27 Strauss R: Sports medicine, Philadelphia, 1984, WB Saunders Co.
28 Szczeklik A: Antipyretic analgesics and the allergic patient, Am J Med 75(A):82–84, 1983.
29 Texter E, Smart D, and Butler R: Antiacids, Am Fam Phy 11(4):111, 1975.
30 Vane J: Inhibition of prostaglandin synthesis as a mechanism of action for aspirin like drugs, Nature (New Biol) 231:232–235, 1971.
31 Weinstein L: Some principles of antibiotic therapy, Ration Drug Ther 11(3):1, 1977.

Rehabilitation of Low Back Injuries

9

Donald A. Chu

OBJECTIVES

Following completion of this chapter, the student will be able to:

- Discuss the importance of the evaluation process in establishing a treatment program for injury to the low back.

- Describe the evaluation sequence used in identifying causes of low back pain.

- Discuss the different philosophical approaches to management of low back pain.

- Explain how manual therapy, therapeutic modalities, and exercise may best be incorporated into a treatment program.

- Be able to differentiate between specific etiologies and causes of low back pain.

- Discuss a specific treatment protocol for dealing with low back pain.

In the general population, four of every five Americans will experience a low back problem in their lifetimes.[59] In the industrial world, low back problems are the single biggest reason for lost time among workers. Nineteen million working days are lost each year, which represents a mean cost of $6000 per back injury.[70, 106] These industrial dollar figures represent an involvement of from 28% to 45% of the working population.[70,88] The United States is not alone in this problem. In the United Kingdom an estimated 20% of all orthopedic referrals are due to backache, and 18 million working days per year are lost.[35,103]

The sports population's low back problems do not appear to be of the same magnitude as those of the general population but do seem to be on the rise. Cannon and James[10] reported a 2% gain in low back cases from 1978 to 1981. Micheli and others,[66] Jackson and others,[51] and Haldeman[41] note the increased incidence of low back problems (LBP) in all age groups. Garrick[30] divided the injuries seen in the last 5 years at a sports medicine facility by location and activity and determined that back injuries comprised 8% of the total injuries seen, with the biggest percentage of cases coming from gymnastics. Micheli and others[66] agree with Garrick[30] but also note that the vast majority of these cases involved females, which might be due to the prevalence of women in gymnastics. Brady[8] also found a 5% back injury rate with runners. This same percentage was reported by Wroble and Albright[111] in their study on wrestling injuries at the University of Iowa. Haldeman[41] stated, however, that 20% of all sports injuries were back related, and Ferguson and others[28] noted a percentage as high as 50 among interior linesmen at a major university. This percentage appears to be rather high compared with the previously mentioned statistics and may possibly be the result of faulty training and/or conditioning techniques. However, the lower percentages reported earlier might be conservative. Not everyone who sustains a low back injury while participating in a sport seeks professional help, especially since 90% of those injuries subside without intervention within 2 months.[106] Also, athletes who injure their backs may not go to a sports medicine center for evaluation.

In spite of the reported discrepancies in the incidence of LBP, clearly they are on the rise. Therefore, the purpose of this chapter is to discuss the low back problems that are most commonly found with sports participation and to investigate current methods of managing these problems. This chapter includes (1) a review of examination sequences, (2) an overview of varied treatment modalities and procedures, and (3) a report on the common pathology and specific treatment available for each condition.

THE EXAMINATION

As with any other area of the body, determining a program of back rehabilitation requires a thorough evaluation of the condition. However, evaluation of back problems takes on special importance and thus requires in-depth discussion. Familiarization with the anatomy and function of the lumbosacral area is paramount for the intelligent interpretation of information found during the examination procedures, which determines the appropriate treatment to be given.[62,63,79] However, Gould[35] states that a knowledge of the pertinent structures is meaningless without an effective tool to interpret the symptoms and complaints reported by the patient. Paris[82] agrees with Gould,[35] stating that the sports therapist must have the visual and palpatory skills necessary for the detection of a special problem. Bosacco and Berman[7] find a detailed history and examination to be the cornerstone of diagnosis. Cyriax and Russell,[17] Maitland,[63] and Paris[79] point out, however, that the role of the sports therapist is not to attempt a differential diagnosis but to identify the nature and extent of the problem so as to be able to determine the appropriate method of treatment. Grimsby[39] notes that the evaluation and treatment determination process does not just precede the treatment but is actually an ongoing process throughout the treatment and afterward. Maitland[63] strongly agrees with this point in a discussion on assessment. Sikorski[99] also believes that reassessment is an integral part of the examination process and even presents a schematic algorithm showing how the assessment-reassessment process could alter the treatment approach (Fig. 9-1).

Because the examination is so critical to the treatment outcome, various styles have been offered.* The common denominator in almost all the examination approaches is that they include the following items: initial observation, history and interview, structural inspection, active and passive movements, palpation, neurological tests, special questions and additional information, correlation of findings, and treatment plan.

Subjective Information

The initial contact affords the sports therapist the opportunity to observe the athlete candidly. Physical and emotional cues can be gotten from the way the athlete responds.[65] Hand shakes, facial expressions, and how athletes get up from their chairs can indicate how comfortable or apprehensive athletes are with their situation and new surroundings. Initial responses can also inform the sports therapist of possible sites of dysfunction or pathology.[79] In the case of an athletic injury, the sports therapist sometimes has the opportunity to see the mechanism of the injury firsthand, which can lead to a more direct evaluatory approach.[76]

A good history is the cornerstone of a good diagnosis and therefore appropriate treatment.[7,63] Maitland[63] further states that an accurate history is imperative if the sports therapist is to have any idea of: (1) the structure(s) involved, (2) the state of those involved structures, (3) the rate of progression of the problem, (4) the present degree of stability of the problem, (5) the likelihood of success with treatment, and (6) the likely prognosis. The order of questioning can vary depending upon the style of the sports therapist, but the basic information needed is: (1) chief complaint, (2) site of symptoms, (3) onset of symptoms, (4) duration of symptoms, (5) nature

*References 17,26,35,39,44,62,63,65,79,89,101.

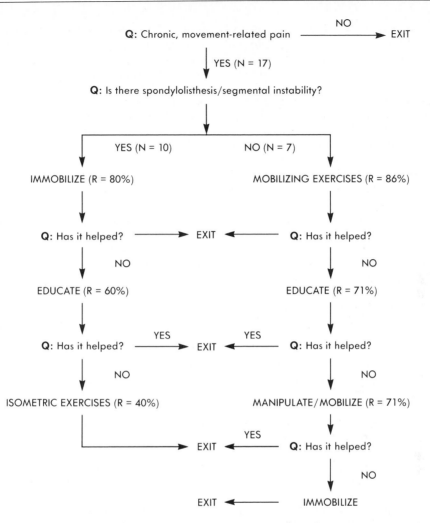

Fig. 9-1. Algorithm showing suggested sequence of treatment.

of symptoms, (6) behavior of symptoms, (7) effect of previous treatment, if any, and (8) special questions.[39,63,65,79,95]

Establishing why the patient is there to see the sports therapist has obvious implications. Thus the first question should be: "In your own words, what is your complaint or problem?"[79,95] This question allows athletes to explain their biggest problems as they see them. It also helps to erase any tension that might be felt by either party, as well as lets the sports therapist know how much of a grip the athlete has on the problem.

The next step is to determine the site of the symptoms. Have the athlete point to the painful area or, if pain is not the problem, to the stiffness, paresthesia, or other problem. Often this area is the actual site of the problem.[65] However, be as exact as possible, as diskogenic conditions as well as systemic pathology refer pain and/or paresthesias into one or both buttocks and lower extremities.[68,90] Paris[79] suggests asking the patient where the pain has been over the last 48 hours to provide the sports therapist with a clearer pain pattern.

Following the location of the problem, the onset of the injury or condition needs to be identified. Here, such information as the mechanism of the injury can be disclosed, as well as the date it happened. If the patient has difficulty pinpointing when the pain started, then a disease entity or a progressive degenerative process might be present.[79,113] Another possibility would be idiopathic conditions, such as Paris's[79] lesion complex and pain arising from scoliosis.[106] Athletes might be very exact as to the date and time because the majority of injuries to their back are sprains and strains.[30] However, Ferguson and others[28] found evidence of spondylolysis and spondylolisthesis among college football linemen. These particular conditions are oftentimes trauma related but without any particular pain at the time of trauma.[51,102,108] Therefore, even in the athlete's case, the onset may be difficult to determine.

Defining the onset to the extent possible enables the examiner to determine the course and duration of the symptoms, which helps to differentiate between acute, subacute, and chronic states of the condition.[95] This knowledge in turn might affect the type of treatment given. An acutely painful muscle strain would be treated much differently than a chronic one.[58,76,91] The status of a condition should not be based on time alone because other factors are involved.[62,63]

The course as well as the duration can point to the direction the problem is going. If symptoms are gradually getting worse since the onset, disease might be present[79] or environmental situations at work, home, or playing field may be aggravating the condition.[65,89] In another instance, patients could present with similar facet joint mechanical restrictions but different time courses, and the delayed time course would be a factor in suspecting synovitis rather than a meniscus-entrapped muscle facet block.[69,79] The nature of the symptoms describes the type of pain or problem perceived. Maitland[63] uses the type of pain as part of the determination of the location of the problem as well as the effectiveness of the treatment. Paris[79] describes in great detail the variety of pain sensations associated with different conditions. Saunders[95] points out that the difference between a sharp, superficial pain and a dull ache is important to the final correlation of findings. If the problem appears to be related to sensation, then differentiating between numbness and pins and needles is important, as numbness may or may not be related to a diminution of sensation.[63,112]

McKenzie[62] emphasizes the behavior of symptoms in the evaluation procedure and has stated that probably the most important question is whether the symptoms are constant or intermittent. This difference can be important in determining the source of the pain and the status of it. According to McKenzie,[62] 70% of low back patients have intermittent pain that is related to postural dysfunction syndromes, whereas the other 30% have constant pain that is of the derangement variety. Different positions and their effect on the symptom are important to ascertain. Increased symptoms while sitting might denote a disk or sacroiliac (SI) problem[23,73] or could be related to posture and dysfunction syndromes or instability from ligamentous insufficiency.[65,82] However, relief of symptoms with sitting might point to spondylolisthesis or facet syndrome.[68,94] Other factors such as the sleeping positions and the effect on the symptoms of walking and standing should be explained. Gracovetsky[36] notes that with right-side torsional injury to either facets or disk, lying on the right side could result in pain due to the axial rotation to the affected side that takes place with the left lateral flexion induced with that position. Symptoms with walking suggest inflammation,[68] SI dysfunction,[23] and even stenosis.[7] The advent of pain on prolonged standing might indicate instability.[82]

The time of day the symptoms are worse or better can also be informative. Early morning stiffness or pain could be the result of an inflammatory or disease process[65] or a disk[63]; later afternoon pain could represent ligamentous insufficiency.[79] Moreover, what relieves or aggravates the symptoms needs to be ascertained. McKenzie[62] notes that this factor, along with some objective observations, might determine the direction the treatment approach might take. The effect, if any, of previous treatments is important to know.[95] If a particular treatment significantly reduced the symptoms in the past, then it should certainly be considered as a means of treatment again.

The special questions category involves information on such things as the result of x-rays, medication taken, general health, recent weight loss or gain, any bowel or bladder problems, occupation of the patient, and any recent illnesses.[95] For example, with spinal stenosis, the clinical symptoms can be misleading and mimic everything from a disk problem to vascular claudication, but the results of a CT scan can be the differentiating factor.[25] This difference certainly would affect the treatment, as exercise and ambulation, normally helpful with a disk situation, might irritate a stenotic problem.[68,79] As another example, bowel or bladder incontinence could represent a disk extrusion or sequestration or a stenotic condition, all of which can result in a cauda equina syndrome, which requires immediate medical attention.[7,12]

Objective Information

The first part of any objective examination should be the structural evaluation,[39,62,79] which involves viewing the client, with the least amount of clothing allowable, from all different angles, thus allowing a more comprehensive integration of structural cues.[95]

Posteriorly, the sports therapist should look at the shoulder level, scapular level, the spinal musculature symmetry, spinal midline position, pelvic level, hip trochanter level, lower extremity musculature, angulation of the knees, and weight distribution of the feet.[23,62,65,95] An uneven shoulder level could represent structural or functional scoliosis or possibly SI dysfunction.[23,79] Uneven scapular levels might also signify scoliosis or muscle atrophy due to neurological impairment, a disease process, or muscle spasm.[79] Asymmetrical spinal musculature could point to segmental instability, spasm, atrophy from a long-standing chronic condition, or nerve root pressure, all depending upon whether the involved side is atrophied or hypertrophied.[6,79,82] A spinal deviation from the midline, or lateral shift, might be a manifestation of a herniated disk on the concave side of the list or a joint dysfunction on the convex side.[17,62,65] However, the lateral shift could be toward (convex side) the side of pain if the herniation is medial to the nerve.[79,89] Pelvic levels can be affected by a number of situations, including anterior or posterior torsion of the innominates,[23] a congenital anomaly of the spine, and a structurally short leg of at least 12.7 to 15 mm.[16,65] Included in the pelvic structural evaluation is palpation of the posterior superior iliac spine (PSIS) and the anterior superior iliac spine (ASIS). These observations help the investigator differentiate between a possible anterior

or posterior torsion of the innominates.[85] The trochanter levels should be examined for possible functional or structural leg-length discrepancies, which could result in torsional injuries at the spine or indicate SI dysfunction or disease.[26,62,85] Leg length can also affect the angulation of the knee on the long side and result in a varus, valgus, or recurvatum deformity.[26] In addition, the weight distribution of the feet needs to be examined, as pronated feet result in a closed chain of events that alters the shock-absorbing mechanism of the legs and SI, results in an overstress situation.[23,26,85]

The posterior view might also reveal possible structural defects such as diastematomyelia and spina bifida occulta via a tuft of hair and/or lumpy, fatty masses.[22,44] These conditions in the athlete may restrict certain types of participation.[76] Other skin signs involve skin tags and café au lait spots, which reflect a possible neurofibroma.[22] This condition could be a source of pain through compression of the spinal cord or nerve roots.[44]

A lateral view can reveal postural abnormalities such as an exaggerated lumbar lordosis or kyphosis, increased or decreased sacral inclination, and the conditions of the knee and abdominal wall.[18,79,95] Increased lordosis may reflect posterior segment instability such as spondylolisthesis, especially if the characteristic step is present.[82,113] It can also signify abdominal weakness and psoas tightness, which can be detrimental to the disks, facets, and SI joints.[1,18,23] The reverse situation, a lumbar kyphosis, can signify a posteriorly migrated nucleus.[37] Hoppenfield[44] states that paravertebral muscle spasm would induce a lumbar kyphosis. Spasm as a primary source of kyphosis was questioned by Paris[79] and does not seem possible based upon the EMG study of Morris and others,[71] unless the posterior musculature were acting in synergy with the flexors, the latter statement being pure speculation. Increased or decreased sacral inclination could either be a sign of tight hip flexors[18] or the result of SI disease pathology such as ankylosing spondylitis.[65] A genu recurvatum might signify a long leg, and abdominal distention might be a sign of overstretched and weak musculature.[18]

An anterior view gives the sports therapist an opportunity to examine the symmetry of the abdominal wall, as well as the levels of the anterior superior iliac spine,[85] which might relate to asymmetrical abdominal weakness[79] and SI dysfunction.[23]

The next step in the examination process concerns active and passive movements. Active movements test the willingness of the individual to move and involve both the contractile and noncontractile tissue.[95] The motions tested consist of flexion, extension, lateral flexion, and rotation[35,79] (Figs. 9-2 through 9-5).

Flexion, or forward bending, should be done with the athlete keeping the knees straight and feet spread slightly apart to involve the hamstrings.[15] During this maneuver, the tester should be looking for deviations in the arc of the movement that could represent hypermobility. A sudden shake or catch indicates that instability is present at that segment.[82] Restriction of flexion with normal spinal curvature might be due to tight hamstrings.[18] Flexion restriction with a flattened lumbar curve denotes tight posterior structures.[63] Diskogenic problems almost always produce pain with forward bending[90] and can result in a deviation either away or toward the side of pain.[62] Structural or functional scoliosis can be detected. Functional scoliosis disappears with flexion, whereas structural scoliosis does not.[22] Palpating the PSIS and detecting a latent motion in the hypermobile joint or an increased excursion on the hypermobile joint can identify dysfunction.[26,82] The athlete who has severe or moderate muscle splinting may be very reluctant to bend forward.[101]

The sports therapist must also be aware of any variations the athlete might make when returning to an upright position from flexion.[38,63] Simple joint dysfunction allows the athlete to assume the upright position mostly the way the flex was accomplished, whereas serious pathology may be present if the upright position is assumed in a tortuous manner.[65]

In addition Mennell and Zohn[65] suggest that tapping the spinous process while the athlete is in the flexed posture could provide information that might differentiate among a disk problem, an inflammatory or disease process, and joint dysfunction. A sharp, short, well-localized pain usually indicates more serious pathology. Disk problems usually are represented by a sharp, short pain that produces a radiating pain.

Extension involves the athlete placing the

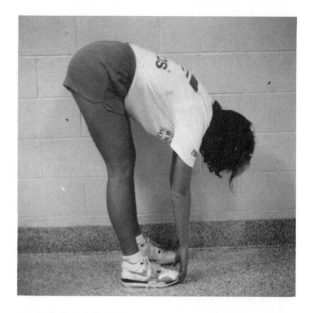

Fig. 9-2. Trunk flexion.

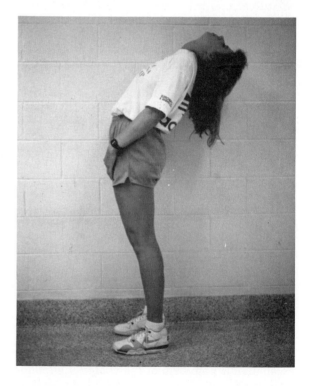

Fig. 9-3. Trunk extension.

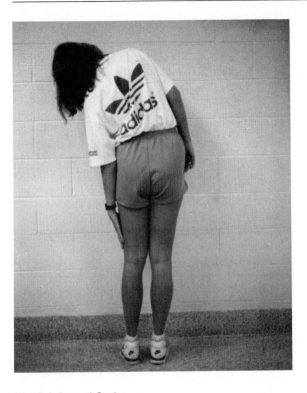

Fig. 9-4. Lateral flexion.

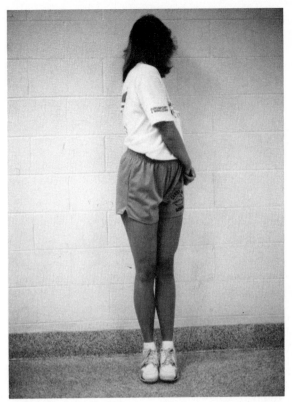

Fig. 9-5. Lateral rotation.

hands slightly posterior to the hips and then
bending backward slowly and as far as possible.
Although sometimes considered of little importance in the examination process,[79] loss of normal
movement may be the result of fluid dynamics
in the disk, which is usually accompanied with
a mild lateral shift.[62] Kissing lamina and SI
dysfunction might also be responsible. If pain
is associated with normal or mildly limited motion, instability of a motion segment or segments could be present, as well as a facet syndrome.[56,113]

Lateral flexion and rotation, the next motions
tested, are interrelated in the lumbar spine,[77] and
one or both are sometimes not specifically
tested.[62,63] Significance here can be in the observation of a hypermobile inferior and hypermobile
superior segment, as witnessed by a flattened
area with a point of sharp angulation during lateral flexion.[79] Rotation is minimal in the lumbar
spine, but the limitation could represent facet
stiffness or block.[83]

McKenzie[63] has chosen not to include lateral

flexion and rotation. Instead, he examines a side
gliding motion that involves simultaneous pelvis
and shoulder movement in opposite directions.
Difficulty with either side motion can signify unilateral impairment on the side that is difficult to
reach.

In some instances, when the active movements yield no reproduction of the symptoms,
overpressure is applied at the end of the range
to try to elicit the symptoms[38,62,63] by stretching
the noncontractile tissue enough to produce
symptoms from the offending tissue. Often this
overpressure is done in quadrant motions
(extension-rotation-lateral flexion) that can even
more precisely elicit a symptom that can specify
a condition.[56,63] This variance of motion has also
been stated to be significant in determining SI
dysfunction[85] (Fig. 9-6).

Repetitive motions can also be informative.
McKenzie[62] states that repeating an active move-

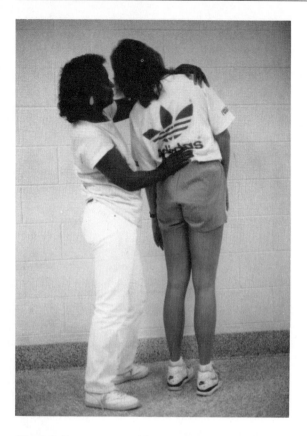

Fig. 9-6. Overpressure with extension and lateral rotation.

ment up to 10 times can elicit either an increase or a decrease in the symptoms, which can determine the type of problem that exists and the direction of movement of the treatment technique.

While the patient is still standing, the sports therapist can test for S1-2 innervation by having the athlete toe stand at least six consecutive times on each foot.[38] Weakness here could point to a spinal nerve root lesion or a sequestered disk.[6,90]

PASSIVE MOVEMENTS AND PALPATION. The next steps in the objective examination involve passive movements and palpation, which are intrinsic to each other.[79,83]

Palpation provides the examiner with information regarding the condition, position, and mobility of skin, subcutaneous tissue, muscles, ligaments, and joint lines[35,38,62,65,79] (Table 9-1).

The skin's temperature and moisture can indicate a chronic or acute situation, usually at that level.[63] The techniques of skin rolling can provide information on the status of subcutaneous tissue.[65,101] Increased tissue fluid tension can accompany problem areas and may be present in acute and chronic conditions.[79,96] Swelling over the sacrum might be associated with a possible SI condition.[23] Deeper palpation can produce information on the muscles and ligaments. The location of trigger points (even though their significance has been questioned[79]) and scarring can be detected. Protective spasm or muscle guarding can be felt along the lesion site[76,79] or could be more diffuse in the case of disease.[23,65]

Some of the benefits of palpation in the standing position were mentioned previously. The prone position allows the determination of joint relationships without weight-bearing stress. Scoliosis found with standing is absent in the prone position if it is functional.[18] Stronger evidence for spondylolisthesis can be found if the step is lost in the prone position.[38,83] Sacral rotation might be suspected with a deepened or shallow sacral sulcus.[85]

Palpation with the athlete supine allows investigations important to SI function. The ASIS locations can be observed for symmetry, and the position of the pubic bones can be noted. These data can suggest innominate torsion.[23,85]

As in the strength test given the plantar flexors while the athlete stands for the active movements evaluation, the supine position allows the orderly and timely examination of the strength of the particular muscle groups that correspond with the appropriate lumbar and sacral (L-S) nerve root levels. This strength is important in a sports situation in which time is limited.[76] Table 9-2 lists the muscles and their corresponding nerve root level. Roy and Irvin[89] recommend that the abdominals be tested while the athlete is still in the supine position. Their importance has already been discussed.[37] Any weakness found in these muscles could be related to nerve root lesion, disk problems, or even a swollen facet.[6,90]

Palpation for mobility involves passive movement testing. Passive movement is divided into physiological and nonphysiological or accessory movements.[35,63]

The accessory movements of the lumbar spine are basically comprised of a posterior-anterior

TABLE 9-1
Palpation

Type	Traumatic Acute	Traumatic Chronic	Reflex Reproduced
Distribution of symptoms	Local to segment	More than one segment	Several segments, often bilateral
Skin feel	Normal, some drag, moisture	Drag, roughened, thickened, dry	Drag, not rough, perhaps moist
Skin temperature	May be raised	Normal reduced	Normal
Muscles	Contracted, protective "guarding"	Contracted postural shortening, fibrosis evident, spasm	Contracted evenly over wider area
Ligaments	Swollen but soft	Thickened and firm or stringy	Usually normal
Joint lines	Sharp and distinct	Blurred or sharp, not distinct	Normal
Subjective tenderness	Local, quite acute	One or more levels, less acute	Normal

TABLE 9-2
Quick Test of Muscle Strength for Nerve Involvement*

Area	Muscle	Innervation Tested
Lumbar	Psoas and iliacus	L1-2
	Rectus femoris	L3-4
	Vastus intermedius, medialis, lateralis	L3-4
	Anterior tibialis	L4
	Extensor hallucis longus	L5
	Extensor digitorum communis	L5 (S1)
	Peroneal	S1 (L5)
	Gastrocnemius—soleus	S1-2
Cervical	Trapezius	C2-4 and spinal accessory
	Deltoid	C5
	Supraspinatus	C5
	Biceps—brachioradialis	C5-6
	Triceps—wrist extensors	C7
	Extensor pollicis longus	C8
	Flexor digitorum sublimis	C8
	Flexor digitorum profundus	C8
	Interosseous and lumbricalis	T1

*Modified from Maitland GD: Vertebral manipulation, ed. 4, Woburn, Mass., 1977, Butterworth Publishers, p. 531.

central pressure (P-A) on the spinous process, a P-A on the transverse process that provides a rotational movement, a transverse pressure on the side of the spinous process, and a distractive traction that decompresses the segments.[35,38,63,79] The first two are best completed prone; the last two could be done standing but probably are done best while the athlete is sitting. These mobility palpations in the prone position should be given with progressive or graded pressure. Maitland[63] has established a grading system from 1 to 4. Grades 1 and 4 are small-amplitude movements at the beginning and end of the range, respectively. Grades 2 and 3 are larger-amplitude movements occupying the middle parts of the available movement (see Fig. 4-2); restriction, from either pain and/or tissue resistance, can be graded with this system. The more acute or involved the segment, usually the more painful and/or restricted the movement. The sitting movements are general motions designed either to produce or to relieve pain and can be helpful in designating a disk condition.[38,79]

Prone accessory tests for the SI joint include the sacral spring test and specific mobility tests. The spring test is a P-A pressure in a small-amplitude quick thrust, on the sacrum.[26] The mobility tests involve palpation of the sacral sulcus with one hand, while the other is providing gentle A-P motion. The reverse test is done by raising the femur in an adducted and extended fashion while palpating the SI joint on the same side.[85] If pain or mobility variances from the norm, which are difficult for the novice to feel,[38] are noted, dysfunction might be present.[23] If pain and restriction are noted and are correlated with other factors throughout the examination, serious pathology such as ankylosing spondylitis might be involved.[65]

While the athlete is still prone, rotation of the hip can be tested as a clearing method.[95]

Passive accessory movements in the supine position comprise mostly SI testing. It is accomplished by applying an approximation and gapping force via the ASIS with the sports therapist's hands.[23] Porterfield[85] suggests testing the subtalar joint, for motion as a dysfunction here could alter the direction of forces focused up to the SI joint.

The passive physiological movements in the supine position involve hip and knee ROM tests and hamstring flexibility. Tightness in these joints can have detrimental effects on both the SI and intervertebral (IV) joints.[5,15,23]

The prone position allows the flexibility of the quadriceps group to be tested. Tightness here could stress the innominates into anterior torsion.[85] Through this an increase in anterior shear upon the IV joints, over time, could result in instability and degenerative changes.[68,102]

Flexion, rotation, and lateral flexion can be passively tested in different ways, depending upon the preference of the sports therapist. Maitland,[63] Grieve,[38] and Porterfield[85] test for these motions with the athlete in the side-lying position. The athlete's knees are on the femoral triangle area, and the sports therapist's hands are palpating the IV joints. A gentle side-to-side motion sequentially gaps the spinous processes and conversely compresses them. Rotation is accomplished with a rocking motion. Lateral flexion is accomplished with the athlete's knees over the edge of the table, and the sports therapist's one hand grasps the lower legs while the other palpates between the spinous process and just lateral to the process. Lowering and raising the feet laterally flexes the spine. Paris[79] uses the prone position in much the same manner as the prone SI accessory test, only palpating the IV joints, for testing rotation. Lateral flexion is accomplished with the knees bent to 90 degrees and rotating them away and toward the examiner. Flexion is done with the athlete lying on one side as described previously.

During the testing of passive motions, special tests should be done to clarify further the examination results.

The straight leg-raising test, or Lasèque's sign, involves raising the leg on the involved side high enough to produce radiating pain, lowering it until pain subsides, and then dorsiflexing the ankle.[44] The return of pain or symptoms is said to be positive for tension signs either of the sciatic nerve, nerve root,[89] or disk.[7] Spinal stenosis may[90] or may not[68] produce a positive Lasèque's sign. What the test is testing is controversial because of the extensive anatomy it affects.[23,38]

Kernig's sign, another tension test, involves passive neck flexion, which if positive produces neck, back, and/or leg pain.[44]

Maitland[63] favors the slump test, which involves long leg sitting in a slumped posture just below any pain level. The sports therapist then flexes the neck and applies pressure to the trunk downwardly. The test can be adapted in the sitting position to account for acute symptoms.

Gaenslen's sign is a test for SI involvement.[44] The athlete's one hip is flexed while the opposite leg is extended over the side of the table. Reproduction of symptoms denotes SI involvement. This test can also be done while the athlete is lying on one side.[89]

Patrick's test is used to detect hip involvement but can also provoke SI symptoms.[44] The hip is flexed, abducted, and extremely rotated, and the ankle is placed on the opposite knee. If needed, a downward pressure is exerted on the knee to clear the joint.

Ober's test should be given to the athlete lying on one side to test the length of the tensor fasciae latae and the iliotibial band.[85] The leg should be flexed, abducted, then extended, and then allowed to adduct to the plinth. If it does not reach the plinth, tightness is present. A short band can develop into SI problems due to its pull on the innominate.[23]

Prone knee flexion can determine any tension problems with the femoral nerve.[38]

NEUROLOGICAL TESTS. The next step in the examination process is neurological tests. To save time, they can be done in coordination with the positions of the other tests or separately. Some of the tests involve muscle testing, which has been previously mentioned. The remainder of the tests are concerned with obtaining information on reflexes and sensation.[79]

The main reflexes to be tested are those of the patella tendon and Achilles tendon.[35] Absent or diminished reflex activity could mean a spinal nerve root lesion of L4 and possibly L5 if it is at the knee, and S1 and/or L5 if at the ankle. Spinal stenosis as well as HNP and well-progressed facet syndrome can affect reflex activity.[33,90,103]

Sensation should be tested if neurological involvement is indicated.[63] The testing should take place along the dermatome of a suspect segment level. The sensations experienced with nerve root irritation are felt as superficial tingling and hypersensitivity along the dermatome. Conversely, sustained pressure, as in stenosis, may produce decreased sensitivity and numbness.[68,83]

At this time in the evaluation, information such as MRI, CT, x-ray, and EMG results should be obtained if applicable. The results of these tests should be used only to substantiate objective findings, as positive findings for HNP are in error up to 50% of the time.[104] However, CT results on spinal stenosis are much more reliable.[105] X-ray findings have been found to have little relationship to lumbar pain.[109]

A correlation or assessment of all the information obtained through the evaluation is made at this point.[38,39,63,79] A treatment plan can then be based on this assessment, and the sports therapist's experience and success with similar findings.

TREATMENT
Manual Therapy

Manual therapy, although its effects are not clearly understood, has been an increasingly popular treatment for L-S problems.[21,41,80] It is broadly defined as including all procedures in which the hands are utilized to massage, mobilize, adjust, or manipulate spinal tissue for therapeutic reasons.[40] More specifically, it is a skilled passive movement to a joint or spinal segment, either within or beyond its active range of motion.[80] Its goal is to increase or improve spinal motion, with implied changes on muscle, ligaments, disks, and neurogenic reflexes.[41] Many different styles and techniques have been developed to accomplish these goals.[17,62,63,79] Table 9-3 summarizes these different schools of thought.

TABLE 9-3
Summary of Principal Theories and Techniques of Schools of Thought

1. BASED ON RELIEVING NERVE ROOT PRESSURE

Chiropractic	- Moves vertebra	- Specific
Cyriax	- Moves disk	- Nonspecific
McKenzie	- Moves disk	- Nonspecific

2. BASED ON RELIEVING PAIN

Maitland	- Oscillates to eliminate reproducible signs
Maigne	- Mobilizes osteopathically; "no pain and contrary motion"

3. BASED ON RESTORING FUNCTION

Osteopathy	- Joint and body systems—specific
Mennell	- Joint play—specific
Kaltenborn	- Arthrokinematics (convex-concave) specific
Paris	- Dysfunction, mechanistic, specific

The different techniques involved in manual therapy consist of nonthrust, thrust, and distraction[17,83] (Table 9-4). Within the nonthrust category, Maitland[63] has delineated four grades of movement based upon amplitude and the portion of the available range of motion. As indicated in Chapter 4, these movements can be either physiological or nonphysiological (accessory).[35] The physiological movements are those that involve motion of the joint beyond the ability of the muscle to perform.[41] The nonphysiological movements are those that are not within the ability of the muscles to perform due to their anatomical positioning.[38,63] Some of the more popular nonthrust movements are cental P-A pressure on the spinous process, unilateral P-A pressure on the transverse process, transverse pressure on the spinous process (difficult in the lumbar spine), rotation using various positions, flexion, and extension.* These techniques would be used in any situation where elongation of the connective tissue, including adhesions, and pain relief are indicated,[79] and perhaps when a repositioning of nuclear material is indicated.[17,63]

Thrust techniques involve a quick, small-amplitude, high-velocity movement, uncontrollable by the client, and delivered at the pathological limit of an accessory movement.[41,63,79] The involvement can be specific or general.[17,41] These

TABLE 9-4

Mobilization: A Classification

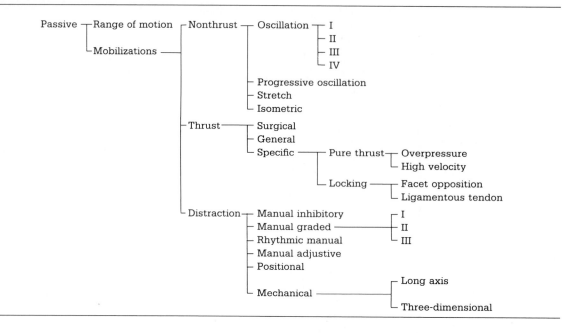

techniques require a high level of skill; they have been known to result in serious injury if done inappropriately and incorrectly.[13] The indication for the techniques, which mostly involve rotation, is desire to alter positional relationships, to snap an adhesion, and to relieve pain.[13,79]

Distraction is defined as the separation of two articular surfaces in a long-axis or longitudinal direction.[79] The most common forms used for the lumbar spine are mechanical and positional, with autotraction gaining in popularity.[94] Mechanical distraction involves the use of a traction machine that can intermittently or statically provide distraction. Positional distraction is done by placing the athlete in a position that provides intervertebral foraminal opening, usually on one side of the segment only. Autotraction uses a special traction bench that can be individually angulated and rotated so that athletes can perform the traction on themselves.[94] Distraction is used to reduce weight bearing on joint surfaces, relieve pressure on an intraarticular structure, to stretch a joint capsule or adhesions, or to help reduce dislocation.[79,94] Cyriax and Russell[17] have also espoused distraction for slow nuclear protrusion

problems and bone-to-bone situations as in advanced scoliosis. Saunders[93] also describes a unilateral mechanical method specific to unilateral facet hypomobility, protective lumbar scoliosis, and lumbar scoliosis caused by unilateral muscle spasm.

Although determining the efficacy of manual therapy is difficult,[13,21,40,41,53] the effects of mobilization are said to be psychological, mechanical, and neurophysiological.* Psychological effects are through the hands-on approach and the recognition of an occasional pop. The mechanical effects involve maintaining the extensibility of the connective tissue and the destruction of intraarticular capsular fiber fatty adhesions, as well as the repositioning of cartilaginous disk material. Neurophysiological effects involve the stimulation of the cutaneous and muscular receptors and the articular mechanoreceptors and the jamming of the transmission from the nociceptors[62,79,112] (Table 9-5).

The contraindications for manual therapy are said to vary according to the skill of the practi-

---

*References 17,23,51,62,63,79.

TABLE 9-5
Synovial Joint Receptors, Location, and the Effects of Mobilization

	Type	Location	Fired by
Type I	Postural	Capsule	Oscillations, progressive or graded
Type II	Dynamic	Capsule	Oscillations, progressive or graded
Type III	Inhibitive	Capsule ligament and ligaments	Stretch or thrust
Type IV	Nociceptive	Most tissues	Injury

tioner.[79] Generally, however, it is not indicated in the presence of disk prolapse, spondylolisthesis, hypermobility, scoliosis, malignancy, tuberculosis, osteomyelitis, osteoporosis, fracture, ruptured ligaments, arthritis, pregnancy (especially in the first and last trimesters), and generally poor health.[38,63,81]

Therapeutic Modalities

Modalities, which are generally more beneficial in the acute phase of an L-S problem,[35,89] consist of heat, ice, and electrotherapy.[86,91,95]

Modalities are generally considered as adjunct therapy for spinal dysfunction or derangement.* However, the soft tissue manifestations of joint dysfunction should not be ignored as they are important to the overall success of treatment.[74,96]

Massage

Massage is a treatment option in L-S conditions that some use extensively.[17,65] Even though it is one of the oldest treatments for musculoskeletal and spinal problems, the exact mechanism of its effects is not fully understood.[20] Its effects may vary, according to the type of massage, but they are generally thought to be either reflexive or mechanical[89] and to result in the relief of pain through relaxation of tissue tension and increase in local circulation.[17,20] The techniques of massage are numerous, with friction massage said to be the most beneficial, especially when applied at right angles to the involved tissue.[17,96] It is indicated for postacute soft tissue trauma,[89] and also suggested for the acute stage of injury.[17]

*References 17,23,38,39,62,63,65,83.
*References 17,23,39,63,68,74,79,95,99.

Massage has also been said to be an important part of myofascial stretching and a preemption of mobilization.[17,65,79] Its contraindications are ongoing hemorrhaging of tissue, infections, thromboses, suspected myositis ossificans, and overuse of the technique.[17,65,89]

Exercise

The use of exercise in back problems is controversial, going from mildly important[83] to extremely important.[90] The therapeutic purpose of low back exercises is to relieve pain, regain range of motion, and strengthen the muscles to restore functional capacity.[58] The mechanisms by which exercise relieves pain are not well understood, especially in idiopathic L-S pain.[48] Nevertheless, exercise is widely prescribed.[58,62,90,92] The type of exercise that should be prescribed is also somewhat controversial. The standard protocol used to be flexion exercises,[107] partly to develop intraabdominal pressure and partly to maintain a posture that would take the pressure or stress off the posterior aspect of the spine, especially L5. This protocol has been severely questioned with the advent of McKenzie extension exercises.[48,84] In contrast to both of these exercise techniques, Saal[90] suggested that L-S exercises should be done in a stabilizing manner to maintain the normal physiological position of the spine while exercising and thus stress the disk and related structures as little as possible. Whichever avenue is taken, the basic aim of any exercise program for the L-S complex should be to increase maximal muscle strength and endurance strength.[58] The important muscle groups within such a program are the abdominals, the back extensors, the hip extensors, the quadriceps, and the latissimus dorsi.[90]

Stretching

Stretching should also be a part of any back rehabilitation program.[60,89] Careful consideration should be given to the type of stretching done, as indiscriminate mobilization of hypermobile segments could be detrimental rather than instrumental to the process.[5,60] Such stretching was found to be a possible source of back pain in 82% of elite lightweight rowers.[46] In most cases, the important structures to check for tightness are the iliotibial tract, hamstrings, hip abductors, internal and external rotators and flexors, ankle plantar flexors, and, depending upon what is found on examination, the trunk extensors and fascia.[2,85,89]

The athlete with L-S problems not only needs to strengthen and stretch the important L-S structures but also needs to maintain, within the confines of the problem, the uninvolved musculature. The importance of program compliance must be stressed to the athlete,[111] who must understand the basic mechanism of L-S function and how it relates to the particular sport.[48,90]

COMMON LUMBOSACRAL INJURIES IN ATHLETES
Sprains

The most common injuries are the L-S sprain and strain,[10] which involve a stress, either sudden or over time, on the ligaments and muscles sufficient to cause injury.[76] Signs and symptoms can vary depending upon the area injured but generally include some restriction in L-S motion, pain either unilateral or bilateral, and tenderness and muscle guarding either over the injury site or opposite to it. Neurological signs are negative, as are nerve root tension signs.[48]

Treatment depends upon the examination findings. If the injury is acute, appropriate modalities should be used to alleviate pain. If rest is necessary for pain relief, the athlete should be positioned so as to not allow further progression of the injury. Maintaining normal erect posture or slightly in hyperextension is usually involved.[62,83] Mobilization, if tolerated and indicated, should start with those movements associated with pain abatement and then progress as tolerated.[63] Activity should be progressed within a pain-free range, and rehabilitation should progress likewise.[48]

Special mention should be made of a sprain of the SI joint. Symptoms can be referred into either the groin, hamstring, or lateral aspect of the thigh or all of these areas.[23] A careful examination is needed to differentiate between an SI sprain and what might look like a herniated disk or nerve root problem at first glance.

Contusions

Contusions to the L-S spine are common.[89] They result from a blow to the spine or sacrum, sometimes sufficient to produce a hematoma.[76] Treatment here involves the usual modalities and procedures for any acute injury.[89] If pain persists, further examination is warranted for joint dysfunction and possible spinous process fracture.[23,76]

Stress Fractures

Stress fractures in the pars interarticularis are sometimes found in the young athlete.[48,51] They are said to be the result of stress from repetitive motions involving compression and hyperextension, especially those involved in football and gymnastics.[28,50] They are recognizable only through a bone scan and present usually unilateral pain with hyperextension and no neurological signs. The treatment is basically rest from the offending activity and manual therapy for any accompanying joint dysfunction.[83,113] Rest from participation can be as long as 6 to 8 months but is usually 3 months.[48]

Spondylolysis

A progressing stress reaction can lead into a spondylolysis.[113] The symptoms are similar to the stress reaction or may be absent.[89] A heredity factor may be involved, especially in those cases evident before the age of 6,[29] as may be a body type relationship.[45]

Spondylolisthesis

Spondylolisthesis is the result of continuing stresses, as described by Troup,[102] that lead to an anterior slippage of the superior vertebrae on the inferior[113] (Fig. 9-7). Clinically, the defect may or may not produce pain. Jackson and Brown[48] state that in many instances the athlete is un-

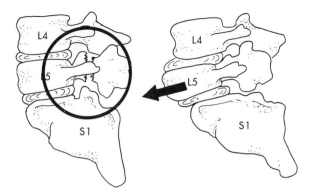

Fig. 9-7. Spondylolisthesis.

aware of any problem. An athlete with an advanced case may complain of pain and usually exhibits significant postural variances. Upon spinal examination, a characteristic shake or catch during forward bending might be evident, along with the step deformity,[82] which Yong-Hing and Kirkaldy-Willis[113] designate as signs of significant instability.

Unlike this spondylitic spondylolisthesis, isthmic spondylolisthesis[89] usually presents in a young teenager, and x-rays show an elongated and thin pars with no defect. The clinical symptoms are usually more significant, and it is more apt to result in surgery. Both of these instability conditions can often lead to a stenotic condition, but eventually stabilize in later years.[7,105]

Treatment involves the usual modalities for pain, if indicated, and stabilization exercises.[68,82] Hyperextension is discouraged and flexion encouraged.[89] Athletic activity is not allowed if pain persists. However, if the sport allows, a modified brace might be used.[66] If the instability is 50% or greater, athletic participation is discouraged. Unfortunately, these problems often result in surgery (fusion).[48]

Disk Problems

Intervertebral disk problems are found more often in college athletes, especially in those involved in football.[48] Disk problems are usually the result of repetitive stresses, especially from rotational activities.[7,37] Eventually these stresses can end in sequestration and instability changes at the three-joint segment complex.[113] This extrusion of disk material can press on pain-sensitive structures and result in certain neurolog-

TABLE 9-6

Differentiating Signs of L4-L5 and L5-S1 Disk Lesions

Signs	L4-L5 Lesion (L5 Signs)	L5-S1 Lesion (S1 Signs)
Power decrease	Extensor hallucis longus (dorsiflexors)	Flexor hallucis longus (plantar flexors)
Sensation decrease	Dorsum of foot and anterior aspect of lower leg	Sole and outer border of leg and foot
Reflexes		Decreased ankle jerk
Plantar stimulation with iliotibial tract response	Iliotibial tract response	No iliotibial tract response
Muscle tenderness	Anterior tibial	Calf muscle
Sciatic nerve stretch tests	Positive	Positive

ical signs (Table 9-6). Structural examination may exhibit a list, usually to the contralateral side.[62] Forward flexion is painful and extension is not, unless significant disk material has encroached into the foramen.[17]

Treatment involves the use of modalities for pain relief, although often no back pain exists.[63,79] Manual correction for listing and extension exercises are indicated if the lower extremity pain does not proceed beyond the knee and weakness is not present.[17,62] Distraction may be used if symptoms are more pronounced.[93,94] If the condition is too acute, rest is indicated.[48] Jackson and Brown[48] note that epidural cortisone injections helped 44% of the athletes treated return to participation.

Idiopathic Pain

Idiopathic L-S pain was found to be the third most common problem seen in a British sports medicine center.[10] Mooney[68] states that pain from unknown origins was the most common clinical syndrome. White and Gordon[106] state that from 20% to 85% of all L-S pain is idiopathic, depending upon whether IV degenerative changes are included. Clinically the symptoms can vary but usually include muscle guarding.

No neurological or significant radiological signs are present.[90]

The treatment in these cases is solely dependent upon the clarifying physical examination.[63,79] Pain is treated with modalities and gentle oscillations. Specific dysfunction is determined and treated accordingly. Rehabilitation is instituted and education is given about proper back management.[68,106] The majority of these people improve within 2 months.[68]

Ankylosing Spondylitis

Ankylosing spondylitis is a relatively rare inflammatory disease that usually occurs in males in their late teens and early twenties.[89] The symptoms involve vague L-S pain associated in the morning with stiffness. Sacroiliac tenderness and pain with compression and Gaenslen's sign are considered the most significant physical findings.[48] Decreased chest expansion and back extension may also be noted. The treatment consists of antiinflammatory medication and extension and postural exercises.[89] Return to participation is dictated by the degree of discomfort and disability.[48]

Fractures

Fractures at the L-S complex mostly consist of transverse process and compression injuries.[76,89] Transverse process fractures are the result of a direct blow or an avulsion due to strong muscle contraction. They are self-limiting and treated symptomatically. In extreme cases, a corset can help manage pain.

Compression fractures involve a forceful flexion and compression of the spine, usually resulting in anterior vertebral involvement.[48] Pain is associated with weight bearing, and initial bed rest is required. As pain decreases, activity increases, with the use of a hyperextension brace. Conditioning exercises can be done with the brace, which is worn for 6 weeks. The athlete usually can return to play in 2 to 3 months.

CONCLUSION

When learning a new sport, one must start with the fundamentals in order before trying more advanced skills. This same principle should be applied to a back rehabilitation program, starting with the neutral postural position and basic stretching. As athletes develop proper technique in the simple exercises, they can progress into more complicated movements and finally apply the same principles in their sport-specific skills.

This chapter has attempted to piece together some of the problems the sports therapist might face when dealing with an athlete or anyone else who complains of L-S pain. The L-S structures are not as evident, so visualization of their functions and biomechanics is imperative. The importance of a detailed clarifying examination and its close relationship with the success of the treatment program were addressed. Through their relationship those conditions discussed and any other conditions that present themselves can be successfully managed.

BACK REHABILITATION PROTOCOL PHASE I

Illustrations of the various back rehabilitation exercises are on pages 170-182.

The exercises included in phase I of a back rehabilitation program are designed to promote the following:

1. Reduction in muscle spasm
2. Increased flexibility
3. Improved posture
4. Strengthened opposite trunk stabilization muscle groups to stabilize the trunk region and to counteract forces of gravity

Three specific muscle groups are important in developing stability of the trunk:

1. The abdominal muscle group, which includes the rectus abdominis, internal oblique abdominals, and external oblique abdominals
2. The back extensor muscle group, which includes the erector spinae muscle group and the intersegmental spinal musculature
3. The gluteal muscles, especially the gluteus maximus

EXERCISES
Neutral stabilization. This positioning exercise should be maintained as best as possible

while performing the following stretching and strengthening exercises.

Stretching exercises (see pages 170-172)
Knee to chest (Fig. 9-9)
Knee to chest with hip rotation (Fig. 9-10)
Lumbar rotation (Fig. 9-12)
Lumbar extension (Fig. 9-13)
Quadriceps stretch (Fig. 9-15)
Hip flexor stretch
Hamstring stretch (Fig. 9-18)

Strengthening exercises
Lower abdominal (Fig. 9-21)
Upper abdominal (Fig. 9-22)
Single arm-leg lift (Fig. 9-32)
Bridge up (Fig. 9-35)

Phase I

Stage	1	2	3	4
Sets	1	1	2	2
Reps	8–10	15	10	15

Phase I Stage 2: Sample program
 1. Neutral positioning (Fig. 9-8)
 2. Knee to chest (Fig. 9-9)
 3. Lumbar rotation (Fig. 9-12)
 4. Lumbar extension (Fig. 9-13)
 5. Quadriceps stretch (Fig. 9-15)
 6. Hamstring stretch (Fig. 9-18)
 7. Lower abdominals (Fig. 9-21)
 8. Bridge up (Fig. 9-35)

As an alternative to sets and reps, exercise can be prescribed for a period of time, for example, starting for 15 seconds and working toward a 2-minute goal.

Phase II

The exercises included in the Phase II rehabilitation program are a progression to the exercises in Phase I, with greater emphasis placed on strengthening the trunk musculature.

EXERCISES
Stretching exercises
Knee to chest with hip rotation (Fig. 9-10)
Hip external rotation (Fig. 9-11)
Hip flexion

Lumbar rotation (Fig. 9-12)
Lumbar extension (Fig. 9-13)
Side-lying quadriceps stretch (Fig. 9-15)
Side-lying hip flexor stretch (Fig. 9-16)
Hamstring stretch (Fig. 9-18)
Calf stretch (Fig. 9-19)
Stretching exercises are continued from Phase
    I if restrictions continue to be present.

Strengthening exercises
Lower abdominals (Fig. 9-21)
Upper abdominals (Fig. 9-22)
Partial sit-ups (Fig. 9-23)
Supine arm-leg bicycling (Fig. 9-27)
Double arm-leg lift (Fig. 9-33)
Kneeling opposite arm-leg lift (Fig. 9-34)
Bridge up with leg raise (Fig. 9-36)
Lat pull downs (Fig. 9-37)
Seated rowing (Fig. 9-39)

Medicine ball exercises
Lateral toss (Fig. 9-49)
Chest pass
Overhead toss (Fig. 9-50)
Reverse sit-up (Fig. 9-51)

Phase II

Stage	1	2	3	4
Sets	1	2	3	3
Reps	10	15	12	15

As an alternative to sets and reps, exercises can be prescribed for a period of time. Start with 20 seconds and work toward a 2-minute goal.

Phase II Stage 3: Sample program
 1. Knee to chest with hip rotation (Fig. 9-10)
 2. Hip external rotation (Fig. 9-11)
 3. Lumbar rotation (Fig. 9-12)
 4. Lumbar extension (Fig. 9-13)
 5. Quadriceps stretch (Fig. 9-15)
 6. Spine arch (Fig. 9-14)
 7. Partial sit-ups (Fig. 9-23)
 8. Supine arm-leg bicycling (Fig. 9-27)
 9. Double arm-leg lift (Fig. 9-33)
10. Bridge up with leg raise (Fig. 9-36)
11. Lat pull downs (Fig. 9-37)
12. Medicine ball exercises (Figs. 9-45
    through 9-56)

PHASE III:

EXERCISE PRESCRIPTION

Stretching
Stretching exercises in Phases I and II are continued if restrictions are noted.
   Hip flexion with external rotation
   Hip external rotation (Fig. 9-11)
   Hip flexion
   Side-lying quadriceps stretch (Fig. 9-15)
   Side-lying quadriceps and hip extension (Fig. 9-16)
   Kneeling lunge stretch
   Hamstring stretch; modified good-morning stretch (Fig. 9-18; Fig. 9-41)
   Thoracic stretch
   Lumbar extension (Fig. 9-13)
   Shoulder flexion
   Shoulder abduction and rotation

Back extension musculature
Prone arm-leg extension
Four-point alternate arm-leg extension (utilizing stick to reinforce staying in neutral)
Bridge up with leg raise (Fig. 9-36)
Prone raise with medicine ball (Fig. 9-45)
Gluet machine—short arc (Fig. 9-42)

Abdominal musculature
Abdominal crunch (Fig. 9-24)
Oblique abdominal crunch (Fig. 9-26)
Supine arm-leg bicycling (Fig. 9-27)
Medicine ball exercises
   Abdominal crunch (Fig. 9-55)
   Reverse sit-up (Fig. 9-51)

Miscellaneous
Posterior split squat with dumbbells
Wall sits (Fig. 9-44)
Lat pull downs (Fig. 9-34)
Straight arm pull down (Fig. 9-38)
Sitting upright row (Fig. 9-39)
Quarter squat with dumbbells
Medicine ball exercises
   Lateral toss (Fig. 9-49)
   Hip rotation
   Trunk rotation (Fig. 9-46)
   Sitting rotation (Fig. 9-47)

Hip crunch (Fig. 9-52)
Back-to-back pass (Fig. 9-48)

Phase III

Stage	1	2	3	4
Sets	2	2	3	3
Reps	10	15	12	15

As an alternative to sets and reps, exercise can be prescribed for a period of time. Start with 15 seconds and work toward a 2-minute goal.

Phase III Stage 4: Sample program
   1. Stretching; include stretching for major muscle groups
   2. Kneeling opposite arm-leg lift (Fig. 9-34) with weights or manual resistance
   3. Bridge up with leg raise (Fig. 9-36); add ankle weight
   4. Gluet machine—short arc (Fig. 9-42)
   5. Oblique abdominal crunch (Fig. 9-26)
   6. Supine arm-leg bicycling (Fig. 9-27) with weights
   7. Posterior split squat with dumbbells
   8. Wall sits (Fig. 9-44)
   9. Lat pull downs (Fig. 9-37)
   10. Sitting upright rows (Fig. 9-39)
   11. Medicine ball exercises (Figs. 9-45 through 9-56)

PHASE IV:

EXERCISE PRESCRIPTION
Exercises in this category are not attempting to eliminate the usage of hip flexor muscles. These muscles are an important part of sports activity, and their stimulation is vital to performance. These exercises are specific to many movement patterns in sports activity. Keep in mind that these exercises are preventive and based on use by the noninjured individual. Also, be aware that many of these are techniques related to skilled activities, and as such they should be performed carefully with attention to control.

Extension
Double arm-leg lift (Fig. 9-33)

Glut-ham back extension
  Parallel
  Hyper
Seated good mornings (emphasis on eccentric
  phase)
Standing good mornings (Fig. 9-41)
Backward medicine ball throw
  Seated
  Standing

Flexion
90-90 sit-ups
Roman chair
Rambo sit-ups
Medicine ball toss
Medicine ball sit-up
Crunch 90-90
Spread and reach crunch
Supine arm-leg bicycling (Fig. 9-27)
Hip crunch (Fig. 9-28)
Alternate knee grab
Seated toe touch with medicine ball (Fig.
  9-56)

Flexion with rotation
90-90 oblique sit-ups
90-degree hip rotation, knee bent (Fig. 9-29)
90-degree hip rotation, leg straight
Medicine ball lateral toss (Fig. 9-49)
  Single pump
  Double pump
Medicine ball throws standing
  Overhead
  Lateral
  Diagonal
Alternate toe touch (spread eagle) (Fig. 9-30)
Medicine ball trunk rotation (Fig. 9-46)
Flexion-rotation with medicine ball

Miscellaneous
45-degree isometrics
45-degree hip crunch (Fig. 9-28)
45-degree hip crunch on diagonal
Stall bar: leg drop
Hanging leg raise (Fig. 9-31)
  Knees bent
  Legs straight
  L sit
V ups
Eccentric sit-up (Fig. 9-25)
"Snatch" sit up with bar

Extension with rotation
Squats
Lat pull down (Fig. 9-37)
Pull ups, behind the neck (Fig. 9-43)
The following format is one method for group-
ing exercises in the "normal" category:

Phase IV: System of Exercise

Stage	1	2	3	4
Sets	1	1	2	2
Reps	10	15	10	15

NUMBER OF EXERCISES FROM EACH GROUP

Flexion	6	5	5	5
Extension	4	5	5	5
Flexion with rotation	0	3	5	5
Miscella-neous				

Phase III Stage 3: Sample program
1. Glut-ham hyperextension (E)
2. Glut-ham hyperextension with rotation (M)
3. Seated good mornings (E)
4. Standing good mornings (Fig. 9-41) (E)
5. 90-90 Crunch (F)
6. Spread leg crunch (F)
7. Supine bicycling (Fig. 9-27) (F)
8. 90-Degree hip rotation (supine) (FR)
9. Medicine ball rotation (FR)
10. Medicine ball lateral throws (FR)
11. Medicine ball hip crunch (Fig. 9-52) (F)
12. Medicine ball backward throw (E)
13. Medicine ball underhand throw (E)
14. Medicine ball lateral toss (Fig. 9-49) (FE)
15. Medicine ball double pump with toss (FR)
16. 45-Degree hip crunch (M)
17. 45-Degree hip crunch on diagonal (M)
18. Squats (M)

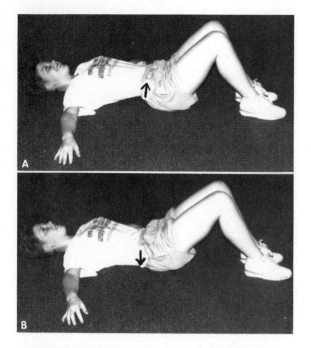

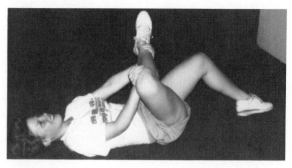

Fig. 9-10. Knee to chest with hip rotation: Lying on back, both knees bent with feet flat on floor, grasp right lower leg and pull toward chest while slightly externally rotating hip. Hold. Switch to opposite side and repeat.

Fig. 9-8. Neutral position: Lying on back, both knees bent and feet flat on the floor. **A,** Arch back and flatten back through full comfortable, pain-free range. **B,** Gradually decrease range of arcs of movement until mid-range trunk stabilization posture is found. This position is not an isometric contraction or static position but a limited range to provide trunk stability.

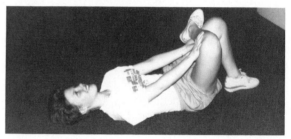

Fig. 9-11. Hip external rotation: Lying on back, both knees bent with feet flat on floor, lift and place right ankle on front of left thigh near the knee. Grasp right ankle with left hand while rotating and abducting leg. Push the knee in a forward direction using the right hand. Switch to opposite side and repeat.

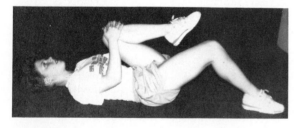

Fig. 9-9. Knee to chest: Lying on back, both knees bent, and maintaining the neutral position, grasp lower leg below the knee and pull toward chest. Keep back flat. Hold. Switch to opposite side and repeat.

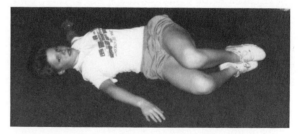

Fig. 9-12. Lumbar rotation: Lying on back, both knees bent with feet flat on floor, keep knees together and let legs and hips rotate to one side. Keep shoulders flat on floor. Switch to the opposite side and repeat.

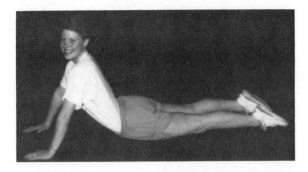

Fig. 9-13. Lumbar extension: Lie on stomach with hands on floor as if ready to do a push-up. Slowly raise upper body, keeping hips on floor. Press shoulders back and down. Extend arms till slight stretch is felt in the lower back. Hips should remain on floor.

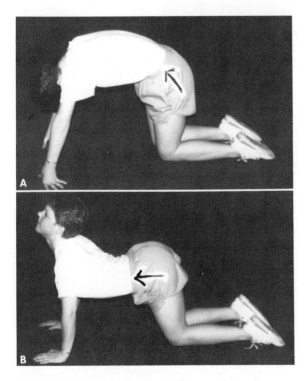

Fig. 9-14. Spine arch: Kneel on all fours, placing knees hip-width apart. **A,** Contract buttocks and allow the back to arch upward. Pelvis will tilt backward. **B,** Relax buttocks and allow pelvis to drop downward, causing the pelvis to tilt forward.

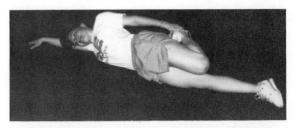

Fig. 9-15. Quadriceps stretch: Lie on right side. Bend left leg and grasp ankle. Pull heel gently toward buttocks. Hold. Switch to opposite side and repeat.

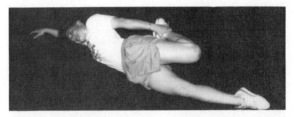

Fig. 9-16. Quadricep and hip flexor stretch: Lie on right side. Bend left leg and grasp ankle. Pull heel gently toward buttock while extending the hip in a backward direction. Hold. Switch to opposite side and repeat.

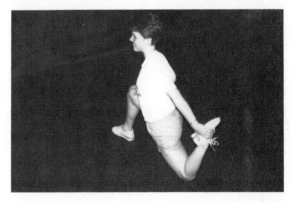

Fig. 9-17. Kneeling hip flexor stretch: Start in a kneeling position with hands on hips. Step right foot forward so that knee is bent at a 90-degree angle. Keeping back in a neutral position, lean forward until the stretch is felt in the hip flexors. Switch to opposite side and repeat.

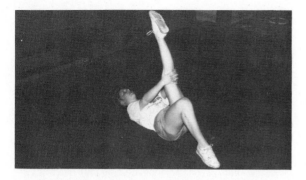

Fig. 9-18. Hamstring stretch: Lie on back with knees bent and feet flat on floor. Lift left foot off floor. Support leg by grasping thigh or by placing a strap around the ball of the foot. Slowly straighten the knee.

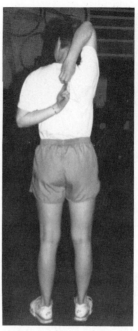

Fig. 9-20. Shoulder rotation: Bend left elbow and walk hand as high up the back as possible. Reach right arm overhead. Attempt to clasp hands behind back. Do not allow ribs to jut forward. A towel may be used if fingers do not touch.

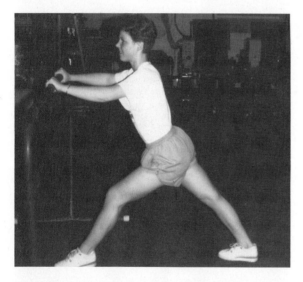

Fig. 9-19. Calf stretch against bar: Stand facing wall with feet approximately 3 feet from bar (or wall). Place hands on wall. Step one foot forward into a lunge position. Lean body toward wall. Keep back heel down and pelvis in neutral.

STRENGTHENING EXERCISES

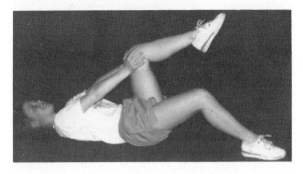

Fig. 9-21. Lower isometric abdominals: Lying on back, flatten lower back on surface. Hold this position while lifting knee up and pushing down on this knee with both hands. Hold this position isometrically. Alternate with opposite leg.

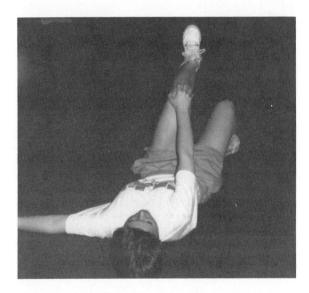

Fig. 9-22. Upper isometric abdominals: Lying on back, both knees bent with feet flat on surface, cross arms on chest to flatten lower back on surface. Hold this position while curling up, bringing one shoulder toward the opposite knee; alternate with opposite side.

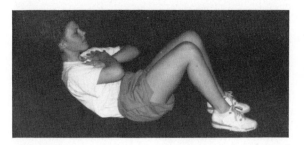

Fig. 9-23. Partial sit-ups: Lying on back, both knees bent with feet flat on surface, cross arms on chest. Curl up, bringing elbows toward thigh, until shoulders are slightly off surface. Exercise can also be performed with hips and knees at 90 degrees. Exhale while curling up, and inhale while returning to starting position.

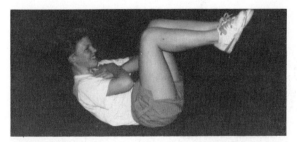

Fig. 9-24. Crunch sit-up: Lying on back, both knees bent with hands grasped behind head, point elbows outward. Keeping low back flat on surface, curl up, keeping elbows pointing outward and moving upper body as a unit until shoulders are slightly off surface. Exercise can also be performed with hips and knees at 90 degrees. Exhale while curling up, and inhale when returning to starting position.

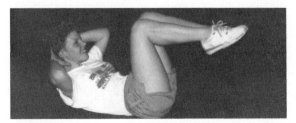

Fig. 9-25. Eccentric sit-up: From the top position of a sit-up, slowly lower upper body to the floor. For more resistance, have a partner provide resistance for the return to the floor.

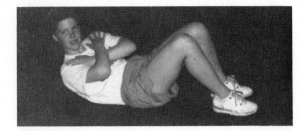

Fig. 9-26. Oblique crunch sit-up: Lying on back, bend both knees with hands grasped behind head and elbows pointing outward. Keeping low back flat on the surface, curl up, keeping elbows pointing outward until shoulders are slightly off the surface. At this point rotate upper body so that right elbow is pointing to left knee. Repeat to opposite side. Exercise can also be performed with hips and knees at 90 degrees. Exhale while curling up, and inhale when returning to starting position.

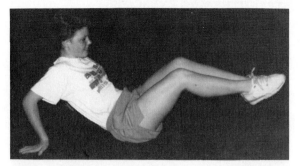

Fig. 9-28. Hip crunch: Sit at 45-degree angle with knees bent, and brace weight on hands behind the hips. Lift feet off the floor and draw the knees toward the chest. This exercise can also be performed off the end of a bench or table so that the trunk muscles can be worked through a greater range of motion.

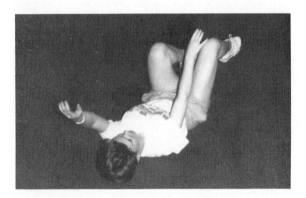

Fig. 9-27. Supine arm-leg bicycling: Lying on back with knees and hips at a 90-degree angle, point arms straight up. Move right knee and arm in a forward direction, while moving left knee and arm in a backward direction, repeating cycle. Keep arms and legs in line, and back flat on the floor.

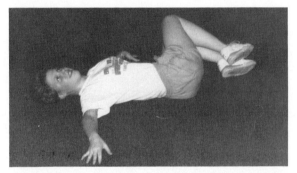

Fig. 9-29. 90-Degree hip rotation: Lying on back, with both knees bent, bring knees toward chest so that hips are at a 90-degree position. Keep knees together and let legs and hips rotate to one side. Keep shoulders flat on floor. Repeat to opposite side. This exercise can also be performed with legs kept straight.

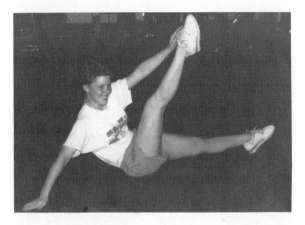

Fig. 9-30. Alternate toe touch (spread eagle): Lying on back with arms straight overhead, begin the movement by raising the torso and right leg at the same time. Touch the right hand to the left leg and return to starting position. Repeat exercise with opposite hand and leg.

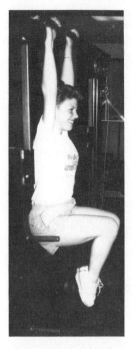

Fig. 9-31. Hanging leg raise: Hanging from pull-up bar or stall bar with knees bent, raise knees toward chest. This exercise can also be performed with legs straight.

TRUNK EXTENSOR LIFTS

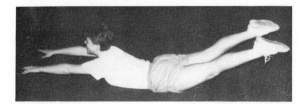

Fig. 9-32. Single arm-leg lift: Lying on stomach, straighten both arms in front of body. Lift one arm and opposite leg off surface about 2 inches. Hold. Repeat with opposite arm and leg.

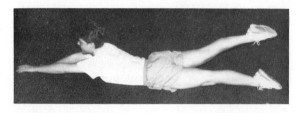

Fig. 9-33. Double arm-leg lift: Lying on stomach, straighten both arms in front of body. Lift both arms and legs off surface about 2 inches. Hold and return to starting position.

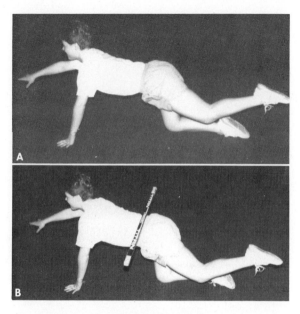

Fig. 9-34. Kneeling opposite arm-leg lift: Get on hands and knees and place knees a hip-width apart. Maintaining the neutral position, straighten one arm in front of body and opposite leg behind body. Hold. Repeat with opposite arm and leg. **A,** A stick can be placed across low back to help monitor maintaining a neutral position. **B,** Add ankle and wrist weights as strength increases.

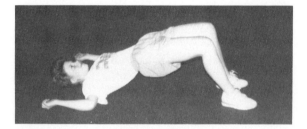

Fig. 9-35. Bridge up: Lying on back, bend knees with feet flat on the surface. Tighten buttocks and abdominals. Lift hips up until the back starts to arch and then return to starting position.

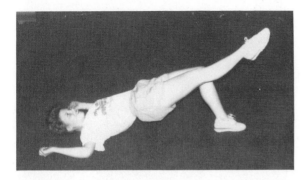

Fig. 9-36. Bridge up with leg raise: Lying on back, bend knees with feet flat on the surface. Tighten buttocks and abdominals. Keeping the neutral position, lift hips off the surface until the back starts to arch. While holding this position, lift right leg off floor straight out in front of body. Repeat, using left leg.

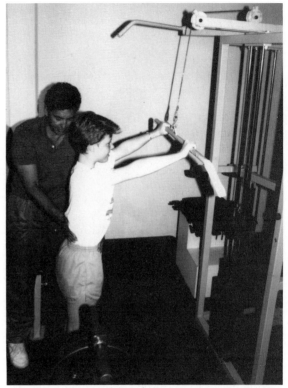

Fig. 9-38. Straight arm pull down: Stand erect with feet a shoulder-width apart. Grasp the bar of the lat machine with a palms-down grip. Keeping the arms straight, pull the bar toward the thigh and return to starting position. Maintain trunk stability while performing entire exercise.

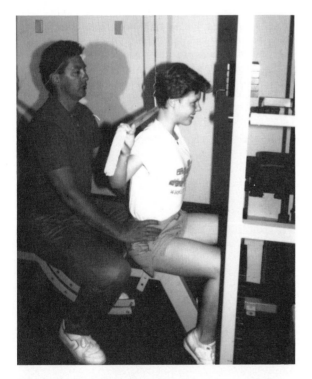

Fig. 9-37. Lat pull down: Start in a kneeling or seated position on a stool. Grasp the bar in a wide palms-down grip with the arms fully extended. Pull the bar down until it touches the base of the neck and then return to the starting position to complete the repetition. The same action can be utilized by pulling the bar in front of the chest.

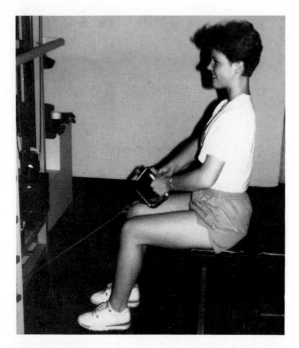

Fig. 9-39. Sitting upright rows: Sitting on bench or stool, grasp bar or cables with arms straight. Feet are supported against machine. Keep back in a neutral position while pulling weight up and toward the body by bending elbows. Return to starting position.

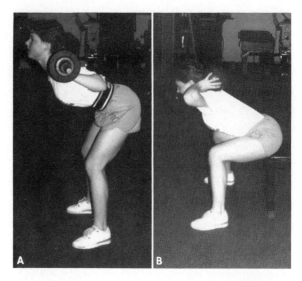

Fig. 9-41 Good mornings: Start with bar behind the neck and resting on the shoulders. Feet are a shoulder-width apart with the legs straight. Bend forward at the waist until the upper torso is parallel with the floor and then return to starting position. Keep the head up and maintain a neutral position. Do not jerk to assist the movement. Exhale while lowering and inhale while raising. Exercise can also be performed in a sitting position.

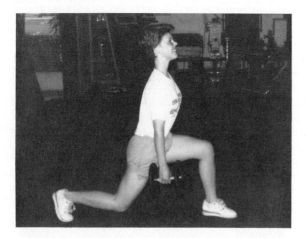

Fig. 9-40. Split squats: Standing with feet a shoulder-width apart, step right foot behind left. Lower buttocks until the left knee is parallel to the floor, pause, and return to starting position. Keep head up slightly and maintain trunk stabilization position.

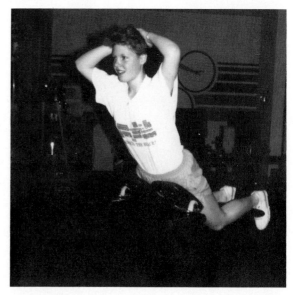

Fig. 9-42. Glut-back extension: Using back extension machine or table with feet and legs supported, allow trunk to drop in a slightly flexed position. Raise trunk into slightly hyperextended position. Return to starting position.

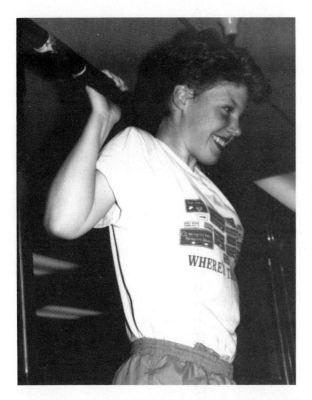

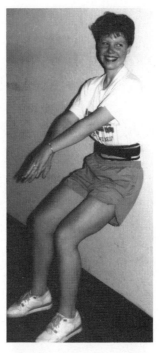

Fig. 9-43. Pull-ups behind the neck: Grasp a pull-up bar with a double overhand grip, slightly wider than shoulder width. Pull body upward, finishing the movement so the bar is positioned behind neck. Slowly lower to starting position and repeat.

Fig. 9-44. Wall sits: Stand with back towards wall. Keeping back against wall, slowly lower yourself until the knees are between 70 and 90 degrees. Hold position and return to starting position.

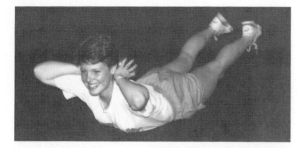

Fig. 9-45. Prone raise: Lying on stomach with ball positioned behind the head, arch back up from floor surface. Hold briefly and lower body to floor surface.

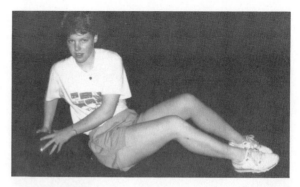

Fig. 9-47. Sitting rotation: Sitting with legs straight out in front of body, place ball behind center of back. Rotate the trunk to the left, using hands grasp the ball, lift and rotate in the opposite direction, and place ball behind center of back. Repeat in opposite direction.

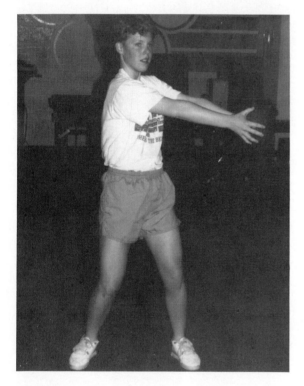

Fig. 9-46. Trunk twister: Standing with feet a shoulder-width apart, ball held directly in front of chest with arms straight. Move ball in a side-to-side fashion with arms straight. Hips should remain facing forward, and twisting motion should occur in the trunk only.

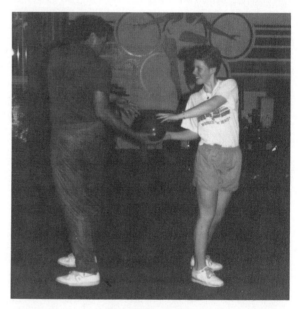

Fig. 9-48. Back-to-back pass: Stand with back to partner. Ball is positioned in front of waist. Rotate the trunk and ball to the left and pass the ball to partner. Twist in opposite direction to receive the ball from partner on the opposite side.

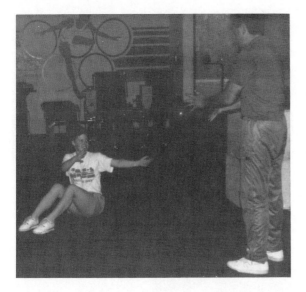

Fig. 9-49. Lateral toss: Sit on the floor with knees bent, feet flat on floor, and partner standing at a diagonal and slightly in front. The ball is rotated from side to side and then tossed up to the standing partner. Exercise can also be done using a double-pump movement prior to tossing the ball.

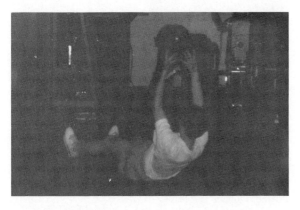

Fig. 9-50. Overhead toss (sitting): Sitting with legs straight in front of body. Partner is standing behind you. Ball held directly in front of chest with arms straight. Keeping arms straight, arch back and throw the ball overhead to partner. Ball can then be rolled on the floor for the return.

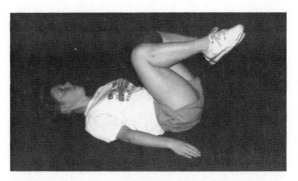

Fig. 9-51. Reverse sit-up: Lying on floor with knees bent, and hold the ball between the knees. Keeping the back flat against the floor, pull knees toward chest and return feet to floor. Exercise can also be performed by pulling the knees on a diagonal toward one shoulder and then repeating to the opposite side.

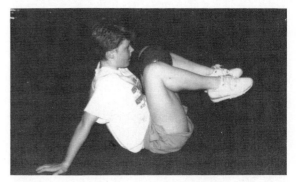

Fig. 9-52. Hip crunch: Sit at a 45-degree angle and brace weight on hands behind hips. Squeezing the ball between knees, lift feet off the floor and draw knees toward the chest. This exercise can also be performed off the end of a bench or table so that the ball can be moved through a longer range of motion.

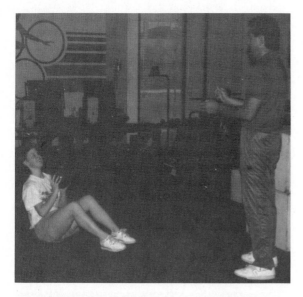

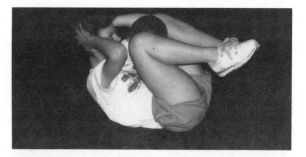

Fig. 9-55. Sit-up crunches: Lying on back, bring knees up to 90 degrees, squeezing the ball between the knees at all times. From this position place the hands behind the head and lift the shoulders up from the floor. Bend head toward chest before starting to avoid jerking off floor. Maintain neutral position.

Fig. 9-53. Sit-up pass: Lying on back with knees bent and ball positioned directly on chest, sit up and push ball off chest in high arching manner toward partner. Partner throws ball back, and the procedure is repeated.

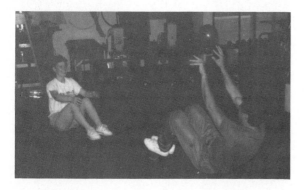

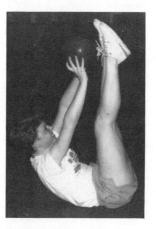

Fig. 9-54. Rocker pass: Sit up with knees bent and ball held directly overhead with arms straight. Partner assumes same position. Rock backward until ball touches floor surface. Use the weight and momentum of the legs to pull body into an upright position and throw the ball to partner.

Fig. 9-56. Seated toe touch: Lying on back, hold medicine ball with both hands. Raise legs straight up in the air and maintain this position. Reach up with the medicine ball and touch the toes. Return to starting position and repeat movement.

SUMMARY

1. Because of the complexity of spinal motion, the sports therapist must be capable of performing a detailed and comprehensive evaluation of low back pain.
2. Hands-on techniques of manual therapy, including nonthrust, thrust, and distraction techniques, have become an increasingly popular treatment for lumbosacral problems.
3. Therapeutic modalities may be effectively used in the treatment of low back pain.
4. Massage techniques are used both to relax tissue tension and to produce an increase in circulation in the injured area.
5. The therapeutic purpose of low back exercise is to relieve pain, regain range of motion, and strengthen muscles to restore functional capacity.
6. The most common low back injuries in the athlete are lumbosacral sprains and strains.
7. Stress fractures in the low back require at least 3 months of rest along with manual therapy.
8. Treatment of spondylolisthesis and spondylolysis involves the use of modalities for pain and stabilization exercises.
9. Disk problems are treated by manual therapy techniques along with modalities for controlling pain.
10. Idiopathic back pain occurs from some unknown origin and is best treated by determining the causes of the pain and then identifying the appropriate postural exercises.
11. Treatment protocols for dealing with low back pain should be based on the traditional stages of healing and include stretching and strengthening exercises.

REFERENCES

1 Adams M and Hutton W: The effect of posture on the lumbar spine, J Bone Joint Surg (Br) 67(4):625–629, 1985.
2 Bach DK and others: A comparison of muscular tightness in runners and nonrunners and the relation of muscular tightness to low back pain in runners, JOSPT 6:315–323, 1985.
3 Bartelink D: The role of abdominal pressure in relieving the pressure of the lumbar intervertebral discs, J Bone Joint Surg (Br) 39(4):718–725, 1957.
4 Belitsky RB, Odam S, and Hubley-Kozey C: Evaluation of the effectiveness of wet ice, dry ice and cryogen packs in reducing skin temperature, Phys Ther 67:1080–1084, 1987.

5 Biering-Sorensen F: Physical measurements as risk indicators for low-back trouble over a one-year period, Spine 9(2):106, 1983.
6 Bohannon R and Gajdosek R: Spinal nerve root compression—some clinical implications, Phys Ther 67(3):376–382, 1987.
7 Bosacco S and Berman A: Surgical management of lumbar disc disease, Radiol Clin North Am 21(2):377–393, 1983.
8 Brady DM: Running injuries: prevention and management, Clin Symp 39(3):2, 1987.
9 Caillet R: Low back pain syndrome, ed 2, Philadelphia, 1968, FA Davis Co.
10 Cannon SR and James SE: Back pain in athletes, Br J Sports Med 18(3):159–164, 1984.
11 Cappozzo A: Force actions in the human trunk during running, J Sports Med 23:14–21, 1983.
12 Choudbury AR and Taylor JC: Cauda equina syndrome in lumbar disc disease, Acta Ortho Scand 51:493–499, 1980.
13 Chrisman D, Mittnacht A, and Snook G: A study of the results following rotatory manipulation in the lumbar intervertebral-disc syndrome, J Bone Joint Surg (Am) 46(3):517–524, 1964.
14 Chusid J: Correlative neuroanatomy and functional neurology, Los Altos, Calif, 1970, Lange Medical Publications.
15 Cibulka M, Delitto A, and Kaldehoff R: Changes in innominate tilt after manipulation of the sacroiliac joint in patients with low back pain, Phys Ther 68(9):1359–1363, 1988.
16 Cummings G and Crowell R: Source of error in clinical assessment of innominate rotation, Phys Ther 68(1):77–78, 1988.
17 Cyriax J and Russell G: Textbook of orthopedic medicine, vol 2, ed 9, Baltimore, 1977, Williams & Wilkins.
18 Daniels L, Williams M, and Worthingham C: Muscle testing: techniques of manual examinations, Philadelphia, 1960, WB Saunders Co.
19 Davis P: Posture of the trunk during the lifting of weights, Br Med J 1:87–89, 1959.
20 Day J, Mason R, and Chesrown S: Effect of massage on serum level of B-endorphin and B-lipotropin in healthy adults, Phys Ther 67:926–930, 1987.
21 DiFabio R: Clinical assessment of manipulation and mobilization of the lumbar spine, Phys Ther 66(1):51–54, 1986.
22 Dixon A: Diagnosis of low back pain—sorting the complainers. In Jayson M, editor: The lumbar spine and back pain, New York, 1976, Grune & Stratton, Inc.
23 DonTigny R: Dysfunction of the sacroiliac joint and its treatment, JOSPT 1(1):23–35, 1979.
24 DonTigny R: Function and pathomechanics of the sacroiliac joint, Phys Ther 65(1):35–44, 1985.
25 Dorwart RH, Vogler JB, and Helms CA: Spinal stenosis, Radiol Clin North Am 21(2):301–317, 1983.
26 Erhard R and Bowling R: The recognition and management of the pelvic component of lowback and sciatic pain, Bull Ortho Section, APTA 2(3):4–15, 1977.

27 Farfan H and others: The effects of tension on the intervertebral joint: the role of torsion in the production of disc dysfunction, J Bone Joint Surg (Am) 52:468, 1970.

28 Ferguson R, McMaster JH, and Stanitski CL: Low back pain in college football linemen, J Sports Med 2(2):63–69, 1974.

29 Fredrickson BE and others: The natural history of spondylolysis and spondylolisthesis, J Bone Joint Surg (Am) 66(5):699–707, 1984.

30 Garrick JG: Characterization of the patient population in a sports medicine facility, Physician Sports Med 13(10):73–75, 1985.

31 Gelabert R: Dancers spinal syndromes, JOSPT 7(4):180–191, 1986.

32 Gersh MR and Wolf SL: Applications of transcutaneous electrical nerve stimulation in the management of patients with pain, Phys Ther 6(3):314–336, 1988.

33 Gonzalez E and others: Lumbar spinal stenosis: analysis of pre- and postoperative somatosensory evoked potentials, Arch Phys Med Rehabil 16:11, 1985.

34 Goss CM: Gray's Anatomy, Philadelphia, 1970, Lea & Febiger.

35 Gould JA: The spine. In Gould JA and Davis GJ, editors: Orthopaedic and sports physical therapy, St Louis, 1985, The CV Mosby Co.

36 Gracovetsky S: The resting spine: a conceptual approach to the avoidance of spinal reinjury during rest, Phys Ther 67(4):549–553, 1987.

37 Gracovetsky S and Farfan H: The optimum spine, Spine 11(6):543–572, 1986.

38 Grieve GP: Mobilization of the spine, ed 3, London, 1980, Churchill Livingstone Inc.

39 Grimsby O: Fundamentals of manual therapy: a course workbook, ed 4, Vagsvygd, Norway, 1985, Sorlandets Fysikalski Institutt.

40 Haldeman S: Spinal manipulative therapy, Clin Orth Related Research 179:62–70, 1983.

41 Haldeman S: Spinal manipulative therapy in sports medicine, Clin Sports Med 5(2):277–291, 1986.

42 Haughton V and others: A prospective comparison of computed tomography and myelography in the diagnosis of herniated lumbar discs, Neuroradiology 142:103–110, 1982.

43 Herkowitz H and Samberg L: Vertebral column injuries associated with tobogganing, J Trauma 18:806–810, 1978.

44 Hoppenfield S: Physical examination of the spine and extremities, New York, 1976, Appleton-Century-Crofts.

45 Hoshina H: Spondylosis in athletes, Physician Sports Med 8:75–79, 1980.

46 Howell D: Musculoskeletal profile and incidence of musculoskeletal injuries in lightweight rowers, Am J Sports Med 12(4):278–281, 1984.

47 Hughston JC and others: Classification of knee ligament instabilities. Part II. The lateral compartment, J Bone Joint Surg 58(2):173–179, 1976.

48 Jackson CP and Brown MD: Analysis of current approaches and a practical guide to prescription of exercise, Clin Orth Related Research 179:46–52, 1983.

49 Jackson CP and Brown MD: Is there a role for exercise in the treatment of patients with low back pain? Clin Orth Related Research 19:39–45, 1983.

50 Jackson D, Rettig O, and Wiltse L: Epidural cortisone injections in the young athletic adult, Am J Sports Med 8(4):239–243, 1980.

51 Jackson DW and others: Stress reactions involving the pars interarticularis in young athletes, Am J Sports Med 9(5):304, 1981.

52 Jorgensen K and Nicolarsen T: Two methods for determining trunk extensor endurance, Eur J Appl Physiol 55:639–644, 1986.

53 Kane R and others: Manipulating the patient: a comparison of the effectiveness of physician and chiropractor care, Lancet 2:1333–1336, 1974.

54 Kapandji IA: The physiology of the joints, ed 8, London, 1982, Churchill Livingstone, Inc.

55 Kelsey J and White A: An epidemiology and impact of low back pain, Spine 10:133–141, 1985.

56 Kirkaldy-Willis WA and Hill RJ: A more precise diagnosis for low back pain, Spine 4(2):102–109, 1979.

57 Knutsson F: The instability associated with disc degeneration in the lumbar spine, Acta Radiol 25:594–608, 1944.

58 Lee CK: The use of exercise and muscle testing in the rehabilitation of spinal disorders, Clin Sports Med 5(2):271–277, 1986.

59 Leff DN: What's new for low back pain and just plain pain, Med World News reprint, June 29, 1980.

60 Liehman W, Snodgrass LB, and Sharpe GL: Unsolved controversies in back management—a review, JOSPT 9(7):239–244, 1988.

61 Luttgren K and Wells K: Kinesiology and scientific basis of human motion, New York, 1982, CBS College Publishing.

62 McKenzie RA: The lumbar spine: mechanical diagnosis and therapy, Waikanae, New Zealand, 1984, Spinal Publications.

63 Maitland GD: Vertebral manipulation, ed 5, London, 1986, Butterworths.

64 Mennell J: The therapeutic use of cold, JAOA 74:81–93, 1975.

65 Mennell J and Zohn OA: Musculoskeletal pain: diagnosis and physical treatment, Boston, 1976, Little, Brown & Co Inc.

66 Micheli LJ, Hall JC, and Miller ME: Use of modified Boston Brace for back injuries in athletes, Am J Sports Med 8:351–356, 1980.

67 Moffett JA and others: A controlled, prospective study to evaluate the effectiveness of a back school in the relief of chronic low back pain, Spine 11(2):121–122, 1986.

68 Mooney V: The syndromes of low back disease, Orthop Clin North Am 14(3):505–515, 1983.

69 Mooney V and Robertson J: The facet syndrome, Clin Orthop 115:149–156, 1976.

70 Morris A: Program compliance key to preventing low back injuries, Occup Health Safety 53:44–46, 1984.

71 Morris JM, Benner G, and Lucas DB: An electromyographic study of the intrinsic muscles of the back in man,

J Anat Lond 96(4):509–520, 1962.

72 Morris JM, Lucas DB, and Bresler B: Role of the trunk in stability of the spine, J Bone Joint Surg (Am) 43(3):327–347, 1961.

73 Nachemson A: The influence of spinal movements on the lumbar intradiscal pressure on the tensile stresses in the annular fibrosus, Acta Ortho Scand 33:183–207, 1963.

74 Nachemson A: Towards a better understanding of low-back pain: a review of the mechanics of the lumbar disc, Rheumatol Rehabil 14(129):129–140, 1975.

75 Nachemson A, Andersson G, and Schultz A: Valsalva maneuver biomechanics. Effects on lumbar trunk loads of elevated intra-abdominal pressures, Spine 11(5):476–478, 1986.

76 O'Donoghue D: Treatment of injuries to athletes, Philadelphia, 1976, WB Saunders Co.

77 Panjabi MM and White AA: Biomechanics of the spine, Neurosurgery 7(1):76–93, 1980.

78 Paris SV: Course notes: introduction to evaluation and manipulation of the spine, Atlanta, 1979, Institute Press.

79 Paris SV: Mobilization of the spine, Phys Ther 8:988–995, 1979.

80 Paris SV: Spinal manipulative therapy, Clin Orth Related Research 179:55–61, 1983.

81 Paris SV: Anatomy as related to function and pain, Ortho Clin North Am 14(3):475–489, 1983.

82 Paris SV: Physical signs of instability, Spine 10(3):277–279, 1985.

83 Paris SV: Course notes: introduction to evaluation and manipulation of the spine, ed 7, Atlanta, 1986, Institute Press.

84 Ponte DJ, Jensen GJ, and Kent BE: A preliminary report on the use of the McKenzie protocol versus Williams protocol in the treatment of low back pain, JOSPT 6(2):130–139, 1984.

85 Porterfield JA: The sacro-iliac joint. In Gould JA and Davies GJ, editors: Orthopaedic and sports physical therapy, ed 1, St Louis, 1985, The CV Mosby Co.

86 Prentice W: Therapeutic modalities for sports medicine, St Louis, 1990, Times Mirror/Mosby College Publishing.

87 Quillen WS: Phonophoresis: a review of the literature and technique, Ath Train 15:109–110, 1980.

88 Rowe M: Low back pain in industry: a position paper, J Occup Med 11:161–169, 1979.

89 Roy S and Irvin R: Sports medicine: prevention, evaluation, management, and rehabilitation, Englewood Cliffs, NJ, 1983, Prentice-Hall.

90 Saal JA: Diagnostic decision making. Paper presented at Lumbar Spine State of the Art '88, San Francisco, Dec 9–10, 1988.

91 Santiesteban AJ: The role of physical agents in the treatment of spine pain, Clin Orth Related Research 179:24–30, 1983.

92 Sarno JE: Therapeutic exercise for back pain. In Basmajian JV, editor: Therapeutic exercise, ed 4, Baltimore, 1984, Williams & Wilkins.

93 Saunders D: Unilateral lumbar traction, Phys Ther 61(2):221–224, 1981.

94 Saunders D: Use of spinal traction in the treatment of neck and back conditions, Clin Orth Related Research 19:31–38, 1983.

95 Saunders D: Evaluation of a musculoskeletal disorder. In Gould JA and Davies GJ, editors: Orthopaedic and sports physical therapy, St Louis, 1985, The CV Mosby Co.

96 Sawyer M and Zbieranek C: The treatment of soft tissue after spinal injury, Clin Sports Med 5(2):387–405, 1986.

97 Schultz A and others: Loads on the lumbar spine, J Bone Joint Surg 64(5):713–720, 1982.

98 Selby K and Paris S: Anatomy of facet joints and its clinical correlation with low back pain, Contemporary Ortho 3(12):312–318, 1981.

99 Sikorski JM: A rationalized approach to physiotherapy for low-back pain, Spine 10(6):571–579, 1984.

100 Stamford B: Using cold for sports injuries, Physician Sports Med 13(1):148, 1985.

101 Travell JG and Simons DG: Myofascial pain and dysfunction: the trigger point manual, Baltimore, 1983, Williams & Wilkins.

102 Troup J: Experimental investigation into the physical properties of the intervertebral disc, J Bone Joint Surg (Br) 33:607, 1976.

103 Waddell S and others: Failed lumbar disc surgery and repeat surgery following industrial injuries, J Bone Joint Surg (Am) 61:201–207.

104 Weinstein JN: The pain receptor system. Paper presented at Lumbar Spine State of the Art '88, San Francisco, Dec 9–10, 1988.

105 Weisz GM and Lee P: Spinal canal stenosis, Clin Orth Related Research 179:134–140, 1983.

106 White A and Gordon S: Synopsis: workshop on idiopathic low-back pain, Spine 7(2):141–149, 1982.

107 Williams P: Examination and conservative treatment for disc lesions of the lower spine, Clin Orthop 5:28–40, 1955.

108 Wiltse L: The etiology of spondylolisthesis, J Bone Joint Surg (Am) 44(3):539–559, 1962.

109 Witt I: Vestergaard A and Rosenklint A: A comparative analysis of x-ray findings of the lumbar spine in patients with and without lumbar pain, Spine 9(3):298–299, 1984.

110 Wolf SL and others: Normative data on low back mobility and activity levels, Am J Phys Med 58(5):217-228, 1979.

111 Wroble RR and Albright JP: Neck and low back injuries in wrestling, Clin Sports Med 5(2):295–303, 1986.

112 Wyke B: Neurological aspects of low back pain. In Jayson M, editor: The lumbar spine and back pain, ed 1, New York, 1976, Grune & Stratton, Inc.

113 Yong-Hing K and Kirkaldy-Willis WH: The pathophysiology of degenerative disease of the lumbar spine, Orthop Clin North Am 14(3):491–504, 1983.

Rehabilitation of Shoulder Injuries

10

Gregory Ott

OBJECTIVES

Following completion of this chapter, the student will be able to:

- Discuss the functional interrelationships among the glenohumeral, scapulo-thoracic, suprahumeral, and clavicular joint mechanisms that are critical for providing full functional range of motion.

- Discuss how pathological conditions of any one of these mechanisms disturbs upper limb function.

- Discuss ligamentous and articular structures of the shoulder complex and their importance in maintaining joint relationships.

- Describe the shoulder complex and its importance for proximal stability for distal mobility.

- Discuss the interrelationships between shoulder complex anatomy and bio-mechanics and how they affect the rehabilitation programs.

- Briefly describe surgical techniques for third-degree shoulder dislocations and acromioclavicular joint separations.

- Outline rehabilitation programs for shoulder complex injuries and discuss the rehabilitation in phase progression.

- Understand the importance of shoulder complex proprioception and normal kinesthesia.

- Outline functional return activities for shoulder pathologies.

- Understand the importance of isokinetic rehabilitation for the shoulder complex.

- Discuss treatment and rehabilitation protocols for specific injuries of the shoulder complex.

- Discuss clinical evaluation findings.

- Briefly discuss specific injuries and the pertinent anatomy of that pathology.

- Understand the concept of total arm strength and how it relates to total rehabilitation of the shoulder complex.

The shoulder girdle is a finely tuned combination of joints that work together in synchronous function. However, the intricacy of this structure, in combination with the versatile range of motions, makes the multijoint shoulder girdle vulnerable to injury (Fig. 10-1). A rehabilitation program of any shoulder injury must be specific to the individual components that, when integrated, result in maximal function of the entire shoulder complex. The program begins with the simplest of movements and progresses toward vigorous combined motions to restore strength, mobility, and the overall function of the shoulder complex and upper extremity.

Jobe[34-37] states that five principles are essential to understanding the shoulder mechanics. First, the shoulder joint is designed more for mobility than for stability. Second, the stability that exists comes from the soft tissue and the positioning of the components of the shoulder complex, particularly the very important scapula. Third, during motion a compromise occurs within the shoulder joint complex to balance the competing demands of stability and mobility. Fourth, the shoulder is not a single joint but a complex scapulothoracic, glenohumeral, acromioclavicular, and sternoclavicular combination of joints. Fifth, a completely rehabilitated shoulder is one that reaches the maximum range of 180 degrees elevation while exhibiting the strength and stability in the soft tissues necessary to meet its particular demands.

At the beginning of a rehabilitation program, rather than looking at the glenohumeral joint individually, the motion of each joint must be assessed. Thus, understanding the interrelation of the components of the shoulder complex is imperative in total shoulder rehabilitation.

As compared to many joints in the body, rehabilitation of the shoulder is extremely important to the successful management of return to normal function for the entire extremity. It is probably the most difficult joint in the body to rehabilitate because of its great range of motion and the complex interaction of muscle functions.

Both the patient and the sports therapist must first understand the goals of rehabilitation:

1. Return of full, unrestricted range of motion
2. Normal strength and function
3. Elimination of pain

Throughout the rehabilitation program, the sports therapist continually needs to explain and reinforce these goals to give the athlete reassurance and confidence. The course of rehabilitation has to consist of a precise and limited number of exercises that are easily understood to avoid confusion, promote total compliance, and lead to a successful outcome. Too many complicated and confusing experiences have a detrimental effect on the total rehabilitation program.

REHABILITATION TECHNIQUES

Throughout this chapter, various protocols and exercise programs are outlined for specific shoulder pathologies. Too often, however, the sports therapist focuses solely on the injured joint and ignores the rest of the upper extremity and trunk musculature.

The concept of **total arm strength** (TAS) was developed as a result of the success seen with knee rehabilitation programs in which trunk, hip, and ankle strengthening and proprioception were incorporated.

Smith and Bronelli[59] support the importance of a total arm rehabilitation program, especially in the area of proprioception. These authors noted a marked decrease in proprioceptive abilities of the upper extremity following shoulder dislocations. With shoulder injuries, programs must not only focus on the shoulder joint but also include strengthening, flexibility, and proprioception of the trunk, elbow, wrist, and hand.

The following section outlines and describes the stretching techniques, strengthening exercises, and treatment protocols that are discussed with each phase of the specific rehabilitation programs.

I. STRETCHING TECHNIQUES FOR THE SHOULDER COMPLEX

Shoulder stretches are essential to the restoration of normal motion of the shoulder complex and efficient use of the musculature structure. These stretches should not cause a painful response but rather a stretching sensation. Each exercise should be held for 10 seconds and repeated 3 to 5 times 3 times a day.

A. Anterior shoulder stretch: Grab the door frame while facing the opposite direction. Pull the arm up as far behind as possible and extend to the

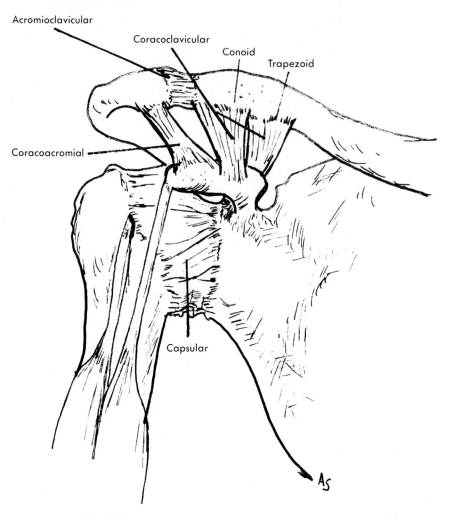

Fig. 10-1. Ligamentous structure of the shoulder complex.

point where a stretch is felt in the front of the shoulder. Then lean away from the door frame to increase the stretch.

B. Posterior shoulder stretch: Standing with arm parallel to the floor, bring the arm horizontally across the body. Using the opposite hand, grasp the elbow and continue to pull across the body until a stretch is felt in the upper back and shoulder.

C. Inferior shoulder stretch: Standing with arm extended overhead, grasp elbow with opposite hand, and pull extended arm behind head until a stretch is felt in the shoulder (Fig. 10-2).

D. Superior shoulder stretch: Reaching behind back with one hand, grasp the opposite arm at the wrist and pull downward while tilting head in the opposite direction to where a stretch is felt in the neck and upper shoulder.

E. Distraction stretch: Standing to the side of the door frame, grab the frame and lean in the opposite direction. A stretch should be felt as body weight separates the shoulder joint.

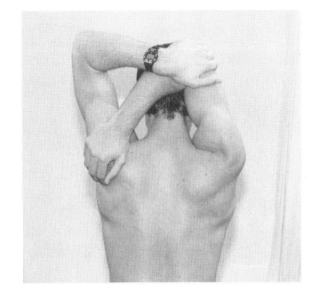

Fig. 10-2. Inferior capsule stretch.

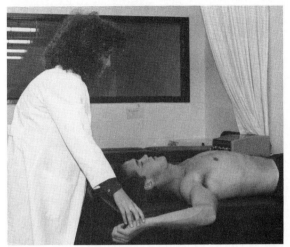

Fig. 10-3. Stretching of anterior capsule in supine position with arm abducted 90 degrees. Excellent stretch for anterior capsule and internal rotators.

F. Rotator cuff stretch at 90 degrees: The capsule around the shoulder joint needs to be stretched before maximum movement can be obtained. Begin these exercises on a table with the shoulder over the table edge and elbow bent to 90 degrees. Allow the weight of the arm to pull down gently in this position. A small weight may be added to increase pull if tolerated and with physician approval (Figs. 10-3 and 10-4).

G. Rotator cuff stretch with arm at 135 degrees: During static flexibility exercises, a particular position is held for a period of time. Static stretching is the best way to initiate a sequence. After stretching, a muscle can be gently moved through the range of motion. In this exercise, raising the arm another 45 degrees (total abduction 135 degrees) stretches more of the anterior musculature surrounding the shoulder.

H. Rotator cuff stretch with arm overhead: Finally, this exercise should be repeated with the arm as far overhead as possible, 180 degrees abduction. The head should remain

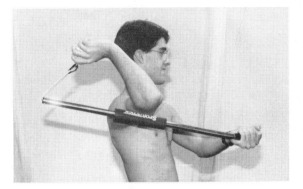

Fig. 10-4. Stretching of internal rotators with assistance of Sports-Stick.

supported while the shoulder itself is over the table edge. Again, just allow the weight of the arm to pull down gently.

II. SHOULDER JOINT MOBILIZATION
To increase movement of a restricted joint, most sports therapists believe that movement must be induced within the patient's available range of motion tolerance.[40] Indications for joint mobilization techniques include joint dysfunction from trauma or prolonged immobiliza-

tion and restriction of joint motion causing pain or restriction of motion during normal physical activity. General contraindications include bacterial infection, recent fracture, joint effusion, inflammation, rheumatoid arthritis, and internal derangement of the joint. Grade I and II techniques are performed to relieve pain and reduce muscle guarding. Specific mobilization techniques for the shoulder complex follow.[40]

A. Techniques for elevation and relaxation of the glenohumeral joint

1. Inferior glide with arm at athlete's side: The athlete is supine, with arm resting at side, and the sports therapist stabilizes the scapula with one hand, the web of the hand contacting the inferior aspect of the neck of glenoid while the other hand grasps the patient's forearm as proximal as possible. The scapula is held fixed while the humerus is moved inferior. Movement is performed initially with the patient's arm at side; as relaxation occurs, move patient's arm gradually toward abduction or flexion. *Note:* This technique is important for relaxation of spasm and relieving pain.

2. Distraction moving toward abduction (Fig. 10-5): The athlete is supine, with arm at side, and the sports therapist stabilizes the inferior neck of glenoid with one hand while the other hand grasps the athlete's humerus above the elbow on epicondyles. The sports therapist stands with body facing away from the athlete. With the scapula held stable, the humerus is moved distally along its long axis. As the athlete relaxes, arm may be gradually moved toward abduction. This movement may be performed up to 80 degrees abduction.

3. Inferior glide moving toward flexion: The athlete is supine, with arm flexed 60 to 100 degrees and

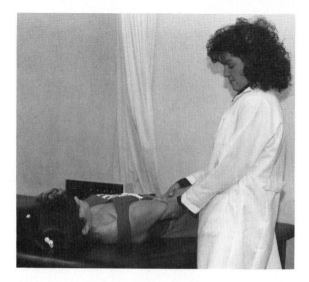

Fig. 10-5. Mobilization technique utilizing long axis distraction; excellent for increasing joint range of motion.

elbow bent. The sports therapist grasps the proximal humerus with both hands and pulls inferior to produce movement of flexion and inferior glide at glenohumeral joint.

4. Inferior glide in abduction: The athlete is supine, with elbow bent and arm abducted and externally rotated but comfortable. The sports therapist supports the elbow with left hand at distal humerus while right hand contacts the superior proximal humerus. Inferior glide of humeral head is produced, and the athlete relaxes. The arm can be gradually abducted. *Note:* This movement may be performed up to 90 degrees. This technique is used to increase abduction and allow stretching into abduction while avoiding impingement of the greater tuberosity on the acromial arch.

B. Techniques for internal rotation of the glenohumeral joint

1. Posterior glide with arm in 10 to

55 degrees abduction: The athlete is supine, with arm slightly abducted. The sports therapist supports the athlete's elbow with one hand while the other hand contacts the upper humerus anterior aspect. Posterior glide is produced by leaning forward slightly and flexing the knees to transmit the force through the straight arm. This technique is used to increase the joint play necessary for internal rotation and flexion.

2. Anterior glide with arm close to limits of internal rotation: The athlete is lying on uninvolved side with arm behind back close to the limits of internal rotation. The sports therapist, standing behind patient, grasps anteriorly with thumb pad of one hand to stabilize acromion and clavicle. The anterior glide is produced by leaning forward to transmit force through the thumbs. Internal rotation is gradually increased by progressively moving the patient's hand up the back. This movement stretches the posterior capsule into internal rotation and avoids posterior impingement of the humeral head on the glenoid labrum.

3. Internal rotation technique with arm close to 90 degrees abduction: The athlete is supine, with arm resting close to 90 degrees abduction and elbow bent 90 degrees and forearm pronated. The sports therapist supports the athlete's wrist with one hand, supports under elbow with finger of other hand on medial side, and positions the upper arm in front and medial to the shoulder. In the movement, the other arm provides enough counterpressure to the shoulder to prevent lifting of the shoulder girdle, the hand maintains the arm in abduction, and the other hand simultaneously rotates the arm internally.

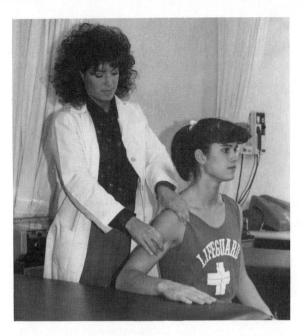

Fig. 10-6. Anterior glide of humerus with arm abducted, used to increase external rotation. Notice hand placement to stabilize scapula.

C. Techniques for external rotation of glenohumeral joint
  1. Anterior glide (Fig. 10-6): The athlete is supine, with arm at side. The sports therapist stabilizes with one hand by grasping the distal humerus just proximal to the elbow and grasps medially around posterior aspect of the humerus with other hand, as far proximal as possible. The anterior glide is effected after the slack in the shoulder girdle has been taken up. This movement is an oscillatory mobilization. This technique is used to increase joint play movement necessary for external rotation.
  2. Posterior glide with arm close to 90 degrees abduction: The athlete is supine, with arm abducted 90 degrees and elbow bent to 90 degrees. The sports therapist supports the athlete's wrist with one

hand and contacts the anterior aspect of the proximal humerus with the other hand. The posterior glide is produced by rotating the arm externally. This method stretches the anterior capsule into external rotation while avoiding anterior impingement of the humerus on the glenoid labrum.

D. Techniques for horizontal adduction and general capsular stretch of the glenohumeral joint

1. Lateral glide with arm at side (glenohumeral distraction): The athlete is supine, with arm at side, elbow bent, and hand resting on stomach. The sports therapist stabilizes with hand at the lateral aspect of the athlete's elbow while the other hand grasps humerus medially, as far proximally as possible. Lateral glide is effected by moving the upper humerus laterally. This technique is used to promote relaxation, relieve pain, and prepare for more vigorous stretching of the capsule.

2. Lateral glide in flexion: The athlete is supine, with arm flexed to 90 degrees. The sports therapist stabilizes the distal humerus with one hand while the other hand is placed against medial surface of the upper end of the humerus. The proximal humerus is moved laterally. This technique is used to restore joint play necessary for horizontal adduction.

Acromioclavicular, sternoclavicular, and scapulothoracic mobilizations may be performed; however, in most cases of glenohumeral tightness these accessory joints become hypermobile and thus contraindicate mobilization. Such mobilization may be needed following prolonged immobilization of the entire shoulder complex.[40]

III. RANGE-OF-MOTION EXERCISES FOR THE SHOULDER COMPLEX

The purpose of range-of-motion exercises is to restore or maintain the range of motion of the shoulder complex. All are done standing with both arms.

A. Warm-up exercises

1. Keeping elbows straight, raise arms forward and upward as far as possible.

2. Keeping elbows straight, take arms straight back as far as possible.

3. Keeping elbows straight and palms turned in, raise arms sideways until they reach shoulder level. At shoulder level, turn palms up and continue raising arms up to touch palms over the head. Keep elbows straight.

4. Bend elbows to 90-degree angles. Keep them tucked into sides and don't let them move. Keeping elbows at 90-degree angles, fold palms across abdomen. Then move hands away from body as far as possible, still keeping elbows tucked in tightly to sides.

B. Codman's pendulum exercises: This exercise is performed in a stooped position to eliminate the force of gravity. The athlete bends forward at the waist and supports the trunk by resting the uninjured hand on a stationary object. The injured arm should be under and perpendicular to the trunk. From this position shoulder flexion, extension, adduction, abduction, and circumduction can be executed. The desired motion is initiated by exerting a minimal muscular effort. Once the arm is in motion, the momentum of the moving limb should be enough to sustain the movement. All work is done within the limits of pain and fatigue. The athlete should start with no weight, but, as pain tolerance increases, the athlete can start with 2½ pounds. A maximum of 10 to 15 pounds should be enough for the purposes of this exercise. Initial movement arcs are small but gradually increase with patient tolerance. The patient should start slowly (10 movements) and strive for 25 to 30 movements in each direction as the goal for this exercise.

1. Position: Lean on unaffected arm, bend over at the waist with support from table, and let the injured arm hang straight down, loose, and relaxed.
   a. Start with small circles to the left and gradually increase in size.
   b. Reverse, and make circles to the right.
   c. Swing forward and backward (shoulder flexion and extension pattern).
   d. Swing arm from side to side in front of the body for shoulder horizontal abduction and adduction (Fig. 10-7).
C. Wall finger-walking exercises: This exercise is specifically designed to increase the range of motion in the shoulder complex. From an erect position and slightly closer than an arm's length from a wall, the athlete slowly "walks" the injured arm up the wall by using the fingers for locomotion. The athlete should attempt full range of motion without substituting by bending the trunk or shrugging the shoulders. This exercise should be done in flexion, abduction, and, if desired, horizontal adduction and abduction. A total of 20 to 25 "walks" in each direction should be the goal. A record of progress should be kept for this exercise.
   1. Stand facing wall and walk fingers up the wall and keep the elbow straight and the shoulders level. Limit motion to 135-degree shoulder flexion unless contraindicated by the pathology (for example, AC sprain).
   2. Stand with side to the wall and walk fingers up the wall. Keep elbow straight and shoulders level. Limit motion to 135-degree shoulder abduction, again, unless contraindicated (Fig. 10-8).
D. Pulley exercises: A reciprocal pulley system is ideal for these exercises. If not available, improvise with some

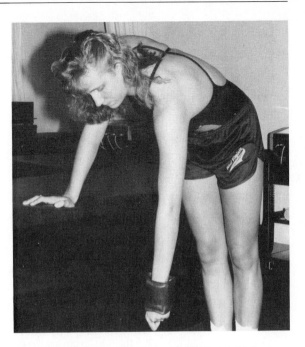

Fig. 10-7. Codman's exercises with light weight for gentle traction of glenohumeral joint.

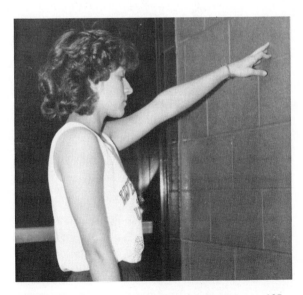

Fig. 10-8. Wall climbing in flexion. Limit motion to 135 degrees to decrease compression in suprahumeral space.

other method that accomplishes the purpose. In these exercises the athlete uses the help of the pulley system to reach a higher level of range of motion by assisting the injured arm through the last degrees of available motion. The athlete is in a seated position, and the exercises are performed in flexion and abduction. Assistance should be provided only after the arm is past shoulder level and the athlete is having difficulty raising the arm any further. The arm should be kept straight, and no substitution should be allowed by bending at the waist or at the elbow. The athlete should work within the limits of pain and strive for a goal of 20 to 25 movements in each direction.

E. Shoulder wheel exercises: The shoulder wheel reconditioning apparatus is useful in the rehabilitation of shoulder injuries. It consists of a metal wheel with an adjustable handle attached to one of the wheel's spokes. Resistance can be applied by tightening a wing nut in the center of the wheel. Before using this apparatus, adjust the wheel's center axis to the shoulder level of the patient and then adjust the handle to approximate the athlete's arm length. In one method of using a shoulder wheel, the athlete does circumduction exercises while facing the wheel and flexion and extension exercises while standing sideways to the wheel. In another method, the circumduction exercises are done while standing sideways to the wheel. No resistance should be applied to the wheel in the beginning but may later be added as the range of motion increases to a level equal to the uninjured shoulder. In early stages, with limited range of motion and weakness, 10 movements in each direction should be the initial goal. Later this figure may be increased to 20 to 25 movements in each direction.

F. Wand, cane, bilateral, or rifle exercises: These exercises are specifically designed to increase the range of motion in the painful shoulder complex. Using the opposite extremity as a guide, specific exercises are designed utilizing a wand, cane, or straight object to assist in increasing the range of motion of the injured shoulder complex (Fig. 10-9).

1. From a standing position, grasp bar with hands a shoulder width apart at mid-thigh level, the starting position for all exercises.

a. Start with bar at thighs, bring up to chest, extend arms straight out and back to chest, and return to thighs.

b. Start with bar at chest, extend arms straight out and back to chest, extend arms to overhead, and return to chest.

c. Start with bar at chest, extend arms up overhead, bring down behind neck to shoulders, extend arms up overhead, and return to chest.

d. Start with bar at chest, extend arms up overhead, front sweep low (keeping arms straight, bend at waist and touch toes), straighten up, and return to chest.

e. Twist: start with bar at thighs, while keeping left hand in place, bring right hand to left shoulder, and return to thigh; then reverse the procedure for the other arm.

f. Diagonal Lunge: start with bar at chest, step diagonally out with the right foot with body weight over that foot, extend arms straight out, bring back to chest, and return to upright position; then follow the same procedure with the left side.

IV. ISOMETRIC EXERCISES FOR THE SHOULDER COMPLEX

These exercises are simple yet highly effective. They can be done at home or in any setting. To be effective they must

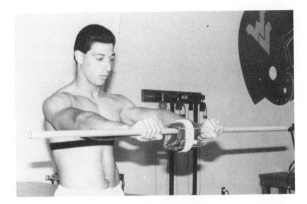

Fig. 10-9. Wand exercise with weight, used to increase range of motion and begin strengthening program.

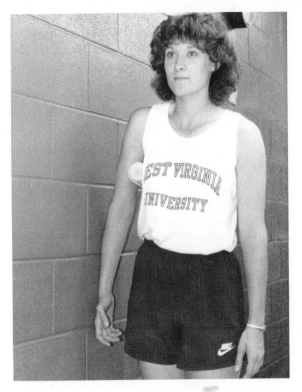

Fig. 10-10. Isometric exercise, with towel roll in axilla, initiates contraction of supraspinatus tendon and deltoid.

be done as instructed. These exercises will provide great benefits in restoring strength to the muscles that control and provide stability to the shoulder complex.

The exercise is done by a maximal contraction of the particular muscle without pain, holding the maximal contraction for a 10-second count, and relaxing; then the contraction-relaxation cycle is repeated. A maximal contraction should be achieved over 2 to 3 seconds rather than as a sudden onset of muscular effort. Likewise, the relaxation should occur in the same fashion. The total time should be 14 to 16 seconds per cycle.

A. Side raises: Standing with affected arm against the wall and the elbow straight, push the arm out to the side against the wall. Hold this position for 10 seconds (Fig. 10-10).

B. Rotations: In a doorway face the open doorjamb. The elbow is bent and kept at the side, with a small towel roll between arm and trunk.
   1. Pull to stomach: Attempt to pull the hand toward the stomach. Hold this position for 10 seconds and then relax. Repeat 10 times, 3 times a day.
   2. Push out to side: Push the hand away from the stomach. Hold this for 10 seconds and relax. Repeat 10 times, 3 times a day. Remem-

ber to keep elbow tucked into the side; the elbow acts as a hinge. It shouldn't move away from the side.

C. Forward raise: Stand facing the wall with arm straight and hand in contact with the wall. Attempt to lift arm forward by pushing against the wall. Hold this position for 10 seconds and relax; then repeat 10 times, 3 times a day.

D. Backward raise: With back to wall and arm straight, attempt to raise arm backward by pushing hand against wall. Hold this position for 10 seconds and relax; then repeat 10 times, 3 times per day.

E. Elbow flexion: Starting with elbow at side bent 90 degrees and palm up, place the noninvolved hand on the wrist of the involved arm. Attempt to bend elbow upward. Push for 10 seconds and relax. Repeat 10 times, 3 times per day.

F. Elbow extension: Starting with elbow at side, bent 90 degrees, and palm vertical, place the noninvolved hand under the involved hand. Attempt to straighten elbow by pushing downward. Push for 10 seconds and relax. Repeat 10 times, 3 times per day.

V. SURGICAL TUBING OR THERA-BAND EXERCISES

These exercises are designed to utilize surgical tubing or Thera-Band as a means of providing resistance to various exercise motions. Each exercise is to be performed much like free weight or weight equipment; that is, the body part should be moved against the resistance provided by the tubing to its maximum point in the range of motion, held for a count, and then returned with a 4 count back to the starting position. In order to increase the resistance, simply shorten the length of the tubing; do the opposite to decrease the resistance. Remember that the body part should not be worked through the painful range of motion and that the tension should be decreased to allow for painless motion.

A. Internal rotation: Keeping arm stabilized, with a small towel roll between chest wall and upper arm, bend elbow 90 degrees and pull tubing straight across body. (Make sure tubing is securely fastened at opposite end.) Do three sets, 10 repetitions, 3 times a day (Fig. 10-11).

B. External rotation: Keeping arm stabilized, with towel roll against chest and elbow bent 90 degrees, pull tubing away from body. Do three sets, 10 repetitions, 3 times a day (Figs. 10-12 and 10-13).

C. Flexion: With arm at side, grip tubing, secure opposite end around foot, and, keeping elbow straight, pull tubing straight in front of body to shoulder level. Do three sets, 10 repetitions, 3 times a day (Fig. 10-14).

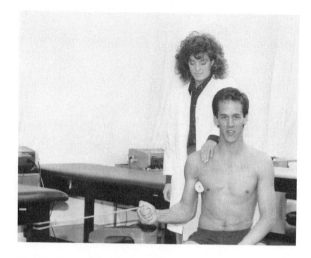

Fig. 10-11. Position for internal rotation exercises with surgical tubing. A small towel roll is used to abduct the arm 10 to 15 degrees to protect the critical zone.

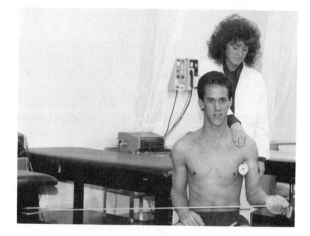

Fig. 10-12. External rotation with tubing. Initially the sports therapist may stabilize scapula with hand to assure joint stability.

D. Extension: With arm at side, grip tubing, secure opposite end, and, keeping elbow straight, pull tubing straight behind body. Do three sets, 10 repetitions, 3 times a day.

E. Horizontal adduction: With arm forward from side 90 degrees, keep elbow straight and pull tubing across

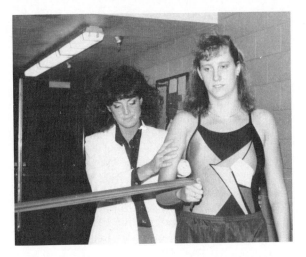

Fig. 10-13. Rotations using Thera-Band for resistance.

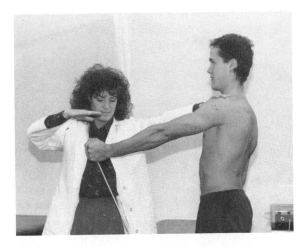

Fig. 10-14. Forward flexion exercise with surgical tubing to a position of 90 degrees, which will minimize joint impingement.

body. Do three sets, 10 repetitions, 3 times a day.

F. Empty can raises: Grip tubing with thumb pointed down and secure opposite end around foot. Bring arm 30 degrees forward from side. Keep elbow straight and raise arm from side to shoulder level. Do three sets, 10 repetitions, 3 times a day.

G. Adduction: Grip tubing in hand, se-

cure opposite end, and, with arm out from side 60 degrees, bring arm toward body, keeping elbow straight. Do three sets, 10 repetitions, 3 times a day.

VI. PROPRIOCEPTIVE NEUROMUSCULAR FACILITATION (PNF) TECHNIQUES FOR THE SHOULDER COMPLEX[41,64]

This technique is a combination of diagonal patterns composed of the three components of motions: (1) flexion-extension, (2) abduction-adduction, and (3) rotation. It is an excellent adjunct to any rehabilitation program and can be used with either bilateral or unilateral extremities. Each pattern provides an optimal contraction of each major muscle group. Allow for a contraction from completely lengthened state to completely shortened state of the muscle. Each contraction works agonists as well as antagonists, with the type of contraction dependent upon the desired movement: isometric or "hold" contraction permitting no joint movement or isotonic contraction allowing motion through an entire range of motion; normal neuromuscular activity requires a combination of both types of contraction (Fig. 10-15). The PNF exercises are an excellent way to provide manually graded resistance. Refer to Chapter 4 for more in-depth discussion.

VII. ISOTONIC STRENGTHENING EXERCISES

Once pain-free full range of motion is achieved, low-intensity weight training can be started. Handweights, sandbags, or dumbbells can be used. These exercises should be done slowly and through a pain-free full range of motion. At the top position of the exercise, hold for a 3 count and then bring back the weight slowly with a 4 count to the starting position. These exercises may be limited at 90 degrees if the shoulder pathology warrants.

A. Forward raises: Standing with the weight to the side, slowly raise the arm forward in shoulder flexion. Keep the elbow straight and palm down.

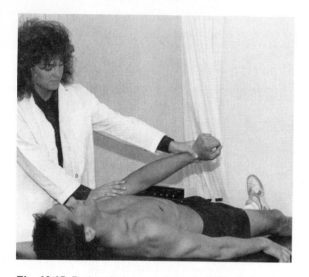

Fig. 10-15. Patient being instructed in PNF pattern for the upper extremity. Proper hand positioning is necessary as a sensory cue.

Hold, slowly return to the starting position, and repeat. Using 2- to 15-pound weights, do three sets, 10 repetitions, twice a day.

B. Lateral raises: Standing with the weight to the side, slowly raise the arm sideways. Keep the elbow straight and palm down. Hold, slowly return to the starting position, and repeat. This exercise should be limited at 90 degrees of shoulder abduction (Fig. 10-16). Using 2- to 15-pound weights, do three sets, 10 repetitions, twice a day.

C. Shoulder rotation: Standing with the weight in hand and elbow bent 90 degrees and into the side of the body with small towel roll next to trunk, move the forearm slowly out away from the body and back toward the stomach. Using 2- to 15-pound weights, do three sets, 10 repetitions, twice a day.

D. Butterfly 1: Lying on back on a table or bench with the arms straight out to the side and palms up, raise both arms overhead where the two weights meet, then slowly lower to the starting position, and repeat. Us-

ing 2- to 15-pound weights, do three sets, 10 repetitions, twice a day.

E. Butterfly 2: Lying face down on table, raise arms to 90 degrees with elbows straight and palms down, raise arms off table as far as possible, hold, slowly lower arms to the table, and repeat. Using 2- to 15-pound weights, do three sets, 10 repetitions, twice a day.

F. Shoulder shrugs: With a barbell or dumbbells in hands, slowly shrug shoulders upward holding for a count of 3, slowly return to the starting position, and repeat. Using 2- to 15-pound weights, do three sets, 10 repetitions, twice a day.

VIII. SPECIFIC ISOTONIC PROGRAMS

A. Hughston exercise program[2,4]: Lie prone (face down) on table, arm abducted to 90 degrees.

1. With thumb pointed toward head, lift at 90 degrees pure abduction, pause for 2 seconds, and repeat. Using 2- to 15-pound weights, do three sets, 10 repetitions, twice a day. This part of the program is a good overall exercise (Fig. 10-17).

2. With thumb pointed toward head, lift arm with hand at eye level, pause for 2 seconds, and repeat. Using 2- to 15-pound weights, do three sets, 10 repetitions, twice a day. This exercise is excellent for the supraspinatus (Fig. 10-18).

3. With thumb pointed up, lift arm at 90 degrees pure abduction, pause for 2 seconds, and repeat. Using 2- to 15-pound weights, do three sets, 10 repetitions, twice a day. This exercise is excellent for supraspinatus, teres minor, and especially infraspinatus (Fig. 10-19).

4. With thumb pointed up, lift arm at eye level, pause for 2 seconds, and repeat. Using 2- to 15-pound weights, do three sets, 10 repetitions, twice a day. This part of the program is an excellent overall exercise (Figs. 10-20, 10-21, and 10-22).

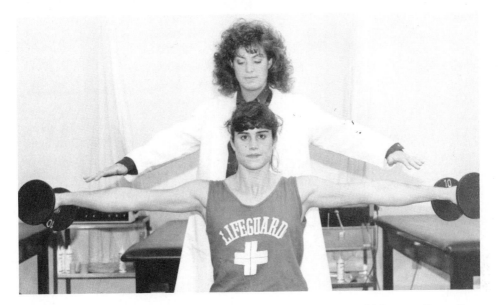

Fig. 10-16. Lateral raises with the sports therapist limiting motion to 90 degrees. Preventing impingement when doing this exercise is important.

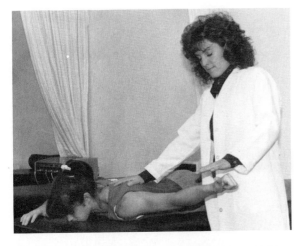

Fig. 10-17. Hughston exercise program: prone on table with arm abducted 90 degrees and thumb pointed to head, lift arm at 90 degrees pure abduction. Hold 2 seconds. (Position 1.)

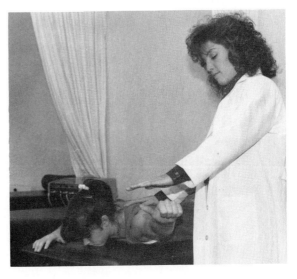

Fig. 10-18. Position 2.

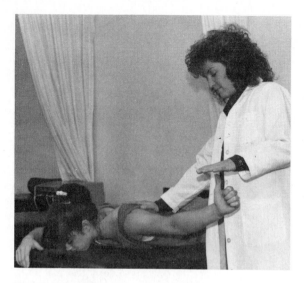

Fig. 10-19. Position 3.

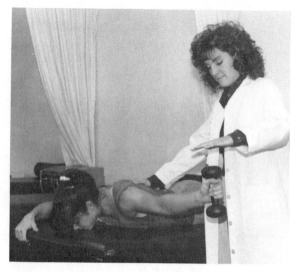

Fig. 10-21. Hughston exercise may be repeated with weight.

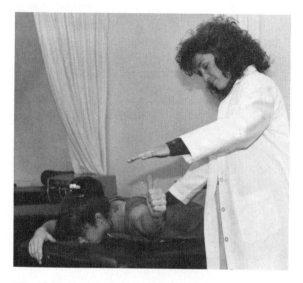

Fig. 10-20. Position 4.

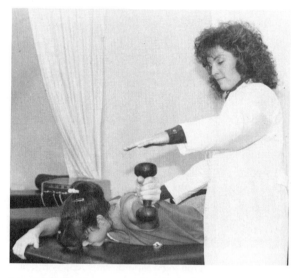

Fig. 10-22. Hughston exercise with weight at eye level.

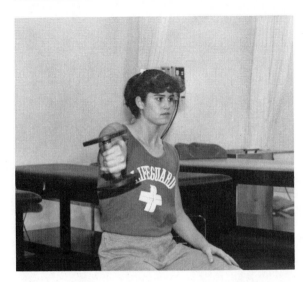

Fig. 10-23. Empty can raise exercise. Thumb pointed down, elbow straight, arm slowly raised outward 45 degrees. Do not raise arm above 90 degrees horizontal.

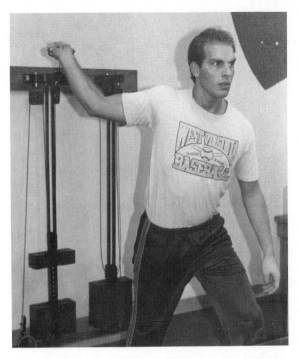

Fig. 10-24. Athlete training on wall pulley system to increase strength on internal rotators.

B. Empty can raise[2,4]
  1. Standing with weight to the side, slowly raise the arm outward at a 45-degree angle with elbow straight and hand inverted (thumb pointing down). Hold at shoulder level, return to the starting position, and repeat. Do not exercise above 90 degrees horizontal (Fig. 10-23). Using 2- to 15-pound weights, do three sets, 10 repetitions, twice a day.
C. Progressive resistive exercises (PREs)
  1. Dumbbell exercises (see isotonic program)
    a. Forward flexion.
    b. Lateral raises.
    c. Butterflies (supine or prone).
    d. Internal rotation.
    e. External rotation.
  2. Stationary wall pulley system (Fig. 10-24).
    a. Forward flexion.
    b. Lateral raises.
    c. Butterflies (supine or prone).
    d. Internal rotation.
    e. External rotation.

  3. Nautilus / Universal / Eagle machines (Figs. 10-25, 10-26, and 10-27).
    a. Strength programs
      (1) Low repetitions and maximum weight.
      (2) Equipment modification may be necessary.
    b. Endurance programs
      (1) High repetitions and minimal to moderate weight.
      (2) Equipment modification may be necessary.
IX. ISOKINETICS
  Isokinetic exercise is defined as exercise with a fixed speed and variable resistance. Isokinetic systems range in cost and complexity, but all meet these basic criteria. Regardless of what type of equipment is used, key points to remember are: (1) isokinetics are usually employed in the third phase of the rehabilitation programs; (2) exercise po-

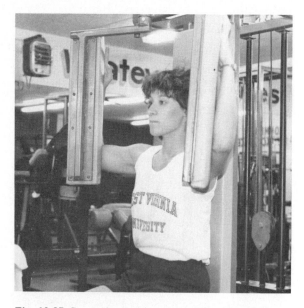

Fig. 10-25. Strengthening for anterior shoulder girdle.

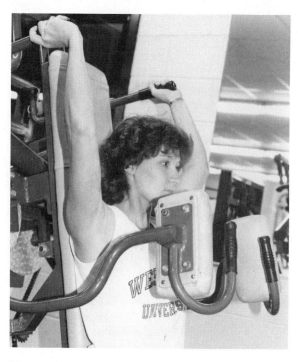

Fig. 10-27. Military press may need modification or elimination from program due to the possibility of impingement.

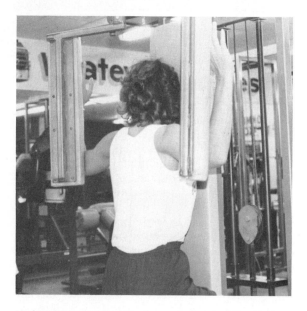

Fig. 10-26. Strengthening for posterior shoulder girdle.

sitions should be varied and include sport-specific joint motions whenever possible; and (3) each muscle group around the joint should be exercised concentrically and eccentrically. Eccentric training was shown to be significant for the throwing shoulder.[18]

Three specific training programs use the velocity spectrum approach with an exercise sequence of ten repetitions at ten different speeds.

A. Slow contractile velocity spectrum program (SCVSP), commonly referred to as a slow-speed program: one set of 10 repetitions at 60, 90, 120, 150, 180, 180, 150, 120, 90, and 60 degrees per second (a total of 100 repetitions).

B. Medium contractile velocity spectrum program (MCVSP): one set of 10 repetitions at 120, 150, 180, 210, 240, 240, 210, 180, 150, and 120 degrees per second (total of 100 repetitions).

C. Fast contractile velocity spectrum program (FCVSP), commonly referred to as a fast-speed program: numerous variations of isokinetic programs may be effective. For the shoulder joint, exercising at speeds above 180 degrees per second has been shown to be most effective. Therefore, all of the protocols given will be fast contractile velocity spectrum programs of one set of 10 repetitions at 180, 210, 240, 270, 300, 300, 270, 240, 210, and 180 degrees per second (total of 100 repetitions).

1. Internal and external rotation positions (Figs. 10-28 and 10-29)
   a. Modified neutral position: arm abducted 30 degrees (FCVSP times three to five sets).
   b. Forward flexed 30 degrees (FCVSP times three to five sets).
   c. Abduction 70 degrees (FCVSP times one to three sets).
   d. Forward flexed 70 degrees (FCVSP times one to three sets).
   e. Abducted 70 degrees and forward flexed 45 degrees (FCVSP times one to three sets).

2. Flexion and extension (Fig. 10-30)
   a. Standing (FCVSP times three to five sets).
   b. Sitting (FCVSP times three to five sets).
   c. Supine (FCVSP times three to five sets).

3. Abduction and adduction (Fig. 10-31)
   a. Short arc
      (1) Submaximal (FCVSP times one to three sets).
      (2) Maximal (FCVSP for one set).
   b. Full ROM
      (1) Submaximal (FCVSP times one to three sets).
      (2) Maximal (FCVSP for one set).

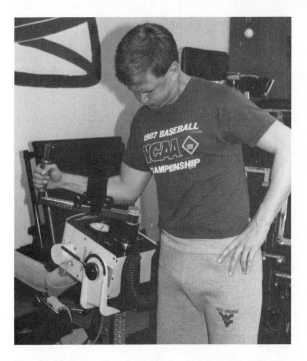

Fig. 10-28. Internal and external rotation using velocity spectrum program.

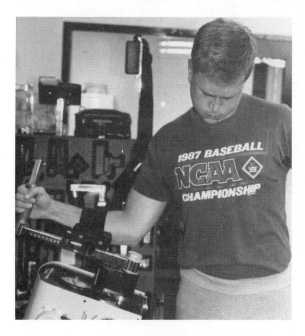

Fig. 10-29. Notice arm abducted 15 to 20 degrees from trunk when performing rotations to decrease irritation at critical zone.

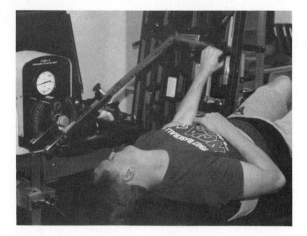

Fig. 10-30. Isokinetic shoulder flexion.

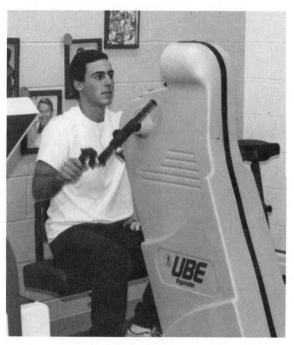

Fig. 10-32. The upper body ergometer (UBE) may be used to increase range of motion as a tool for muscle strength gains.

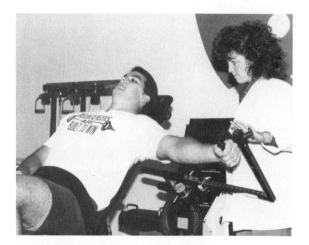

Fig. 10-31. Patient exercising on isokinetic device while sports therapist limits abduction to 90 degrees.

4. Supraspinatus isolation: abducted, forward flexed 45 degrees (FCVSP times one to three sets).
5. Diagonals
   a. D1 pattern (FCVSP times one to five sets). See Chapter 7.
   b. D2 pattern (FCVSP times one to five sets). See Chapter 7.
6. Prone: external rotation (FCVSP times one to five sets).

X. ENDURANCE PROGRAMS
   A. Upper body ergometer (UBE; Fig. 10-32).

1. Used as warm-up and cool-down during exercise.
2. Increase strength with varying resistance.
3. Increase muscular and cardiovascular endurance.
   Example: muscular endurance—"Muscular Workout":
      120 degrees—5 minutes at 2½ minute sprint for 30 seconds
      90 degrees—5 minutes at 4½ minute sprint for last 30 seconds
      90 degrees—5 minutes at 4½ minute sprint for last 30 seconds
   The vascular endurance program "Bout Workout" consists of:
      60 degrees—3 minutes, 1 minute rest
      60 degrees—3 minutes, 1 minute rest

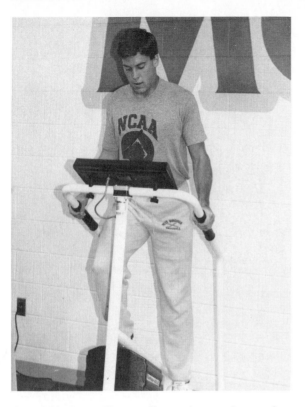

Fig. 10-33. An excellent cardiovascular exercise may be the Stairmaster.

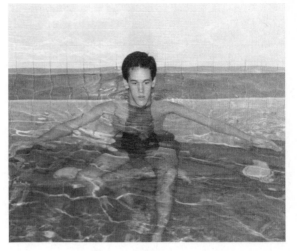

Fig. 10-34. Aquatic therapy can be added to the program for exercise or cardiovascular endurance.

         60 degrees—3 minutes, 1 minute rest

         90 degrees—3 minutes, 1 minute rest

         90 degrees—3 minutes, 1 minute rest

         90 degrees—3 minutes, 1 minute rest

B. Hydrafitness equipment: allows resistance at variable speeds based on dialed levels of resistance controlled by fluid pushed through hydraulic cylinders.

C. Stairmaster (Fig. 10-33).

D. Fitron, stationary bicycle.

E. Swimming (Fig. 10-34).

F. Chest row, excellent for chest and upper back musculature.

G. Shoulder press (exercise caution with inflammatory conditions).

XI. FUNCTIONAL PROGRESSIONS

    A. Throwing program[45]: The goal of this return-to-throwing program is safely and efficiently reconditioning the arm to normal functional ability. The program gradually increases the intensity and volume of throwing each week. Intervals of brief throwing combined with short rest periods help the athlete adjust to a normal game situation. Parts of the program may need to be revised based on the injury, progress, or playing position. A well-designed strength and flexibility program should be followed in conjunction with the throwing program.

    B. Begin program: start throwing with approximately 10 to 15 light warm-ups of only about 30 feet. Mimic the throwing motion prior to using the ball.

       1. Long toss consists of very gentle high lobs between 90 and 180 feet. The throw should be done in a rainbow fashion with minimal cocking effort. Proper follow-through should be utilized.

2. Short toss is the most important phase of the program. It will progress from 30 to 60 feet. Level throwing should be attempted prior to throwing from the mound.

C. Return-to-throwing program

1. *Phase I*

LONG TOSS	Rest 10 minutes	SHORT TOSS
90 feet		30 feet
10 to 12 throws		15 to 20 throws
50% intensity		50% intensity

(During rest phase, stretch arm, shoulder, trunk, and legs.)

2. *Phase II*

LONG TOSS	Rest 10 minutes	SHORT TOSS
90 to 120 feet		60 feet
10 to 12 throws		15 to 20 throws
50% intensity		50% intensity

LONG TOSS	Rest	SHORT TOSS
90 to 120 feet		60 feet
10 to 20 throws		25 to 30 throws
50% intensity		50% intensity

LONG TOSS	Rest	SHORT TOSS
90 to 120 feet		60 feet
10 to 12 throws		30 to 40 throws
50% intensity		50% intensity

3. *Phase III*

LONG TOSS	Rest	SHORT TOSS
120 to 150 feet		60 feet
10 to 12 throws		25 to 30 throws
50% intensity		50% intensity

LONG TOSS	Rest	SHORT TOSS
120 to 150 feet		60 feet
10 to 12 throws		25 to 30 throws
50% intensity		Work to 75% intensity

LONG TOSS	Rest	SHORT TOSS
120 to 150 feet		60 feet
10 to 12 throws		30 to 40 throws
50% intensity		Work to 75% intensity

4. *Phase IV* (interval sequence: begin off the mound)

SHORT TOSS
60 feet

10 to 12 throws	Rest	10 to 20 throws

Work to 75% intensity

(This phase may need to be repeated for 3 to 5 days.)

5. *Phase V* (interval sequence: begin off the mound and include breaking balls).

SHORT TOSS
60 feet

15 throws	Rest	10 throws	Rest	5 throws

Work to 75% intensity

SHORT TOSS
60 feet

15 throws	Rest	15 throws	Rest	10 throws

SHORT TOSS
60 feet

15 throws	Rest	15 throws	Rest	15 throws

6. *Phase VI* (off the mound)

SHORT TOSS
60 feet
20 to 30 throws
75% to full intensity

SHORT TOSS
60 feet
30 to 40 throws
75% to full intensity

SHORT TOSS
60 feet
75% to full intensity

Simulate game situation with work-rest intervals, approximately 15 throws per inning and a 10-minute rest. Progress innings as tolerated and check endurance and throwing speed.

D. Throwing progression[2]

Day 1: Lob toss: From deep center field, throw ball so that it will roll to a stop at second base. Number of throws depends on athlete comfort, but permit no more than 80 throws. If no pain develops by 24 to 48 hours after throwing, increase activity.

Day 2: Lob toss: From deep center field to second base on one hop

Day 3: Lob toss: From deep center field, a long toss to second base. The athlete may take 3 days to a week to progress. Move to 60-foot distance and increase intensity. Place a continued emphasis on good form and mechanics.

REHABILITATION PROGRAMS

Incorporating the stretching, strengthening, and rehabilitation principles, rehabilitation programs have been designed for a number of shoulder pathologies. These programs combine various exercise and stretching techniques for optimum results.

The specific rehabilitation content of this chapter is divided into four specific sections: injuries to joint structures, injuries to the musculotendinous unit, inflammation of shoulder joint structures, and isolated associated pathologies of the shoulder complex. Each section includes etiology, resulting pathology, specific clinical evaluation techniques, and a comprehensive discussion of treatment protocols for each associated injury.

Injuries to the Shoulder Joint Structures

CONTUSIONS. The most common mechanism of injury in this classification occurs from direct blunt force trauma. Corley[12] states, "The significant problem of blunt trauma to the shoulder is the formation of *heterotopic bone* or *myositis ossificans* which may significantly limit shoulder motion and rehabilitation." In athletic participation this problem is an increased area of concern for the athlete.

Contusions to the shoulder girdle can be of different degrees of magnitude. Normally, they occur to the AC joint or to the deltoid area. The cause is simple: a direct blow results in localized pain, swelling, and hemorrhage, which leads to decreased range of motion and radiating pain. Standard treatment of choice is to treat symptomatically and to increase range of motion as quickly as pain allows.

Acromioclavicular contusions. Injuries to the AC joint seem to have the highest incidence of the contusion-related etiologies. The AC joint bruise causes localized pain and swelling; however, no ligamentous damage has occurred. This area may need to be protected during the initial 3 to 5 days with sling immobilization, sling and swath, or a shoulder immobilizer that should be removed three to four times a day for treatment and followup rehabilitation. The first principle with AC contusions is early, gentle, pain-free

range of motion, with a return to normal motion as quickly as possible. These athletes may need to be protected upon return to sports participation. If needed, an AC contusion pad can be modified and manufactured to provide optimal protection.

Acromioclavicular contusion rehabilitation program

PHASE I: This phase emphasizes decreasing the inflammatory response and initiating a pain-free ROM exercise program. Immobilization may be necessary until symptoms subside. The exercises included in this phase are:

1. Isometrics.
2. Codman's.
3. Gentle ROM activities.
4. Wall climb.
5. Shoulder wheel.
6. Pulley system.
7. Wand exercise.

PHASE II: Once the acute inflammation subsides, isometrics are pain free, and ROM improves, low-intensity resistance exercises may begin. Included in this phase are:

1. Wand exercises with weight.
2. Surgical tubing.
3. PNF.
4. Early PREs.

PHASE III: Pain-free ROM must be achieved to progress to this phase. More aggressive isotonic strengthening includes:

1. Specific *isotonics.*
2. Swimming.
3. UBE.
4. Isokinetics.

PHASE IV: In this phase, the athlete has returned to the desired activity, and should be on a program to maintain strength and ROM. Protective padding may be necessary for those returning to contact athletics.

Deltoid contusions. Contusions to the deltoid musculature can result in referred pain to the deltoid tuberosity. These contusions need to be treated in the same manner as an AC contusion. However, a contusion to the axillary nerve complex must be ruled out with AC and/or deltoid contusions. Axillary nerve injuries are discussed later in this chapter.

Deltoid contusion rehabilitation program. The deltoid contusion rehabilitation program is the same as that for AC contusions, given above.

SPRAINS. Approximately 80% of the injuries to the shoulder girdle are sprains,[3] usually of three types: AC sprains, SC sprains, or glenohumeral sprains.

Acromioclavicular sprains. The AC joint is the most frequently sprained area of the shoulder complex. Here the etiologies vary from a direct blow to falling on the elbow to drive the humerus superiorly into the acromial arch space, resulting in injury to the two ligaments that support the AC joint. With increasing severity, the length of time in the four phases of rehabilitation increases.

	SYMPTOMS	PHASE I LENGTH	THROUGH PHASE IV
First degree	No joint laxity Minimal swelling No deformity	1-5 days	7-10 days
Second degree	Joint laxity Moderate swelling Observable deformity	5-7 days	21 days
Third degree	Complete ligament laxity Gross swelling Obvious step-off deformity	7-10 days	3-6 weeks
Third degree	With surgery	14 days	6-8 weeks

AC sprain rehabilitation

PHASE I (acute): Immobilization and inflammation control are the key components of this stage. Subthreshold isometrics and ROM below 90 degrees may begin if tolerated.

PHASE II (subacute): Once weaned from immobilization, continue with increasing mobility and strength.*

1. Codman's pendulum, wall climbing, shoulder wheel.
2. Isometrics.
3. UBE.

---

*A key to AC injury rehabilitation during a strengthening program is 90-degree limitations. Do not exercise above the 90-degree horizontal shoulder plane, 90 degrees abducted and 90-degree flexion. Exercising above this plane in early-stage rehabilitation causes irritation to the surrounding structures and leads to early degenerative joint disease. Strengthening below the 90-degree horizontal plane decreases the chance of initiation of an inflammatory response.

4. Wall pullies, PREs below 90 degrees with light weight.
5. Maintain conditioning.

PHASE III (strengthening): Full range of motion should be obtained before progressing to the strengthening phase.

1. PNF.
2. ROM exercises for all shoulder motions with cuff weights, progressing to dumbbells.
3. Modified weightroom activities including shoulder shrugs, upright rows, bicep curls, and abduction and flexion to 90 degrees.
4. Isotonic strengthening for internal and external rotation.
5. Isokinetics.
6. Running activities.

PHASE IV: Includes functional progression exercises. The program must proceed slowly at this point. A throwing progression is advisable to minimize the inflammatory response. Protective padding may be necessary to return to active contact participation.

Grade III AC sprains may require surgical stabilization by physician preference. Common surgical techniques for the AC joint include:

Loop fixation procedure: Performed on grade III AC separations by looping a Dacron wire around the coracoid process and clavicle.

Kirschner wiring: Performed on grade III AC separations by placing a Kirschner wire through the acromion and into the clavicle to reduce the separation.

Weaver-Dunn procedure: The coracoacromial ligament is detached at the acromial end. The lateral end of the clavicle is sheared at an oblique angle so that the inferior portion is directly above the coracoid. The coracoacromial ligament is then reattached, and any excess ligament is removed.

Bosworth screw fixation: Performed on grade III separations for fixation of the coracoid to the clavicle. The clavicle is held down on the coracoid, and a hole is drilled through the clavicle and into the coracoid. A Bosworth coracoclavicular screw is inserted.

Rehabilitation programs following AC joint surgeries vary according to the particular surgical method used. Therefore, guidelines for exercise must be established that do not stress the surgical constraints.

Sternoclavicular joint injuries. Sternoclavicular sprains can be classified as first, second, or third degree. These injuries are infrequent but may result in a great deal of discomfort and decreased movement of the associated shoulder girdle and extremity. Also, third-degree SC injuries, especially associated posterior displacement of the clavicle, must be recognized acutely. Again, treatment of first-, second-, and third-degree SC sprains is symptomatic to alleviate pain and initiates range-of-motion exercises as soon as possible to return to normal function. Most physicians believe that no period of immobilization is necessary with this type of injury. Rehabilitation also should include strengthening of the anterior chest muscles, as the SC joint has little musculature support. Protective padding may be effective in relieving symptoms for return to participation.

GLENOHUMERAL DISLOCATIONS AND SUBLUXATIONS WITH RESULTANT INJURIES TO ASSOCIATED AREAS. To differentiate between dislocation and subluxation, the glenohumeral subluxation is a partial slipping or sliding of the humeral head from the glenoid fossa with a spontaneous reduction that requires no external force for reduction; the glenohumeral dislocation is a complete removal of the humeral head from the associated glenoid fossa, requires external force for reduction, and may result in a chronic laxity that warrants possible surgical intervention. The capsular ligament has been extenuated or torn which results in gross laxity.

Dislocations are usually classified in one of four directions[20]:

1. Anterior displacement—subacromial (results in 95% of all dislocations).
2. Inferior dislocations—subglenoid.
3. Posterior dislocations.
4. Global or multidirectional dislocations—instability in more than one plane.

Common complications with anterior dislocations are[20,29]:

1. Severe stretching and tearing of the anterior capsule.
2. Possible axillary nerve damage to its innervation of the deltoid muscle.
3. Limited or no tensile strength of the resultant musculature associated with the glenohumeral joint.
4. Tear of the inferior glenohumeral ligament.

5. The rotator cuff, specifically the subscapularis tendon, may be damaged or torn.
6. Repeated dislocation will be from progressively less force.
7. Fracture of the greater tuberosity, which is relatively frequent in older athletes and most commonly caused by a shearing force against the acromion process and coracoclavicular ligament.
8. A possible isolated labrum tear from an anterior dislocation.
9. Compression fracture occurring at the posterior lateral humeral head—referred to as a Hill Sack lesion.

Specific exercise programs are outlined for anterior dislocations, posterior dislocations, and multidirectional instabilities. The sports therapist has the responsibility to be aware of the direction of instability and not elicit an apprehensive response from the patient.

Direct force to the arm while it is positioned in abduction and external rotation causes 95 to 98% of anterior dislocations. Of these, 85 to 90% of anterior dislocations recur. A direct relationship exists between age and recurrence: those younger than 20 have a 92% recurrence rate; those 20 to 40 have a 60% rate; those older than 40 have a 15% rate.[32]

Shoulder subluxations are identified by the direction of the instability. Again, anterior, posterior, inferior, and multidirectional subluxations are the four classifications. Principally, anterior subluxations comprise 95%, and only 2 to 3% are classified as posterior or inferior instabilities. Instabilities in more than one plane are classified as multidirectional or global instabilities. Rehabilitation programs for the subluxing glenohumeral joint are comparable to that of the dislocation.

To implement a successful rehabilitation program, the sports therapist must remember that the anatomy of the glenohumeral joint is such that it has both static and dynamic stabilizers. The static stabilizers, however, provide a minimal amount of support to the glenohumeral joint. The coracohumeral ligament, superglenohumeral ligament, middle glenohumeral ligament, and inferior glenohumeral ligament constitute the anterior joint capsule. Minimal stability is provided by the glenoid labrum associated with the anterior capsule. The dynamic stabilizers of this joint—the subscapularis, supraspinatus, infraspinatus, teres minor and deltoid muscles—provide the majority of the associated protection.

Concerning the rehabilitation program, Grana and others[21] point out that "throughout the rehabilitation period, patient must be instructed to avoid positions of hyperflexion, external rotation, and shoulder abduction combined with external rotation."

Following the initial acute glenohumeral dislocation, most physicians agree that a period of immobilization is necessary to allow the acute symptoms to subside and capsular healing to take place. This immobilization may be anywhere from 10 days to 6 weeks, depending on physician choice. The following is an aggressive rehabilitation program for an acute glenohumeral dislocation.

Acute glenohumeral dislocation rehabilitation

PHASE I: In this phase, concentrate on isometrics and gentle range of motion when the sling is removed to promote return to normal joint mechanics and motion. Also, initiate a light exercise program to retard muscular atrophy during this immobilization period. Exercises in this phase would include:

1. Codman's.
2. Wand exercises.
3. Wall climbing to 90 degrees horizontal.
4. Accessory joint mobilization techniques.
5. Isometric exercises in all planes.
6. Active elbow motions.

PHASE II: In this phase, approximately 4 to 6 weeks after the injury, the athlete has obtained at least 30 degrees of external rotation and is slowly returning to functional activity. The exercises in this phase include:

1. Isometric exercises in all planes.
2. Light weight added to range-of-motion activities.
3. Isotonic exercises.
4. Specific isotonic exercises, including Hughston, empty can, and PREs.
5. PNFs.
6. UBE to increase range of motion.

Once normal pain-free range of motion has returned, the athlete patient may progress to the next phase.

PHASE III: This stage is denoted by the return of normal joint range of motion, beginning return to limited activity. Exercises in this phase include progressing the isotonic exercises of phase II by increasing weight and the progressive-resistive exercise regime. Caution should be exercised when concentrating on external rotation. Limitation of movement may be necessary to avoid stress of the anterior capsule. Of particular importance in this phase are:

1. Shoulder shrugs, internal rotation, external rotation to 45 degrees, abduction, adduction, and flexion.
2. PNF patterns.
3. Weight training equipment can be used at this time with modification.
4. Isokinetic exercises are generally initiated at low speeds, followed by high-speed velocity spectrum programs. Particular attention is given to rotation (internal), adduction, and horizontal adduction.

PHASE IV: Return to complete activity. A maintenance program must be defined to continue strengthening internal rotators, adductors, and horizontal adductors. This program is based on a three-times-a-week conditioning and strengthening program that follows a progressive-resistive exercise regime either isotonically, isokinetically, or in combination. Protective devices may be necessary to return to activity, depending on physician preference.

Even with rehabilitation, some risk factors do remain for recurrence, principally the age, activity level, traumatic dislocation, and type of instability. To return to competition without apprehension or recurrent instability, the athlete should have significant strength of the internal and external rotators equaling approximately 20% of the body weight or 90% of the opposite shoulder. In addition, those returning to contact sports may be treated with a functional brace or harness, which is well tolerated by athletes playing certain positions in football but not necessarily applicable to other sports.

When recurrence does occur, a chronic glenohumeral subluxation leads to joint instability. Physician opinion on the method of treatment varies in accordance to the type and frequency of the subluxation. Most physicians continue a conservative treatment program until functional disability occurs. An aggressive rehabilitation program for chronic glenohumeral subluxation would include the following:

Chronic glenohumeral subluxation rehabilitation

PHASE I: Immobilization during this phase varies greatly; Henry and Genung[29] report that:

1. The prognosis of recurrent dislocations was not affected significantly by immobilization.
2. The amount of time between injury and recurrence was not related to immobilization or the length of immobilization.
3. There is a high recurrence rate for this injury among high school students.
4. Immobilization for 3 to 6 weeks does not alter the recurrence rate.

Therefore, most immobilization for the chronic subluxing shoulder has minimal effect on glenohumeral stabilization. Thus exercises during this phase would include:

1. Isometrics in all planes.
2. All range-of-motion exercises to return to normal, pain-free motion as quickly as possible.
3. Surgical tubing, concentrating on rotations.
4. UBE for motion.

Once pain-free normal range of motion has returned, the athlete can progress to the next phase.

PHASE II: This phase may start only a few days after the subluxation. In this phase concentrate on strength and limitation of external rotation with abduction.

1. Continue isometrics and range-of-motion activities.
2. Surgical tubing.
3. Isotonic exercises: these exercises are performed like progressive-resistive exercises in the controlled range. Exercise caution with external rotation with abduction. Concentrate on internal rotation, adduction, and horizontal adduction.
4. UBE programs for strength and motion.
5. PNF patterns.

PHASE III: This stage is devoted to the return of normal joint range of motion, limitation of external rotation to 45 degrees, and return to full activity. Continue to increase the program with the following exercises:

1. PNF.
2. Surgical tubing for rotations.
3. Isotonic exercises concentrating on shoulder shrugs, internal and external rotation, adduction and flexion, specific concern with horizontal adduction. Weight equipment may be modified to limit external rotation and abduction.
4. Isokinetic exercises are generally initiated at low speeds and develop to a high-speed program.

PHASE IV: Again, in this phase the athlete has returned to complete activity and is now on a maintenance program. This program is based on a three-times-a-week strengthening program that combines all aspects of phases I through III. Protective devices may be employed, depending on physician preference.

When the conservative program has failed, surgical intervention may be necessary to stabilize the glenohumeral joint. Numerous surgical procedures are available for reconstruction of the anterior joint capsule, including:

DuToit staple capsulorrhaphy: This procedure's main purpose is to staple the shoulder joint capsule to the neck of the scapula when a separation of the capsule and glenoid cavity has occurred. An incision is made to expose the anterior capsule and the neck of the scapula. A staple is driven through the capsule and the neck of the scapula.

Modified Bristow: A technique designed to stabilize the shoulder yet allow for an excellent range of motion. A portion of the coracoid process is transferred and placed at the anterior glenoid.

Bankart procedure: The main purpose of this technique is to reinforce the anterior capsule and increase the efficiency of the subscapularis and anterior rim of the glenoid to the neck of the scapula.

Putti-Platt procedure: This surgery reinforces the anterior capsule and increases the efficiency of the subscapularis muscle. The lateral flap of the subscapularis is attached to the glenoid labrum by suturing. The medial portion of the subscapularis is then overlapped over the lateral flap.

Postsurgical rehabilitation. This nonspecific program is based on the athlete's progress following surgery.

PHASE I: This phase concentrates on the return of normal joint mechanics in terms of regaining range of motion and a light exercise program to retard muscular atrophy in the immobilization period. The exercises included in this stage are:

1. Pendulum exercises.
2. Wand exercises.
3. Wall climbing exercises.
4. Accessory joint mobilization techniques.
5. Isometric exercises.

PHASE II: In this phase, the athlete is approximately 4 to 6 weeks out of the sling, has obtained at least 30 degrees of external rotation, and is slowly returning to functional activity. The exercises in this phase include:

1. Isometric exercises (continue as previously outlined).
2. Pendulum exercises and wand exercises can now be performed with the use of light weight and can be performed for approximately 30 repetitions.
3. Isotonic exercises are performed upon a progressive-resistive exercise basis in the range that the athlete has achieved.
4. Accessory joint mobilization may be continued based on the return of normal joint mechanics and end feels.

PHASE III: This stage is denoted by the return of normal joint range of motion, limitation of external rotation to 45 degrees, and return to full activity by the patient. Exercises in this phase include isotonic exercises that are now begun on weight machines or by using an increasing progressive-resistive exercise regimen. Of particular importance are:

1. Shoulder shrugs.
2. Internal rotation.
3. External rotation.
4. Abduction.
5. Flexion.
6. Proprioceptive neuromuscular facilitation patterns.
7. Weight training equipment can be used at this time depending on accessibility; its use can be guided by the athlete's pain.
8. Accessory joint motion may be continued only if scapulothoracic mechanics have not yet returned.
9. Isokinetic exercises are generally initiated at high speeds with particular attention to rotation and abduction.

PHASE IV: In this stage the athlete has returned to complete activity and is now on a maintenance program. This program is based on a 3-times-a-week conditioning basis following a progressive-resistive exercise regime. Protective devices may be employed, depending on physician preference.

More specific guidelines have been established for the modified Bristow procedure and the Putti-Platt. The modified Bristow technique is used more often in athletics because it stabilizes yet allows for more shoulder external rotation. Putti-Platt surgery gives maximum anterior stability but limits external rotation.

Modified Bristow procedure rehabilitation protocol. The modified Bristow procedure is a surgical technique designed to stabilize the shoulder. The shoulder muscles are transferred so that they may stabilize the anterior shoulder and prevent future dislocations. A portion of the coracoid process is transferred and placed at the anterior glenoid rim. A limitation of 10 to 15 degrees in external rotation should be expected as a trade-off for this added stability (Figs. 10-35 and 10-36).

PHASE I: Sling and swath are worn continuously 2 to 4 weeks. At 2 weeks, adjustments may be made for personal hygiene. After 2 weeks, the elbow may be freed from the sling three times during the day to perform active motion. Isometrics may be performed at the shoulder while in the sling except for forward flexion and external rotation.

1. Passive and active elbow ROM.
2. Isometrics, except shoulder flexion and external rotation.
3. Gentle Codman's.

PHASE II: Remove sling (2 to 4 weeks) and begin active and resistive elbow exercises with small weight. Shoulder exercises are performed to increase ROM.

1. Codman's.
2. Active wall climb.
3. Active ROM, all planes.
4. Isometrics, all planes.
5. Resistive ROM elbow motions.
6. Begin stationary bicycle, stairmaster, other aerobic activity.

PHASE III: Strengthening program may now begin (6 to 12 weeks).

1. Codman's with weight.
2. Continue ROM in all planes.
3. Begin PREs with 2 to 4 pounds of weight.
4. PNF.

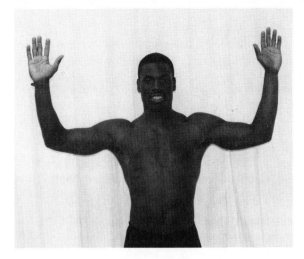

Fig. 10-35. Patient with bilateral Bristow procedures.

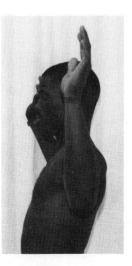

Fig. 10-36. Side view of patient shows 10- to 15-degree limitation in external rotation that should be expected.

5. Continue wrist resistive exercises.
6. Continue elbow resistive exercises.
7. Isotonic program.
8. Begin isokinetic exercises.

No passive motion, only active motion to regain external rotation and abduction, should be attempted. Continue stationary bicycle, swimming, stairmaster, and other cardiovascular conditioning exercises.

PHASE IV: Evaluate isokinetically (12 weeks)

before considering return to participation. Continue previously determined exercise program to increase strength and ROM, if indicated. Nearly full ROM and at least 90% strength of shoulder must be attained prior to returning to unrestricted activity.

Putti-Platt procedure rehabilitation protocol. This program calls for 2 weeks of postoperative immobilization.

WEEK 3
1. Begin Codman's exercises with no weight.
2. Begin active wall climbs: flexion and abduction.
3. Begin active range of motion: flexion, abduction, and extension.
4. Begin passive range of motion: bicep curls.
5. Begin isometric exercises: adduction, internal rotation, external rotation, elbow flexion, and elbow extension.

WEEKS 4 AND 5
1. Continue Codman's exercises with 3 to 5 pounds.
2. Continue active wall climbs.
3. Continue active range of motion and add external rotation and prone horizontal abduction.
4. Continue resistive bicep curls.
5. Begin resistive range of motion; wrist flexion and wrist extension.
6. If active flexion and/or abduction is 90 degrees, begin resistive flexion and/or abduction through the use of surgical tubing.
7. Begin stationary bicycle, swimming, or other aerobic activity.

WEEKS 6 TO 8
1. Continue Codman's exercises with weight.
2. When active flexion and/or abduction reach 180 degrees, begin progressive-resistive exercise (flexion, extension, abduction, adduction, internal rotation, external rotation, horizontal abduction) with weights of 2 to 3 pounds.
3. If active flexion and/or abduction reach 180 degrees, begin PNF.
4. Begin resistive range of motion; shoulder shrugs.
5. Continue resistive range of motion; wrist flexion and wrist extension.
6. Continue resistive bicep curls.
7. Continue stationary bicycle, swimming, etc.

WEEKS 9 TO 11

1. Continue PNF.
2. Continue resistive range of motion: bicep curls, shoulder shrugs, wrist flexions, and wrist extension.
3. Continue progressive-resistive range of motion: shoulder flexion, abduction, extension, horizontal abduction, internal rotation, and external rotation.
4. Continue stationary bicycle, swimming, or rowing.

WEEKS 12 AND 13

1. Continue progressive-resistive range of motion: horizontal abduction.
2. Continue PNF patterns.
3. Begin isokinetic exercises such as Cybex, abduction-adduction, flexion-extension, and internal-external rotation.
4. Continue stationary bicycle, swimming, or rowing.
5. Begin passive range of motion: external rotation with arm adducted and with arm abducted to 90 degrees.

WEEK 14 TO MONTH 4

1. Continue passive range of motion within end of range.
2. Continue isokinetic exercises with gradually increasing resistance and high speeds (300 degrees/second to 240 degrees/second) progressing toward slow speeds (90 degrees to 60 degrees/second).
3. Continue PNF patterns.
4. Continue progressive resistance exercise with free weights.
5. Continue stationary bicycle, rowing machine, or other cardiovascular conditioning exercise.

END OF MONTH 4

1. Isokinetic evaluation, bilateral.
2. Consideration of return to participation.
3. Continue previously noted regimen if strength increase is indicated.

Arthroscopic shoulder reconstruction rehabilitation protocol. These guidelines are specifically for an arthroscopic reconstruction of the anterior inferior glenohumeral ligament with a fascia lata graft[46] (Fig. 10-37). These guidelines are also usable for glenoid labrum reattachments, but the time frame may be accelerated. Athletes react differently, and the treatments and guidelines should be changed according to the athlete's signs and symptoms.

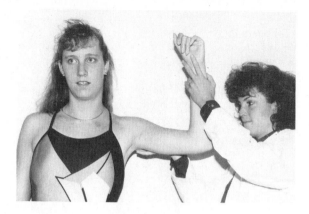

Fig. 10-37. Patient following arthroscopic shoulder reconstruction with minimal cosmetic changes.

PHASE I

1. Sling through first 3 weeks.
2. Start Codman exercises at 1 to 2 weeks.
3. Start isometric exercises at 1 to 2 weeks.
4. Start mobilization out of sling, passive ROM, and supine wand exercises at 3 weeks.
5. Start active assistive ROM against gravity at 3 to 4 weeks.
6. Start active ROM against gravity at 4 weeks.
7. Start limited resistive exercises at 4 to 5 weeks.

NOTE: Strength of the graft is weakest at about 4 to 5 weeks, at which time the athlete and the sports therapist need to be cautious.

PHASE II

1. Start progressive ROM at 5 to 6 weeks.
2. Increase strengthening exercises at 6 weeks.
3. Mobilize into external rotation with arm abducted at 8 weeks.

PHASE III: Stress strengthening exercises, neuromuscular control, and functional progression.

1. Start resistive exercises with large arcs of motion at 10 weeks.
2. Start isokinetics at 10 to 12 weeks.
3. Start isotonic exercises at 10 to 12 weeks.
4. Start functional progression at 12 weeks.
5. Vigorous strengthening.

PHASE IV: Return to functional activity.

1. Maintain strengthening and proprioception programs.
2. Isokinetic maintenance.

GLENOID LABRUM TEAR. The **glenoid labrum tear** usually results from shoulder instabilities. A conservative rehabilitation program initiated 4 to 6 weeks after a labrum tear would include a progression of range-of-motion exercises (including Codman's, wall climbing, wand exercises), progressive-resistive exercises, surgical tubing, isokinetic programs, and then a functional progression protocol. However, labrum tears are difficult to manage from a rehabilitation standpoint. These programs do not result in a reversal of the pathology. Controlling the symptoms and generally strengthening the shoulder complex may decrease the effects of the tear. However, failure to control labrum tears usually results in surgical intervention arthroscopically with excision of the tear, repair of the tear, and/or a capsulorrhaphy. The torn labrum associated with anterior instabilities has been referred to as a **Bankart lesion**[32] (Fig. 10-38). With injury to the glenoid rim and anterior capsular ligaments, these structures become detached from the anterior glenoid and no longer function as an anterior constraint to the humeral head, and a dislocation occurs. In addition, often a compression fracture occurs at the posterior lateral portion of the humeral head; it is often referred to as a **Hill-Sachs** lesion[32] and is associated with recurrent instability in the anterior direction. It can also be noted in the posteriorly unstable shoulder and is appropriately named **posterior Bankart lesion** and **reverse Hill-Sachs lesion.**[32]

Pappas, Zawacki, and McCarthy[52] state that "achieving normal glenohumeral and scapulothoracic motion is an absolute necessity before strengthening programs are begun." Thus a complete rehabilitation program for glenohumeral instabilities includes a progression for strengthening all the dynamic stabilizers of the upper extremity after normal range of motion is obtained. However, emphasis must be placed on specific muscle strengthening according to the type of instability.

With an anterior instability, the exercise program must emphasize strengthening the internal rotators, subscapularis, pectoralis major, coracobrachialis, and long head of the biceps. Contraindicated acutely are movements above 90 degrees of abduction with external rotation to avoid stressing the anterior capsule, as well as exercises that would stretch the anterior musculature. Also, mobilizations with the arm abducted to 90 degrees are to be avoided.

For posterior instabilities, emphasis is placed on strengthening the infraspinatus, teres minor, and the posterior deltoid. This program requires limiting movement into full horizontal adduction and internal rotation to avoid stretching the posterior capsule and musculature.

A conservative program for the multidirectional instability would emphasize strengthening the muscles on the side of the major instability; however, alleviating pain is the most important factor for these athletes. Some athletes who exhibit multidirectional instabilities require strengthening of the entire shoulder girdle complex, principally the rotator cuff muscles, deltoid, and scapula stabilizers. Most physicians agree that the early emphasis in the case of a multidirectional instability is on tightening the surrounding tissues and strengthening the muscles on the involved side. However, optimum tightening or shortening of the muscles is accomplished by immobilization. Exercising in a limited range of motion strengthens muscles and can contribute to their tightening. Stretching exercises to increase range of motion, however, are instituted only when adequate strength has been regained and only if functional motion deficits need to be addressed. Mobilization techniques are good for the anterior joint dislocations; however, anterior glides must be avoided for they promote external rotation. Rigid restrictions of activities and aggressive muscle rehabilitation are important in decreasing the number of recurrences; however, the most important factor of any recurrent instability is prevention by a proper and comprehensive exercise program.

CLAVICLE FRACTURES. Fractures of the shoulder complex are usually isolated to one specific area, the clavicle. Normally, clavicle fractures occur in the middle third of the bone and are easily identifiable; they are usually treated with a figure eight sling or splint for a period of 4 to 6 weeks. However, unstable fractures may require surgical stabilization.

Rehabilitation during immobilization is usually isolated to shoulder range of motion bilaterally and symptomatic treatment at the fracture site. Once normal healing has occurred and the splint is removed, strengthening of the entire shoulder girdle complex must be initiated. This rehabilitation should include all proximal and

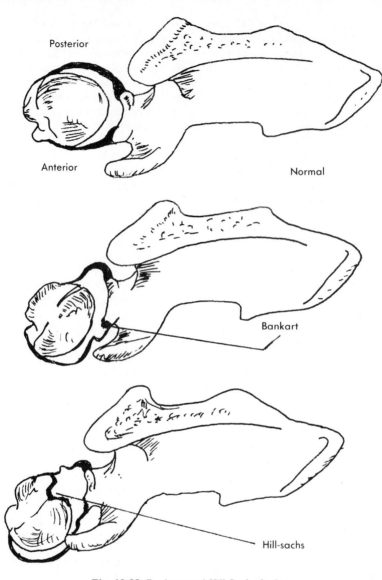

Posterior

Anterior

Normal

Bankart

Hill-sachs

Fig. 10-38. Bankart and Hill-Sachs lesions.

distal musculature. Full glenohumeral range of motion must be achieved, particularly normal AC and SC joint function. Remember that the shoulder complex works in harmonious fashion; therefore, a fractured clavicle with a prolonged period of immobilization causes reduction in normal motion at both SC and AC joints. Also, the scapulothoracic joint must be considered after prolonged immobilization.

Fractured clavicle rehabilitation program

PHASE I: In this phase, the athlete is immobilized 4 to 6 weeks in a figure eight splint (Fig. 10-39). Isometrics and gentle ROM exercises are performed to retard atrophy. Maintain cardiovascular endurance with the stationary bicycle.

PHASE II: Once the splint is removed, continue isometrics and begin ROM exercises such as:

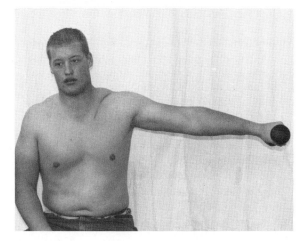

Fig. 10-39. Surgical stabilization of the clavicle may be necessary with severe fractures. Caution must be used when beginning the rehabilitation program.

1. Codman's.
2. Wall climb.
3. Wand exercises.
4. Shoulder wheel.
5. Low-intensity strengthening below 90 degrees.
6. Mobilization of glenohumeral and scapulothoracic joint.
7. Fitron for cardiovascular endurance.

PHASE III: Pain-free ROM must be achieved to progress to phase III. Low-intensity strengthening may then begin, including:

1. Wall pulleys.
2. Wand exercises with weight.
3. PREs.
4. Surgical tubing.
5. PNF.
6. UBE.
7. Specific isotonic and isokinetic programs 6 to 8 weeks after the injury.
8. Cardiovascular exercises may include swimming, stairmaster, and UBE.

PHASE IV: Return to activity highlights this phase. The strengthening program emphasizes anterior and posterior chest musculature. Protective padding over the clavicle may be warranted for contact athletics.

HUMERUS AND NECK FRACTURES. Fractures of the proximal third of the humerus or surgical neck fractures must be identified immediately upon initial examination and evaluation. These fractures are treated acutely with immobilization in sling and swath or shoulder immobilizer for periods of 4 to 6 weeks. This injury relates directly to associated frozen shoulder syndrome or adhesive capsulitis. Early motion is absolutely necessary to prevent such disorders. The specific rehabilitation protocol for a fractured proximal third of the humerus or associated epiphyseal fracture is outlined next.

Fractured proximal third of humerus or surgical neck fracture rehabilitation program

PHASE I: In this phase, the athlete is immobilized for 2 to 6 weeks. Physicians' opinions vary on motions allowed during this period. If permitted, isometrics in all planes and elbow ROM may begin to prevent atrophy. Adhesive capsulitis or frozen shoulder may develop during this phase, and the sports therapist should be aware of its signs and symptoms.

PHASE II: Once the patient is out of immobilization, ROM exercises may begin.

1. Continue isometrics.
2. Gentle stretching.
3. Low-intensity PREs as ROM returns.
4. UBE.
5. Mobilization of all shoulder joints except glenohumeral.

PHASE III: In this phase, weight training increases for the entire shoulder complex, keying on the scapular stabilizers.

1. PREs; wand with weight.
2. PNF.
3. Wall pulleys.
4. Surgical tubing.
5. Isokinetics.
6. Swimming.

PHASE IV: This phase marks the return to desired activity once pain-free, normal ROM and comparable strength are achieved. Continue a maintenance program.

NOTES: Maintenance of cardiovascular endurance in phases 1 and 2 is important, but caution is necessary to avoid displacement of the fracture site with exercise.

Avulsion fractures of the head of the humerus, scapula fractures, and acromial fractures are rare shoulder complex injuries but need to be ruled out by x-ray.

DEGENERATIVE JOINT DISEASE. Degenerative joint disease (DJD) can be present in any of the shoulder area joints, particularly the sternoclavicular and acromioclavicular joints. It is seen mainly in synovial AC joints.

PHASE I: Progressive degeneration of the articulating surfaces causes pain, limited motion, and decreased function. In the acute stage, DJD is treated symptomatically with modalities of choice. Isometrics may be initiated.

PHASE II: Strengthen the surrounding musculature for joint protection and improved flexibility. In this phase, a low-intensity, pain-free strengthening program may begin. Avoid exercise above 90 degrees.

PHASE III: Increase strength via isokinetics below 90 degrees by using high repetitions and low weight, surgical tubing, PNF, UBE, and aquatic therapy.

PHASE IV: Return to activity via functional progression. As with all programs for the shoulder complex, this progression should be sport-specific. If conservative management fails, surgical intervention, most commonly distal clavicle resection and/or acromioplasty, may be necessary.

Injuries to the Musculotendinous Units of the Shoulder Complex

These injuries involve the contractile structures of the shoulder complex. Dysfunction in this area leads to proximal instability, decreases the efficiency of the distal arm segment, and results in insufficient arm mobility. This section is divided into three components: muscular strains, dislocation of the biceps tendon, and injuries to the rotator cuff.

MUSCULAR STRAINS. Muscular strains of the shoulder complex are a specific injury to an isolated muscle or muscle group. They must be determined with an accurate evaluation. From the evaluation, a specific protocol can be designed that includes range of motion, flexibility, and strengthening at midrange with both high-speed and low-speed programs.

Muscle strains rehabilitation program

PHASE I: In this phase immobilization may be necessary to protect the injured area from spasm. The exercises that may be included are:

1. Gentle stretching.
2. Codman's.

3. Early ROM exercises, wall climb, wand exercise.
4. UBE.
5. Isometrics.
6. Maintain cardiovascular conditioning through use of exercise bike.

PHASE II: This phase begins when isometrics are painless and ROM is full.

1. Wall pulleys.
2. Wand exercise with weight.
3. Early PREs.
4. Isolate injured area with isometrics.

PHASE III: Pain-free motion signifies the beginning of a more aggressive strengthening program, including:

1. Surgical tubing.
2. Specific isotonics.
3. PNF.
4. UBE.
5. High-speed isokinetics.
6. Swimming.

PHASE IV: Return to normal activity with a maintenance strengthening and ROM program. External support with strapping or an elastic wrap may be necessary.

BICEPS TENDON DISLOCATION. An acute injury to the musculotendinous unit that results from direct trauma or a forceful contraction of the biceps complex may result in a dislocation of the biceps tendon. Normally this injury has a specific history and mechanism that is described by the patient during the evaluation. The tendon itself may dislocate from the bicipital groove, usually from overhead activity, repetitive hard throwing, or forceful contraction of the arm into external rotation from a position of shoulder abduction external rotation. A tear of the transverse humeral ligament allows this dislocation to occur. A positive Vergason test confirms the evaluation. The Vergason test is performed with the individual sitting or standing. The elbow is flexed to 90 degrees and the arm at 0 degrees abduction. The athlete attempts to rotate the arm externally and flex the elbow, which produces pain and possible dislocation of the tendon over the lesser tubercle of the humerus. A positive test would suggest instability of the tendon and rupture of the transverse ligament.

Following the acute episode a period of immobilization with a strengthening program is the normal rehabilitation protocol. Chronic instability may lead to surgical stabilization to repair the transverse ligament or rupture of the tendon.

The following rehabilitation program is for the acute dislocation but may be altered for chronic instability.

Acute dislocation rehabilitation program

PHASE I: Short period of immobilization (7 to 14 days). ROM should be easily attained. Strength and motion can begin. Emphasize regaining motion without stressing healing tissues. Avoid any significant pain and stress.
1. ROM exercises.
2. Isometric exercises.
3. Passive ROM and supine wand exercises.
4. Active assistive ROM against gravity.
5. Full flexibility exercises.

PHASE II: Begin to increase strength and quality of motion.
1. Multiple-angle isometrics.
2. PNF and manual resistance.
3. Low-intensity isotonics.
4. UBE.
5. Surgical tubing.

PHASE III: Continue strengthening and begin functional return.
1. Obtain full, pain-free ROM.
2. Specific isotonics.
3. UBE and PNF programs.
4. Submaximal isokinetic program for shoulder abduction and IR/ER.
5. Begin functional return program (swimming, throwing progression).

PHASE IV: Return to activity.
1. Full-range isokinetic program all planes— velocity spectrum program.
2. UBE and PNF patterns.
3. Aquatic therapy.
4. Throwing progression.
5. Sport-specific exercise.

INJURIES TO ROTATOR CUFF. The rotator cuff injury to the shoulder complex is the most commonly missed diagnosis at the shoulder. The typical patient is the 40- to 50-year-old male worker who is participating in recreational athletics. The mechanism associated with a fall onto the outstretched arm, a rapid, forced abduction of the arm against resistance, or overuse microtrauma leads to tendonitis or acute rupture of a specific rotator cuff tendon. Classically, this athlete feels a sharp pain or snap, cannot abduct the arm, and cannot sleep due to night pain, and the injury involves the dominant shoulder in most cases. A first-degree rotator cuff strain is a mild strain, a second-degree strain is a moderate disability, and a third-degree strain is a complete rupture and disability (Table 10-1).

The following treatment program for rotator cuff injuries was designed by Keith Erb.[19] This protocol should be incorporated with an exercise program that focuses on postural training, cuff strengthening, and total arm strength and proprioception. The section on supraspinatus tendonitis (impingement syndrome) contains a more detailed rehabilitation program.

Rotator cuff treatment protocol
1. All treatments must be done with the humerus abducted and supported at approximately 45 degrees of abduction to facilitate circulation to the avascular zones.
2. Ultrasound is applied for approximately 5 minutes to the supraspinatus fossa.
3. Interrupted pulsed electrical stimulation is applied with 3-inch electrodes. One electrode should be applied over the supraspinatus fossa. The other electrode should be placed on the deltoid muscle, with the upper border of the electrode just distal to the acromion and coracoacromial arch. The intensity of the current should be turned up to a level that gets a contraction showing some depression of the humeral head. Be careful not to cause too strong a contraction and thereby too much tension on the supraspinatus lesion. Also, the level of current should be at a comfortable setting for the athlete; it should not hurt.
4. Apply a cold pack to the supraspinatus and infraspinatus fossa with the athlete lying supine in the abducted position for 20 minutes.
5. Wait 5 minutes.
6. With the patient sitting in the supported abducted position, apply a deep, lubricated effleurage massage proximal to distal to the supraspinatus and infraspinatus muscles with emphasis to the supraspinatus. The clinician should be careful to release pressure when approaching the "V" made by the junction of the clavicle and acromium process.

TABLE 10-1

Findings in a Rotator Cuff Strain

Degree of Strain	Severity	Symptoms	Rehabilitation
First degree	Mild strain	Tenderness over tendon insertions Mild weakness Loss of normal shoulder rhythm Limited AROM	Conservative management Modalities of choice Flexibility Strengthen involved structures
Second degree	Incomplete or partial thickness Tear, resulting in scar tissue for development	Decreased muscle strength Loss of shoulder rhythm Tenderness at insertion Tenderness at musculotendinous junction	Antiinflammatory medication Sling/swath Flexibility
Third degree	Complete tendon rupture Scarring tissue	Weakness with inability to abduct shoulder actively Tenderness at insertion Possible drop arm test Possible muscle isolation tests Crepitus Possible lesion Atrophy of affected muscle Positive anothogram or MRI	Modalities Conservative management Surgery Immobilization

General instructions

1. Never allow the arm to rest at the side. This position cuts the blood supply off the tendon and retards healing. Instruct the athlete always to prop the arm and support it at about 45 degrees of abduction when sitting. When the athlete is standing, the arm is in use, and the abducted position can be disregarded; however, when standing for prolonged periods, the athlete should be instructed to support the hand in a pants pocket or waistband.
2. Avoid any activity above waist level.
3. Avoid any heavy lifting, pushing, or pulling.
4. Instruct the athlete to avoid excessive use of the arm for any activity; it needs rest and protection to heal. In general, any activity causing pain should be avoided.
5. Instruct the patient to apply a cold pack twice daily for at least 30 minutes to the top and back of the shoulder in the area of the supraspinatus and infraspinatus. The arm must be supported out to the side on a table or pillow in the abducted position.
6. When the athlete is free of pain and has no painful arc in shoulder flexion and abduction and when resistive tests are negative for pain, the athlete can begin a more definitive exercise program.

Inflammation of Shoulder Complex Structures

Although numerous injuries to the shoulder with resultant pain and disability arise from acute injuries, a process of repeated microtraumas sometimes is associated with secondary conditions such as tendonitis.[49,50] Most literature has been unable to identify clearly the exact etiological factors that may cause a disease process or overuse to the shoulder complex (Fig. 10-39). However, most inflammations can be classified into five categories:

1. Supraspinatus tendonitis.
2. Bicipital tendonitis.
3. Infraspinatus and teres minor tendonitis.
4. Bursitis, subdeltoid and subacromial.
5. Adhesive capsulitis.

Proper planning of the rehabilitation program requires further delineation as to the extent of the disability and the nature of the inflammation. Acute inflammatory conditions are characterized by pain that is present at rest, diffuse in its distribution, and often referred from the site of the primary condition. Any passive movement restriction usually is a result of soft tissue impingement and muscle guarding in response to pain.

People with chronic shoulder conditions typically do not complain of pain at rest, although specific activities usually elicit pain, particularly at the end of range of motion. The hallmark sign of a chronic inflammatory condition is the loss of range of motion, both actively and passively, which implies soft tissue shortening of the associated structures. Palpable tenderness may be noted in a distinct area, although not always at the site of the soft tissue shortening. Treatment procedures to eliminate tendonitis are varied. Immobilization, hot and cold therapy, phonophoresis, and even drug therapy associated with some forms and lengths of rest all have been effective procedures in the treatment of shoulder tendonitis. Likewise, procedures to reduce pain are also varied. Transcutaneous electrical nerve stimulation, hot and cold therapy, and early mobilization have had positive benefits on the pain associated with tendonitis. Friction massage is another key element that can be added to the treatment program of shoulder tendonitis. Cyriax and Cyriax[13] point out a number of different massage techniques that are used by sports therapists for the treatment of shoulder tendonitis. However, deep friction massage seems to be the most effective. It may be used in conjunction with orthopedic manual therapy techniques of mobilization.

SUPRASPINATUS TENDONITIS. Inflammation of the supraspinatus tendon of the rotator cuff is believed by many authors to be the single most common cause of shoulder pain. Rotator cuff tendonitis is now commonly classified as impingement syndrome when isolated to supraspinatus tendonitis. Hawkins and Kennedy[27] classify the impingement syndrome in three categories:

Stage I: Usually occurs to athletes 25 years old or younger, with symptoms of a toothachelike discomfort or pain, primarily involving the supraspinatus tendon. It features point tenderness over the greater tuberosity and the anterior acromion, a painful arc of abduction to a maximum of 90 degrees, pain initiated with forced flexion, and resultant edema and hemorrhaging. Usually this condition is reversible.

Stage II: Greatly affects the population between 25 and 40 years old. Again, symptoms present with toothachelike pain or discomfort, somewhat heightened at night, and severe pain with the drop arm test. This condition is somewhat irreversible and caused by a fibrosing and thickening of the supraspinatus tendon, biceps tendon, and the subacromial bursa, which cause a painful arc syndrome.

Stage III: Seen in the general population of 40 years old and over, with a prolonged history of shoulder problems. Wearing and attrition of the supraspinatus and/or biceps tendons are present and may result in a secondary rotator cuff tear. Pain is much worse at night and prohibits any form of athletic endeavor. Surgical intervention may be warranted. Again, a thorough evaluation to identify the exact problem with impingement syndromes is absolutely necessary.

Impingement has been defined by Neer[49,50] as the impingement of the anterior portion of the acromion with its attached coracoacromial ligament on the critical area of the rotator cuff and biceps tendon. A very positive impingement test with point tenderness at the critical zone occurs in all cases. Poor blood supply to this area is cited as reason for susceptibility of this area to injury (Fig. 10-40). The critical zone is defined by Hill and Simon as: "when the shoulder is abducted, the vessels of the supraspinatus are completely filled."[30] When the arm is adducted, a constant area of avascularity extends to within 1 cm of the insertion of the tendon into the greater tuberosity. Chronic irritation of the supraspinatus in the avascular region could lead to an inflammatory response, which is clinically referred to as **tendonitis.** This process may spread to the biceps tendon, the subacromial bursa, and even to the AC joint. With time and the progression of wearing and attrition, microtears and partial-thickness rotator cuff tears may result. If this process continues, secondary bony changes that potentially lead to complete-thickness rotator cuff tears may occur. **Impingement syndrome** is the term used to describe this process (Fig. 10-41). Limited active range of motion and full passive range of motion may be identified. The rehabilitation protocols for impingement syndrome are varied; however, general consideration must

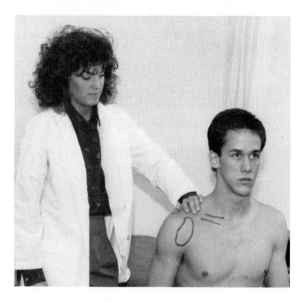

Fig. 10-40. Identifying the critical zone of the subacromial area.

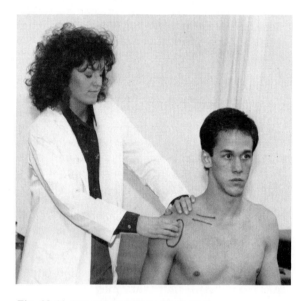

Fig. 10-41. Palpation of the critical zone.

be given to decreasing the symptoms, increasing strength, and increasing flexibility. Postural corrections, a key area often overlooked, may be necessary.

Many factors can contribute to the etiology of the impingement syndrome, including a natural degeneration of this critical zone due to the aging process, repetitive action or ringing out of the supraspinatus tendon, a generalized weak rotator cuff, weak trapezoids and serratus anterior, limited internal rotation, a hypertrophic coracoid process, and many related postural dysfunctions.[7,27,49,50] Also, amateur incoordination and fatigue expose the rotator cuff to impingement. Naturally, overuse from a particular sport such as throwing, tennis, and swimming must also be considered. The conservative trial treatment for impingement syndrome suggested by most literature is 8 to 12 weeks of controlling inflammation, increasing range of motion, increasing strength, modifying posture and activity, and a modified functional progression. If the rehabilitation program is ineffective, however, surgical procedures to modify the coracoid acromial arch may be necessary. Surgical procedures designed to alleviate these problems include the subacromial bursectomy, coracoid acromial ligament resection, anterior acromioplasty, and distal clavicle resection.

Impingement syndrome rehabilitation program

PHASE I: Decrease the inflammatory response and begin exercise to improve proximal stabilization in the acute phase. Exercise should always be performed within the pain-free range of motion.

1. Increase strength of serratus anterior, latissimus dorsi, rhomboid, trapezius, and levator scapulae. That these muscles provide maximum stability is crucial.
2. Rotator cuff isometrics. Functional rehabilitation exercises are very important with these muscle groups.
3. Postural training.

Once pain-free range of motion is established, progression to phase 2 may begin. Lengthen any shortened structures that have been identified, such as anterior musculature, shoulder elevators, and the biceps tendon. Strengthen any weakened structures below 90 degrees horizontal to avoid compromising the subacromial structures.

PHASE II:

1. Low-intensity PREs for supraspinatus (empty can raise).
2. Teres minor tendon strengthening.
3. Functional patterns of the rotator cuff using surgical tubing and PNF.
4. Specific isotonic exercises: Hughston and empty can raise.

NOTE: Avoid positions of shoulder abduction with moderate to heavy weight and/or mechanical machines.

Next, postural corrections must be initiated. The serratus anterior, the protractors, the rhomboids, and the middle trapezius all need to be taken into consideration in the strengthening program. Stabilization and retraction of the scapula are vital in the elimination of rounded shoulders.

PHASE III:

1. Strengthening: increase the isotonic program to include progressive PREs and a high-speed program on isokinetic devices. Change any postural problems, looking again at the shoulder elevators, tightness of the anterior chest, and strengthening of the posterior musculatures of the back for gradual return to modified activity.
2. Velocity spectrum training of the rotator cuff (internal and external rotation). This exercise may require velocity speed of upwards of 600 degrees per second.
3. Velocity spectrum training for strength of shoulder complex musculature.

PHASE IV: Return to activity may take up to 8 weeks. The importance of complying with the program of gradual return should be emphasized to the athlete. A frequent error is returning to activity too quickly.

BICIPITAL TENDONITIS. Another overuse syndrome at the shoulder complex that is often misinterpreted as impingement is bicipital tendonitis or tenosynovitis. The etiology is often overuse or trauma to the anterior aspect of the shoulder that causes irritation to either the tendon itself or the sheath that protects it. Commonly this syndrome is secondary to repetitive hard throwing or overhead activity, for example, swimming, tennis, and baseball. For athletes with bicipital tendonitis, pain is present on palpation of the bicipital groove, with passive stretch of the tendon, and with resistive movement from the stretched position. Shoulder flexion, internal rotation, and shoulder abduction to 90 degrees with external rotation may also be weak and painful. Continued irritation to this tendon may well lead to persistent disability and/or tendon rupture.

Treatment programs for this condition have included conservative management, antiinflammatory medication, ice, electrical stimulation, ul-

trasound, and phonophoresis. The rehabilitation protocol may incorporate any of these treatment modalities. Cross friction massage may be indicated.

PHASE I: Decrease inflammatory response and begin a gentle stretching program.
1. Stretching anterior shoulder musculature.
2. Isometrics.
3. Strengthen posterior shoulder structures.
4. Postural training.

PHASE II: Once the acute condition has subsided, begin low-intensity PREs and continue to stretch the anterior structure.
1. Continue anterior muscle stretching.
2. Low-intensity PREs.
3. Empty can raise.
4. Infraspinatus and teres minor strengthening for external rotation.
5. Surgical tubing program.
6. UBE.
7. PNF.
8. Postural strengthening to retract shoulders.

PHASE III: Pain-free motion should be the guide to progress to this phase for specific strengthening.
1. Low-intensity PREs.
2. UBE and PNF.
3. Begin isokinetic program: submaximal velocity spectrum program for shoulder abduction, IR, ER.
4. Aquatic therapy.
5. Begin functional return activities, swimming, a throwing program, and sport-specific exercises.

PHASE IV: Return to activity may take up to 8 weeks. The importance of gradual return should be reinforced.
1. Maximal isokinetic program: all planes, shoulder abduction-adduction, IR-ER, flexion-extension, and horizontal abduction-adduction, velocity spectrum program.
2. PNF exercises.
3. UBE program.
4. Functional return activities.

OTHER TENDONITIS PATHOLOGIES. Rehabilitation programs of other specific tendonitis pathologies of the shoulder joint can also be classified into four phases.

PHASE I: The rest and antiinflammatory phase, with particular attention to decreasing the inflammatory response, initiating isometrics to retard atrophy, and beginning gentle range-of-motion exercises.

PHASE II: Reestablishing pain-free range of motion and beginning low-intensity strengthening exercises.

PHASE III: Strengthening with concentration on high number of repetitions and low amount of weight in the unaffected planes. Also, deep friction massage may be instituted, along with continued stretching, ROM, and strengthening exercises.

PHASE IV: Functional progression return, the key being program specificity.

Conservative management of overuse syndromes may be ineffective in some instances. Surgical procedures may be necessary to relieve symptoms.

BURSITIS. There are numerous bursae around the shoulder complex. All play a very important role in decreasing friction between two or more structures and lubricating the articular surfaces. The bursae most frequently inflamed are the subacromial and subdeltoid. Each has a significant role in the anatomy of the suprahumeral space, with their primary function as that of providing lubrication to decrease friction of contractile structures. Unfortunately, the subacromial and subdeltoid bursae are irritated quite easily. Specific examination and evaluation of the shoulder girdle complex should allow the sports therapist to identify these structures as to the specific pathology. Bursitis can be recognized by:

1. History of overuse.
2. Intermittent pain in dominant shoulder.
3. Pain after activity.
4. Night pain.
5. History of trauma.
6. Limited AROM.
7. Limited PROM and/or noncapsular pattern.
8. Pain on palpation.
9. Empty end feel.
10. Late-onset painful arc.

Immediately decreasing the acute symptoms with medication, injection, and modalities of choice—ice, electrical stimulation, or phonophoresis—can significantly improve these athletes. The addition of transverse friction massage may be appropriate in the subacute state. Once the acute symptoms have subsided, a more detailed rehabilitation program may be initiated.

PHASE I
1. The rest and antiinflammatory phase, with the objective of decreasing the inflammatory response.
2. Isometrics.
3. PROM techniques.
4. Gentle AROM in nonpainful range.

PHASE II: Progression to this phase may move very quickly, 2 to 3 days, after the acute symptoms have been controlled.
1. Pain-free AROM.
2. Low-intensity PREs.
3. Surgical tubing.
4. Wand exercises.
5. UBE, self ROM.
6. Cross friction massage.

PHASE III: Once pain-free, normal ROM has occurred, concentration on strengthening measures is necessary.
1. Continued stretching of shortened structures.
2. Normal, pain-free ROM exercises.
3. PREs (low weight and high repetitions) specific to shoulder stabilizers and posterior shoulder muscles.
4. Surgical tubing.
5. PNF techniques.
6. Specific isotonics.
7. Submaximal isokinetic program.

PHASE IV: Return to normal activity, maintenance of strength, normal ROM and stretching techniques. Postural control exercise may be significant.

ADHESIVE CAPSULITIS. Usually a resulting factor secondary to a primary pathological condition of the shoulder complex, adhesive capsulitis has a very debilitating effect on shoulder girdle motion and thus affects the functional ability of the upper extremity. The joint capsule of the glenohumeral joint becomes adhered to itself due to a lack of motion, and adhesions develop in contractile structures. Adhesive capsulitis develops secondary to rotator cuff injuries or tears, prolonged immobilization, and proximal humeral fractures; however, this condition may develop from other pathologies that limit glenohumeral motion. Primarily this condition is seen in people who are more sedentary, who are older than 50, and who have previously sustained a shoulder complex injury. This condition is rarely seen in younger, more active people.

Normally, treatment goals are very elementary: decrease pain, increase range of motion, increase muscle strength, endurance, and coordination, educate patients, and improve function. Following an evaluation of the shoulder girdle, the sports therapist can assess the treatment and rehabilitation plan. Critical information that should be gained from evaluation includes:

1. History.
2. Active ROM.
3. Passive ROM.
4. Palpation.
5. Mobility testing of accessory joints.

The sports therapist may find restrictions in motion that commonly are referred to as **capsular patterns.** Two patterns that may be restricted are:

$$ER > ABD > IR \quad or \quad ER > IR > ABD$$

Normally the first example is the most common, with the greatest limitations in external rotation, followed by abduction, and the least restriction of motion in internal rotation.

Once the evaluation and assessment has been made, a detailed, comprehensive treatment and rehabilitation program can be developed.

PHASE I: In this phase, emphasis is placed on decreasing the inflammatory response and initiating a pain-free ROM program. No immobilization is indicated in this phase. It may be the most challenging phase of the entire program because of the restrictions in motion.

1. Medications to control inflammation (*NSAIDs*) and modalities of choice (ice or heat). Ultrasound may be effective in breaking adhesions.
2. Active stretching techniques.
3. Passive stretching techniques; care must be used in passive techniques to the glenohumeral joint.
4. Mobilization techniques: AC, SC, GH, and scapulothoracic joint.
5. Patient education in self-mobilization techniques: wall pulleys, inferior glide technique, rotation, chinning bar (straight hang), and prone on all fours.

PHASE II: Once the acute inflammation subsides, isometrics and low-intensity resistance exercises may begin. Continue to concentrate on ROM and normal function.

1. ROM exercises.
2. Mobilization techniques.
3. PNF exercises.
4. Wand exercises.
5. Surgical tubing.
6. Low-intensity PREs.
7. Swimming.
8. UBE.

PHASE III: Progression to this phase must not begin until pain-free, normal ROM is achieved. Once this improvement has occurred, a more aggressive isotonic and isokinetic strengthening program can be initiated.

1. Specific isotonics.
2. PNF.
3. Swimming.
4. UBEs.
5. Isokinetics.
6. Functional activities.

PHASE IV: In this phase the patient has returned to the desired normal activity and should be on a program to maintain ROM and strength.

Associated Pathologies of the Shoulder Complex

The varied associated pathologies of the shoulder complex include thoracic outlet syndrome, axillary nerve contusion or neuropathies, winging scapula due to injury to the long thoracic nerve, and brachial plexus syndromes. The following are example programs for those associated injuries.

THORACIC OUTLET SYNDROME REHABILITATION. The etiology of a thoracic outlet syndrome is compression of the subclavian artery and/or vein, possibly with associated compression of the brachial plexus nerve bundle, primarily the ulnar nerve. The mechanism can be associated with a cervical rib, compression from the scalene musculature, costoclavicular joint irritation, a clavicle fracture, or hyperabduction in the sleeping position. Even some postural deformities can be associated with the thoracic outlet syndrome (Fig. 10-42). Lutz and Gieck[42] state that rehabilitation should be directed at correcting postural problems as well as stretching and strengthening specific neck, upper trapezius, and other suspensory muscles of the shoulder girdle. A period of 4 to 6 weeks may be needed to achieve significant results from rehabilitation. Rehabilita-

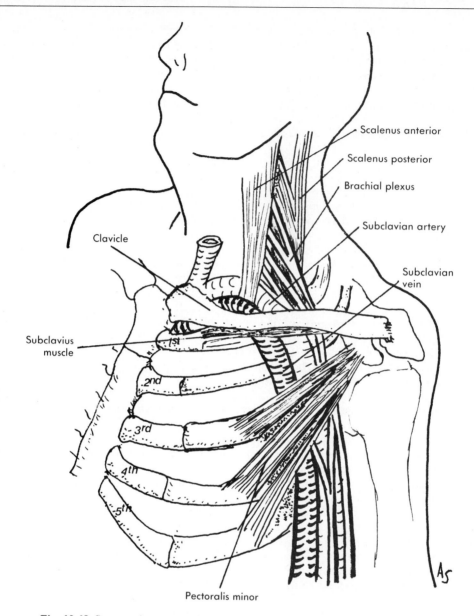

Fig. 10-42. Structural components to be considered in thoracic outlet syndrome.

tion procedures include (Fig. 10-43):

PHASE I (acute phase): Treat symptomatically with antiinflammatories, heating modalities, ultrasound, and electrical stimulation in combination. Cervical traction may be employed if a spastic neck musculature exists. Severe cases may require some form of immobilization while in the ambulatory state.

PHASE II (subacute): Stretching of the associated musculature, focusing on the lateral neck stretch, pectoralis major stretch, and stretching for flexibility of the scaline musculature, is of primary importance. Specific postural programs, described at the end of this section, should be implemented.

PHASE III (strengthening of surrounding areas):

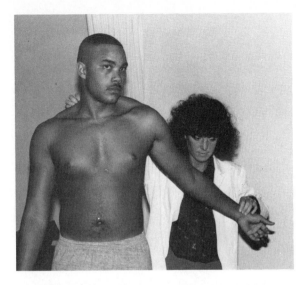

Fig. 10-43. Examination for thoracic outlet syndrome using Adson's test: when patient turns head, an absent or diminished pulse indicates compression of the subclavian artery.

Normally strengthening is concentrated in the posterior aspect of the shoulder complex: serratus anterior, posterior deltoid, middle trapezius, rhomboids, upper and lower trapezius, and levator scapular group.

PHASE IV (functional progression return): Avoid slouching position with forward shoulder and head. Educate the patient in correct posture awareness and avoidance of overarm activities.

Shoulder girdle exercises for thoracic outlet syndrome. At the beginning, each exercise is done 10 times in succession twice a day. As the shoulders and neck gain strength, the number of times each exercise is done consecutively can be increased.

1. Stand erect with the arms at the sides, holding in each hand a 2-pound weight (sandbags or bottles, jars, or sacks filled with sand). Shrug the shoulders forward and upward, and relax. Shrug the shoulders backward and upward, and relax. Shrug the shoulders upward, relax, and repeat.

2. Stand erect with the arms out straight from the sides at shoulder level while holding a 2-pound weight in each hand (palms should be down). Raise the arms sideways and up until the backs of the hands meet above the head (keep elbows straight). Relax and repeat.

As strength improves and exercises 1 and 2 become easier, weights should be made heavier; increase to 5 and later to 10 pounds.

3. Stand facing a corner of the room with one hand on each wall, arms at shoulder level, palms forward, elbows bent, and abdominal muscles contracted. Slowly let the upper part of the trunk lean forward and press the chest into the corner. Inhale as the body leans forward. Return to the original position by pushing out with the hands. Exhale with this movement.

4. Stand erect with arms at sides. Bending the neck to the left, attempt to touch the left ear to the left shoulder without shrugging the shoulder. Bending the neck to the right, attempt to touch the right ear to the right shoulder without shrugging the shoulder. Relax and repeat.

5. Lie facedown with the hands clasped behind the back. Raise the head and chest from the floor as high as possible while pulling the shoulders backward and the chin in. Hold this position for a count of 3. Inhale as the chest is raised. Exhale and return to the original position. Repeat.

6. Lie down on the back with arms at sides and a rolled towel or small pillow under the upper part of the back between the shoulder blades and no pillow under the head. Inhale slowly and raise the arms upward and backward overhead. Exhale and lower the arms to the sides. Repeat 5 to 20 times.

AXILLARY NERVE CONTUSIONS OR NEUROPATHY. The etiology is often a contusion to the posterior deltoid musculature or lateral flexion of the neck to the same side resulting in a neuropraxia of the axillary nerve. Contusion to this nerve results in motor weakness and associated decreased sensory distribution on the lateral aspect of the deltoid and humerus, seen as weakness of abduction, external rotation, and shoulder extension.

Rehabilitation protocol

PHASE I (acute): Treat symptomatically with moist heat and antiinflammatories. Electrical stimulation may be necessary by treating a denervated nerve with galvanic current. Maintain ROM in affected shoulder and begin isometric program.

PHASE II (subacute): Strengthening and flexibility programs must be initiated. For strengthening of associated musculature, internal rotators, adductors, and forward flexors of the shoulder, concentrate initially on abduction to 90 degrees and external rotation. Flexibility should be maintained for general range of motion in all planes of the shoulder joint.

PHASE III (strengthening): Working on progressive resistive exercises in all planes, dumbbells, wand exercises, surgical tubing, wall pulleys, and even an isokinetic program if possible.

PHASE IV (functional return): Return to participation depends on achieving equal bilateral strength. In severe cases of axillary nerve contusions, EMG studies may be necessary, and prolonged periods of rehabilitation may be required.

WINGING SCAPULA. A winging scapula involves an injury to the long thoracic nerve. The etiology is usually associated with neck injury and/or shoulder injury from a compression force, lateral flexion of the neck, or direct blow to the long thoracic nerve that causes partial or total paralysis of the serratus anterior musculature and thus the winging of the effected scapula (Fig. 10-44).

PHASE I (acute stage): Treat symptomatically with moist heat, electrical stimulation, and heating modalities of choice. Increase range of motion without immobilization. Begin isometric program, Codman's, and wand exercises.

PHASE II (strengthening and stretching programs): Strengthen associated musculature, trapezius, rhomboids, and latissimus dorsi by using wand exercises with weight, surgical tubing, wall pulleys, isotonic programs, and PNFs. Stabilization of the scapula is of primary importance for any shoulder motion; thus, injury to the serratus anterior musculature disrupts the total shoulder complex rhythm, especially over-the-head activities.

PHASE III (increased strengthening): Begin an isokinetic program, progressing from a slow-

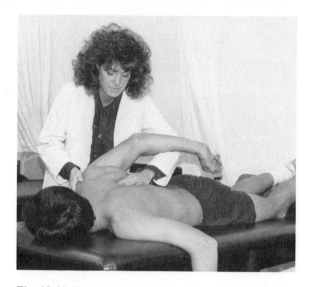

Fig. 10-44. Palpating for winging of scapula, which can be a result of injury to the long thoracic nerve.

speed velocity spectrum program to a high-speed program. Concentration is on serratus anterior muscle and its actions.

PHASE IV (functional program): Return to active participation via a functional program.

BRACHIAL PLEXUS INJURIES TO THE SHOULDER COMPLEX. Although not necessarily an isolated shoulder joint or complex injury, brachial plexus injuries do have a significant effect on the shoulder complex and upper extremity. The normal etiology of brachial plexus lesions involves lateral flexion of the neck to the opposite side with resultant shoulder depression on the same side as the force, resulting in the stretching or traction force of the brachial plexus nerve bundle. This resultant stretching gives pain, numbness, tingling, and a dead arm effect down the affected extremity. Normally, this feeling goes away in a matter of seconds; however, with repeated brachial plexus syndromes, these symptoms are prolonged and result in muscular weakness of the associated area. With all brachial plexus injuries, prevention is a key component in the rehabilitation protocol for brachial plexus lesions.

PHASE I: Immobilization is not necessary unless the strength of the associated extremity significantly decreases. A sling or sling and swath may be necessary to provide this immobilization. Treatment of choice in this phase is to treat symptomatically to reduce the related muscle spasms and associated pain.

PHASE II: In this phase, concentrate on achieving pain-free range of motion in the shoulder and neck. Once free of pain, begin low-intensity isotonics that focus on the neck musculature, upper trapezius, and anterior and posterior shoulder musculature. Surgical tubing, wand exercises with weight, PNF, and specific isotonics may all be incorporated in this phase.

PHASE III: Begin aggressive PRE exercises and isokinetics in all planes. Concentrate on strengthening the neck musculature to prevent repeated lateral flexion stretch injuries. Strengthening the associated muscles is imperative because normal strength gains must be achieved before return to unrestricted participation can be allowed.

PHASE IV: Begin functional progression prior to return. Protection with a neck collar may be necessary if the patient participates in football or wrestling.

Suggestions have been given in this chapter to assist the sports therapist in developing protocols for a wide variety of shoulder pathologies. Once a thorough evaluation has determined the structures involved, individualization of the rehabilitation programs is the key to optimum recovery, with consideration given to the patient's goals, age, activity level, and surgical procedures.

Shoulder injuries alone are usually not life-threatening; with shoulder involvement, however, the effectiveness of the movement of the entire upper extremity is decreased. Whether the patient is a recreational or world-class athlete, a laborer or housewife, daily living activities are suddenly compromised with shoulder disability. Quality of life can be greatly improved by early recognition and individualized treatment of the particular shoulder pathology.

SUMMARY

1. The effects of articular surfaces of the glenohumeral joint contribute minimally to stability, and the dynamic relationship of the joint is largely the function of the soft tissue structures.

2. The shoulder complex soft tissue structures and rotator cuff mechanism have significant roles in maintaining joint stability and range of motion.

3. Management of rotator cuff injuries remains varied because of the opinions among physicians and sports therapists regarding the cause of rotator cuff pathology.

4. Conservative management appears to be favorable for the treatment and rehabilitation of shoulder complex pathologies.

5. Examination and interpretation should enable the clinician to identify movement disorders of the shoulder complex.

6. Disorders can be divided into dysfunction of contractile tissues and dysfunction of non-contractile structures.

7. Appropriate treatment and rehabilitation goals may be established on the basis of shoulder complex evaluation.

8. Sports therapists should consider rehabilitation with proprioception and kinesthesia in the treatment of patients with glenohumeral dislocations.

9. Rehabilitation protocols must be able to implement all components of the treatment program to assure functional return to activity.

10. The multijoint shoulder girdle is vulnerable to injuries that require decisions by the sports therapist for appropriate evaluation, treatment, and followup rehabilitation that allows the patient to return to normal motion, strength, endurance, and proprioception.

REFERENCES

1 Anderson J: Grant's atlas of anatomy, ed 8, Baltimore, 1983, Williams & Wilkins.
2 Andrews R and Blackburn TA: Throwing injuries to the shoulder: pathomechanics, diagnosis and treatment, professional presentation.
3 Arnheim DD: Modern principles of athletic training, ed 6, The CV Mosby Co.
4 Beckett M: Rotator cuff and associated injuries of the pitcher's mechanism, professional presentation.
5 Bergfeld JA, Andrish JT, and Clancy WG: Evaluation of the acromioclavicular joint following first- and second-degree sprains, Am J Sports Med 16(4):153–159, 1978.
6 Booher J and Thibodeau G: Athletic injury assessment, St Louis, 1985, The CV Mosby Co.
7 Bowling R, Rockar P, and Erhard R: Examination of the

shoulder complex, Phys Ther 66(12):1866–1877, 1986.

8   Bream T: Putti-Platt rehabilitation program, professional presentation.

9   Brunet M: Rotator cuff impingement syndrome in sports, Physician Sports Med 10(12):86–94, 1982.

10   Cain P and others: Anterior stability of the glenohumeral joint (dynamic model), Am J Sports Med 15(2):144–148, 1987.

11   Carmichael S and Hart D: Anatomy of the shoulder joint, J Ortho Sports Phys Ther 6(4):225–228, 1985.

12   Corley F: Shoulder injuries in contact sports, professional presentation.

13   Cyriax J and Cyriax P: Illustrated manual of orthopaedic medicine, Butterworth Publishing, 1974.

14   Davies GJ: A compendium of isokinetics in clinical usage, ed 35, Lacrosse, Wisc, 1987, S & S Publishers.

15   Donatelli R and Greenfield B: Case study: rehabilitation of a stiff and painful shoulder: a biomechanical approach, J Ortho Sports Phys Ther 67(10):118–126, 1987.

16   Duda M: Prevention and treatment of throwing arm injuries, Physician Sports Med 13(6):181–186, 1985.

17   Einhorn A: Shoulder rehabilitation: equipment modification, J Ortho Sports Phys Ther 6(4):247–253, 1985.

18   Ellenbecker TS, Davies GJ, and Rowinski MJ: Concentric versus eccentric isokinetic strengthening of the rotator cuff, Am J Sports Med 16:64–69, 1988.

19   Erb K: Physical therapy rotator cuff treatment protocol, professional presentation.

20   Foster CR: Multidirectional instability of the shoulder in the athlete, Clin Sports Med 2(2), 1983.

21   Grana W, Holder S, and Schelberg-Karnes E: How I manage acute anterior shoulder dislocations, Physician Sports Med 15(4), 1987.

22   Greipp J: Swimming shoulder: influence of flexibility and weight training, Physician Sports Med 13(8):92–105, 1985.

23   Grimsby O: Arthokinetics of the shoulder complex, professional presentation.

24   Hart D and Carmichael S: Biomechanics of the shoulder, J Ortho Sports Phys Ther 6(4):229–234, 1985.

25   Hawkins R: Shoulder instability, professional presentation.

26   Hawkins R and Hobeika P: Physical examination of the shoulder, Orthopedics 6(10), 1983.

27   Hawkins RJ and Kennedy JC: Impingement syndrome in athletes, Am J Sports Med 8:151–158, 1980.

28   Heckman T: Proprioceptive neuromuscular techniques in the shoulder, Cincinnati Sportsmedicine/The Midwest Institute of Orthopaedics, 1984.

29   Henry JH and Genung JA: Natural history of glenohumeral dislocation—revisited, Physician Sports Med 10(3), 1982.

30   Hill J and Simon ER: Rotator cuff injuries, Sports Medicine Update 1(2):1–6, 1988.

31   Hoppenfeld S: Physical examination of the spine and extremities, New York, 1976, Appleton-Century-Crofts.

32   Hurley J: Shoulder instability, paper presented at Cleveland Clinic Sports Symposium, July 27, 1986.

33   Jackson DW: Chronic rotator cuff impingement in the throwing athlete, Am J Sports Med 4(6):231–240, 1976.

34   Jobe F, editor: Clinics in sports medicine: symposium on injuries to the shoulder in the athlete, vol 2, number 2, Philadelphia, 1983, WB Saunders.

35   Jobe FW and Jobe CN: Painful athletic injuries of the shoulder, Clin Ortho Related Research 173:117–124, 1983.

36   Jobe FW and Moynes DR: Delineation of diagnostic criteria and a rehabilitation program for rotator cuff injuries, Am J Sports Med 10(6):336–339, 1982.

37   Jobe F, Moynes D, and Brewster C: Rehabilitation of shoulder joint instabilities, Orthop Clin North Am 18(3):473–482, 1987.

38   Johnson J, Sim F, and Scott S: Musculoskeletal injuries in competitive swimmers, Mayo Clin Proc 62:289–304, 1987.

39   Keene JS: Anatomy and saliant biomechanical aspects of the shoulder, May 1988.

40   Kessler R and Hertling D: Management of common musculoskeletal disorders, New York, 1985, Harper & Row, Publishers Inc.

41   Knott M and Voss DE: Proprioceptive neuromuscular facilitation, ed 2, New York, 1968, Harper & Row, Publishers Inc.

42   Lutz FR and Gieck JH: Thoracic outlet compression syndrome, Ath Train 21:302, 1986.

43   McLeod WD and Andrews JR: Mechanisms of shoulder injuries, Phys Ther 66(12):1901–1904, 1986.

44   McMaster W: Painful shoulder in swimmers: a diagnostic challenge, Physician Sports Med 14(12):108–122, 1986.

45   Madden T: Return to throwing program, professional presentation.

46   Meador R: Rehabilitation following arthroscopic reconstruction, professional presentation.

47   Meador R: Rehabilitation following arthroscopic rotator cuff debridement, professional presentation.

48   Myers K: Rehabilitation of the chronic anterior glenohumeral dislocation, professional presentation.

49   Neer CS: Impingement lesions, Clin Orthop 173:70–77, 1979.

50   Neer CS and Welsh RP: The shoulder in sports, Orthop Clin North Am 8(3):583–590, 1977.

51   Nitz AJ: Physical therapy management of the shoulder, Phys Ther 66(12):1912–1915, 1986.

52   Pappas AM, Zawacki RM, and McCarthy CF: Rehabilitation of the pitching shoulder, Am J Sports Med 13:225–235, 1985.

53   Peat M: Functional anatomy of the shoulder complex, Phys Ther 66(12):1855–1865, 1986.

54   Penny JN and Welsh RP: Shoulder impingement syndrome in athletes and their surgical management, Am J Sports Med 9(1):11–15, 1981.

55   Roy S and Irvin R: Sports medicine prevention, evaluation, management and rehabilitation, Englewood Cliffs, NJ, 1983, Prentice Hall.

56   Schenkman M and Decartaya V: Kinesiology of the shoulder complex, J Ortho Sports Phys Ther 8(9):438–450, 1987.

57   Simonet W and Cofield R: Prognosis in anterior shoulder

dislocation, Am J Sports Med 12(1):19–23, 1984.

58 Singleton MC: Functional anatomy of the shoulder, Phys Ther 46(10):1043–1051, 1966.

59 Smith R and Brunolli J: Shoulder kinesthesia after anterior glenohumeral joint dislocation, Phys Ther 69(2):106–112, 1989.

60 Springer S: Examination and evaluation of the painful shoulder, professional presentation.

61 Taber's Cyclopedic Medical Dictionary, ed 15, Philadelphia, 1987, FA Davis.

62 Tank R and Halbach J: Physical therapy evaluation of the shoulder complex in athletes, J Ortho Sports Phys Ther 3(3):108–120, 1982.

63 Timm K: Isokinetics in shoulder rehabilitation, paper presented at International Isokinetic Congress, Ft Lauderdale, Fla, April 24–27, 1988.

64 Voss DE, Ionta MK, and Myers BJ: Proprioceptive neuromuscular facilitation, ed 3, New York, Harper & Row, Publishers Inc.

65 Walsh D: Shoulder evaluation of the throwing athlete, HealthSouth, Sportsmedicine Update 4(2):1–7, 1989.

66 Walsh W and others: Shoulder strength following acromioclavicular injuries, Am J Sports Med 13(3):153–158, 1985.

67 Zarins B and Rowe C: Current concepts in the diagnosis and treatment of shoulder instability in athletes, Med Sci Sports Exer 16(5), 1984.

Rehabilitation of Elbow Injuries

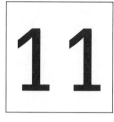

Danny T. Foster

OBJECTIVES

Following completion of this chapter, the student will be able to:

- Discuss important rehabilitation concepts for treating injuries to the elbow.

- Discuss treatment of acute inflammations, injuries involving the joint structures, and injuries involving the musculotendinous units of the elbow.

- Discuss conventions of exercise techniques in the management of elbow soft tissue recovery.

- Recognize and explain the differences between rehabilitation procedures for elbow joint restrictions and joint laxities.

- Outline a plan of therapeutic exercise designed to manage common elbow trauma.

As presented here, elbow rehabilitation follows a scheme identifying general clinical problems for which a variety of exercise techniques may be applied. Basic therapeutic indications and applications, with examples of specific sports injuries that commonly occur at the elbow, are reviewed in detail, and the general protocols are outlined for a guide to rehabilitation progression.

As with most joint trauma, the major clinical problems seen at the elbow (Fig. 11-1) are pain, swelling, reduced range of motion (ROM), and muscular weakness. These features usually follow an acute onset and are interrelated in that, once present, one precipitates another during the inflammatory period.

INFLAMMATIONS

Whether each of the features above are attributed to inflammation or remain following an acute response, common management for inflammation may be effective in enabling an op-

timal resolution of damaged tissue. Common initial techniques designed to reduce inflammation to wounded or injured tissue are (1) cryotherapy, (2) local compression, (3) stress reduction, (4) at least hand elevation, and (5) nonsteroidal antiinflammatory drugs (NSAIDs). Although any injury, to some extent, becomes acutely inflamed, those resulting from acute, excessive mechanical trauma and most likely to demonstrate these signs and symptoms are subluxations and dislocations of the **ulnohumeral joint** (medial elbow), strains of the **wrist flexor mass,** and strains of the **elbow flexor group.** The medial elbow dislocations are most commonly **valgus** but a high proportion are posterior. Less commonly, fractures of the distal humerus, olecranon, **physes,** midradius and/or ulna, and radial head elicit obvious deformity and weakness, usually reduced range of motion (ROM), and acute localized swelling at the site of the fracture. Pain under these circumstances may not be informative, but usually a history and patient perception are good early indicators. Acute in-

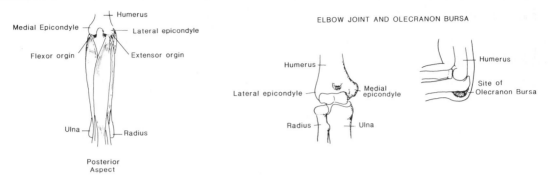

FLEXORS AND EXTENSORS ATTACHMENTS OF FOREARM

ELBOW JOINT AND OLECRANON BURSA

Fig. 11-1. Elbow joint complex.

flammations from chronic and repetitive forces at or through the elbow generally indicate significant degenerative pathology; in a young athlete, such inflammations represent difficult management cases. Among this category of trauma, the sports therapist commonly sees medial epicondylitis (little leaguer's elbow, golfer's elbow, baseball elbow), lateral epicondylitis (tennis elbow, epicondylagia lateralis, extensor carpi radialis brevis tendonitis), **radial head degeneration, traction spurs,** olecranon fossitis, and triceps tendonitis.

Cryotherapy

Cryotherapy in elbow rehabilitation is a common modality universally applied in acute trauma management; however, the sports therapist must be aware of the physiological and psychological responses to cold in the elbow region. Circulation here is usually very good and limb density is low. These factors may be considered in modifying the time and/or temperature of the cooling agent when treating the elbow. Tolerable but vigorous local icing is commonly applied for 15 to 30 minutes as soon after an initial evaluation as possible, preferably within the hour. Some clinical practices expand the treatment time considerably, but the sports therapist should be concerned about the effective skin temperature and the depth of tissue damage. Because condylar ridges are very superficial in this area, acute tissue damage, such as fractures, posterior and/or medial dislocations, and flexor mass strains may be **exacerbated** by the inflam-

matory effect of the ice. Adjustments of the effective skin temperature can be made with wet or dry toweling or cloth. Some sports therapists have used glycerol or skin protectants in this area, especially for sensitive patients. Unless open wounds are present, acute applications of ice or cold are combined with external compression and elevation of the limb. Following the initial cold treatment, icing throughout the inflammatory period is standard procedure. Cold can be applied periodically after the onset of injury, over the wrapping, as often as is feasible. Each session may last from 15 to 30 minutes once the perception of cold is felt. If the temperature of the skin and cooling agent is close to 85B F, then extended cooling is usually tolerated well, as well as vigorous cooling through a wet wrapping. If the effective skin temperature is closer to 60B F, then the 15- to 30-minute time limit appears prudent for superficially placed tissue damage. A possible guide might be one treatment every 2 waking hours during the acute stage (1 to 7 days, usually) so that if some hours are missed, the maximum expected benefit would still be achieved. Optimal directed care is, practically, three to four times daily. Adjunctive care with cold during immediate care or shortly thereafter is frequently used to enhance antiswelling and antipain effects. Some of these adjunctive therapies for the elbow region, as reported in the literature and used in clinical practice, are galvanic stimulation (high voltages, interferential or standard), microcurrent stimulation, and cold pressure or other pressure devices. Because the effectiveness of these adjunctive approaches is still a matter of clinical judgement, the sports therapist is directed to texts by Prentice for further discussion.

Local Compression

Circulation is definitely diminished by elbow flexion above 90 degrees because of soft tissue compression; the effect is even more pronounced in the well-developed athlete. That type of compression may be effective immediately after an injury but loses its cost-benefit ratio with many bony and soft tissue injuries. External compression with an Ace-type elastic wrap, elastic stockinette, or full-arm mesh sleeve may be applied to the elbow either singly or in combination with elbow flexion. When applying Ace-type wraps to this area, attempt to place the elbow in the **resting position** or position of least joint compression or the position in a sling (Table 11-1) before application because moving to this position once the wrap is applied usually results in increased compression at the proximal forearm and elbow and then distal arm **stasis,** swelling, or numbness. Full elbow flexion, used as compression, should be avoided following dislocations, fractures, and **joint compression injuries.** Instructions to the athlete concerning skin color, feelings of numbness and tingling, throbbing, and other signs of circulatory distress should be made clear. Some practical instructions for a variety of problems for which the above symptoms may develop during treatment by compression include: (1) first, elevate the hand, and if this is not helpful in 2 to 3 minutes,

lie down and elevate the entire arm with pillows; (2) if not relieved within 5 minutes, apply ice to the wrapped area; (3) again, if not relieved within 5 minutes, loosen the wrap or compression; and (4), should none of this work to relieve the signs of excessive compression, use a referral protocol. **Ischemic Volkmann's contracture,** whether from **iatrogenic,** excessive, and prolonged compression or as a secondary entity to forearm and humeral fractures, is a devastating problem to anyone, let alone to a throwing or upper extremity-dominant athlete.

Stress Reduction and Elevation

Because elevation is the only exercise component (that is, rest) in the above list, a short consideration of specifics is warranted. Elevation of the hand, such as provided by a sling, Velpeau, or immobilizer, offers little to the understanding of optimal positioning, other than to produce a bent elbow, usually so that the hand is at or above the level of the heart. Kinesiology shows that the resting or loose-packed position of the elbow is about 70 degrees of flexion and 10 to 20 degrees of supination. Barring further complications such as surgical procedures, fractures, and the like, this position allows for a maximum volume of inflammatory joint swelling and for midrange posture to facilitate relaxation. A sling that supports the forearm and extends to the metacarpophalangeal joints would most effectively promote inflammatory resolution through controlled joint and supported limb positioning, which together serve to reduce pain and enhance muscular relaxation. The hand might be best placed to rest gently with the ulnar edge of the palm next to the abdomen. True elevation is most effective when the athlete is being treated and when at home by lying supine with pillows supporting the affected arm. Decreasing stress at the site of tissue damage may not be as easy as placing the arm in a sling. **Close-packed** positions of the elbow vary among the three joints in the **elbow complex.** Additionally, tension at the wrist and hand, such as when gripping or writing, produces joint compression forces at the elbow through muscular action. When extensive swelling or joint surface injuries are present, wrist and hand activities may have to be minimized.

TABLE 11-1

Resting (Loose-Packed) and Close-Packed Positions of the Elbow

Joint	Position
Ulnohumeral	
Loose	70° flexion, 10° supination
Close	Extension
Radiohumeral	
Loose	Full extension, full supination
Close	90° flexion, 5° supination
Proximal Radioulnar	
Loose	70° flexion, 35° supination
Close	5° supination

CARE FOR ACUTE INFLAMMATION

IMMEDIATE CARE (Within 4 Hours of the Injury)

1. Cold (never in a dependent position; rest the cold agent on the arm, not the reverse)
2. Compression (Ace)
3. Elevation and/or protection (sling)
4. Rest (effective, full-limb inactivity)
5. Antiinflammatory medication
6. Instructions on care and compliance

POST-IMMEDIATE CARE (1 to 7 Days, Usually)

1. Symptomatic care
   Cold (3 to 4 times daily)
   Compression (24 hours)
   Elevation and/or protection (24 hours, except during exercise)
   Rest (the elbow, hand, shoulder as needed)
   Antiinflammatory (take as prescribed, until finished)
2. Controlled exercises for the elbow, wrist, hand, and shoulder, pain free and as indicated by the condition. Controlled exercises may have to be limited if the patient is in a cast, and symptomatic care may be restricted to elevation, rest, and antiinflammatory medication. No restrictions need be placed on the other components, however.
3. Cardiovascular training; usually no restrictions exist for this type of exercise. However, biking is strongly preferred to running if jostling is a concern.
4. General body exercises: as long as shoulder and arm stabilization is not used in the exercise, these activities are unlimited and indicated for sport-specific progressions.

MEDICATIONS

Antiinflammatory nonsteroidals (such as naproxen and sulindac) and certainly steroidal antiinflammatories (dexamethasone) have their greatest effect in the long term by early administration, less than 4 hours after an injury. However, tissue healing responses (as measured by tissue strength) may be diminished during a window period early in recovery. This effect holds the sports therapist to a steady progression in rehabilitation, even in the face of significant pain relief and apparent full function. Despite the recent and widespread use of NSAIDs, research evidence is not clear whether blocking cyclooxygenase activity with nosteroidals or blocking arachidonic acid synthesis by the use of steroids results in enhanced or diminished healing rates.

Until this issue is resolved, the dramatic results often seen with NSAIDs need to be assessed in light of a false confidence factor, denoted in the terminology "combating inflammation"; therefore, timing in rehabilitation must still be based on knowledge of healing rates and evaluation parameters. This process of rehabilitation timing for the elbow appears relatively straightforward in the literature.

The sports therapist may picture the mnemonic the three Cs for cool, calm, and collected when treating acute pathological conditions about the elbow: **cool** for effective tissue temperatures ranging from 60° to 85° F, **calm** for low stresses and only tolerable (pain-free) motion, and **collected** for the circulatory and limb support provided by elastic wraps and slings or immobilizers.

JOINT STRUCTURES AND MUSCULOTENDINOUS UNIT INJURIES
Motion Restrictions

Limited ranges of normal motion following surgery, long-term immobility, and trauma represent subacute or chronic complications of many elbow pathologies. They may be produced by soft tissue **dysfunction** and related to underlying contractures, adhesions, and muscle spasm. Muscle weakness may also be a factor in the limitation of ROM but is not considered in this discussion until the protocol for this problem and then again in the section on joint laxity. Late stages of tissue healing or scar maturation with clinically assessed limited motion may be prevented by early and tolerable physiological motion if the sports therapist pays attention to the stresses placed on surgical repair sites, on stabilizing structures, and on joint surfaces. As Fred Allman has so aptly stated, "the main effort in treatment should be directed to the cause of the condition rather than the resultant effect."[43] Clinically, the athlete may present with flexion limitation more often than extension and supination as equally affected as pronation. Progressive stages of medial collateral ligament tears in pitchers, fractures, and dislocations are common examples of injuries that develop motion restrictions. The following techniques may be appropriately used when (1) active but limited ROM is pain free and (2) when passive physiological overpressure is pain free or mildly painful after resistance is felt. Additional criteria for the indications of joint and soft tissue mobilization in this region can be found in several resources.[11,18,19,21,42] Common motion goals for these patients may involve maintaining available motion or retarding progressive mechanical restrictions, stimulating neurophysiological mechanoreceptors, inhibiting nociceptive stimuli, encouraging synovial fluid motion, maintaining nutrient exchange, and elongating hypomobile structures. Should the hypomobile structures represent the new and major stabilizing structures of the elbow complex following significant joint injury, the following techniques may not be indicated.

Soft Tissue Mobilization

As usual, an assessment of the underlying cause should progress from superficial (skin) to deep (joint capsule) with palpation and motion assessment techniques.[18,21,24,25,42] Soft tissue mobilization techniques such as **directional shear, tension oscillations, scissoring,** and deep friction massage may be effectively applied either singly or in combination to increase elbow flexion or rotations. Following these techniques, the sports therapist should attempt to retain and enhance active ROM with at least submaximal isometric resistance in the new available range or hold-relax-active motion and slow reversal-hold-relax proprioceptive neuromuscular facilitation (PNF) techniques for emphasis on shoulder and elbow and then emphasis on wrist and hand (Fig. 11-2). Other strengthening and stretching techniques may be effective for those not trained in PNF techniques and for those who do not have the luxury of extended one-on-one time. Although stretching is a nuclear component to retaining normal function, inappropriate and

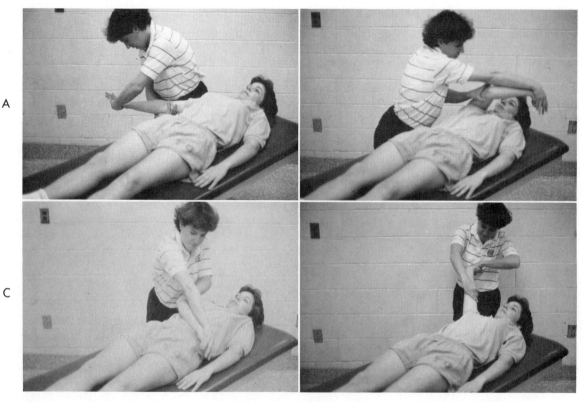

Fig. 11-2. Proprioceptive neuromuscular facilitation patterns. **A,** D1 flexion; **B,** D1 extension; **C,** D2 flexion; **D,** D2 extension.

overexuberant technique severely compromises the final result if the underlying problem is other than muscle adaptive shortening from immobility.

Stretching

Athletes can easily be taught simple stretching techniques with a partner or with the use of apparatus but must be educated, observed, and given feedback early and regularly in order to avoid ineffective, overzealous, and sometimes disastrous results. Partner techniques can be used to obtain the most desirable results and are generally used early in the progression of rehabilitation. For stretching the triceps, medial and lateral heads, and the anconeus, the athlete is best situated to begin supine, arm slightly abducted, with the elbow flexed and slightly supinated (Fig. 11-3). Facing the head of the athlete at the side, the sports therapist's hand furthest from the athlete should grasp the dorsal forearm just

proximal to the wrist; the other hand should stabilize the proximal humerus. Gradual flexion is pursued in an arclike motion in an attempt to reach the athlete's fingers to the shoulder. Flexion agonist action can be resisted to facilitate triceps relaxation. The long head of the triceps may be ideally stretched with the athlete lying prone, shoulder fully flexed, and the pillow or table situated for full shoulder adduction (Fig. 11-4). The sports therapist faces the athlete at the head and grips the forearm just proximal to the wrist with the hand closest to the head and stabilizes the athlete's shoulder posteriorly with the other hand. From a flexed and slightly supinated position, the forearm is moved gradually to full flexion.

Stretching into supination primarily involves the pronators and flexors of the wrist and hand, whereas stretching into pronation involves the

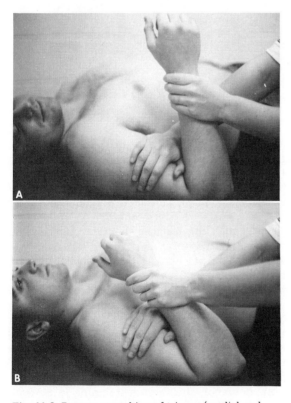

Fig. 11-3. Partner stretching of triceps (medial and lateral head) and anconeus. **A,** Starting position; **B,** terminal position.

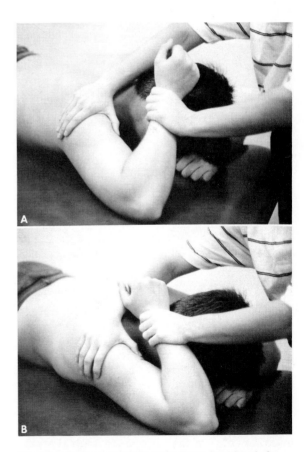

Fig. 11-4. Partner stretching of triceps, long head. **A,** Starting position; **B,** terminal position.

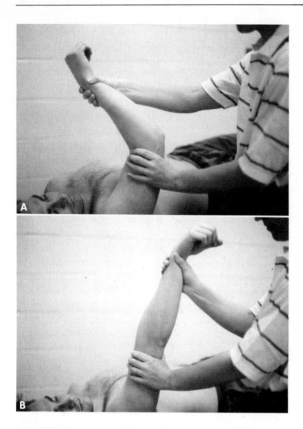

Fig. 11-5. Partner stretching of supinator. **A,** Starting position; **B,** terminal position.

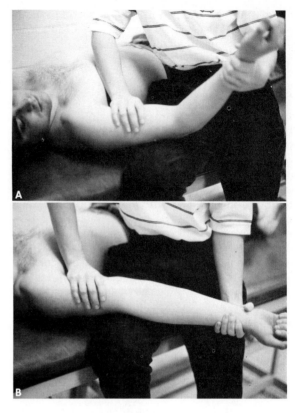

Fig. 11-6. Partner stretching of pronator teres and quadratus. **A,** Starting position; **B,** terminal position.

supinator and extensors of the wrist and hand (Fig. 11-5). Only the supinator and pronators (teres and quadratus) are presented here. For supination, the athlete lies supine with the arm flexed to about 90 degrees and fully medially rotated; the forearm is slightly flexed and fully pronated. The sports therapist should face the athlete, standing at the side and gripping the distal arm dorsally with the hand closest to the athlete while the other hand stabilizes the upper arm dorsally just proximal to the elbow. The sports therapist gradually and fully extends the elbow and simultaneously draws the forearm further ulnarward.

The pronator teres may be stretched by two methods: one primarily for the humeral head and one primarily for the ulnar head with the pro-

nator quadratus. Humeral head stretching of the pronator is performed with the athlete supine, arm flexed to about 90 degrees and fully laterally rotated (Fig. 11-6). The ulnar head and pronator quadratus are also stretched in this position. Additionally, the forearm is slightly flexed and fully supinated for the starting position. The sports therapist should sit at the athlete's side, holding the forearm in the lap and facing the hand. Then grip the dorsal and distal forearm with the hand toward the head and stabilize the upper ventral arm, proximal to the elbow, with the other hand. Gradually and fully extend the elbow while drawing the forearm maximally in the ulnar direction. The second stretching maneuver involves the same flexed starting position; however, the forearm remains in neutral.

The therapist this time retains a flexed elbow and draws the forearm into a maximum ulnar direction.

Each of the stretching maneuvers can be modified to use wands, poles, walls, tables, and changes in body position. The stretch should not be painful and should be sustained statically for at least 30 seconds, whether in continuous or intermittent time periods. The available evidence suggests that stretches lasting less than 30 seconds diminish the potential elongation gains, and stretches lasting greater than 30 seconds add no additional benefit to stress resistance.[44] Because the stretch is directed at tendinous and collagen-rich fascial components, damping of these tissues occurs over a matter of hours, and stretching once per day appears to be sufficient; any gains in motion should be followed by active shortening of the antagonistic muscle group(s). This followup, active resistance exercising is designed to retain control and motion through subsequent treatment times.

Joint Mobilization

Joint mobilization techniques have been shown to be very effective in combating joint restrictions but must follow detailed evaluations and constitute skilled technical performance; otherwise, the neurophysiological and mechanical effects promoted with these techniques may be nullified by resulting joint trauma and hypermobility. This technique can be relatively safe if basic principles are followed. Although joint mobilization requires potentially extensive one-on-one time, it is definitely within the time frame and capabilities of the sports therapist.

To increase flexion of the ulnohumeral joint, sustained or early oscillatory traction commonly precedes other accessory motions (Fig. 11-7). For traction of the ulnohumeral joint, the athlete lies supine with the wrist resting against the sports therapist's outside shoulder to allow the elbow to be in the resting position. The sports therapist uses the medial aspect of the inside hand over the proximal ulna on the volar surface and then reinforces this placement with the outside hand. Force through the hand is directed against the proximal ulna at a 45-degree angle to the ulnar shaft, which is parallel to the angulation of the

joint surfaces. Mobilization in this manner can begin at physiological elbow flexion angles less than the resting angle of 70 degrees but should progress by taking up the end of the available range and always applying a 45-degree direction to the pull along the shaft of the ulna. A distal glide also assists ulnohumeral joint flexion, during which the traction position and maneuver is started and then a pull is directed along the long axis of the ulna. The sustained or oscillatory mobilization grades range in their length of application; however, sustained pulls of over 1 minute without results indicate that another maneuver or technical adjustment may be more effective. Some experience is needed to gain an appreciation of tissue end feel, but the end result is objectively measured by gains in flexion ROM.

Radiohumeral joint restrictions infrequently limit flexion or extension but may be involved with rotation restrictions. Traction of the radiohumeral joint proceeds axially along the radial shaft, and distraction glides are applied perpendicular to the head of the radius, either in a volar direction for flexion, or a dorsal direction for extension (Fig. 11-8). Further clarification of these maneuvers can be found in Kisner and Colby, Kessler and Hertling, or Wadsworth.[18,19,42] Likewise, to increase pronation and supination, the proximal radius is mobilized dorsally to increase pronation and volarly to increase supination (Fig. 11-9). The resting position of the supported forearm is 70 degrees of flexion and about 35 degrees of supination. The treatment hand may rest on a table or plinth, with this position being maintained by the palm of the other hand. The direction of motion is in the plane of the radial notch of the ulna, parallel to the long axis of the ulna. The sports therapist needs to stabilize the humerus and proximal ulna medially with a hand coming from underneath the arm. The other hand is placed around the head of the radius with the fingers on the volar surface and the palm on the dorsal surface. Volar forces are accomplished by pushing through the palm, and dorsal forces by pulling through the fingers.

Joint restrictions may occur from a variety of elbow traumas. Early attention to acute inflammatory treatment and subsequently early, active, pain free ROM may produce full and optimal results. Subacute use of soft tissue mobilization

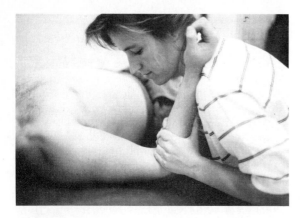

Fig. 11-7. Position for ulnohumeral joint traction.

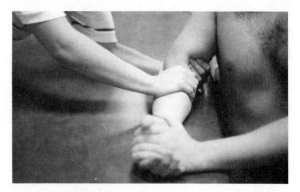

Fig. 11-9. Position for radioulnar joint volar and dorsal glides.

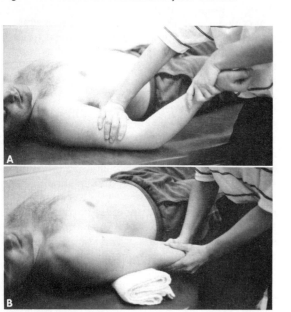

Fig. 11-8. Positions for **A,** radiohumeral joint traction and **B,** volar and dorsal glides.

and stretching is frequently effective for motion restrictions involving adhesions and muscle spasm. Where these procedures are ineffective, joint mobilization techniques may serve to elongate adhesions and subsequently to diminish muscle spasm. In any case, gains in ROM should be followed by exercise attempts at muscular control in order to take up the new available range and thus provide neural feedback for the controlled muscular pattern that will be needed

for the athlete to progress back to normal function.

Joint Laxity

Acute, pathological laxity of joint-stabilizing structures represents an entirely different circumstance from chronic, pathological laxity following elbow trauma. Resolution of nearly normal **joint play** may be anticipated in acute hypermobile conditions, even those that may extend for months. Subsequently, the major goals for joint laxity problems become (1) to maintain a shortened physiological position of ligamentous tissue, (2) to increase tissue stress progressively without abnormal mechanical strain, (3) to strengthen the secondary muscular stabilizers, and (4) to retrain **automatic reflex joint control.** For chronic laxity, surgical treatment is frequently proposed. Conservative goals, however, concentrate on (1) increasing tissue hypertrophy by directly applying oscillatory tension, (2) strengthening the secondary muscular stabilizers, and (3) retraining automatic reflex joint control.

STRENGTHENING. Because medial laxity affects the anterior oblique portion of the medial collateral ligament, early-stage exercise is often restricted to the resting position at 70 degrees of elbow flexion with slight supination. In this position isometric tension can be directed toward flexion and extension. Also in this position, shoulder and wrist exercises are encouraged. Maintaining forearm position has been promoted to impart stress to the surrounding musculature and joint structures without producing elongation or tension mechanical strain within the medial collateral ligament. Progression of these exercises usually follows a lack of symptoms during or following each session of exercise. Endurance-type exercise intensity, frequency, and duration appear to enhance the metabolic functions in healing ligaments. Isometric exercises that progress in 10- to 20-degree positions from resting are promoted early as tolerated; submaximal isometric tension is tolerated earlier than maximal (Fig. 11-10). As long as pre- and post-stress testing reveal no comparable change in valgus laxity, full supination and pronation appear to progress to full range before progression to full flexion and extension ranges. Usually, limits of strengthening exercises fall within 10 to 90 degrees of elbow flexion because this range provides the least valgus deformity and tension on the medial collateral ligament. Isotonic exercise, with both concentric and eccentric components in an endurance mode, likewise facilitates the healing response. These exercises can be performed manually with the sports therapist or with the athlete's other hand or performed with dumbbells, weights, or sandbags, but working with a bar or stationary weight machines should be avoided until full, pain-free and stable supination is gained.

Exercise in any direction of motion remains isolated, planar, and not coordinated with other joints until **proximal control** and fatigue resistance are gained. Pronation and supination exercises may need special stabilization, for example, placing the elbow and medial proximal forearm next to the trunk and maintaining shoulder internal rotation (Fig. 11-11). By placing the palm of one hand over the dorsal aspect of the distal forearm and wrist and the other hand over the matching ventral aspect, the sports therapist can interlace the fingers to control resistance to both rotation motions of the elbow and control movement of the shoulder. If the shoulder were allowed to move into adduction and external rotation, the elbow becomes vulnerable to valgus stress. Isokinetic exercise (Fig. 11-12), if available, yields a dimension of controlled motion more specific to the functional aspects of a slow-onset *U*-shaped torque curve in flexion and a rapid onset but slowly decreasing torque curve in extension.

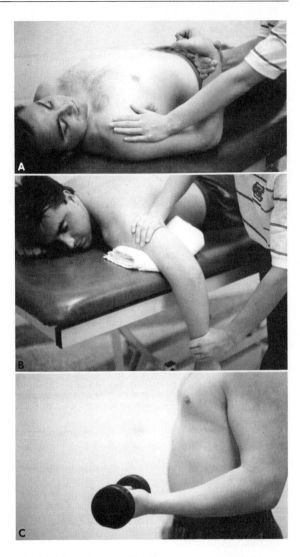

Fig. 11-10. Partner position for isometric exercise resistance for **A**, elbow flexion, **B**, elbow extension, and **C**, isotonic flexion and extension.

REFLEX CONTROL. Not only the strength aspect but also the rapidity with which the athlete gains peak torque or power serve to retrain muscular control for secondary stabilization. Other exercise methods that promote repeated muscular contractions through the available range of motion can be utilized to promote automatic reflex control of joint surface tension from the congruent apposition of the bony members within

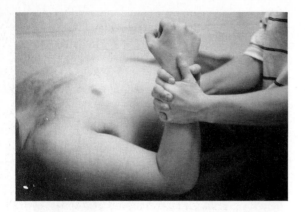

Fig. 11-11. Partner position for resisted pronation and supination.

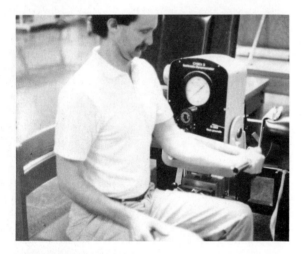

Fig. 11-12. Isokinetic setup for **A,** elbow flexion, extension and **B,** pronation, supination.

the elbow complex. By stimulating a variety of proprioceptors in muscle, tendon, and fascia, reflex patterns develop, even if those serving the joint capsule are compromised. This new position awareness may take days to months to become automatically controlled but appears very promising for most cases. Further clarification of this concept is developed in the next section.

Chronic Laxity

Chronic laxity usually presents with other pathological conditions; however, this discussion focuses on singular laxity, which may be present following an acute episode and where muscular control fails to be sufficient. Physicians and sports therapists identify the major feature of this problem as hypermobility in valgus with a firm, pain-free end feel. Note also that with sustained valgus stress or vigorous elbow flexion exercise, the examiner observes no increase in laxity over what occurs in the opposite extremity. At first glance, oscillatory tension placed through the medial collateral ligament may appear contraindicated. With other ligaments, such as the anterior cruciate, exercise that places a joint shear stress is encouraged during later stages of ligament repair (for example, knee extensions). An elongation tension stresses the collagen matrix and thereby stimulates the alignment of these fibrils.[38,44] In a chronic situation, the ligamentous tissue is expected to be fully repaired but elastically deformed. Direct stress to a lax medial collateral ligament may not occur as a result of activity within the normal ROM. To stimulate hypertrophic changes in this instance, gentle oscillatory valgus stress maneuvers may be effective. Valgus stress may be accomplished by grade III mobilization traction or distal glide as described earlier (Fig. 11-13). Medial-lateral ulnar oscillations (valgus with some rebound varus) may be introduced by cradling the athlete's wrist and hand next to the sports therapist's side with one elbow and supporting the arm close to the athlete's elbow with the opposite hand so that the fingers wrap around the dorsal and medial sides (see Fig. 11-13). The sports therapist's other hand wraps around the proximal forearm from dorsal to lateral so that a force through the fingers can provide a straight medial shear or, with a slight body adjustment, a valgus angulation stress. Counterforce is applied by directly opposing the medial stress at the elbow with the hand at the arm.

MUSCLE REEDUCATION. Strengthening exercises can be similarly performed as described in the acute case; however, the goal in this instance is toward early strength gains. Further, the strength levels must be maintained throughout an athlete's career and beyond because weakness and fatigue are the major factors allowing abnormal stresses to be focused on joint tissue instead of being attenuated by muscle. Regardless of the amount of strength or the ability of

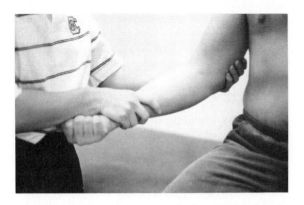

Fig.11-13. Position for gentle oscillatory valgus stress.

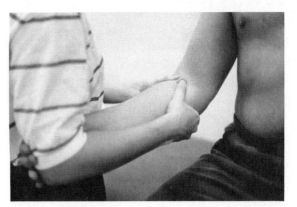

Fig. 11-14. Position for initial subluxation reduction.

the arm and forearm muscles to withstand fatigue, abnormal joint mechanics, allowed by loose capsular reinforcements, can progress to further debilitating injury. In the chronic laxity case, muscle reeducation for control of proper joint mechanics seems to play its greatest role. Initial recognition of subluxation (dynamic valgus laxity, or instability) has proven to be very difficult at the elbow compared to other joints but is still the first step in the development of neurophysiological feedback control. When the elbow is subluxed by the sports therapist with the method of the maneuver producing the most hypermobility, the athlete may be instructed to attempt to rotate the shoulder medially or possibly extend the elbow (Fig. 11-14). This position and maneuver should be so weak as to elicit the fear of something being wrong and an inability to generate significant tension. The athlete should recognize this position as the position of most vulnerability or the position of weakness. Reducing the subluxed position by contracting specific musculature should allow the athlete to feel comfortable and strong with shoulder medial rotation or elbow extension. One way to accomplish this reduction is to make a fist or extend the fingers fully. No objective EMG data clarify any further detail. Once recognized, the athlete should perform isometric-type contractions to "reduce" the mildly subluxed joint in alternately reduced and then subluxed positions. Another approach is to distract the joint surfaces by traction and have the athlete actively contract medial flexors or the biceps to reduce into a stable position for further exercise. As the athlete gains

control of the preceding maneuver, a variety of body positions and stresses can be applied either at the elbow or from the hand (Fig. 11-15). Body positions might include kneeling on all fours and push-up positions next to the wall or on the floor. The sports therapist can assist the progression by providing external forces to the body or arms that are novel in direction and unanticipated by the athlete. These exercises finally progress to skills and tumbling activities associated with specific sports. Early retraining should go through a movement from flexion to extension in a functional range that surrounds the subluxation positions (area) so that progression of control becomes voluntarily smooth and then both smooth and automatic, with attempts at distracting the athlete's attention.

With the exception of elbow dislocations, lateral laxity is rare among athletes. When this laxity is present on examination, the same principles regarding medial laxity apply with both acute and chronic cases. However, pronation and supination play a more prominent role in the protection and control of the radius. Apparently few acute radial head dislocations develop residual laxity; however, the radioulnar joint is always affected to some degree. Maintaining a pronation alignment of the forearm should assist in the stability of the joint while performing elbow flexion and extension exercises.

Joint laxities commonly arise acutely from joint injuries but also chronically from repeated valgus stress, as in throwing. Early management of these cases can result in a joint that is fully

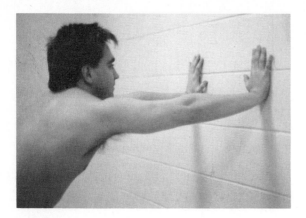

Fig. 11-15. Novel positions from which automatic reflex joint control can be practiced.

functioning if not entirely normal in anatomic relationships. Attention to possible painless stretching of ligamentous tissue during the critical recovery period can protect against residual laxity in many cases. When laxity is present following wound maturity, muscular strength and proprioception can play integral roles in stability of the elbow joint complex for sport skills. The long-term caution is that these individuals need to maintain a high level of strength and awareness if they are to avoid or reduce significant degenerative changes.

TREATMENT OF SUBACUTE JOINT AND MUSCULOTENDINOUS INJURIES

SUBACUTE CARE: *1 to 2 Weeks*
1. Symptomatic Treatment
   a. Heat packs
   b. Whirlpool
   c. Ultrasound or phonophoresis (1 to 10% steroid cream)
   d. Diathermy
   e. Cryotherapy
   f. Cold following activity
   g. Compression and/or protection as long as swelling and functional ranges are limited by pain
   h. Elevation at night or with a sling when uncomfortable from being dependent for long periods
   i. Antiinflammatory medication
2. Controlled exercises (if a cast is continued, omit passive, active, or active assistive exercises with immobilized parts and perform

brief but rhythmic contractions) AROM and strengthening
   a. Stabilizing exercises with the shoulder and wrist (limited to the resistance tolerated by elbow position and contraindications)
      (1) shoulder shrugs
      (2) shoulder flexion, abduction, extension, external rotation
      (3) wrist flexion, extension, supination, pronation
      (4) grip exercises (see Chapter 12)
      (5) finger extensions
   b. Elbow flexion and extension in a pain-free range
   c. Elbow supination and pronation in a painfree range
   d. PNF patterns
   e. Soft tissue mobilization
   f. Cryokinetics
3. Cardiovascular training: jogging and aerobics can usually be tolerated well in this stage.
4. General body exercises: exercises involving minimal resistance through the shoulder and arm, such as leg presses and sit-ups, may be tolerated for stabilization and positioning.
5. Goals
   a. Increase ROM
   b. Decrease pain
   c. Decrease swelling
   d. Regain normal ADLs
   e. Gain athlete's full compliance
   f. Maintain strength and viability in joints and muscles above and below the elbow
6. Criteria to increase activity
   a. 80% pain-free ROM
   b. Mild to no swelling
   c. Functional ADLs

CHRONIC CARE: *2 Weeks to 3 Months* (Usually uncomplicated fractures, Dislocations, Tendonitis)
1. Symptomatic care
   a. Heat before exercise or cryokinetics
   b. Cold after exercise
   c. Other adjunctive care as needed or desired (electrical therapies, ultrasound)
   d. Compression, protection, and/or elevation as needed

Continued on p. 246

THROWING AND TENNIS PROTOCOLS

THROWING

This program may be instituted for throwers following a recovery period from surgery, injection, or acute inflammation. Typical resting periods for the above conditions may be 2 weeks to 18 months. The athlete should have full, pain-free ROM and comparable strength to the uninvolved side for the shoulder, elbow, and wrist. Stretching *and* upper extremity warmup should be performed prior to the routine. Icing should be routine following each workout. Progression is based on 24-hour symptoms, but, particularly in postsurgical cases where circulation may not be optimal, forced rest for 48 hours may be needed to establish a tissue stress response. Throwing occurs every other day and conditioning with weight training on off days. The early routine consists of both short and long tosses.

For the short toss, start tossing the ball for 30 feet for 10 repetitions so that control feedback and technique can be gauged. The toss should be a three-quarter overhead style.

Increase every other day by 10 repetitions until 30 repetitions are reached. Then move up to half speed. Next increase to 40 feet, but drop back to 20 repetitions at half speed. Move progressively to 30 repetitions as tolerated. Finally move to 60 feet, starting back at 20 repetitions. Once reaching 30 repetitions with comfort, move to three-quarter speed.

For the long toss, start at 50 feet and 10 repetitions. Use the same gauge as in the short toss, and increase every other day if no symptoms occur. Use an overhead high toss only. Once reaching 30 repetitions at 50 feet, move to 70 feet and 20 repetitions and progress to 30 repetitions. Move from 70 feet to 100 feet and then to 130 feet as above. Optimal progression is 2 to 3 weeks.

The late routine also consists of short and long tosses. For the short toss, progress up to three-quarter speed. When comfortable, go to the mound. Then progress to half-speed breaking ball. Three-quarter to full-speed fast and breaking balls can be worked into games so that no more than 50 balls are thrown.

For the long toss, pitchers may want to stay with the early routine, whereas fielders may add more distance.

TENNIS

Lateral epicondylitis may be recognized when the elbow is extended by extensor tendon pain, especially on isolated middle finger extension. Assuming other entities have been ruled out, this condition arising from playing tennis may be treated effectively through stretching, deep friction massage, or mobilization at the proximal attachment of the extensor carpi radialis brevis muscle. Other wrist extensors have been implicated in this general syndrome. A host of preventive measures can be applied to prevent recurrences.

1. Players should receive advice about or pay attention to excessively tight strings, wet balls, and excessively small grip size.
2. Counterforce bracing may be used to aid in comfort early and when absence from the sport is not desirable.
3. Adequate conditioning decreases the chances of general body fatigue setting up poor stroke technique from poor positioning for the stroke.
4. Players should assess their stroke technique for errors.
5. Strengthening the grip and wrist extensors is paramount.
6. Periodic stretching of the extensors is important.
7. Especially when hitting a lot of backhands, follow the workout with ice for 15 to 30 minutes.

When the acute symptoms subside, specific resistance exercises should focus on wrist flexion and extension, ulnar and radial deviation, and supination and pronation. These should be performed through a tolerable ROM, preferably full, for at least six repetitions. Progress to 15 to 25 repetitions at a given resistance or isokinetically. Isotonic resistances should increase by about 2½ pounds and work up to 10 pounds.

This procedure appears desirable for many athletes, using three sets of 10 to 15 repetitions each set. Wrist- and finger-stretching techniques in full elbow extension should be used in conjunction with gripping exercises (handheld springs or tennis ball).

2. Controlled exercises
   a. Shoulder and wrist progressions
   b. Elbow resistance exercises and ROM, if needed
   c. Shoulder, wrist, and elbow stretching as indicated
   d. PNF patterns
   e. Muscle reeducation (chronic laxities)
   f. Sport-patterned movement manually or with elastic cords or cables. The preference is to develop endurance early in the plan, later concentrating on strength as control is gained, and then once again working on endurance at increasing levels of strength. Patterned movement with skilled activities, response time, and speed of movement are late stage types of activities.
3. Cardiovascular training: any activity that the athlete wishes to participate in for this development is usually tolerated well.
4. General body exercises: weight lifting and sport-specific drills are usually progressed until full return evaluation is obtained.
5. Sport protection: ideally no protection would be needed; however, elbow sleeves (for heat and increased resting muscle tone), counterforce bracing, taping, and other devices have been used.
6. Goals
   a. Increase or maintain ROM
   b. Increase strength and endurance
   c. Decrease or eliminate pain
   d. Decrease or eliminate swelling
   e. Increase sport function
   f. Increase cardiovascular efficiency
   g. Develop physical and mental readiness for sport
7. Criteria to increase activity
   a. 80 to 100% strength at 300 feet/second and 60 feet/second
   b. 90 to 100% endurance
   c. Full ROM, pain free
   d. 90 to 100% sports skills assessment
      (1) Throwing motion
      (2) Push-ups
      (3) Pull-ups
      (4) Visual-motor control
      (5) Accuracy drills
      (6) Total body movement drills
      (7) Sport and position drills (low to high risk)
   e. No pain on tissue stress
   f. No increasing laxity (if present) before to after activity

FULL RECOVERY: *3 Months to 1 Year or More*

1. Symptomatic care (as needed for recurrent pain and swelling from overexuberant activity)
2. Controlled exercises (ROM and selective strengthening may need to be maintained in order to maintain a low risk of reinjury)
3. Cardiovascular training (provided by sport or directed by the training staff)
4. Total body exercises (provided by sport or directed by the training staff)
5. Goals
   a. 100% comparable strength, allowing for dominance
   b. 100% sports skills assessment
   c. 100% preseason cardiovascular and weight status
   d. No evidence of continuing pathology from the primary lesion
   e. Full recovery of anatomical and biomechanical function may not be expected in this group of patients

SUMMARY

1. The elbow plays a critical role with the shortening and lengthening of the upper extremity in the task of adjusting to an infinite placement of the hand.
2. The three joints of the elbow complex act independently between flexion and extension and supination and pronation, both in joint surface movement and in muscular activity; therefore, application of this information aids in the use and positioning of the elbow segments in rehabilitation.
3. Acute care of inflammatory conditions about the elbow might follow the concepts of "cool, calm, and collected" for appropriate temperatures, limited but allowable motion, and proper support for circulation and conditioning.
4. Among the most frequent problems facing the sports therapist from injuries about the elbow are motion restrictions due to long-

term immobility, such as with fractures, chronic, repetitive microtears, such as with chronic medial epicondylitis, and joint laxities due to acute dislocations or chronic repetitive valgus loading.

5. To treat motion restrictions about the elbow, soft tissue mobilization, stretching, active ROM, active-assistive ROM, and joint mobilization in the physiological and accessory planes of the three elbow joints are techniques that have proved beneficial.

6. Elbow injuries should be considered for return to throwing in a progression of specific workloads once full ROM is pain free and flexion-extension strength is comparable to the opposite side.

7. Tennis injuries may be reduced in frequency and severity with attention to racket string tension, racket size, proper stroke technique, and general body conditioning.

8. Residual elbow joint laxity problems may be treated conservatively by selectively strengthening the surrounding musculature, gaining automatic reflex joint control, gaining proximal and distal joint control, and developing hypertrophy of the ligamentous restraints.

9. Attention to symptomatology and the changing status of inflammation and repair in a rehabilitation regimen for the elbow allows the sports therapist to plan long-term treatment goals and ensures conscious monitoring, not only of progress but also of appropriate return criteria in a joint complex frequently subject to overuse; minimal time away from sports participation is ensured.

10. Controlled exercises for the elbow during the various phases of a rehabilitation program provide a basis for strength, endurance, proprioception, and synergistic improvement prior to more complicated and demanding tasks, related not only to ADLs but also to the more involved tasks of sport activity.

REFERENCES

1 Arnheim D: Modern principles of athletic training, St Louis, 1989, Times Mirror/Mosby College Publishing.

2 Baker C: Evaluation, treatment, and rehabilitation involving submuscular transposition of the ulnar nerve at the elbow, JNATA 23(1):10–12, 1988.

3 Birrer R: Sports medicine for the primary care physician, Norwalk, Conn, 1984, Appleton-Century-Crofts.

4 Booher J and Thibodeau G: Athletic injury assessment, St Louis, 1989, Times Mirror/Mosby College Publishing.

5 Bowling R and Rockar P: The elbow complex. In Gould J and Davies G, editors: Orthopaedic and sports physical therapy, St Louis, 1985, The CV Mosby Co.

6 DeLisa J: Rehabilitation medicine, Philadelphia, 1988, JB Lippincott Co.

7 Ellison A and others: Athletic training and sports medicine, Chicago, 1984, American Academy of Orthopaedic Surgeons.

8 Evjenth O and Hamberg J: Muscle stretching in manual therapy, Milan, 1984, New Intherlitho Spa.

9 Fahey T: Athletic training, Palo Alto, Calif, 1986, Mayfield Publishing.

10 Grabiner M, Robertson R, and Campbell K: Effects of fatigue on activation profiles and relative torque contribution of elbow flexor synergists, Med Sci Sport Exercise 20(1):79–84, 1988.

11 Halar E and Bell K: Contracture and other deleterious effects of immobility. In DeLisa J, editor: Rehabilitation medicine, Philadelphia, 1988, JB Lippincott Co.

12 Hartley A: Elbow assessment, Printed in Toronto, Canada, 1988.

13 Harvey J: Rehabilitation of the injured athlete, Clinics in sports medicine 4(3):405–438, 1985.

14 Herrick R and Herrick S: Ruptured triceps in powerlifting presenting as cubital tunnel syndrome, Am J Sports Med 15(5):514–516, 1987.

15 Hoppenfeld S: Physical examination of the spine and extremities, New York, 1982, Appleton-Century-Crofts.

16 Joynt R: Therapeutic exercise. In DeLisa J, editor: Rehabilitation medicine, Philadelphia, 1988, JB Lippincott Co.

17 Kapandji I: The physiology of the joints, London, 1980, Churchill Livingstone.

18 Kessler R and Hertling D: Management of common musculoskeletal disorders, Philadelphia, 1983, Harper & Row Publishers, Inc.

19 Kisner C and Colby L: Therapeutic exercise, Philadelphia, 1985, FA Davis Co.

20 Kulund D: The injured athlete, Philadelphia, 1988, JB Lippincott Co.

21 Kushner S and Reid D: Manipulation in the treatment of tennis elbow, AM JOSPT 7(5):264–272, 1986.

22 McAuliffe T and others: Early mobilization of colles' fractures: a prospective trial, JBJS 69B(5):727–29, 1987.

23 McCue F: Injuries to the elbow, forearm, and hand, Clin Sports Med 5(4):681–700, 1986.

24 Magee D: Orthopedic physical assessment, Philadelphia, 1987, WB Saunders Co.

25 Maitland G: Peripheral manipulation, London, 1983, Butterworth & Co.

26 Micheli L: Pediatric and adolescent sports medicine, Boston, 1984, Little, Brown & Co.

27 Morrey B, An K, and Stormont T: Force transmission through the radial head, JBJS 70(2):250–256, 1988.

28 Norkin C and Levangie P: Joint structure & function, Philadelphia, 1987, FA Davis Co.

29 O'Donoghue D: Treatment of injuries to athletes, Philadelphia, 1987, WB Saunders Co.

30 Pedegana L and others: The relationship of upper extremity strength to throwing speed, Am J Sports Med 10(6):352–354, 1982.

31 Robbins S and Kumar V: Basic pathology, Philadelphia, 1987, WB Saunders Co.

32 Roy S and Irvin R: Sports medicine, Englewood Cliffs, NJ, 1983, Prentice-Hall.

33 Schneider R, Kennedy J, and Plant M: Sports injuries, Baltimore, 1985, Williams & Wilkins.

34 Scott W, Nisonson B, and Nicholas J: Principles of sports medicine, Baltimore, 1984, Williams & Wilkins.

35 Sisto D and others: Electromyographic analysis of the elbow in pitching, Am J Sports Med 15(3):260–263, 1987.

36 Smith N: Sports medicine: health care for young athletes, Evanston, Ill, 1983, American Academy of Pediatrics.

37 Snijders C and others: Provocation of epicondylagia lateralis (tennis elbow) by power grip or pinching, Med Sci Sport Exer 19(5):518–523, 1987.

38 Soderberg G: Kinesiology, Baltimore, 1986, Williams & Wilkins.

39 Tehranzadeh J, Labosky D, and Gabriele O: Ganglion cysts and tear of triangular fibrocartilage of both wrists in a cheerleader, Am J Sports Med 11(5):357–359, 1983.

40 Torg J, Vegso J, and Torg E: Rehabilitation of athletic injuries, Chicago, 1987, Year Book Medical Publishers.

41 Voss D, Ionta M, and Myers B: Proprioceptive neuromuscular facilitation, Philadelphia, 1985, Harper & Row Publishers, Inc.

42 Wadsworth C: Manual examination and treatment of the spine and extremities, Baltimore, 1988, Williams & Wilkins.

43 Welsh R and Shephard R: Current therapy in sports medicine 1985–1986, St Louis, 1985, The CV Mosby Co.

44 Woo S and Buckwalter J: Symposium on injury and repair of the musculoskeletal soft tissues, Savannah, Ga, 1987, American Academy Orthopaedic Surgeons.

45 Zarins B, Andrews J, and Carson W: Injuries to the throwing arm, Philadelphia, 1985, WB Saunders Co.

Rehabilitation of Hand and Wrist Injuries

12

Scott M. Lephart

OBJECTIVES

Following completion of this chapter, the student will be able to:

- Describe common sports-related injuries of the wrist and hand.

- Describe the mechanism and pathology associated with hand and wrist injuries.

- Understand and implement management protocols for the injuries.

- Describe rehabilitation objectives, including flexibility and strength goals.

- Implement appropriate rehabilitation protocols for the various injuries.

- Apply appropriate protective devices to decrease incidence of recurrent injury to hand and wrist.

The wrist and hand are exceedingly susceptible to injury in most sports. Sports requiring throwing, catching, grabbing, and falling constantly place the athlete's wrist and hand in positions that can result in injury. Injuries to the wrist and hand vary in degree of severity and range from soft tissue contusions to injuries requiring prolonged immobilization. Furthermore, the debilitation of an injury to the wrist and hand can vary from athlete to athlete and often depends on the athlete's position and reliance on the function of the wrist and hand for performance.

This chapter will outline the commonly encountered wrist and hand injuries in sports. Its purpose is to provide appropriate management and rehabilitation guidelines to protect, rehabilitate, and prevent recurrent injury to the region. The function of the hand is essential to daily activities outside athletic participation, and the functional integrity of the hand must never be compromised during care of these injuries.

WRIST INJURIES
Tendon Injuries

Repetitive utilization of the forearm, wrist, and hand in sports activity can result in tendinitis injuries, most of which can be classified as overuse inflammatory conditions. Tendon injuries are most prevalent in those sports in which throwing or a racket is used. Tendinitis and stenosing tenosynovitis are the most common sports-related tendon conditions of the wrist.[19] Both the flexor and extensor mechanisms can be involved, depending on the mechanism inducing the stress.

As is true of all overuse injuries, acute management must include both the discontinuance of the activity responsible for the inflammatory condition and the use of conservative measures to reduce inflammation. In severe cases splinting may be indicated to reduce further irritation to the involved tendons. Once the inflammatory condition is stabilized, the next step in the rehabilitation program is to restore flexibility. This is essential to prevent the formation of tendon adhesions that can result in further inflexibility and the recurrence of the tendinitis upon return to sports activity. Once a sound flexibility program has been implemented, a resistive exercise program should be utilized emphasizing the development of strength and endurance of the involved musculature. Additionally, in such sports as tennis and racquetball, stroke mechanics must be analyzed to determine whether improper mechanics may have been responsible for producing the tendinitis.

DE QUERVAIN'S TENOSYNOVITIS. The most common stenosing tenosynovitis reported is De Quervain's, which is a result of repetitive ulnar deviation and of the wrist.[15,17—19] De Quervain's stenosing tenosynovitis occurs at the radial styloid process where the abductor pollicis longus and the extensor pollicis brevis pass through a fibroosseous canal.[19] Chronic irritation caused by ulnar deviation during tennis and golf swings produces the tenosynovitis within the fibroosseous canal. The condition presents pain with thumb use and gripping, inflammation at the radial styloid process, and crepitation when the wrist is extended and radially deviated.[19]

Most cases of De Quervain's tenosynovitis can be managed successfully with conservative measures including ice, antiinflammatory agents, and, in severe cases, immobilization until the acute pain subsequent to the inflammation subsides. A flexibility and strengthening protocol for the abductor pollicis longus and the extensor pollicis brevis should be implemented once the pain and inflammation have subsided. Additionally, a thumb spica can be applied when returning the athlete to activity to prevent extreme ranges of thumb opposition and wrist ulnar deviation (Fig. 12-1).

EXTENSOR MECHANISM TENOSYNOVITIS. The most common overuse injuries of the extensor mechanism occur in the radial extensor tendons of the wrist, the extensor carpi radialis and brevis.[12,19] Athletes who perform wrist extension—radial deviation maneuvers, including tennis and racquetball players, weight lifters, and rowers, are particularly susceptible to developing insertional tenosynovitis. These tendons are also susceptible to overstretching during the deceleration phase of wrist flexion in such sports as golf, shot putting, and other throwing activ-

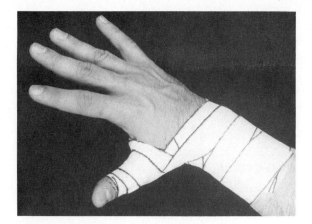

Fig. 12-1. Thumb spica taping for De Quervain's tenosynovitis to prevent extreme ranges of thumb opposition and wrist ulnar deviation.

ities.[12] Clinically, pain is reproduced with passive flexion and active extension and/or radial deviation of the wrist and with direct palpation of the tendon insertion into the radial carpals.

The extensor carpi ulnaris is housed within a separate fibroosseous tunnel and is more superficial than the radial extensors of the wrist.[12] Furthermore, fluid commonly accumulates within the tendinous sheath, which is a common site of tenosynovitis resulting from overuse for golfers and tennis players.[3,9,19] Because of the tendon's superficial proximity, the thickened synovial sheath and tendon can be seen and palpated during forearm rotation.

Like most overuse inflammatory conditions, extensor tenosynovitis is acutely managed with rest and antiinflammatory measures. Immobilization may be indicated in severe cases to remove the stressful mechanism of chronic extension, or overstretching due to chronic flexion of the wrist (Fig. 12-2). Strength and flexibility measures can be implemented for the extensor tendons once the acute inflammation has subsided.

FLEXOR MECHANISM TENDINITIS. Sports requiring sudden or chronic wrist flexion maneuvers can lead to flexor carpi ulnaris (FCU) irritation. The tendon insertion of the FCU includes the pisiform bone and the hypothenar fascia.[12] Irritation to the FCU tendon results in pain and strength deficits with gripping and flexion of the wrist owing to inflammation within the tendon.

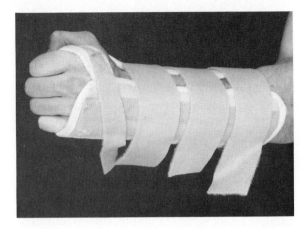

Fig. 12-2. Wrist immobilizer to prevent wrist flexion and extension.

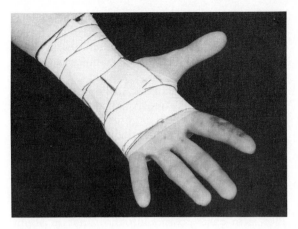

Fig. 12-3. Plamar checkrein taping to prevent wrist hyperextension.

The FCU dominates wrist flexion activity. Maneuvers such as curling dumbbells, releasing a ball during throwing, and swinging a golf club commonly induce tendinitis. Pain is normally dispersed throughout the ulnar aspect of the wrist owing to the broad tendinous insertion, although pain can usually be elicited upon palpation of the pisiform when it is inflamed.[12] Immobilization is usually suggested with FCU tendinitis due to the frequent use of the wrist flexor muscles in normal daily activities. In addition to immobilization, antiinflammatory measures are indicated until pain and swelling subside. Wrist flexion flexibility and strengthening measures should be implemented once the acute symptoms have subsided.

CARPAL TUNNEL SYNDROME. Carpal tunnel syndrome is one of the most common wrist conditions associated with sports.[17,20,25] The condition is usually subsequent to an overuse wrist flexion activity such as golf or tennis that results in a flexor tenosynovitis. Swelling of the flexor tendons within the enclosed carpal tunnel space compresses the median nerve and results in pain or paresthesia in the radial aspect of the hand. Chronic carpal tunnel syndrome can result in thenar muscular atrophy due to the deinnervation caused by compression of the median nerve. Conservative management includes immobilization and antiinflammatory measures in an attempt to relieve compression on the median nerve. In severe cases the decompression is performed surgically by releasing the transverse carpal ligament that bounds the anterior aspect of the tunnel.

Ligament Injuries

The major stabilizing ligaments of the wrist are the palmar intracapsular ligaments on the volar aspect of the wrist.[5] These intracapsular ligaments extend from their radial or ulnar origin to insert into their respective proximal row of carpal bones. The ligaments are sprained when the wrist is hyperextended and deviated, usually a result of falling when the hand attempts to break the athlete's fall.

Conservative management of wrist sprains involves antiinflammatory measures and supporting the wrist acutely for comfort. Surgery is usually indicated only in severe ligament injury resulting in instabilities of the carpal bones.[5] Rehabilitation of the overlying tendons is indicated to enhance dynamic stability in the region. Supportive taping is usually required when the athlete returns to activity to prevent hyperextension and terminal ranges of ulnar and radial deviation (Fig. 12-3).

Fractures

SCAPHOID. The scaphoid is located in the lateral-distal carpal row. The lateral aspect of the scaphoid possesses a shallow waist that is directly impinged by the distal radius when the wrist is extended and radially deviated. The most common mechanism of fracture of the scaphoid is falling on the outstretched arm while the wrist is extended. The force of the fall impinges the radius into the scaphoid and can fracture the bone at its narrow waist.

Differentiation between a scaphoid fracture and a soft tissue injury is often difficult. Therefore, a radiographic evaluation is usually warranted, given tenderness over the anatomical snuffbox and diminished grip power.[15,17,18] With early diagnosis, most scaphoid fractures can be managed with immobilization for approximately 3 months.[26] Immobilization usually consists of a short-arm cast, positioning the wrist in slight flexion with the thumb immobilized in abduction and opposition. The rules of sports such as intercollegiate football allow the athlete to wear an unyielding splint, thus allowing the athlete to return to competition while the scaphoid is healing. A protective silicone rubber short-arm thumb spica splint can be simply devised to immobilize the fracture during sports activity.[26] The silicone splint should be removed and the plaster cast reapplied immediately after the athletic event. Mobilization of the wrist is usually not warranted until complete fracture healing has occurred. Therefore, flexibility and strengthening must include the entire hand and wrist region once the fracture has healed due to the prolonged period of immobilization.

HAMATE. The hamate is located in the medial-dorsal aspect of the wrist. The hamate possesses a hooklike projection that protrudes into the base of the hypothenar eminence. This protrusion can be fractured when a clublike device is in the palm of the hand and the wrist is ulnarly deviated during swinging.[26] Such sports as golf, tennis, baseball, and squash may elicit the mechanism of a hamate fracture.[24,26] Normal wrist functions are unaffected by the fracture, and possibly the only signs of fracture may include tenderness to palpation and forceful ulnar deviation.

If the fracture is not displaced, a short-arm cast that extends to the little finger is applied.[15,17,18] If the fracture is displaced, surgical excision of the fractured hook seems to be the most efficient management of hamate fractures in athletes.[26] After surgery the wrist is immobilized for 3 weeks, after which active motion can begin if pain is not present. The athlete can usu-

ally return to activity 6 weeks after surgery with protective taping.[26]

REHABILITATION OF WRIST INJURIES

The basic goals of rehabilitation of the wrist, which include arresting inflammation and restoring and enhancing flexibility and strength, are the same for both soft tissue injuries and fractures. Modifications and precautions may be indicated, depending on the particular pathology of the injury, but the protocols tend to be similar.

Rehabilitation following fracture and immobilization of the wrist must initially focus on regaining active range of motion (ROM) and then progress to restoring muscular strength, power, and endurance. Precaution should be taken to protect the fracture when the athlete returns to activity, and protective support is necessary following removal of the cast.

Most tendon inflammatory conditions of the wrist are a result of chronic irritation and can be classified as overuse injuries. To address the consequences of overuse, it is important to discontinue the activities responsible for the inflammatory condition. In addition to rest, the conservative measures of ice, antiinflammatory agents, and, in severe cases, immobilization are necessary. The following list outlines the treatment and rehabilitation protocol.

TREATMENT AND REHABILITATION OF WRIST INJURIES
PHASE I: *Acute*
1. Rest/immobilization (Fig. 12-2).
2. Ice (submersion or packs).
3. Oral antiinflammatory.

PHASE II: *Inflammation stabilized*
1. Cryokinetic techniques.
2. Active/active-assisted flexibility (Fig. 12-5).
3. Active ROM.

PHASE III: *Painfree ROM*
1. Warm whirlpool/active ROM.
2. Ultrasound.
3. Active/active-assisted flexibility.
4. Progressive resistance flexion, extension, supination, pronation, and deviation exercises (dumbbell, elastic tubing, etc.) (Figs. 12-6, 12-7, and 12-8).

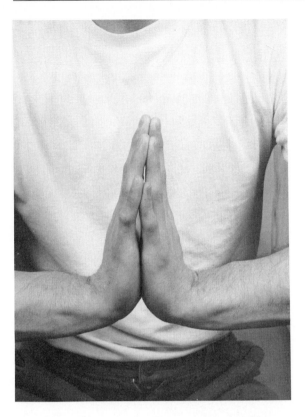

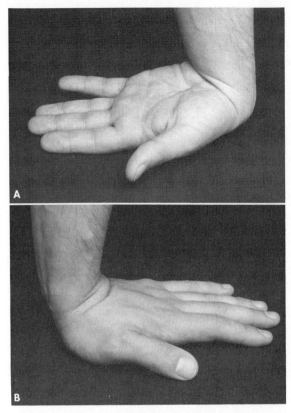

Fig. 12-4. Active-assisted wrist extension stretching with the athlete utilizing the uninvolved hand to assist stretching the involved wrist to terminal extension.

Fig. 12-5. Static stretching using a table to assist terminal **A**, flexion; **B**, extension.

PHASE IV: *Near normal strength and ROM*
1. Warm whirlpool/ROM.
2. Active/active-assisted flexibility.
3. Progressive resistance exercises.
4. Sport-specific exercises (Fig. 12-9).

Flexibility

Fractures and soft tissue overuse injuries of the wrist require rest and often prolonged immobilization. Following this period of rest or immobilization, restoring and enhancing flexibility of the wrist flexor and extensors are necessary. The mechanism of wrist tendon involvement can be either eccentrically or concentrically induced: thus both flexion and extension exercises are necessary in the rehabilitation protocol, regardless of the specific condition. The use of a warm whirlpool, with the athlete performing active motion while in the whirlpool, will facilitate the goal of increased flexibility by increasing tissue temperature and elasticity.[21] Because the terminal ranges of flexion or extension may elicit pain at a fracture site upon removal of the casting, the athlete should be encouraged to exercise within pain-free ranges of motion.

The flexibility program should include both active and active-assistive stretching exercises. The stretching exercises should be performed actively to the pain-free terminal range of motion. Upon reaching the terminal range of active motion, the athlete should perform an active-assisted stretch using the uninvolved hand (Fig. 12-4). The terminal range of the active-assisted stretch should be held statically for 3 to 5 seconds (Fig. 12-5). In addition to wrist flexion and

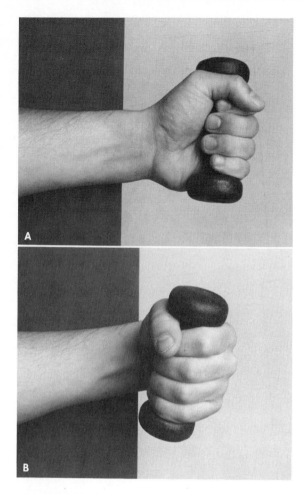

Fig. 12-6. Wrist flexion dumbbell strengthening exericises.

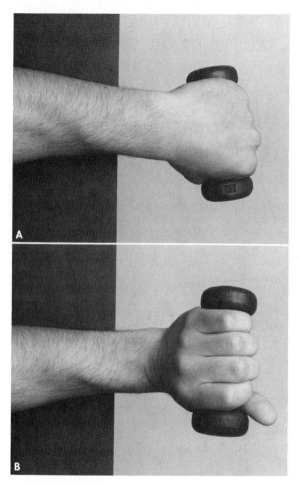

Fig. 12-7. Wrist extension dumbbell strengthening exercises.

extension, ulnar and radial deviation stretching should be integrated into the rehabilitation program.

Strengthening

Rehabilitation of wrist tendon injuries must be monitored closely by the sports therapist to prevent recurrence of the inflammation. The exercise program must develop both strength and endurance without inducing excessive irritation to the tendon. This result can be achieved only if the athlete is willing to modify the exercises so that pain is not induced during the rehabilitation exercises. A protocol of progressive resis-

tance exercise[13] using dumbbell weights, elastic tubing, or other modalities is recommended to provide resistance to the exercising muscle. Three to four sets of 10 repetitions are generally recommended with increasing resistance incrementally from set to set or from session to session.

Wrist flexion and extension exercises should be performed with the elbow and forearm stabilized. This position can easily be achieved with the elbow flexed to 90 degrees and positioning the forearm on a table with the hand and wrist extending beyond the table's end. Stabilization can be achieved by securing the elbow tightly to the side while performing the exercises. All

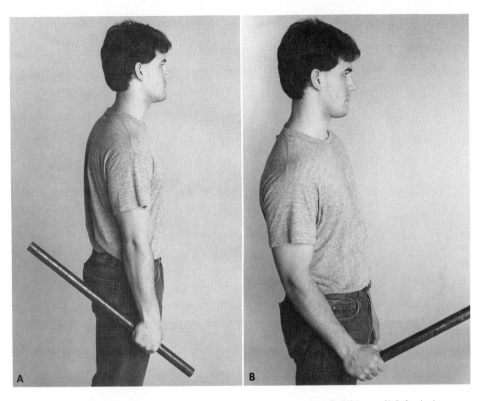

Fig. 12-8. A, Wrist ulnar deviation strengthening exericise. **B,** Wrist radial deviation strengthening exericise.

exercise should be performed throughout the entire range of motion and should be performed without pain in the involved tendon or bone (Fig. 12-6). Ulnar and radial deviation and pronation-supination exercises should also be performed. Deviation exercises are easily performed with steel bar or hammerlike devices (Fig. 12-7, Fig. 12-8). Resistance can be modified by hand position. Rubber tubing can be devised to exercise the pronator and supinator muscles and tendons.

The final stage of rehabilitation should include strengthening the musculature in the patterns that are required upon return to sports activity. With creativity the sports therapist can devise strengthening programs for the wrist and hand that are sport specific and thus decrease the potential for recurrent injury upon return to competition. Examples of sport-specific exercises include releasing a baseball (Fig. 12-9, *A, B*), the acceleration phase of a golf swing (Fig. 12-9, *C, D*), and releasing a football.

HAND INJURIES
Tendon Injuries

EXTENSOR MECHANISM. Injuries to the extensor mechanism are common in sports that require catching a ball. Commonly, football receivers, baseball, basketball, and volleyball players are susceptible to having the ball hit the extended distal phalanx and forcefully flexing the distal interphalangeal joint (DIP) or the proximal interphalangeal joint (PIP).[18]

One of the most common athletic injuries to the extensor mechanism is a rupture of the insertion of the extensor digitorum tendon from the distal phalanx resulting in a **mallet finger** or **drop finger.**[16] The athlete with a mallet finger is unable to extend actively the flexed DIP. The DIP is in a flexed position as a result of the flexor digitorum profundus tendon being unopposed when the extensor tendon has ruptured.

The exact involvement of a mallet finger can

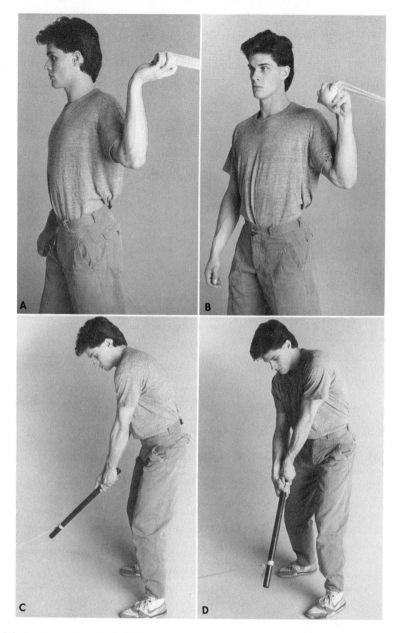

Fig. 12-9. Sport-specific rehabilitation exercises using resistance of elastic tubing: **A, B,** wrist flexion during baseball throwing; **C, D,** wrist flexion, extension, and deviation during a golf swing.

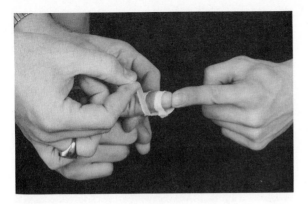

Fig. 12-10. The athlete maintains slight DIP hyperextension while the splint is positioned on the volar aspect of the mallet finger.

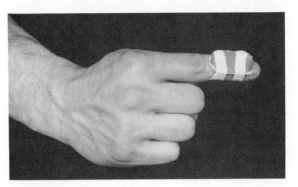

Fig. 12-11. Mallet finger splinting on the dorsal aspect of the finger for athletic participation.

vary from stretching or rupturing the tendon, to the tendon avulsing a piece of the distal phalanx.[16] Conservative management of the mallet finger involves immediate splinting of the DIP into a slightly hyperextended position to allow healing. Splinting the PIP along with the DIP, which would result in stiffness to the PIP, is not necessary. McCue and others suggest 8 to 10 weeks of immobilization after injury and encourage the athlete to wear the splint during athletic activities for an additional 6 to 8 weeks to prevent reinjury. Active motion is initiated during the 6 to 8 weeks with the splint reapplied following exercise.[16–18]

The splint must be regularly moved from the dorsal and volar surfaces of the finger. When the splint is moved, the athlete must stabilize the DIP and maintain the hyperextended position while the splint is being reapplied (Fig. 12-10). Cases of full-thickness skin necrosis have been reported as a result of impeded blood supply when the splint has been positioned on the dorsal surface of the finger for prolonged periods.[22] Therefore, the splint should be alternated from the dorsal surface of the finger to the volar surface regularly. During athletic participation, the splint should be positioned on the dorsal aspect of the finger if the athlete needs to catch or grasp during the event (Fig. 12-11).

The **boutonniere deformity** is also a common injury to the hand in athletics. As with the mallet finger, a boutonniere deformity is usually the result of forceful flexion of the finger while the hand is extended. Forced flexion of the finger with the DIP extended results in flexion of the PIP and can rupture the central slip of the extensor digitorum communis. The lateral bands of the flexor digitorum communis slide to the volar surface of the PIP and cause flexion of the interphalangeal joint (15 to 30 degrees) and extension of the DIP.[18] Rupture of the central slip renders the athlete unable to extend the PIP, thus resulting in the boutonniere deformity.

Management of the boutonniere deformity includes splinting of PIP joint in an extended position for 6 to 8 weeks. The splint does not need to immobilize the metacarpal phalangeal joint (MCP) or the DIP. Active motion is initiated at 6 to 8 weeks. Additional splinting should occur for 6 to 8 weeks during athletic competition.[18]

FLEXOR MECHANISM INJURIES. Although injury to the flexor mechanism is not as common as injury to the extensor mechanism in the athletic population, forced extension of the finger can strain or rupture the flexor digitorum profundus (FDP) tendon. The most common mechanism of FDP rupture occurs when an athlete is grabbing an opponent's jersey and forcefully extends the finger to result in a **jersey finger**.[19] Differentiating between a strain and complete rupture is often difficult for the clinician due to the mass of soft tissue and swelling in the volar aspect of the finger.

Management of the ruptured flexor tendon depends on the exact pathology involved. Tendon ruptures vary in degree of tendon retraction, volar plate involvement, and vinculum involvement. In most cases the tendon must be surgically repaired and the finger immobilized, with the MCP flexed to 30 degrees and the interphalangeal joints flexed to 10 degrees for a minimum of 3 weeks.[18] Active motion is started at approximately the third week with the protective splint reapplied immediately following the exercise. The splint is worn protectively up to 12 weeks after surgery but can be replaced with a mitten-type splint for some athletic competition if active gripping is not essential for performance.[18]

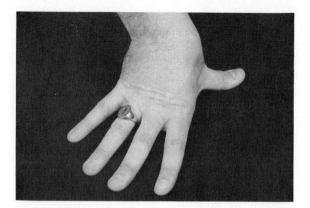

Fig. 12-12. Extension-abduction mechanism of gamekeeper's thumb.

Ligament Injuries

Capsular and ligament sprains of the fingers are frequent injuries in sports. The fingers are vulnerable whenever they are hyperextended or have axial, lateral, or rotary forces applied. Athletes refer to the hyperextension and axial compression injuries as "stoved" or "jammed" fingers. This type of injury usually results in a hemarthrosis to the proximal interphalangeal joint.

A lateral force to the finger can result in a collateral ligament sprain that compromises joint stability. However, a significant amount of laxity may not be evident if swelling is present to stabilize the joint. Conservative management of collateral sprains and severe capsular sprains includes splinting the finger in 30 degrees of flexion for 3 to 4 weeks. Active motion can begin 10 to 14 days after injury, and a protective splint should be worn for 4 to 6 weeks after injury during athletic competition.[11,15]

Injury to the ulnar collateral ligament (UCL) of the thumb, also referred to as **gamekeeper's thumb** or **skier's thumb,** is a common athletic injury that results from the thumb being forcefully extended and abducted.[4,6,7,23] The pole of a skier extending the skier's thumb while falling or an opponent's jersey forcefully extending an athlete's thumb are frequent mechanisms resulting in a sprain or rupture of the UCL at the level of the proximal phalanx of the thumb (Fig. 12-12).

Gamekeeper's thumb generally presents a sprain or partial rupture to the UCL combined with a mild to moderate strain of the adductor and flexor pollicis muscles. Diminished strength, swelling, and pain are associated with the injury, although instability is difficult to assess unless a complete rupture of the UCL has occurred. The condition is managed conservatively with a thumb spica to support and protect the injury.[15,17] The spica is applied with the thumb adducted and slightly opposed for protection in athletic activities. In severe sprains or when the thumb is minimally used during the activity, further stabilization can be achieved by taping the thumb to the index finger (Fig. 12-13).[15]

Fractures and Dislocations

FRACTURES. The metacarpals of the hand are vulnerable to fracture any time a substantial force is applied to the bone in an axial loading fashion while the MCP joint is flexed. Typically boxers sustain metacarpal neck fractures known as a **boxer's fracture.**[2] In most cases, metacarpal fractures are treated with closed reduction and immobilization in a short-arm cast for 3 to 6 weeks, and immobilization of the PIP and DIP are not included.[15]

Proximal phalanx fractures are commonly the result of a hyperextension mechanism. Improper reduction of this fracture can result in significant adhesions of the extrinsic tendons in this region.[15] The adhesions can severely restrict active

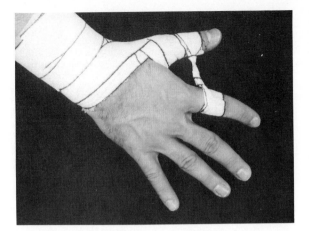

Fig. 12-13. Thumb spica with checkrein to prevent extension and abduction of the thumb during athletic participation.

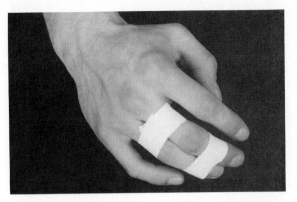

Fig. 12-14. Finger splinting to the adjacent finger for athletic participation.

motion at the PIP and DIP, which can be devastating to an athlete. Management involves closed reduction in most cases. The PIP is immobilized in 30 degrees of flexion, which tends to relax the extrinsic tendons and prevent significant tension adhesions. The collateral ligaments assist in stabilizing the MCP and thus maintain control of the fractured proximal portion of the phalanx.[15]

Active motion can begin approximately 3 weeks after injury, and sports activity can also begin at this time if significant healing has occurred. Wearing the splint can be discontinued for athletic participation at approximately 9 weeks and replaced by taping it to an adjacent finger for stabilization of the fracture for an additional 3 weeks (Fig. 12-14).[15]

Oblique and transverse fractures through the cortical bone in the waist of the shaft of the middle phalanx are characteristic of sports-related finger injuries.[2,15] The dorsal insertion of the central slip of the extensor tendon into the base of the phalanx of the two slips of the flexor digitorum sublimis makes these fractures anatomically susceptible to deformity.[2] Longitudinal traction applied with or without flexion, depending on the site of injury, is used to reduce these fractures. The fractures usually respond slowly to healing; thus, traditionally they are splinted until completely healed. Stable fractures are splinted for 3 weeks before exercises are initiated. Un-

stable fractures may require percutaneous fixation with K-wires and protection.[2,15]

DISLOCATIONS. The most common finger dislocation involves the PIP joint due to a hyperextension mechanism resulting in a dorsal dislocation.[2,15] This dislocation is easily reduced. In fact, athletes themselves often reduce the dislocation on the field. Once reduced and fracture and volar plate involvement have been ruled out, the joint should be immobilized in 20 to 30 degrees of flexion for 3 weeks.[15] The athlete can generally return to competition at approximately 3 weeks, although the finger should be splinted by taping it to an adjacent finger for an additional 2 weeks. Active motion should be encouraged at 2 to 3 weeks after injury.

REHABILITATION OF THE HAND

The primary goal during rehabilitation of the hand is to restore active range of motion. Immobilization typically results in stiffness of the joints of the fingers, which then results in a lack of terminal ranges of flexion and extension. Treatment and rehabilitation depend upon the pathology, and thus immobilization times differ. In some cases joint motion can be initiated during the healing phase, but other injuries require strict immobilization for specified periods of time. A thorough understanding of the unique action of the hand musculature is necessary to isolate joint movements and enhance motion in all of the involved joints. See Table 12-1 for treatment and immobilization guidelines.

TABLE 12-1

Treatment and Immobilization of Finger Injuries

Injury	Constant Splinting (weeks)	Begin Motion (weeks)	Additional Splinting for Competition (weeks)	Joint Position
Mallet finger	6–8	6–8	6–8	Slight DIP hyperextension
Collateral ligament sprains	3	2	4–6	30° flexion
DIP and PIP dislocations	3	3	3	30° flexion
Boutonniere deformity	6–8	6–8	6–8	PIP in extension; DIP, MCP not included
DIP, PIP fractures	9–11	3	3	30° flexion
MCP fractures	3	3	4–6	30° flexion
FDP repair	3–5	3	3–5	Depends on repair

Modified from Gieck JH and McCue FC III: Splinting of finger injuries, Ath Train 17:215, 1982.

During the acute stage of rehabilitation of those conditions, such as capsular sprains, allowing for early mobilization of the joints, active motion can be enhanced by utilizing cryokinetic techniques.[14] Cryotherapy assists in controlling the inflammation subsequent to the hand trauma, reduces pain, and thus facilitates active exercise (Fig. 12-15).[10] Once the inflammation has been stabilized, heating modalities such as warm whirlpools and paraffin should be implemented to enhance tissue elasticity and assist with the restoration of active motion.[21] Paraffin has also proven to be effective in reducing chronic edema and hemarthrosis in the interphalangeal regions of the hand (Fig. 12-16). The treatment and rehabilitation protocol is outlined as follows:

TREATMENT AND REHABILITATION OF HAND INJURIES

PHASE I: *Acute*
1. Immobilization (dependent upon pathology; Table 12-1).
2. Ice packs; retain immobilization and keep splint dry.
3. Oral antiinflammatory.

PHASE II: *Begin Motion* (Table 12-1)
1. Warm whirlpool/active range of motion.
2. Isolated joint passive and active motion.
3. Reapply splint.

PHASE III: *Removal of Splint* (Table 12-1)
1. Warm whirlpool/active ROM or paraffin

followed by active ROM.
2. Gripping strength exercises (Fig. 12-18).
3. Isolated resistance exercises (Figs. 12-19, 12-20).
4. Dexterity exercises (Fig. 12-21).

Flexibility

Active motion exercises for the hand must include both gross motor exercises and isolated joint motion. All exercises of the hand should be performed gently and must be performed pain free. Gross motor exercises should be performed during a warm whirlpool or immediately following paraffin or cold application, as indicated. Both flexion and extension exercise are encouraged regardless of the particular pathology. Generally the arm should be positioned in 90-degree flexion and stabilized against the athlete's torso or on a table. Active motion protocols for the hand should be consistent with the principles of rehabilitation with regard to technique and duration. All exercises should be performed throughout the entire range of active motion for three to four sets of eight to ten repetitions. Pain, other than that induced by muscle fatigue, should terminate the exercise session. Flexion and extension exercises of the entire hand should be performed, and then each involved finger should be exercised and each involved joint isolated.

Isolating each involved finger and each in-

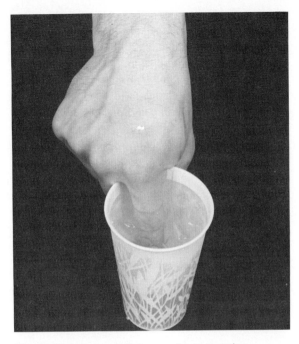

Fig. 12-15. Finger cryotherapy prior to exercise.

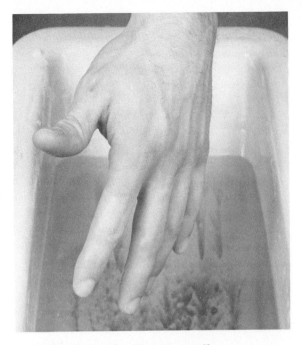

Fig. 12-16. Hand being dipped in paraffin.

volved joint motion is necessary, particularly when the flexor digitorum profundus (FDP) and flexor digitorum superficialis (FDS) tendons are involved. The FDP tendon inserts into the distal phalanx, and the tendon of the FDS inserts into the middle phalanx. In order to exercise the FDP, the DIP must be flexed while the MCP and PIP are stabilized (Fig. 12-17).

Following a period of immobilization, the hand intrinsic muscles must also be reconditioned. The palmar and dorsal interosseous and the lumbrical muscle assist in flexion of the MCP and extension of the PIP joints while the interosseous muscles are primarily responsible for abduction and adduction of the fingers. Active abduction and adduction exercises should be performed similar to flexion and extension exercises. beginning with exercising the hand as a whole and followed by isolating each finger.

Strengthening and Dexterity Exercises

Active range-of-motion exercises will initiate strengthening of the hand musculature but are not sufficient to regain both dexterity and power in the selected tendons and hand intrinsic mus-

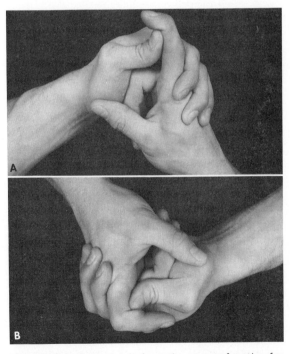

Fig. 12-17. Isolating joints for active range of motion for exercises: **A,** stabilizing the MCP and PIP to exercise the DIP; **B,** stabilizing the MCP to exercise the PIP.

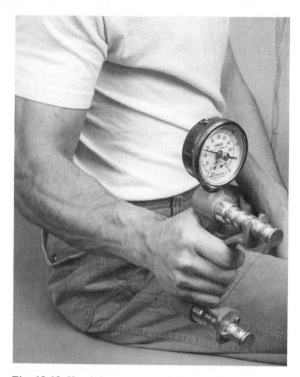

Fig. 12-18. Hand dynamometer for isometric exercise and measuring grip strength.

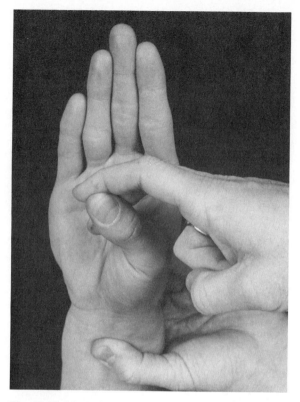

Fig. 12-19. Manual resistance for thumb opposition exercises.

cles following immobilization. The principles of muscle strengthening in the injured hand are consistent with rehabilitation protocols for any injury. However, as compared with the technology available to rehabilitate other injuries, limited resistance modalities exist specifically for the purpose of hand strengthening. Grip strength can be regained using gripping putty, a rubber ball, and hand grip coils. A hand dynamometer can be used to measure isometric grip strength (Fig. 12-18). Gripping exercises should consist of a maximal and sustained voluntary contraction for 3 to 5 seconds in sets of 10 repetitions. Graded resistance protocols are difficult to achieve with gripping exercises; thus repetitions are usually increased as strength increases.

The strengthening needs of the thumb are unique due to the variety of thumb intrinsic muscles that need to be exercised. Active motion of the thumb must include adduction, abduction, flexion, extension, opposition, and circumduction. Once active ROM is achieved, manual re-

sistance exercises can easily be implemented. Manual resistance can be performed either by the sports therapist or by the athlete (Fig. 12-19). In addition to manual resistance, rubber bands can be utilized as a mode of progressive resistance (Fig. 12-20). Strengthening of the finger intrinsic muscles and tendons similarly can be achieved via manual resistance or using rubber bands for resistance.

Dexterity exercises should also include pinching, tearing, and other activities that are essential not only for athletics but also for daily activities. Such activities include picking up coins, tearing tape, and gripping clubs, balls, or other objects requiring dexterity and tactile senses (Fig. 12-21).

Support and Protection for Return to Sports

Often the athlete can return to activity prior to complete healing of hand injuries. The injuries

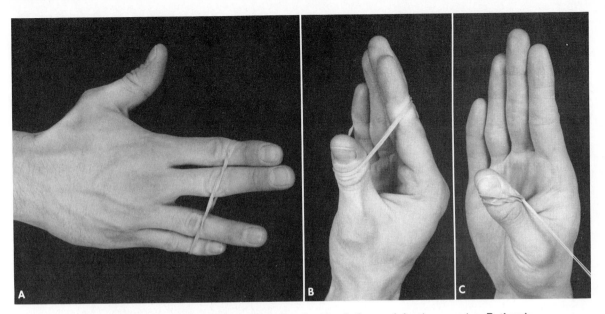

Fig. 12-20. Resistance exercises using rubber bands: **A,** finger abduction exercise; **B,** thumb abduction exercise; **C,** thumb opposition exercise.

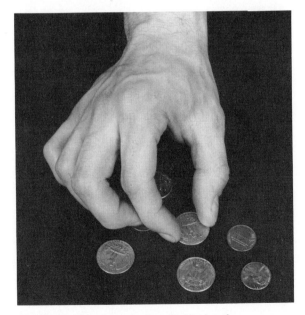

Fig. 12-21. Dexterity exercises for the hand.

must be supported and protected during this period to prevent recurrent injury to the hand. Finger splints can be modified to allow gripping by moving the splint to the dorsal surface of the hand or in some cases using a flexible support device. Joint instability of the finger can be splinted to adjacent fingers for support or can be splinted to prevent unwanted motion. Finally, the thumb can be supported to prevent any or all motions, depending on the needs of the particular athlete.

SUMMARY

1. Injuries to the wrist and hand are common in sports that require the athlete to throw, catch, or grab, or when the hand is involved in breaking the athlete's fall.
2. Wrist injuries are often subsequent to overuse activities that result in inflammation of the tendons in the region. Thus management of wrist inflammatory conditions must include rest from the sport for a period of time and in some cases immobilization.
3. Rehabilitation objectives following wrist injuries must initially focus on regaining active range of motion and then progress to restor-

ing muscular strength, power, and endurance.

4. Hand injuries are generally a result of trauma induced by a ball, an opponent's jersey, or falling. These injuries include tendon and ligament disruptions, fractures, and dislocations.

5. The hands are relied on for dexterity during most daily activities as well as for athletics. Therefore, normal motion and function must be reestablished after injury. Active motion exercises seem to be the most successful modality to rehabilitate the hand from such injuries.

6. The hand and wrist must be protected upon returning to athletic competition once rehabilitation is complete. Many taping, bracing, and supportive devices are available to decrease the incidence of recurrent injury upon the athlete's return to sports participation.

REFERENCES

1 Bassett FH and others: A protective splint of silicone rubber, Am J Sports Med 7(3):358–360, 1979.
2 Brunet ME and Haddad RJ: Fractures and dislocations of the metacarpals and phalanges, Clin Sports Med 5(4):773–781, 1986.
3 Burkhart SS, Wood MB, and Linscheid RL: Post-traumatic recurrent subluxation of the extensor carpi ulnaris tendon, J Hand Surg 11A:519, 1986.
4 Commandre F and Viani JL: The football keeper's thumb, J Sport Med Phys Fitness 1(6):121–122, 1976.
5 Culver JE: Instabilities of the wrist, Clin Sports Med 5(4):725–740, 1986.
6 Curtin J and Kay NR: Hand injuries due to soccer, Hand 8:93–95, 1976.
7 Ganel A and others: Gamekeeper's thumb: injuries of the ulnar collateral ligament of the metacarpo-phalangeal joint, Br J Sports Med 14(2–3):92–96, 1980.
8 Gieck JH and McCue FC: Splinting of finger injuries, Ath Train 7:215, 1982.
9 Hajj AA and Wood MB: Stenosing tenosynovitis of the extensor carpi ulnaris, J Hand Surg 11A:519, 1986.
10 Hocatt JE and others: Cryotherapy in ankle sprains, Am J Sports Med 10(5):316–319, 1982.
11 Isani A and Melone CP: Ligament injuries of the hand in athletics, Clin Sports Med 5(4):757–772, 1986.
12 Johnson RK: Soft tissue injuries of the forearm and hand, Clin Sports Med 7(2):329–348, 1988.
13 Kisner C and Colby LA: Therapeutic exercises: foundations and techniques, Philadelphia, 1985, FA Davis Co.
14 Knight KL: Cryotherapy in sports medicine. In Schubner K and Burke EJ, editors: Relevant topics in athletic training, New York, 1978, Movement Publications.
15 Kuland DN: The injured athlete, ed 2, Philadelphia, 1988, JB Lippincott Co.
16 McCue FC and Abbott JL: The treatment of mallet finger and boutonnaire deformities, Va Med Mon 94:623, 1966.
17 McCue FC and others: Hand and wrist injuries in the athlete, Am J Sports Med 7(5):275–286, 1979.
18 McCue FC and Wooten SL: Closed tendon injuries of the hand in athletics, Clin Sports Med 5(4):741–755, 1986.
19 Osterman LE, Moskow L, and Low DW: Soft tissue injuries of the hand and wrist in racquet sports, Clin Sports Med 7(2):329–348, 1988.
20 Phalen GS: The carpal-tunnel syndrome: seventeen years experience in diagnosis and treatment of six hundred fifty-four hands, J Bone Joint Surg 48A:211, 1966.
21 Prentice WE: Therapeutic modalities in sports medicine, St Louis, 1986, Times Mirror/Mosby College Publishing.
22 Rayan GM and Mullins PT: Skin necrosis complicating mallet finger splinting and vascularity of the distal interphalangeal joint overlying skin, J Hand Surg 12A(4):548–551, 1987.
23 Rovere GD and others: Treatment of "gamekeeper's thumb" in hockey players, Am J Sports Med 3:147–151, 1975.
24 Stark HH and others: Fracture of the hook of the hamate in athletics, J Hand Surg 59A:575–582, 1977.
25 Woods MB and Dobyns JH: Sport-related extraarticular wrist syndromes, Clin Orth Related Res 202:95–101, 1986.
26 Zemel NP and Stark HH: Fractures and dislocations of the carpal bones, Clin Sports Med 5(4):709–724, 1986.

SUGGESTED READINGS

Burton RI and Easton RG: Common hand injuries in the athlete, Orthop Clin North Am 4:809–838, 1973.
Ellsasser JC and Stein AH: Management of hand injuries in a professional football team, Am J Sports Med 7:178–182, 1979.
Kalenak A and others: Athletic injuries of the hand, Am Fam Physician 14:136–142, 1976.
Kelly DW and others: Index metacarpal fractures in karate, Physician Sports Med 8(3):103–106, 1980.
Leddy JP and Packer JW: Avulsion of the profundus tendon insertion in athletes, J Hand Surg 2:66–69, 1977.
McCue FC III and others: The coach's finger, Am J Sports Med 2:270–275, 1974.
Raymond P: Care of the hands, Oarsman 9(2):40–41, 1977.
Reef TC: Avulsion of the flexor digitorum profundus: an athletic injury, Am J Sports Med 5:281–285, 1977.

Rehabilitation of Hip and Thigh Injuries

13

Bernard DePalma

OBJECTIVES

Following completion of this chapter, the student will be able to:

- Understand the functional anatomy of the hip and thigh.

- Discuss athletic injuries to the hip and thigh.

- Describe functional injury evaluation of the hip and thigh.

- Recognize abnormal gait cycles as they relate to hip and thigh injuries.

- Explain the behavioral approach to rehabilitation of the hip and thigh, including short-term goals and rehabilitation timetables.

- Discuss the role of functional evaluation in when to return an athlete to competition, based on rehabilitation timetables.

This chapter describes functional rehabilitation programs that follow hip and thigh injuries. The behavioral approach, which utilizes short-term goal setting and rehabilitation timetables, characterizes these rehabilitation programs. The sports therapist and athlete together should develop the rehabilitation program with an emphasis on the sports therapist's functional evaluation and clinical findings, and each exercise program in this chapter should be presented to the athlete in terms of short-term goals. One objective for the sports therapist is to make the rehabilitation experience challenging for the athlete in order to promote adherence to the rehabilitation program. No matter how good the rehabilitation program is, it will not be effective if the athlete does not follow through.

The chapter presents a comprehensive review of injuries that commonly occur to the hip and thigh. Discussion of each injury includes a brief review of the literature, the functional evaluation and clinical findings pertinent to that injury, and a specific treatment and rehabilitation program. Keep in mind that the time sequences for programs presented in this chapter are approximations; shortening or lengthening the time sequences may be necessary, depending upon the degree of injury.

HIP POINTER

A **hip pointer** can best be described as a subcutaneous contusion caused by a direct blow to the iliac crest and/or the anterior superior iliac spine. In most cases, the contusion can cause separation or tearing of the origins or insertions of the muscles that attach to these two prominent bony sites.[10] Usually the athlete has no immediate concern, but within an hour of the injury bleeding, swelling, and pain can severely limit the athlete's movement. In rare cases, a fracture of the crest may occur.[21] An x-ray should be taken

I would like to thank Jim Case, M.A., A.T.C., Assistant Athletic Trainer at Cornell University, for his contribution to various portions of this chapter.

to rule out iliac crest fractures and/or avulsion fractures, especially in younger athletes.[10] If the hip pointer is not treated early, within approximately 2 to 4 hours, the athlete may experience severe pain and limited range of motion of the trunk due to the muscle attachments involved.

More serious injuries must also be ruled out. One athlete who reported all the signs and symptoms of a hip pointer on the field later was determined to have a ruptured spleen.

A strain of the abdominal muscles at their attachment to the anterior and inferior iliac crest can easily be differentiated from a contusion by obtaining a good history of the mechanism of injury at the time it occurs. A forceful contraction of the abdominal muscles while the trunk is being passively forced to the opposite side may cause a strain of the muscles at their insertion to the iliac bone.[17]

Evaluation and Clinical Findings

GRADE I HIP POINTER. An athlete with a grade I hip pointer may have both a normal gait cycle and normal posture. The athlete may complain of slight pain on palpation with little or no swelling. This athlete may also present full range of motion of the trunk, especially lateral side bending to the opposite side of the injury. A grade I hip pointer usually does not prevent competition.

GRADE II HIP POINTER. An athlete with a grade II hip pointer may have moderate to severe pain on palpation, noticeable swelling, and an abnormal gait cycle. The gait cycle may be changed due to a short swing through phase on the affected side; the athlete may take a short step and be reluctant to keep the foot off the ground. The athlete's posture may be slightly tilted to the side of the injury. Active hip flexion and trunk flexion may cause pain, especially if the anterior superior iliac spine is involved, due to the insertion of the sartorius muscle. Range of motion may be limited, especially lateral side bending to the opposite side of the injury and trunk rotation in both directions. This athlete could miss 5 to 14 days of competition time.

GRADE III HIP POINTER. An athlete with a grade III hip pointer may have severe pain on palpation, noticeable swelling, and possible discoloration. The athlete's gait cycle could be abnormal, with very slow, deliberate ambulation and extremely short stride length and swing through phase. The athlete's posture may present a severe lateral tilt to the affected side. Trunk range of motion may be limited in all motions. Active hip flexion and trunk flexion may reproduce pain. This athlete could miss 14 to 21 days of competition time.

Treatment and Rehabilitation

Ice, compression, and rest should be started immediately. Subcutaneous steroid injection has been found to decrease inflammation and enable early range-of-motion exercises. Oral antiinflammatory medication is also beneficial in the early stages to reduce pain and inflammation. Transcutaneous electrical nerve stimulation (TNS) may be helpful on the day of injury to decrease pain and promote range-of-motion exercises.

To speed recovery, use ice massage for 10 minutes, followed by pain-free trunk active range of motion exercises. Concentrate on lateral side bending to the opposite side of the injury (Fig. 13-1). When active swelling and inflammation stop, on approximately the second or third day, ultrasound is very beneficial for gaining range of motion following ice massage. Pain-free active range-of-motion exercises are vital to the recovery process. Active motion, usually started on the second day, helps promote healing and decreases the time the athlete is prohibited from practice and competition. On approximately days 3 to 5, hip abduction, flexion, and extension

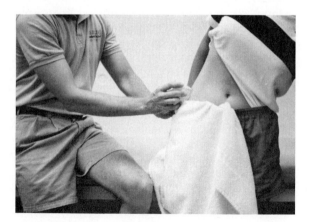

Fig. 13-1. Ice cup massage to hip pointer with side bending to opposite side.

progressive resistive strengthening exercises (using an ankle cuff or weight boot) may be performed, as long as this activity does not cause pain (Figs. 13-2 through 13-7). Trunk-strengthening exercises may also be added. Compression should be maintained throughout the period with practice or competition. On returning to competition, the athlete should wear custommade protective doughnut padding.

TREATMENT OF HIP POINTERS
PHASE I: *Days 1–2*
  1. Ice (massage).
  2. Rest.
  3. Compression.
  4. Subcutaneous steroid injection.
  5. Oral antiinflammatory medication.
  6. TNS.
PHASE II: *Days 2–3*
  7. Ultrasound.
  8. Pain-free hip and trunk active range-of-motion exercises (concentrating on lateral

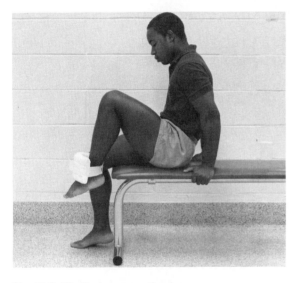

Fig. 13-2. Hip flexion strengthening.

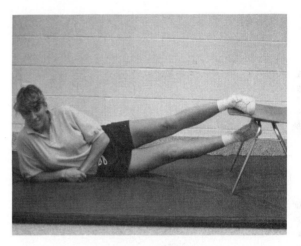

Fig. 13-4. Hip adduction strengthening.

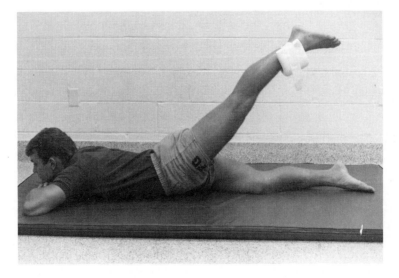

Fig. 13-3. Hip extension strengthening.

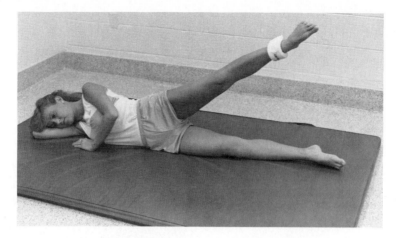

Fig. 13-5. Hip abduction strengthening.

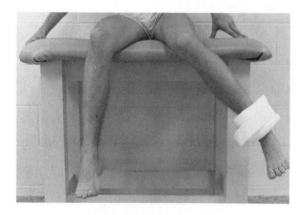

Fig. 13-6. Hip internal rotation strengthening.

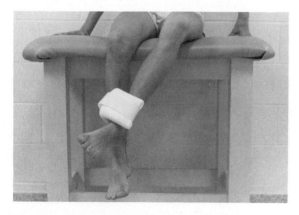

Fig. 13-7. Hip external rotation strengthening.

side bending to the opposite side). Slow stretch held for 15 to 30 seconds times 3 to 5 sets daily.

PHASE III: *Days 3–5*

9. Pain-free hip abduction progressive resistive strengthening exercises: 3 sets of 10–15 repetitions daily.

10. Pain-free hip flexion progressive resistive strengthening exercises: 3 sets of 10–15 repetitions daily.

11. Pain-free hip extension progressive resistive strengthening exercises: 3 sets of 10–15 repetitions daily.

12. Pain-free active trunk flexion and extension strengthening exercises: 3 sets of 10–15 repetitions daily.

PHASE IV: *Day 5*

13. Functional sport-specific activities.

14. Custom-made, protective doughnut pad.

INJURY TO THE ILIAC SPINE
Anterior Superior Iliac Spine

The anterior superior iliac spine serves as an attachment for the sartorius muscle. Pain at this site may indicate apophysitis, an inflammatory response to overuse.[1] Severe pain associated with disability requires an x-ray to rule out an avulsion fracture.[1] Apophysitis and/or a contusion to the anterior superior iliac spine may accompany a hip pointer and should be treated as such.

Anterior Inferior Iliac Spine

The anterior inferior iliac spine serves as an attachment for the rectus femoris. As with the anterior superior iliac spine, apophysitis and/or a contusion may be treated as a hip pointer (see Treatment for Hip Pointer). An avulsion fracture caused by a violent, forceful contraction of the rectus femoris or a violent, forceful passive stretch of the hip into extension should be ruled out by x-ray. These injuries are seen more often in younger athletes.

Posterior Superior Iliac Spine Contusion

Contusions to the posterior superior iliac spine must be differentiated from vertebral fractures and more serious internal organ injuries.[1] Depending upon the athlete's pain and range of motion, an x-ray should be taken to rule out vertebral fractures and vertebral transverse process fractures. Other injuries to this area are not common due to the lack of muscle attachments.[17] Avulsion fractures may not be seen in this area, but a fracture of the posterior superior iliac spine should be ruled out. This injury may be painful but usually does not cause disability.

EVALUATION AND CLINICAL FINDINGS. An athlete with a contusion to the posterior superior iliac spine may complain of pain on palpation and have swelling that is usually not extensive. The athlete's gait cycle may look normal except in severe cases, when the athlete may take short choppy steps to avoid the pain associated with landing at heel strike. In severe cases, the athlete's posture may show a slight forward flexion tilt of the trunk. This athlete may show full active range of motion of the trunk, with mild discomfort. In moderate to severe cases, up to 3 days of rest may be needed before return to competition.

TREATMENT AND REHABILITATION. Ice massage may be used for the first 3 days, followed by pulsed ultrasound in the less severe cases. The athlete may usually begin hot packs with pain-free stretching exercises within the first 3 days, as long as the active swelling has been controlled (Figs. 13-8 through 13-13). Exercises should include active and passive trunk and hip flexion and extension. A protective doughnut pad should be worn for competition.

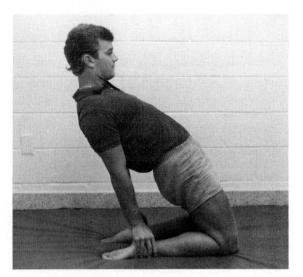

Fig. 13-8. Hip flexor stretching.

TREATMENT OF CONTUSIONS TO THE POSTERIOR SUPERIOR ILIAC SPINE

PHASE I: *Days 1–3*

1. Ice (massage).
2. Ultrasound (pulse).
3. Hot packs.
4. Pain-free active and passive range-of-motion exercises of the trunk and hip. Stretches held for 30 seconds times 5 repetitions daily. Active exercises performed as 3 sets of 10 repetitions daily.

PIRIFORMIS SYNDROME SCIATICA

The sciatic nerve is a continuation of the sacral plexus as it passes through the greater sciatic notch and descends deeply through the back of the thigh. Hip pain is often diagnosed as sciatic nerve irritation. The sciatic nerve may be irritated by a low back problem, but it is also subject to trauma where the nerve passes underneath or through the piriformis muscle, in which case sciatic nerve irritation is also called *piriformis syndrome*. In approximately 15% of the population, the sciatic nerve passes through the piriformis muscle, separating it into two. This condition is seen in more women than men, and the cause may be a tight piriformis muscle.[7]

Injury to the hamstring muscles may also

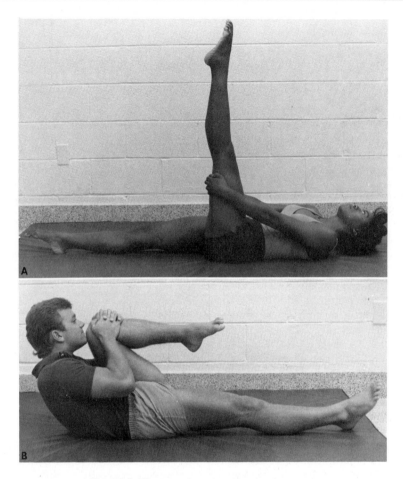

Fig. 13-9. Hip extensor stretching techniques.

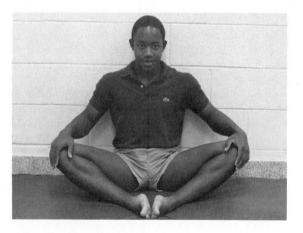

Fig. 13-10. Hip adductor stretching.

cause sciatic nerve irritation, as can irritation from ischial bursitis.[7] In a traumatic accident that causes posterior dislocation of the femoral head, the sciatic nerve may be crushed or severed and require surgery.[7]

The most common cause of sciatic nerve irritation in athletics, especially contact sports, is a direct blow to the buttock. Owing to the large muscle mass, this injury is not usually disabling when the sciatic nerve is not involved. When the sciatic nerve is involved, however, the athlete may experience pain in the buttock, extending down the back of the thigh, possibly into the lateral calf and foot.[17] Sciatic pain is usually a burning sensation.

With sciatica, the sports therapist must rule

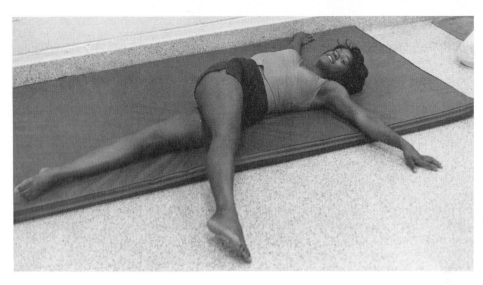

Fig. 13-11. Hip abductor stretching.

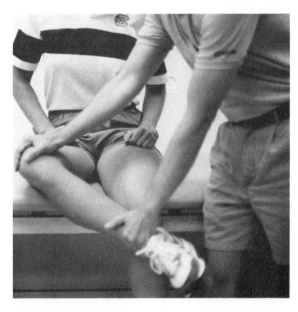

Fig. 13-12. Hip internal rotator stretching.

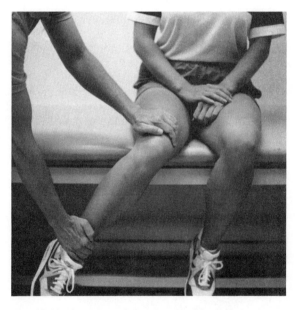

Fig. 13-13. Hip external rotator stretching.

out disk disease before starting any exercise rehabilitation program. Stretching exercises that are indicated for sciatica, such as trunk and hip flexion, may be contraindicated for disk disease. To differentiate low back problems (disk disease) from piriformis syndrome as the cause of sciatica, determine if the athlete has low back pain with radiation into the extremity. Back pain is most likely midline, exacerbated by trunk flexion, and relieved by rest.[20] Coughing and straining may also increase back pain and possibly the radiation. Muscle weakness and sensory numbness may also be found in an athlete with disk disease.[20] Athletes with piriformis syndrome may have the same symptoms without low back pain.

If, after treatment and rehabilitation, the athlete still maintains neurological deficits, further evaluation should be performed and disk disease should be ruled out again.

Evaluation and Clinical Findings

In the case of piriformis syndrome, the athlete may report a deep pain in the buttock without low back pain and possibly radiating pain in the back of the thigh, lateral calf, and foot, also indicating sciatica.[7] The sports therapist's evaluation should include the low back, as well as the hip and thigh. The athlete's gait cycle could present a lack of heel strike, landing in the foot-flat phase, a shortening of the stride, and possible

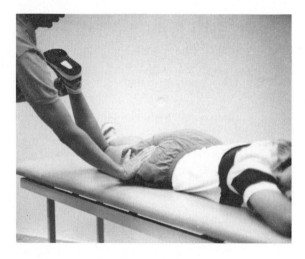

Fig. 13-14. Evaluating tightness of the piriformis.

ambulation with a flexed knee. The athlete's posture, in severe cases, may show a flexed knee with the leg externally rotated. Palpation in the sciatic notch could also produce pain.

With the athlete lying supine and the hip in a neutral position with the knee in extension, active resistive external rotation and passive internal rotation of the hip may reproduce the pain[7] (Fig. 13-14). Straight leg raises performed passively or actively may also cause symptoms.

With the athlete in the same position as above and relaxed, a decrease in passive internal rotation of the hip joint as compared to the uninjured side may indicate piriformis tightness.

Severe sciatica caused by piriformis syndrome may put the athlete out of competition for 2 to 3 weeks.

Treatment and Rehabilitation

If the sciatic nerve is irritated and the athlete complains of radiation into the extremity, the first 3 to 5 days should consist of modalities to decrease the pain associated with sciatica. Ice and/or heat, in contrast form or alone, at the sciatic notch and hamstring areas may decrease symptoms. Deep-heat modalities may cause irritation to the sciatic nerve and should be avoided.

After the acute pain has been controlled, the athlete may perform pain-free stretching exercises for the low back, hip, and hamstring muscles, as long as disk disease has been ruled out. The piriformis muscle is stretched by passive internal rotation of the hip (Fig. 13-15). Contract-relax techniques (PNF) may aid in lengthening the piriformis muscle. The athlete should also concentrate on hamstring-stretching exercises, performed pain-free while maintaining a lordotic curve in the lumbar area as the athlete stretches. Piriformis strengthening may be accomplished through resistive external rotation of the hip (see Fig. 13-10).

Reviewing a normal gait cycle may also aid in gaining range of motion if the athlete has been ambulating with a flexed knee. The hamstrings, as well as the sciatic nerve, may have shortened in this case.

The athlete should be capable of performing pain-free activity such as running and cutting before being allowed to return to competition.

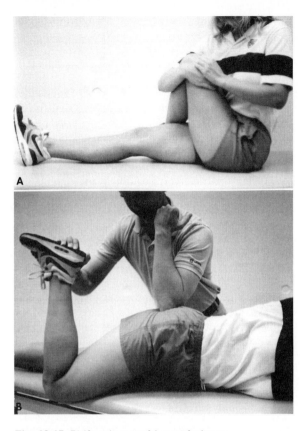

Fig. 13-15. Piriformis stretching techniques.

Developing chronic problems poses danger if the athlete participates with radiation into the extremity. The best method of treatment is prevention by instituting a good flexibility exercise program for athletes.

TREATMENT OF PIRIFORMIS SYNDROME SCIATICA

PHASE I: *Days 1–3*

1. Ice.
2. Heat (superficial).

PHASE II: *Days 3–5*

3. Pain-free piriformis stretching exercises in internal rotation. Hold stretch for 30 seconds times 5 repetitions twice a day.
4. Pain-free hamstring stretching exercises maintaining lumbar lordotic curve. Hold stretch for 30 seconds times 5 repetitions daily twice a day.
5. Pain-free low back stretching exercises

knee to chest. Hold stretch for 30 seconds times 5 repetitions twice a day.

PHASE III: *From day 5*

6. Jogging.
7. Sport-specific activities.

BURSITIS OF THE HIP

Bursitis and other disorders of the bursa are often mistaken for other injuries due to the location of numerous other structures around the bursa. The bursa is a structure that normally lies within the area of a joint and produces a fluid that lubricates the two surfaces between which it lies.[18] It has also been known to attach, very loosely, to the joint capsule, tendons, ligaments, and skin. Therefore, it is indirectly involved with other close structures.[18] The bursa function is to dissipate friction caused by two or more structures moving against one another.

Bursitis is usually caused by direct trauma and/or overuse stress. Bursitis associated with bleeding into the bursa is the most disabling form of bursitis. Swelling and pain may limit motion with a hemorrhagic bursitis.[18]

The sports therapist must also consider the possibility of an infected bursa. If it is suspected, the athlete should be referred for blood tests.

Trochanteric Bursitis

The most commonly diagnosed hip bursitis is greater trochanteric bursitis. The greater trochanter bursa lies between the gluteus maximus and the surface of the greater trochanter.[7]

One possible cause for trochanteric bursitis may be irritation caused by the iliotibial band, as the gluteus maximus inserts into it.[7] Repetitive irritation, such as running with one leg slightly adducted (as on the side of a road), may cause trochanteric bursitis on the adducted side. Trochanteric bursitis caused by overuse is mostly seen in women runners who have an increased Q angle and/or a possible leg-length discrepancy.[1] Tight adductors may cause a runner's feet to cross over the midline and thus put an exceptional amount of force on the trochanteric bursa.[10]

Lateral heel wear in running shoes may also cause excessive hip adduction, which may indirectly cause trochanteric bursitis. In contact sports, a direct blow may result in a hemorrhagic bursitis, which could be extremely painful to the athlete.[18]

EVALUATION AND CLINICAL FINDINGS. Traumatic trochanteric bursitis is more easily diagnosed than overuse trochanteric bursitis. Palpation produces pain over the lateral hip area and greater trochanter. In both cases the athlete's gait cycle may be slightly abducted on the affected side to relieve pressure on the bursa. An athlete's attempt to remove weight from the affected extremity may cause a shortened weight-bearing phase. The athlete may report an increase in pain on activity, and active resistive hip abduction may also reproduce the pain.

This athlete could miss 3 to 5 days of competition, depending on the severity of the bursitis.

TREATMENT AND REHABILITATION. A complete history must be taken to determine the cause of trochanteric bursitis. The athlete's gait cycle, posture, flexibility, and running shoes should be examined.

Oral antiinflammatory medication usually helps decrease pain and inflammation initially. For the first 2 to 3 days, ice in conjunction with compression (especially with hemorrhagic bursitis) should be used. When active swelling has been controlled, ultrasound may be used, with pain-free hip adduction stretching exercises for the iliotibial band. The hip-stretching exercises should be performed with the knee extended and with the knee flexed. With all bursa injuries, ice and compression are the keys to decreasing swelling, inflammation, and pain.

An orthotic evaluation should be performed to check for any malalignment that may have caused disfunction and/or leg-length discrepancy. Hip abduction progressive resistive strengthening exercises may be performed when the athlete is free of pain. For contact sports, a pad should be worn upon return to competition (see Treatment for Hip Bursitis on page 275).

Ischial Bursitis

The ischial bursa lies between the ischial tuberosity and the gluteus maximus. Ischial bursitis is often seen in people who sit for long periods.[7] In athletes ischial bursitis is more commonly caused by direct trauma, such as falling or a direct hit when the hip is in a flexed position that exposes the ischial area.

EVALUATION AND CLINICAL FINDINGS. The athlete may report trauma to the area. With the hip in a flexed position, palpation over the ischial tuberosity may reproduce the pain. The athlete may experience pain on ambulation when the hip is flexed during the gait cycle. Also, stair climbing and uphill walking and running may reproduce pain. Depending on injury severity, this athlete need not miss competition time.

TREATMENT AND REHABILITATION. Treatment for ischial bursitis consists of positioning the athlete with the hip in a flexed position to expose the ischial area (i.e., lying on the side with hip flexed). Ice is used for 2 to 3 days, followed by heat. Hip and trunk flexion stretching exercises may be performed when they are free of pain. Oral antiinflammatory medication may help decrease the pain and promote range of motion. Avoiding direct trauma to the area usually allows healing within 3 to 5 days. For contact sports, a pad should be worn (also see the Treatment for Hip Bursitis on page 275).

Iliopectineal Bursitis

Rarely seen in athletics, iliopectineal bursitis could potentially be caused by a tight iliopsoas muscle.[7] Osteoarthritis of the hip may also cause iliopectineal bursitis.[7] It may often be mistaken for a strain of the iliopsoas muscle and can be difficult to differentiate.

EVALUATION AND CLINICAL FINDINGS. Resistive hip flexion—sitting with knee bent or lying supine with the knee extended—may reproduce the pain associated with iliopectineal bursitis. Also, passive hip extension with the knee extended may produce pain. Palpable pain in the inguinal area may also help in evaluating the athlete. In some cases, the nearby femoral nerve may become inflamed and cause radiation into the front of the thigh and knee.[7] Osteoarthritis must be ruled out in evaluating iliopectineal bursitis.

TREATMENT AND REHABILITATION. Oral antiinflammatory medication may be helpful initially. A form of deep heat and/or ice massage may be used to aid in decreasing inflammation and pain. The iliopsoas tendon must be stretched, and progressive resistive strengthening exercises to the hip flexors may be performed within a pain-free range of motion.

TREATMENT OF HIP BURSITIS

PHASE I: *Days 1–3*

1. Ice.
2. Compression.
3. Pain-free hip-stretching exercises to the muscles involved. Hold stretch for 30 seconds times 5 repetitions twice a day.
4. Protective pad.
5. Oral antiinflammatory medication.

PHASE II: *From day 3*

6. Ultrasound.
7. Pain-free hip flexion progressive resistive strengthening exercises: 3 sets of 10 repetitions performed 3 days a week.

PUBIC INJURIES

Pain in the area of the pubic symphysis may be difficult to diagnose. Unless the athlete reports being hit or experiencing some kind of direct trauma, pubic pain may be caused by osteitis pubis, fractures of the inferior ramus (stress fractures and avulsion fractures), and groin strains.

Osteitis Pubis

Because an overuse situation predisposes an athlete to this injury, osteitis pubis is seen mostly in distance running, football, wrestling, and soccer. Repetitive stress on the pubic symphysis, caused by the insertion of muscles to the area, creates a chronic inflammatory condition at the site.[1] Constant movement of the symphysis in sports such as football and soccer produces inflammation and pain. Direct trauma to the symphysis may also cause periostitis. Symptoms develop gradually, may be mistaken for a muscle strain, and can be difficult to differentiate. Exercises that aid muscle strains may cause more irritation to the symphysis; thus early active exercises are contraindicated.[10]

Referral to a physician to rule out hernia problems and prostatitis may be helpful in evaluating osteitis pubis.[10] X-ray changes may take 4 to 6 weeks to show. The athlete should be treated symptomatically in the meantime.

EVALUATION AND CLINICAL FINDINGS. An athlete with osteitis pubis may have pain in the groin area and may complain of an increase in pain with running, sit-ups, and squatting.[1] The athlete may also complain of lower abdominal pain with radiation into the inner thigh. Differentiating osteitis pubis from a muscle strain may be confusing.

Palpation over the pubic symphysis may reproduce pain. In severe cases, the athlete may show a waddling gait due to the shear forces at the symphysis.[21] Infection should be ruled out before treatment is begun.

In most cases, the athlete may miss 3 to 5 days of competition. In severe cases, from 3 weeks up to 3 months of rest and treatment may be necessary.

TREATMENT AND REHABILITATION. Rest is the main course of treatment. The lower body must be protected from shear forces to the symphysis area. Ice with ultrasound may be used to decrease inflammation and pain. Oral antiinflammatory medication may also help to relieve pain.

Hip adductor stretching exercises may be performed as soon as pain has decreased. Strengthening exercises for the abdominal muscles, low back muscles, hip abductors, hip adductors, hip flexors, and hip extensors may be performed within a pain-free range of motion. Strengthening, in the later phases, helps develop stability at the pubic symphysis.

Treatment of pubic injuries

PHASE I: *Days 1–3*

1. Rest.
2. Ice.
3. Ultrasound.
4. Oral antiinflammatory medication.

PHASE II: *Days 3–5*

5. Pain-free hip adductor muscles stretching exercises. Hold the stretch for 30 seconds times 5 repetitions twice a day.

PHASE III: *From day 5*

6. Pain-free abdominal strengthening exercises, 3 sets of 10 repetitions daily.
7. Pain-free low back strenthening exercises, 3 sets of 10 repetitions daily.
8. Pain-free hip abductor strengthening exercises, 3 sets of 10 repetitions daily.
9. Pain-free hip adductor strengthening exercises, 3 sets of 10 repetitions daily.

10. Pain-free hip flexors strengthening exercises, 3 sets of 10 repetitions daily.
11. Pain-free hip extensors strengthening exercises, 3 sets of 10 repetitions daily.

Fractures of the Inferior Ramus

Stress fractures and avulsion fractures should be ruled out before treating the pubic area for injury. Avulsion fracture of the inferior ramus is usually caused by a violent, forceful contraction of the hip adductor muscles or forceful passive movement into hip abduction, as in a split. The extent of the avulsion must be diagnosed by x-ray. A palpable mass may be detected under the skin. In some cases, surgical repair should be considered.

Stress fractures may occur from overuse. The patient may report the same symptoms as in osteitis pubis. X-rays may appear normal until the third or fourth week. Taking a good history may aid in diagnosing a stress fracture.

An athlete with a stress fracture may miss 3 to 6 weeks of competition. An avulsion fracture may keep an athlete out of competition for up to 3 months.

TREATMENT AND REHABILITATION. Rest is the key in treating fractures of the inferior ramus. Ice and/or heat may be used to decrease pain. The timetables presented in Treatment of Pubic Injuries on page 275 should be lengthened accordingly. Hip stretching and strengthening exercises may be performed within a pain-free range of motion. Return to activity should be gradual, deliberate, and, by all means, free of pain.

Groin Strain

A groin strain may occur to any muscle in the inner hip area. Whether it is to the sartoris, rectus femoris, the adductors, or the iliopsoas, the muscle and degree of injury must be determined and the injury treated accordingly.[3]

A groin strain may develop from overextending and externally rotating the hip or from forcefully contracting the muscles involved, as in running, jumping, twisting, and kicking. Diagnosis and treatment may be difficult because of the number of muscles in the area.

Discomfort may start as mild but develop into moderate to severe pain with disability if not treated correctly. A chronic strain may cause bleeding into the groin muscles. Myositis ossificans could form in the groin area (see the section on myositis ossificans); in chronic groin strains, it may be palpated and should be treated accordingly (see section on thigh injuries). If a groin strain is treated correctly, myositis ossificans can be avoided.

EVALUATION-CLINICAL FINDINGS

Grade I groin strain. The athlete may complain of mild discomfort with no loss of function and full range of motion and strength. Point tenderness may be minimal, with negative swelling. The gait cycle may be normal. Depending upon the severity of the injury, this athlete need not miss competition time.

Grade II groin strain. Palpation may reproduce pain, and a noticeable defect as well as moderate swelling may be detected. This athlete may show an abnormal gait cycle. Ambulation may be slow, and the stride length may be shortened on the affected side. The athlete may tend to hike the hip rather than drive the knee through during the swing through phase. Range of motion may be severely limited, and resistance could cause an increase in pain. This athlete may miss 3 to 14 days of competition, depending on the severity of injury.

Grade III groin strain. This athlete may need crutches to ambulate. A noticeable defect may be detected in the involved muscle or tendon. Point tenderness may be severe, with noticeable swelling. Range of motion may be severely limited. The athlete may splint the legs together and be apprehensive about allowing movement in abduction. Resistance may not be tolerated. The athlete could potentially miss 3 weeks to 3 months of competition, depending on the severity of the injury.

Differentiating a hip adductor strain from a hip flexor strain is the first step in treating this injury. Resistive adduction while lying supine with the knee in extension may significantly increase pain if the hip adductors are involved. Flexing the hip and knee and resisting hip adduction may also increase pain. If the injury is a pure hip adductor strain, the supine position with the knee extended may reproduce more discomfort than flexing the hip and knee. If resistive adduction with the hip and knee flexed produces more discomfort, the hip flexor may also be involved.

With the athlete lying supine, resistive hip flexion with the knee in extension tests for an iliopsoas strain. Resistive hip flexion with the knee flexed tests for a rectus femoris strain.

After determining the muscle or muscles involved and the degree of the injury, treatment and rehabilitation is the next step.

TREATMENT AND REHABILITATION

Grade I groin strain. Ice and ultrasound should be started immediately, with pain-free hip adductor stretching exercises (Fig. 13-7). Pain-free progressive resistive strengthening exercises may also be performed (see Fig. 13-6). Care must be taken not to further aggravate the injury.

Treatment of Grade I groin strain

PHASE I: *From day 1*
1. Ice.
2. Ultrasound.
3. Pain-free progressive resistive strengthening exercises, 3 sets of 10 repetitions daily.
4. Pain-free hip stretching exercises. Hold the stretch for 30 seconds times 5 repetitions daily.

Grade II groin strain. Ice should be started immediately, with gentle, pain-free active range-of-motion exercises of the hip. Electrical muscle stimulation modalities can be very useful in the early stages to decrease inflammation and pain and to promote increases in range of motion.[19] Isometrics should also be performed as soon as they can be managed without pain. A normal gait cycle should be taught to the athlete, even if it involves using crutches for 1 to 3 days. After the third day ultrasound may be used. The athlete may perform pain-free hip adductor stretching exercises and also perform progressive resistive strengthening exercises within a pain-free range of motion, progressing in motion and weight as discomfort decreases. On approximately day 5 the athlete may be able to start biking, swimming, and possibly jogging. Activities should be gradually increased without pain to full activity.

Hip adductor strains usually take longer to treat and rehabilitate than hip flexor strains of the same grade. Treatment and rehabilitation should be modified accordingly.

Treatment of Grade II groin strain

PHASE I: *Days 1–3*
1. Ice.
2. Compression.
3. Electrical muscle stimulation modalities.
4. Crutches.
5. Pain-free isometric exercises.
6. Pain-free active range-of-motion exercises.

PHASE II: *Days 3–5*
7. Ultrasound.
8. Pain-free progressive resistive strengthening exercises, 3 sets of 10 repetitions daily.

PHASE III: *From day 5*
9. Biking.
10. Swimming.
11. Jogging.
12. Sport-specific activities.

Grade III groin strain. Grade III groin strains should be iced, compressed, and immobilized, and the athlete should be using crutches. Electrical muscle stimulation modalities are useful in the acute stage to decrease inflammation and pain and to promote range of motion.[19] Rest for 1 to 3 days is recommended, with compression at all times.

After surgery has been ruled out, the athlete may perform pain-free isometric exercises between days 3 and 5. Slow, pain-free active range-of-motion exercises may also be performed during days 3 to 5. A normal gait cycle should be emphasized by using crutches. Crutches should not be eliminated until the athlete can ambulate with a normal, pain-free gait cycle.

Heat modalities in the form of ultrasound, hot packs, or diathermy, should be used before exercise on approximately day 5.

During days 7 to 10, the athlete may perform progressive resistive strengthening exercises without pain, progressing in weight and motion. Gentle, pain-free stretching exercises should also be performed. The athlete needs to achieve a good strength level, usually within 10 days of starting progressive resistive strengthening exercises, to perform functional activities such as biking, swimming, and jogging.

Treatment and rehabilitation timetables may be modified. The modifications should be based on the degree of injury within the grade presented.

Treatment of Grade III groin strain

PHASE I: *Days 1–3*

1. Rest.
2. Ice.
3. Compression.
4. Electrical muscle stimulation modalities.
5. Crutches and immobilization.

PHASE II: *Days 3–5*

6. Pain-free isometric exercises.
7. Pain-free active range-of-motion exercises.
8. Crutches continued if necessary.

PHASE III: *Days 5–14*

9. Heat modalities.
10. Pain-free progressive resistive strengthening exercise, 3 sets of 10 repetitions daily.
11. Pain-free stretching exercises. Hold stretch for 30 seconds times 5 repetitions twice a day.

PHASE IV: *Days 14–21*

12. Biking.
13. Swimming.
14. Jogging.
15. Sport-specific activities.

HIP DISLOCATION

Dislocation of the hip joint takes a considerable amount of force due to the deep-seated ball-in-socket joint. When dislocation does occur, it is generally a posterior dislocation that takes place with the knee in a flexed position. Fractures may be associated with a dislocation and should always be considered. However, this injury is extremely rare in athletics. If it should occur, it should be treated as a medical emergency. The athlete should be checked for distal pulses and sensation. The sciatic nerve should be examined to see if it has been crushed or severed.[17] Do this by checking sensation and foot and toe movements. If the sciatic nerve is damaged, knee, ankle, and toe weakness may be pronounced.

Hip dislocations may also lead to avascular necrosis, which is a degenerative condition of the head of the femur due to a disruption of the blood supply during dislocation.[1]

Evaluation and Clinical Findings

The athlete may be totally disabled, in severe pain, and usually unwilling to allow movement of the extremity. The trochanter may appear larger than normal with the extremity in internal rotation, flexed, and adducted.[17] X-rays should be performed before anesthetized reduction.

Treatment and Rehabilitation

Two to three weeks of immobilization and bed rest is initially needed. Rehabilitation of the thigh and ankle may also be included at this time. Pain-free hip isometric exercises may be performed. Electrical muscle stimulation modalities may be used initially to promote muscle reeducation and retard muscle atrophy.[19]

At approximately 3 to 6 weeks, pain-free active range-of-motion exercises can be performed. Crutch walking is progressed and performed until the athlete can ambulate with a normal gait cycle and without pain. At approximately 6 weeks, the athlete may perform gentle progressive resistive strengthening exercises with a weight cuff or weight boot. All six movements of the hip should be included in the progressive resistive strengthening exercises (hip flexion, abduction, extension, adduction, internal rotation, and external rotation; see Figs. 13-2 through 13-7). Pain-free stretching exercises should not be performed for 8 to 12 weeks.

At approximately 12 weeks, the athlete may perform Nautilus hip and low back, abduction and adduction, and possibly leg press exercises. Swimming and biking may also be performed at 12 weeks. At 16 weeks, the athlete may progress to functional activities such as jogging and possibly light squats.

TREATMENT OF HIP DISLOCATION

PHASE I: *Weeks 2–3*

1. Immobilization.
2. Bed rest.
3. Thigh and ankle rehabilitation. Quadriceps and hamstring isometrics performed all day daily. Ankle isometrics and progressive resistive strengthening exercises performed with Theraband (dorsiflexion, plantarflexion, eversion, inversion) daily.
4. Electrical muscle stimulation modalities.
5. Hip isometrics in all six movements (hip flexion, abduction, extension, adduction, internal, and external rotations) throughout the day, daily.

PHASE II: *Weeks 3–6*

6. Pain-free active range-of-motion exercises in all six movements, 3 sets of 10 repetitions daily.
7. Crutch walking, teaching normal gait.

PHASE III: *Weeks 6–12*

8. Pain-free progressive resistive strengthening exercises in all six movements, 3 sets of 10 repetitions 3 days per week.
9. Pain-free hip stretching exercises at approximately weeks 8 to 12. Stretching in all six movements, holding the stretch for 30 seconds times 3 to 5 repetitions for each movement daily.

PHASE IV: *Weeks 12–16*

10. Nautilus (hip and low back, abduction and adduction, leg press), 3 sets of 10 repetitions 3 days per week.
11. Biking.
12. Swimming.

PHASE V: *From week 16*

13. Jogging.
14. Light squats, 4 sets of 6 to 8 repetitions 2 days per week.
15. Sport-specific activities.

HAMSTRING INJURIES
Ischial Tuberosity

The ischial tuberosity is a common site of injury to the hamstring muscle group (the biceps femoris, semitendinosus, and semimembranosus). All three hamstring muscles originate from the ischial tuberosity.

The most common ischial injury, as it relates to the hamstring group, is an avulsion fracture of the tuberosity. This injury usually results from a violent, forceful flexion of the hip, with the knee in extension.[17] A less severe irritation of the hamstring origin at the ischial tuberosity may also develop.

LESS SEVERE INJURY

Evaluation and clinical findings. An athlete with the less severe injury or irritation of the hamstring origin at the ischeal tuberosity may complain of discomfort on sitting for extended periods and discomfort on palpation. The athlete may ambulate with a normal gait cycle. This athlete may also complain of pain while walking up stairs or uphill. Resistive knee flexion and resistive hip extension with the knee in an extended

position may reproduce the pain. Passive hip flexion with the knee in extension may also cause discomfort. This athlete may not miss competition time.

Treatment and rehabilitation. Ice and ultrasound may be started on day 1, with gentle, pain-free hamstring-stretching exercises. Also, heat in the form of hot packs may be used before competition while the athlete is stretching. To isolate the hamstring muscles while stretching, the athlete should maintain a lordotic curve in the lumbar back area while flexing at the trunk to stretch the hamstrings (Fig. 13-16). Pain-free hamstring muscle progressive resistive strengthening exercises may also be performed on day 1.

Treatment of hamstring injuries

PHASE I: *From day 1*

1. Ice.
2. Ultrasound.
3. Hot packs.
4. Pain-free hamstring-stretching exercises. Maintain a lumbar curve and hold stretch for 30 seconds times 5 repetitions daily.
5. Pain-free hamstring progressive resistive strengthening exercises, 4 sets of 10 repetitions 3 days a week.

AVULSION FRACTURE

Evaluation and clinical findings. The more severe ischial tuberosity avulsion fracture presents a different clinical picture. Palpation may produce moderate to severe pain, and the athlete may be in moderate to severe pain with a very abnormal gait cycle. The athlete's gait cycle may lack a heel strike phase and have a very short swing through phase. The athlete may attempt to keep the injured extremity behind or below the body to avoid hip flexion during the gait cycle. Resistive knee flexion and resistive hip extension with the knee in an extended or flexed position may reproduce the pain. Passive hip flexion with the knee extended and with the knee flexed may cause moderate to severe pain at the ischial tuberosity. X-rays may or may not show the injury.[17]

Treatment and rehabilitation. Surgery is usually not necessary. Immobilization and limiting physical activity are usually enough to allow healing. Ice and limited physical activity that involves hip flexion and forceful hip extension and knee flexion for the first 3 weeks is usually all that is

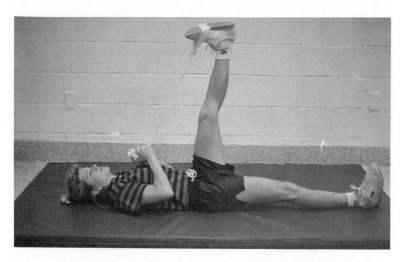

Fig. 13-16. Hamstring stretches maintaining lordotic curve.

necessary. Crutches may be needed for the first 3 weeks while a normal gait cycle is taught.

During weeks 3 through 6, the athlete may begin heat modalities (hot packs, ultrasound, diathermy, whirlpool), with pain-free active range of motion, lying prone and sitting. Pain-free hamstring-stretching exercises may also be performed. Regaining full range of motion during the rehabilitation program is very important. Many athletes never regain full hip flexion range of motion following this injury.

Weeks 6 through 12 are a progressive phase for hamstring progressive resistive strengthening exercises (Fig. 13-17). Swimming, biking, and jogging may also be performed in this phase, but the athlete should avoid forceful knee and hip flexion and forceful hip extension.

After week 12, the athlete without pain may progress to sport-specific activities.

Further treatment for injuries to the hamstrings
PHASE I: *Weeks 1–3*
1. Ice.
2. Immobilization (avoid hip and knee flexion and active hip extension).
3. Crutch walking.
PHASE II: *Weeks 3–6*
4. Heat modalities.
5. Pain-free hamstring active range-of-motion exercises. Lying prone and sitting, flex the knee through a pain-free range of motion, 3 sets of 10 repetitions daily.
6. Pain-free hamstring-stretching exercises

maintaining a lumbar lordotic curve. Hold the stretch for 30 seconds times 5 repetitions daily.
PHASE III: *Weeks 6–12*
7. Pain-free hamstring progressive resistive strengthening exercises, 4 sets of 10 repetitions 3 days per week.
8. Swimming.
9. Biking.
10. Jogging.
PHASE IV: *From week 12*
11. Sport-specific activities.

Hamstring Strains

Hamstring strains are common, and the causes are numerous. A quick, explosive contraction of the hamstrings, while the hip is in flexion with the knee extended, bringing the hip into extension and flexing the knee, could lead to a strain of the hamstring muscles. Many theories try to explain the cause of hamstring strains. Imbalance with the quadriceps is one theory, according to which the hamstring muscles should be 60% to 70% of the quadriceps muscles strength. Other possibilities are hamstring muscle fatigue, running posture and gait, leg-length discrepancy, decreased hamstring range of motion, and an imbalance between the medial and lateral hamstring muscles.[1]

EVALUATION AND CLINICAL FINDINGS
Grade I hamstring strain. With a grade I ham-

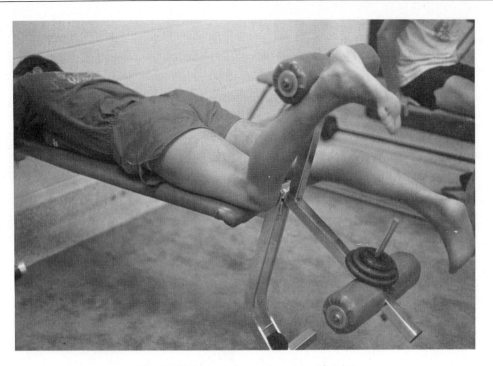

Fig. 13-17. Isotonic hamstring strengthening.

string strain, the athlete may complain of sore hamstring muscles, with negative pain on palpation and negative swelling. The athlete's gait cycle may be normal. Hip flexion range of motion is probably normal, with a tight feeling reported at the extreme range of hip flexion. Resistive knee flexion and resistive hip extension with the knee extended is probably free of pain or possibly produce a tight feeling with good strength present.

This athlete may not miss competition time but should be watched closely. Rehabilitation and strengthening should begin immediately to avoid further injury.

Grade II hamstring strain. With a grade II hamstring strain, the athlete may report having heard or felt a pop during the activity. The athlete usually ambulates with an abnormal gait cycle. The athlete may lack heel strike and land during the foot flat phase of the gait cycle. Swing through phase may be limited due to the athlete's unwillingness to flex the hip and knee. The athlete may tend to ambulate with a flexed knee.

Palpation may produce moderate to severe pain, and a defect in the muscle belly may be evident, with noticeable swelling. Resistive knee flexion and resistive hip extension with the knee extended may cause moderate to severe pain. The athlete may also have a noticeable weakness on resistive knee flexion and resistive hip extension with the knee extended and flexed. Resistive hip extension with the knee flexed also tests the strength of the gluteus maximus muscle.

Passive hip flexion with the knee extended may also produce moderate to severe pain. The athlete's range of motion may be moderately to severely limited in hip flexion with the knee extended and moderately limited in hip flexion with the knee flexed.

An athlete with a grade II hamstring strain could miss 5 to 21 days of competition.

Grade III hamstring strain. With a grade III hamstring strain, the athlete may be unable to ambulate without the aid of crutches. The athlete may report having heard or felt a pop during the activity. The sports therapist may detect swelling and severe pain on palpation. A noticeable defect in the muscle belly may be present. The athlete may have poor strength and be unable to resist knee flexion and hip extension with the knee extended. The athlete may have fair strength upon resistive hip extension with the knee flexed, due to the gluteus maximus muscle. Resisting these motions usually causes pain. Passive hip flexion, knee extended, may not be tolerated due to pain. Passive hip flexion, knee flexed, may be moderately to severely limited.

An athlete with a grade III hamstring strain could miss 3 to 12 weeks of competition.

TREATMENT AND REHABILITATION

Grade I hamstring strain. On the first day, the athlete may begin ice and compression, with gentle, pain-free hamstring-stretching exercises while maintaining a lumbar lordotic curve to isolate the hamstring muscles. Heat, in the form of hot packs and/or whirlpool, may be used before activity with stretching exercises. Pain-free hamstring progressive resistive strengthening exercises may also be performed immediately in order to prevent further injury to the hamstring muscles during activity.

Ultrasound may be used after ice or hot packs and before strengthening exercises. Utilizing an NK table is preferable for hamstring progressive resistive strengthening exercises (Fig. 13-18) because the sitting position gives the hamstring muscles a biomechanical advantage in working the hamstring muscles through a full range of motion. By sitting (the hip is flexed) and using an NK table, the hamstrings are stretching at the buttock and they are allowed to be more efficient during knee flexion exercises, in comparison to lying prone and performing hamstring progressive resistive strengthening exercises. Isokinetic exercises, in the form of an orthotron or cybex, may be used in conjunction with the NK table isotonic exercises (Fig. 13-19).

Treatment of Grade I hamstring strain

PHASE I: *From day 1*
1. Ice.
2. Compression.
3. Heat (hot packs, whirlpool, ultrasound).
4. Pain-free hamstring stretching exercises. Hold stretch for 30 seconds times 5 repetitions daily. Always maintain a lumbar lordotic curve while stretching the hamstrings.
5. Pain-free hamstring progressive resistive strengthening exercises. Isotonics performed on the NK table, 4 sets of 10 rep-

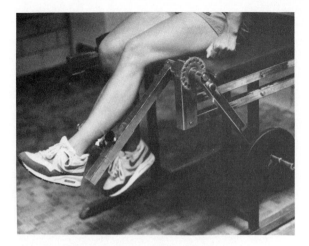

Fig. 13-18. NK table hamstring exercise.

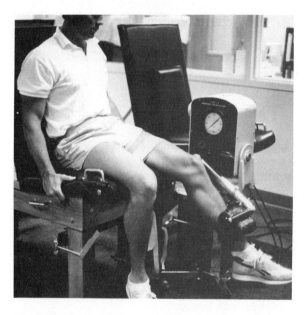

Fig. 13-19. Isokinetic exercise of the hamstrings and quadriceps.

etitions 3 days per week.
6. Isokinetics 3 days per week.

Grade II hamstring strain. An athlete with a grade II hamstring strain should be treated conservatively due to the potentially chronic nature of this injury.

A pain-free normal gait cycle should be taught

as soon as possible, and crutches should be used to accomplish a normal gait cycle. Ice, compression, and gentle, pain-free hamstring-stretching exercises, making sure the athlete maintains a lumbar lordotic curve to isolate the hamstring muscles, are performed on day 1. Electrical muscle stimulation modalities may be used to promote range of motion and to decrease pain.[19] Active range of motion while lying prone may also be performed between days 1 and 3, if the athlete can do so without pain. Hamstring isometric exercises may be taught as soon as possible, again within pain-free limits. Pain-free motion is very important and usually decreases the length of time an athlete misses competition. At approximately day 3, the athlete may begin heat in the form of hot packs and whirlpool, combined with pain-free stretching exercises, or ultrasound followed by pain-free stretching exercises. Utilizing the NK table, hamstring progressive resistive strengthening exercises may also be performed on day 3, if pain free. Isokinetics may be valuable in conjunction with isotonics (NK table). Swimming and biking may be added between days 3 and 6. Jogging and sport-specific activities may be added accordingly, beginning with day 6.

In the later phases of all three grades of hamstring muscle strains, the athlete should be educated in performing full range-of-motion leg press exercises on Nautilus, and light weight squats (Fig. 13-20). These two exercises are very helpful in strengthening the hamstrings in a weight-bearing position.

All activities should be followed by ice treatments to decrease inflammation and discomfort.

Treatment of Grade II hamstring strain

PHASE I: *Days 1–3*

1. Ice.
2. Compression.
3. Electrical muscle stimulation modalities.
4. Pain-free hamstring-stretching exercises. Hold for 30 seconds times 5 repetitions daily. Maintain lumbar lordotic curve.
5. Pain-free hamstring active range-of-motion exercises lying prone, 3 sets of 10 repetitions daily.
6. Pain-free hamstring isometric exercises.

PHASE II: *Days 3–6*

7. Heat (hot packs, whirlpool, ultrasound).
8. Pain-free hamstring progressive resistive

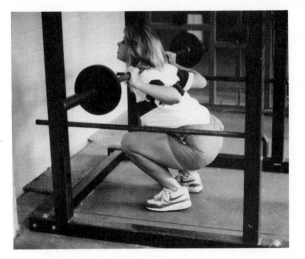

Fig. 13-20. Squats below parallel.

strengthening exercises. Isotonics on the NK table, 4 sets of 10 repetitions 3 days per week.
9. Isokinetics 3 days per week.
10. Swimming 2 days per week.
11. Biking 2 days per week.

PHASE III: *From day 6*

12. Jogging.
13. Sport-specific activities.
14. Leg press exercises, 3 sets of 10 repetitions 2 days per week.
15. Squats, 4 sets of 6 to 8 repetitions 2 days per week.

Grade III hamstring strain. After surgery has been ruled out, an athlete with a grade III hamstring strain may take 3 to 8 weeks to rehabilitate and in more severe cases up to 3 months.

Ice, compression, and crutches should be started immediately. Electrical muscle stimulation modalities may be used in the early stages to decrease inflammation and pain and promote range of motion.[19] The athlete should remain on crutches for 3 to 14 days in order to rest the injury and learn a normal gait cycle. Resting the injury for at least 3 to 5 days is usually necessary to decrease inflammation, pain, and splinting and to prepare the athlete for active range-of-motion exercises.

On approximately day 5, the athlete may perform pain-free active range-of-motion exercises lying prone, with gentle, pain-free hamstring-stretching exercises. Ice or heat, in the form of hot packs and ultrasound, may be used before or during stretching. Pain-free hamstring isometric exercises may be performed on approximately day 5.

Between days 10 to 14, the athlete may perform pain-free hamstring progressive resistive strengthening exercises by utilizing the NK table and isokinetic machines. The athlete who can do so without pain may swim and bike. This athlete needs to develop good (and preferably excellent) hamstring strength before progressing to jogging and sport-specific activities after 14 days. This conservatism is because of the possibility of reinjury.

The athlete should be educated in performing full range-of-motion leg press exercises on Nautilus and light weight squats. Especially with this injury, the time parameters presented have to be modified depending on the degree of injury within its grade.

Treatment of Grade III hamstring strain
PHASE I: *Days 1–5*
1. Ice.
2. Compression.
3. Electrical muscle stimulation modalities.
4. Crutches.
5. Rest.

PHASE II: *Days 5–10*
6. Pain-free hamstring active range-of-motion exercises lying prone daily.
7. Heat (hot packs, whirlpool, ultrasound).
8. Pain-free hamstring-stretching exercises while maintaining a lumbar lordotic curve. Hold stretch for 30 seconds times 5 repetitions daily.
9. Pain-free hamstring isometric exercises daily.

PHASE III: *Days 10–14*
10. Pain-free hamstring progressive resistive strengthening exercises. Isotonics on NK table, 4 sets of 10 repetitions 3 days a week.
11. Isokinetics 3 days a week.
12. Swimming 2 days a week.
13. Biking 2 days a week.

PHASE IV: *From day 14*
14. Jogging.
15. Sport-specific activities.

16. Leg press exercises, 3 sets of 10 repetitions 2 days per week.
17. Squats, 4 sets of 6 to 8 repetitions 2 days per week.

Hamstring Tendon Strains

Another injury that occurs to the hamstring muscles is a strain of the hamstring tendons near their attachments to the tibia and fibula. This injury has also been diagnosed as tendinitis. The athlete may report pain but may not experience disability. An athlete with a hamstring tendon strain or tendinitis may present a history of overuse and chronic pain for a few days.

EVALUATION AND CLINICAL FINDINGS. Palpation helps to isolate which tendon or tendons are involved, and resistive knee flexion, with the tibia in internal and external rotation, aids in the evaluation. The gastrocnemius muscle tendons in the same area must be ruled out. If resistive ankle plantar flexion with the knee in extension does not reproduce symptoms, gastrocnemius involvement may be ruled out.

TREATMENT AND REHABILITATION. An athlete who presents this condition responds nicely to 1 to 2 days of rest with oral antiinflammatory medication. Ice massage and ultrasound are helpful in decreasing inflammation and pain. Gentle hamstring-stretching exercises with the hip in internal and external rotation help to isolate the tendon or tendons involved and should be performed on day 1. Hamstring progressive resistive exercises can be performed on day 1 if they can be done without pain.

TREATMENT OF HAMSTRING TENDON STRAINS
PHASE I: *From day 1*
1. Ice.
2. Rest.
3. Ultrasound.
4. Pain-free hamstring-stretching exercises with the leg in internal and external rotation held for 30 seconds times 5 repetitions daily.
5. Pain-free hamstring progressive resistive strengthening exercises. Isotonics on the NK table, 4 sets of 10 repetitions 3 days a week.
6. Isokinetics 3 days a week.

FEMORAL FRACTURES

Fractures of the femur may be classified as stress fractures, avulsion fractures, or traumatic fractures.

Stress Fractures

Stress fractures of the femur are rare but may be seen due to repetitive microtrauma.[7] Young athletes are more likely to develop this injury.

EVALUATION AND CLINICAL FINDINGS. The athlete may complain of pinpoint pain that increases during activity. The initial x-rays are usually negative. Obtaining a good history is very important and should include activities, change in activities, and running gait analysis.[7]

TREATMENT AND REHABILITATION. As with all stress fractures, finding the cause is the first step in treatment and rehabilitation. While the athlete is in the non-weight-bearing phase of rehabilitation, non-weight-bearing activities should be utilized. Biking, swimming, and upper body ergometers may be used. The athlete may perform pain-free thigh-strengthening exercises and progress as shown in the lists outlining treatment of grades II and III hamstring strain (pages 283-284) and grades II and III quadriceps strain (pages 288-289).

Avulsion Fractures

Athletes may suffer an isolated avulsion fracture of the femoral trochanters. When the greater trochanter is involved, the cause is usually a violent, forceful contraction of the hip abductor muscles. An avulsion fracture of the lesser trochanter occurs due to a violent, forceful contraction of the iliopsoas muscle.[7]

EVALUATION AND CLINICAL FINDINGS. Palpation may produce pain and possibly a noticeable defect of the greater trochanter. Resistive movements and passive range of motion of the hip may reproduce pain. X-rays must be taken to confirm the injury.

TREATMENT AND REHABILITATION. Immobilization may be the treatment of choice for an incomplete avulsion fracture. With a complete avulsion fracture, internal fixation is usually required.

The athlete performs isometric hip exercises on the first day of rehabilitation, with isometric quadriceps exercises and ankle-strengthening exercises. Crutches are used for at least 6 weeks until a pain-free normal gait cycle can be accomplished. After 6 weeks, the athlete may perform pain-free active range-of-motion exercises and pain-free straight leg raise exercises involving hip flexion, abduction, extension, and adduction. During approximately week 8, the athlete may perform hip progressive resistive straight leg raises in all four movements (flexion, abduction, extension, and adduction).

Biking and swimming are performed when range of motion allows. The athlete is then progressed to jogging and sport-specific activities.

TREATMENT OF AVULSION FRACTURES

PHASE I: *Weeks 1–6*
1. Immobilization.
2. Crutches.
3. Isometric exercises daily (hip, thigh, and ankle exercises).

PHASE II: *Weeks 6–8*
4. Pain-free hip active and passive range-of-motion exercises daily (hip flexion, abduction, extension, adduction, internal and external rotation).

PHASE III: *From week 8*
5. Pain-free hip progressive resistive exercises daily in (hip flexion, abduction, extension, adduction, internal and external rotation).
6. Biking.
7. Swimming.
8. Jogging.
9. Sport-specific activities.

Traumatic Fractures

A femoral neck fracture is associated with osteoporosis and is rarely seen in athletics.[7,11,22] However, a twisting motion combined with a fall may produce this fracture. Because the femoral neck fracture may disrupt the blood supply to the head of the femur, avascular necrosis is often seen later. This injury must receive proper treatment.

TREATMENT AND REHABILITATION. After surgery or during immobilization, isometric hip exercises are started immediately. Athletes, especially younger athletes, are progressed slowly. Within 2 to 3 months, gentle active and passive hip range-of-motion exercises are performed. Muscle-strengthening exercises (see Treatment of Avulsion Fractures) and a normal gait cycle should be taught to the athlete.

In some cases, exercise has been shown to increase bone density and reverse the rate of osteoporosis.[7,22,23]

QUADRICEPS MUSCLE STRAIN

A strain to the large quadricep muscles in the front of the thigh may be very disabling, especially when the rectus femoris muscle is involved. With no history of direct contact to the quadriceps area, the injury can be treated as a muscle strain.

A quadriceps strain usually occurs due to a sudden violent, forceful contraction of hip and knee flexion, with the knee initially extended. An overstretch of the quadriceps, with the hip in extension and the knee flexed, may also cause a quadriceps strain.

Tight quadriceps, imbalance between quadricep muscles, and leg-length discrepancy, may also cause a quadriceps strain.[21]

Evaluation and Clinical Findings

GRADE I QUADRICEPS STRAIN. With a grade I quadriceps strain, the athlete may complain of tightness in the front of the thigh. The athlete may be ambulating with a normal gait cycle and present a history of the thigh feeling fatigued and tight. Swelling may not be present, and the athlete usually has negative discomfort on palpation or very mild discomfort when the rectus femoris is involved.

With the athlete sitting over the edge of a table, resistive knee extension may not produce discomfort. If the athlete is lying supine with the knee flexed over the edge of a table, resistive knee extension may produce mild discomfort, if the rectus femoris is involved. With the athlete lying prone, active knee flexion may produce a full pain-free range of motion, with possible tightness at extreme flexion.

An athlete with a grade I quadriceps strain may not miss competition time but should be watched closely and started on a rehabilitation and strengthening program immediately.

GRADE II QUADRICEPS STRAIN. With a grade II quadriceps strain, the athlete may have an abnormal gait cycle. The knee may be splinted in extension. The athlete may present an externally rotated hip to use the hip adductors to pull the leg through during the swing through phase, especially when the rectus femoris is involved. In severe cases, it may also be accompanied by hiking the hip during the swing through phase.

The athlete may have felt a sudden twinge and pain down the length of the rectus femoris during activity.[21] Swelling may be noticeable, and palpation may produce pain. A defect in the muscle may also be evident in a grade II strain. Resistive knee extension, when both sitting and lying supine, may reproduce pain. Lying supine and resisting knee extension may be more painful when the rectus femoris is involved. With the athlete lying prone, active knee flexion range of motion may present a noticeable decrease, in some cases a decrease up to 45 degrees. With a quadriceps strain, any decrease in knee flexion range of motion should classify the injury as a grade II or III strain.

This athlete may miss 7 to 21 days of competition, depending on the amount of active range of motion present. The lack of range of motion and the number of competition days missed are usually directly correlated.

GRADE III QUADRICEPS STRAIN. An athlete with a grade III quadriceps strain may be unable to ambulate without the aid of crutches and may be in severe pain, with a noticeable defect in the quadriceps muscle. Palpation may not be tolerated and swelling may be present almost immediately. The athlete may not be able to extend the knee actively and against resistance. An isometric contraction may be painful and may produce a bulge or defect in the quadriceps muscle, especially the rectus femoris. With the athlete lying prone, active knee flexion range of motion may be severely limited and may not be tolerated.

This athlete may miss 3 to 12 weeks of competition. In severe cases, surgery may be a consideration.

Treatment and Rehabilitation

GRADE I QUADRICEPS STRAIN. Ice, compression, active range of motion, and isometric quadriceps exercises may be performed immediately. Pain-free quadriceps progressive resistive strengthening exercises may be performed within the first two days (Fig. 13-21). Compression should be used at all times until the athlete is free of pain and no longer complaining of a tight feeling.

TREATMENT OF GRADE I QUADRICEPS STRAIN

PHASE I: *Days 1–2*

1. Ice.
2. Compression.
3. Quadriceps muscle active range of motion performed lying prone, sitting, and lying supine, 3 sets of 10 repetitions daily.
4. Quadriceps isometric exercises all day daily.

PHASE II: *From day 2*

5. Pain-free quadriceps progressive resistive strengthening exercises. Isotonic exercises using the NK table, 4 sets of 10 repetitions 3 days per week.
6. Isokinetics 3 days per week.

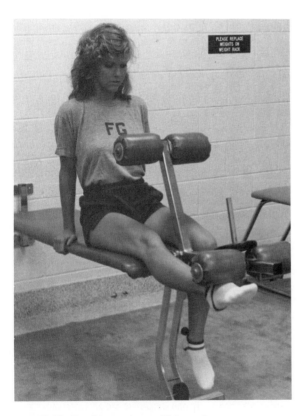

Fig. 13-21. Quad isotonics on Universal.

GRADE II QUADRICEPS STRAIN. Ice, compression, and crutches may be used immediately for 3 to 5 days. Electrical muscle stimulation modalities may be used acutely to decrease swelling, inflammation, and pain and promote range of motion.[19] At approximately day 3, the athlete may perform quadriceps isometric exercises and pain-free quadriceps active range-of-motion exercises. These exercises are performed lying prone and sitting and then progressing to the supine position to allow more efficiency to the rectus femoris muscle (Fig. 13-22). Ice used in conjunction with active range of motion is very helpful in regaining motion and strengthening the quadricep muscles pain free. Passive stretching exercises to the quadricep muscles are not recommended until later phases of the rehabilitation program. Compression is continued throughout the rehabilitation period. A pain-free normal gait cycle is reviewed and emphasized, with and without crutches.

During approximately days 3 to 7, the athlete may begin heat (hot packs, whirlpool, ultrasound) before exercise. During this phase of rehabilitation, pain-free straight leg raises without weight, progressing to straight leg raises with weight, are performed (Fig. 13-23).

Days 7 through 14 are pain-free quadriceps progressive resistive strengthening exercise

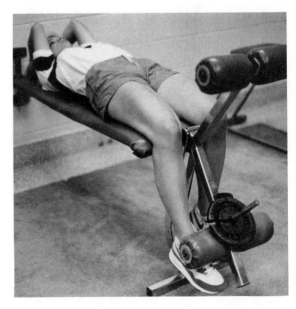

Fig. 13-22. Quadriceps strengthening for rectus femoris.

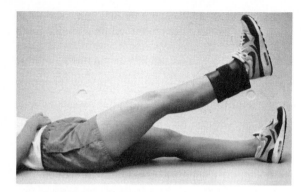

Fig. 13-23. Straight leg raises with weight boot.

days. The NK table is used due to its ability to change the force on the quadricep muscles by changing the lever arms and torque (Fig. 13-24). Isokinetics are also performed in this phase. Pain-free leg press exercises and squats may be performed in the later part of this phase. Training the quadriceps eccentrically and in a weight-bearing position by using leg press exercises and squats is very helpful in the rehabilitation program and in preventing reinjury. Swimming and biking can also be performed as long as the athlete avoids forceful kicking. The bike seat should be adjusted to accommodate a pain-free range of motion. Pain-free quadriceps-stretching exercises are not performed until days 7 to 14.

When the athlete has full pain-free range of motion, jogging and sport-specific activities may be added to the rehabilitation program.

TREATMENT OF GRADE II QUADRICEPS STRAIN

PHASE I: *Days 1–3*

1. Ice.
2. Compression.
3. Crutches.
4. Electrical muscle stimulation modalities.

PHASE II: *Days 3–7*

5. Pain-free quadriceps isometric exercises all day daily with and without ice.
6. Pain-free quadriceps active range-of-motion exercises lying prone, sitting, and lying supine, 3 sets of 10 repetitions daily with and without ice.
7. Heat (hot packs, whirlpool, ultrasound).
8. Straight leg raises daily progressing to weights, 4 sets of 10 repetitions 3 days a week.

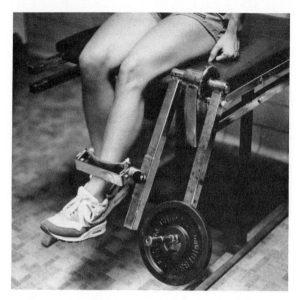

Fig. 13-24. NK table quad exercises.

PHASE III: *Days 7–14*

9. Pain-free quadriceps progressive resistive strengthening exercises. Isotonics using the NK table, 4 sets of 10 repetitions 3 days a week.
10. Isokinetics 3 days a week.
11. Swimming 2 to 3 days a week.
12. Biking 2 to 3 days a week.
13. Begin quadriceps-stretching exercises. Hold stretch for 30 seconds times 5 repetitions daily.
14. Leg press exercise, 3 sets of 10 repetitions 2 days a week.
15. Squats, 4 sets of 6 to 8 repetitions 2 days a week.

PHASE IV: *From day 14*

16. Jogging.
17. Sport-specific activities.

GRADE III QUADRICEPS STRAIN. An athlete with a grade III quadriceps strain should be on crutches for 7 to 14 days to allow for rest. Compression, ice, and electrical muscle stimulation modalities may be used immediately. Quadriceps-stretching exercises are not performed until later phases. Compression is maintained until the athlete has full pain-free range of motion.

On approximately day 7, the athlete may begin pain-free quadriceps isometric exercises.

Gentle, pain-free quadriceps active range-of-motion exercises while the athlete is lying prone may be performed if special attention is paid to avoiding overstretching the quadricep muscles. Ice, in conjunction with active range of motion while sitting over the end of a table, is very useful in regaining range of motion. Heat (hot packs, whirlpool, ultrasound) may be used on approximately days 7 to 10.

Pain-free straight leg raises without weight may be performed. Weight may be added after days 10 to 14.

Depending upon active range of motion, pain-free quadriceps active progressive resistive strengthening exercises may be performed after the third week. Isokinetics may also be added to the rehabilitation program, along with swimming and biking. The bicycle seat height should be adjusted to accommodate the athlete's available range of motion.

At approximately 4 to 5 weeks, leg press exercises and squats may be performed pain free. Depending on the severity of the injury, the athlete should have full active range of motion by the fourth week. Only when full active range of motion is accomplished should quadriceps-stretching exercises be performed. The athlete is then progressed to jogging and sport-specific activities.

TREATMENT OF GRADE III QUADRICEPS STRAIN

PHASE I: *Week 1*

1. Ice.
2. Compression.
3. Electrical muscle stimulation modalities.
4. Crutches.

PHASE II: *Week 2*

5. Pain-free quadriceps isometric exercises daily.
6. Pain-free quadriceps active range of motion exercises daily (see Treatment of Grade I Quadriceps Strain, page 287).
7. Heat (hot packs, whirlpool, ultrasound).
8. Straight leg raises with no weights daily, 4 sets of 10 repetitions.

PHASE III: *Week 3*

9. Straight leg raises with weights, 4 sets of 10 repetitions 3 days a week.

PHASE IV: *Week 4*

10. Pain-free quadriceps progressive resistive exercises. Isotonics using the NK table, 4 sets of 10 repetitions 3 days a week.

11. Isokinetics 3 days a week.
12. Swimming 2 to 3 days a week.
13. Biking 2 to 3 days a week.
14. Quadriceps-stretching exercises. Hold stretch for 30 seconds times 5 repetitions daily.

PHASE V: *Week 5*

15. Leg press exercises, 3 sets of 10 repetitions 2 days a week.
16. Squats, 4 sets of 6 to 8 repetitions 2 days a week.

PHASE VI: *Week 6*

17. Jogging.
18. Sport-specific activities.

QUADRICEPS CONTUSION

Because the quadricep muscles is in the front of the thigh, a direct blow to the area that causes the muscle to compress against the femur can be very disabling.[1] A direct blow to the anterior portion of the muscles is usually more serious and disabling than a direct blow to the lateral quadriceps area, due to the differences in muscle mass present in the two areas. Blood vessels that break cause bleeding in the area where muscle tissue has been damaged.[21]

At the time of injury, the athlete may develop pain, loss of function to the quadriceps mechanism, and loss of knee flexion range of motion. How relaxed the quadriceps were at the time of injury and how forceful the blow was determine the grade of injury.

Evaluation and Clinical Findings

GRADE I QUADRICEPS CONTUSION. With a grade I quadriceps contusion, the athlete may present a normal gait cycle, negative swelling, and only mild discomfort on palpation. The athlete's active knee flexion range of motion while lying prone may be within normal limits. Resistive knee extension while sitting and lying supine may not cause discomfort.

This athlete may not miss competition time, but compression and protective padding should be worn during competition until the athlete is symptom free.

GRADE II QUADRICEPS CONTUSION. Before notifying the trainer, this athlete may attempt to continue to participate as the injury progressively becomes disabling. The athlete's gait cycle may be abnormal. The knee may be splinted in extension and the athlete may avoid knee flexion while bearing weight, due to the feeling of the knee wanting to give out. This athlete may also externally rotate the extremity to use the hip adductors to pull the leg through during the swing through phase. This move may be accompanied by hiking the hip at push off.

Swelling may be moderate to severe, with a noticeable defect and pain on palpation. While the athlete is lying prone, active range of motion in the knee may be limited, with possibly 30 to 45 degrees of motion lacking. Resistive knee extension while sitting and lying supine may be painful, and a noticeable weakness in the quadriceps mechanism may be evident.

This athlete may miss 3 to 21 days of participation, depending upon the severity of injury.

A grade II quadriceps contusion to the lateral thigh area is usually less painful due to the lack of muscle mass involved in the injury. The athlete may experience pain on palpation but may not be disabled. While the athlete is lying prone, knee flexion range of motion may be within normal limits, with possibly a small decrease in range present. Resistive knee extension while the athlete is sitting and lying supine may cause mild discomfort with good strength present.

The athlete with a grade II quadriceps contusion to the lateral thigh area may not miss competition time.

GRADE III QUADRICEPS CONTUSION. With a grade III quadriceps contusion, the muscle may herniate through the fascia to cause a marked defect, severe bleeding, and disability.

The athlete may not be able to ambulate without crutches. Pain, severe swelling, and a bulge of muscle tissue may be present on palpation. When the athlete is lying prone, knee flexion active range of motion may be severely limited. Active resistive knee extension while the athlete is sitting and lying supine may not be tolerated, and severe weakness may be present.

An athlete with a grade III quadriceps contusion may miss 3 weeks to 3 months of competition time.

Treatment and Rehabilitation

GRADE I QUADRICEPS CONTUSION. The athlete may begin ice and compression immediately.

Compression should be continued until all signs and symptoms are absent.

Gentle, pain-free quadriceps-stretching exercises may be performed on the first day. Quadriceps progressive resistive strengthening exercises may also be performed pain free. Isokinetics may be utilized with isotonic exercises.

The athlete's active range of motion should be carefully monitored. If motion decreases, the injury should be updated to a grade II contusion and treated as such.

Compression and protective padding should be worn at all times during competition.

TREATMENT OF GRADE I QUADRICEPS CONTUSION
PHASE I: *From day 1*
1. Ice.
2. Compression.
3. Pain-free quadriceps-stretching exercises. Hold for 30 seconds times 5 repetitions daily.
4. Pain-free quadriceps progressive resistive strengthening exercises. Isotonics using the NK table, 4 sets of 10 repetitions 3 days a week.
5. Isokinetics 3 days a week.

GRADE II QUADRICEPS CONTUSION. This athlete should be treated very conservatively. Crutches should be used until a normal gait can be accomplished free of pain. Ice, compression, and electrical muscle stimulation modalities may be started immediately to decrease swelling, inflammation, and pain and to promote range of motion.[19] Compression should be applied at all times to counteract bleeding into the area.

Pain-free quadriceps isometric exercises may be performed as soon as possible, usually within the first 3 days. Between days 3 and 5, ice is continued with pain-free active range of motion, while the athlete is sitting and lying prone. Passive stretching is not used until the later phases of rehabilitation. Massage and heat modalities are also contraindicated in the early phases, due to the possibility of promoting bleeding.

At approximately day 5, the athlete may perform straight leg raises without weights and then progress to weights, pain free. As active range of motion increases to approach 95 to 100 degrees of knee flexion, biking may be performed if the seat height is adjusted to the athlete's available range of motion.

Between days 7 and 10, heat in the form of hot packs, ultrasound, and/or whirlpool may be used as long as swelling is negative and the athlete is approaching full active range of motion while lying prone. Pain-free quadriceps progressive resistive strengthening exercises may be performed with the NK table. Isokinetics may be performed in conjunction with isotonic exercises. Ice and/or heat modalities, with active range of motion, may be continued before all exercises.

Swimming and jogging are performed on approximately days 10 to 14. Pain-free quadriceps-stretching exercises may be added at approximately the fourteenth day. The athlete may progress to leg press exercises and squats, also after the fourteenth day. Jogging and sport-specific activities may be used in the last phase to prepare the athlete for competition.

Compression and protective padding are continued during competition to avoid reinjury.

TREATMENT OF GRADE II QUADRICEPS CONTUSION

PHASE I: *Days 1–3*
1. Rest.
2. Crutches.
3. Ice.
4. Compression.
5. Electrical muscle stimulation modalities.
6. Quadriceps isometric exercises daily.

PHASE II: *Days 3–5*
7. Pain-free active range-of-motion exercises lying prone and sitting.
8. Straight leg raises without weights daily.

PHASE III: *Days 5–7*
9. Straight leg raises with weights, 4 sets of 10 repetitions 3 days a week.
10. Biking 2 days a week.

PHASE IV: *Days 7–14*
11. Heat (hot packs, ultrasound, whirlpool).
12. Pain-free quadriceps progressive resistive strengthening exercises. Isotonics using the NK table, 4 sets of 10 repetitions 3 days a week.
13. Isokinetics 3 days a week.
14. Swimming 2 days a week.
15. Pain-free quadriceps-stretching exercises. Hold for 30 seconds times 5 repetitions daily.

PHASE V: *From day 14*
16. Leg press exercises, 3 sets of 10 repetitions 2 days a week.
17. Squats, 4 sets of 6 to 8 repetitions 2 days a week.
18. Jogging.
19. Sport-specific activities.

GRADE III QUADRICEPS CONTUSION. With a grade III quadriceps contusion, the athlete should use crutches, rest, ice, compression, and electrical muscle stimulation modalities immediately to decrease pain, bleeding, and swelling and counteract atrophy.[19]

After surgery has been ruled out, the athlete may begin pain-free isometric quadriceps exercises between days 5 and 7. Ice and compression may be continued after day 7, with pain-free active range-of-motion exercises while the athlete is lying prone and sitting. At approximately day 10, the athlete may perform straight leg raises without weights and then progress to weights by day 14. Electrical muscle stimulation modalities may be very helpful in this phase to counteract muscle atrophy and reeducate muscle contraction.

After day 14, the athlete may utilize heat in the form of hot packs and/or whirlpool, as long as the swelling has decreased and the athlete has gained active range of motion. At approximately the third week of rehabilitation, pain-free quadriceps progressive resistive strengthening exercises may be performed in conjunction with isokinetics.

Swimming and biking may be added; adjust the bicycle seat height to accommodate the athlete's range of motion. Pain-free quadriceps stretching may also be performed if the athlete is careful not to overstretch the quadricep muscles.

Leg press exercises and squats may be performed after the fourth week, and the athlete can then progress to jogging and sport-specific activities. Compression and protective padding should be worn at all times during competition.

The rehabilitation timetables presented for grade II and grade III quadriceps contusions may be modified, depending upon the severity of the injury within its given grade.

TREATMENT OF GRADE III QUADRICEPS CONTUSION

PHASE I: *Days 1–5*
1. Crutches.
2. Rest.
3. Ice.

4. Compression.
5. Electrical muscle stimulation modalities.

PHASE II: *Days 5–7*

6. Pain-free quadriceps isometric exercises daily.

PHASE III: *Days 7–14*

7. Pain-free quadriceps active range-of-motion exercises while lying prone and sitting daily.
8. Straight leg raises first without weights and progressing to weights, 4 sets of 10 repetitions 3 days a week.
9. Electrical muscle stimulation modalities continued.

PHASE IV: *Days 14–21*

10. Heat (hot packs, whirlpool).

PHASE V: *Week 3*

11. Pain-free quadriceps progressive resistive strengthening exercises. Isotonics using the NK table, 4 sets of 10 repetitions 3 days a week.
12. Isokinetics 3 days a week.
13. Pain-free quadriceps-stretching exercises. Hold for 30 seconds times 5 repetitions daily.
14. Biking 2 days a week.
15. Swimming 2 days a week.

PHASE VI: *Week 4*

16. Leg press exercises, 3 sets of 10 repetitions 2 days a week.
17. Squats, 4 sets of 6 to 8 repetitions 2 days a week.
18. Jogging.
19. Sport-specific activities.

MYOSITIS OSSIFICANS

With a severe direct blow or repetitive direct blows to the quadricep muscles that cause muscle tissue damage, bleeding, and injury to the periosteum of the femur, ectopic bone production may occur.[1,13] In 3 to 6 weeks, calcium formation may be seen on x-ray. If the trauma was to the quadricep muscles only and not the femur, a smaller bony mass may be seen on x-ray.[1]

If quadriceps contusion and quadriceps strain are properly treated and rehabilitated, myositis ossificans may be prevented. Myositis ossificans can be caused by trying to "play through" a grade II and grade III quadriceps contusion and/or strain and by early use of massage, stretching

exercises, ultrasound, and other heat modalities for grade II and grade III quadriceps contusion and/or strain.[1]

Treatment and Rehabilitation

After 1 year, surgical removal of the bony mass may be helpful. If the bony mass is removed too early, the trauma caused by the surgery may actually enhance the condition.

After diagnosis by x-ray, treatment and rehabilitation should follow that of a grade II or grade III quadriceps contusion and/or quadriceps strain. (See treatments for grade II and grade III quadriceps contusions and strains.)

The bony mass usually stabilizes after the sixth month.[10] If the mass does not cause disability, the athlete should be closely monitored and follow the rehabilitation programs outlined in Treatment of Grade II Quadriceps Contusion (page 291) and Treatment of Grade III Quadriceps Contusion (page 291).

SUMMARY

1. Injuries to the hip and thigh can be extremely disabling and often require a substantial amount of time for rehabilitation.
2. Hip pointers are contusions of the soft tissue in the area of the iliac crest and must be treated aggressively during the first 2 to 4 hours following injury.
3. Sciatica and piriformis syndrome should be specifically differentiated from other problems that produce low back pain or radiating pain in the buttocks and leg. Rehabilitation programs are extremely variable for different conditions and may even be harmful if used inappropriately.
4. Trochanteric bursitis is relatively common in athletes, as is ischial bursitis. Treatment involves efforts directed at protection and reduction of inflammation in the affected area.
5. Strains of the groin musculature, the hamstring, and the quadriceps muscles can require long periods of rehabilitation for the athlete. Early return often exacerbates the problem.
6. Protection is the key to treatment and rehabilitation of quadriceps contusions and accompanying myositis ossificans.

REFERENCES

1   Arnheim DD: Modern principles of athletic training, St Louis, 1985, The CV Mosby Co.
2   Coole WG and Gieck JH: An analysis of hamstring strains and their rehabilitation, J Ortho Sports Phys Ther 9(2):77–85, 1987.
3   Daniels L and Worthingham C: Muscle testing, techniques of manual examination, ed 3, Philadelphia, 1972, WB Saunders Co.
4   DeLorme TL and Watkins AL: Progressive resistive exercises: technique and medical application, New York, 1952, Appleton-Century-Crofts, Inc.
5   DePalma BF and Zelko RR: Knee rehabilitation following anterior cruciate ligament injury or surgery, Ath Train 21:3, 1986.
6   Gordon EJ: Diagnosis and treatment of common hip disorders, Med Tral Tech Q 28(4):443, 1981.
7   Gould JA III and Davies GJ: Orthopedic and sports physical therapy, St Louis, 1985, The CV Mosby Co.
8   Hollinshead WH: Functional anatomy of the limbs and back, Philadelphia, 1976, WB Saunders Co.
9   Hoppenfield S: Physical examination of the spine and extremities, New York, 1976, Appleton-Century-Crofts, Inc.
10 Kulund DN: The injured athlete, Philadelphia, 1982, JB Lippincott Co.
11 Lewinneck G: The significance and comparison analysis of the epidemiology of hip fractures, Clin Orthop 152:35, 1980.
12 Lewis A: Normal human locomotion, Quinnipiac College, Hamden, Conn, 1977.
13 Lipscomb AB: Treatment of myositis ossificans traumatica in athletes, Am J Sports Med 4:61, 1976.
14 Magee DJ: Orthopedic physical assessment, Philadelphia, 1987, WB Saunders Co.
15 Moore KL: Clinical oriented anatomy, Baltimore, 1985, Williams & Wilkins.
16 Norkin L and LeVange P: Joint structure and function, Philadelphia, 1983, FA Davis Co.
17 O'Donoghue DH: Treatment of injuries to athletes, Philadelphia, 1976, WB Saunders Co.
18 Overuse injuries: clinics in sports medicine, Philadelphia, 1987, WB Saunders Co.
19 Prentice WE: Therapeutic modalities in sports medicine, St Louis, 1986, Times Mirror/Mosby College Publishing.
20 Rehabilitation of the injured athlete: clinics in sports medicine, Philadelphia, 1985, WB Saunders Co.
21 Roy S and Irvin R: Sports medicine: prevention, evaluation, management, and rehabilitation, Englewood Cliffs, NJ, 1983, Prentice-Hall Inc.
22 Stevens J: The incidence of osteoporosis in patients with femoral neck fractures, J Bone Joint Surg (Fr) 44:520, 1962.
23 Tinker R, editor: Ramamurti's orthopaedics in primary care, Baltimore, 1979, Williams & Wilkins.
24 Torg J, Vegso J, and Torg P: Rehabilitation of athletic injuries: a guide to therapeutic exercise, Chicago, 1987, Year Book Medical Publishers Inc.
25 Tortora GJ: Principles of human anatomy, New York, 1980, Harper & Row, Publishers Inc.

SUGGESTED READINGS

Antich TJ and Brewster CE: Modification of quadriceps femoris muscle exercises during knee rehabilitation, Phys Ther 66(8):1246–1250, 1986.

Arnheim DD: Modern principles of athletic training, St Louis, 1985, The CV Mosby Co.

Carter TA: Piriformis syndrome: a hidden cause of sciatic pain, Ath Train 23(3):243–245, 1988.

Coaches Roundtable: The squat and its application to athletic performance, National Strength and Conditioning Association Journal 68:10–22, 1984.

Combs JA: Myositis ossificans traumatica: pathogenesis and management, Ath Train 22(3):193–196, 1987.

Coole WG and Gieck JH: An analysis of hamstring strains and their rehabilitation, J Ortho Sports Phys Ther 9(2):77–85, 1987.

Daniels L and Worthingham C: Muscle testing, techniques of manual examination, ed 3, Philadelphia, 1972, WB Saunders Co.

DeLorme TL and Watkins AL: Progressive resistive exercises: technique and medical application, New York, 1952, Appleton-Crofts, Inc.

Gieck J, McCue F, Stoller S, and Lephart S: Fracture dislocation of the hip while playing football, Ath Train 21(2):124–126, Summer 1986.

Gould JA III and Davies GJ: Orthopedic and sports physical therapy, St Louis, 1985, The CV Mosby Co.

Hollinshead WH: Functional anatomy of the limbs and back, Philadelphia, 1976, WB Saunders Co.

Lewis A: Normal human locomotion, 1977, Quinnipiac College, Hamden, Conn.

Magee DJ: Orthopedic physical assessment, Philadelphia, 1987, WB Saunders Co.

Mann RA, Moran GT, and Dougherty SA: Comparative electromyography of the lower extremity in jogging, running, and sprinting, The Am J Sports Med 14(6):501–509, 1986.

O'Shea P: The parallel squat, National Strength and Conditioning Association Journal 78:4–6, 1985.

Prentice WE: Therapeutic modalities in sports medicine, St Louis, 1986, Times Mirror/Mosby College Publishing.

Rehabilitation of the injured athlete: clinics in sports medicine, Philadelphia, 1985, WB Saunders Co.

Torg J, Vegso J, and Torg P: Rehabilitation of athletic injuries: a guide to therapeutic exercise, Chicago, 1987, Year Book Medical Publishers Inc.

Rehabilitation of Knee Injuries

14

J. Marc Davis

OBJECTIVES

Following the completion of this chapter, the student will be able to:

- Understand the injury mechanism of the most common knee injuries.

- Be able to explain the five phases of rehabilitation and how each phase relates to a specific pathology.

- Understand specific rehabilitation protocols for the various knee pathologies.

- Be able to discuss the functional parameters for a safe return of the athlete to activity.

The growth of scientific knowledge has been exponential since the beginning of the twentieth century, and fortunately for the athlete the treatment of knee injuries has advanced rapidly also. For example, the introduction of arthroscopic techniques has greatly reduced the actual trauma of many reparative and reconstructive procedures, not to mention the accuracy of the diagnosis. Research into biomechanics has furthered the knowledge of knee kinematics illuminating the functions of the supporting structures of the knee, and computer technology and manufacturing have allowed the development of myriad devices for research, testing, and exercise. Yet all this equipment and knowledge is of marginal benefit if the people involved do not make optimum use of the information available and if lines of communication are limited or restricted.

The sports therapist has an obligation to the injured athlete to understand the nature of the injury, the function of the structures damaged, the technique of repair or reconstruction, and the different methods available to rehabilitate the athlete safely. The sports therapist must understand the treatment philosophy of the athlete's physician and be careful in applying different treatment routines—what may be a safe but outdated technique to one physician may be dogma to another. Again, communication is crucial to prevent misunderstandings and a subsequent loss of rapport with either the athlete or the physician. The successful sports therapist must be able to rehabilitate the injured athlete using techniques that are safe and sound yet may vary from patient to patient and from physician to physician.

Hence, the purpose of this chapter is to present different approaches to knee rehabilitation. Clinics differ in treatment philosophy, equipment, and expertise of staff yet may produce equally gratifying results.

The restoration of normal knee function is the goal of the rehabilitation process and is quantified by a full range of motion, normal strength, no swelling, a relatively pain-free state with activity, and normal patterns of sport-specific movements.[6,14] The rehabilitative process should be designed with these parameters in mind and with the realization that attaining these goals is affected by the type of injury treatment option chosen (surgical versus nonsurgical), length of immobilization, and the availability and quality of therapy.

Under ideal conditions, the physician, the sports therapist, the athlete, and the athlete's family communicate freely and function as a team. This group is intimately involved with the rehabilitative process beginning with patient assessment, treatment selection, and implementation and ending with functional exercises and return to activity. The sports therapist directs the postacute phase of rehabilitation, and the athlete must understand that this part of recovery is just as crucial as surgical technique to the return of normal joint function and the subsequent return to athletic competition. This area is the sports therapist's specialization and link in the treatment chain.

Two basic principles must be followed to develop a safe and successful rehabilitation program: the effects of immobilization must be minimized and healing tissues must never be overloaded.[10] Giving these two principles equal and even consideration allows the therapist to develop a safe program and the athlete to complete the process with as healthy and functional a knee as is currently possible.

GENERAL PRINCIPLES OF REHABILITATION
Range of Motion

Following injury a decrease in motion is likely. This loss may be due to the effects of the injury, the trauma of surgery, and/or the effects of immobilization. Waiting for ligaments to heal completely is a luxury that cannot be afforded in an effective rehabilitation program. Ligaments do not heal completely for 18 to 24 months, yet periarticular tissue changes can begin within 4 to 6 weeks of immobilization.[10] These changes are marked histologically by a decrease in water content in collagen and by an increase in collagen cross-linkage.[2,10] The institution of an early range-of-motion (ROM) program can prevent these harmful changes, provided that early motion is restricted to passive motions that do not overload the healing tissues. Active motions are initiated later in the recovery process and progress toward a normal range of approximately 0 to 130 degrees.

Pitfalls that can slow or prevent the regaining of a normal range of motion include imperfect surgical technique (improper placement of an anterior cruciate replacement), development of joint capsule or ligament contracture, and muscular resistance due to pain.[7,10,19] The surgeon must address motion lost as a result of technique, but the sports therapist can successfully deal with motion lost due to soft tissue contracture or muscular resistance.

To alleviate lost motion effectively, the cause of the limitation must be identified. An experienced sports therapist can detect soft tissue resistance to motion by the quality of the feel of the resistance at the end of the range. Muscular resistance to motion has a firm end feel and can be treated by utilizing muscle tendon techniques such as heat, ice, spray and stretch, and PNF techniques.[7] Joint capsule or ligamentous contracture has a leathery end feel and may not respond to conventional motion exercises of simple passive, active assistive, and active motion.[7] These contractures can limit the accessory motions of the joint; until the accessory motions are restored, conventional exercises do not produce positive results.

Accessory motions are movements that occur at a joint and are necessary for normal joint function but are not under the active or voluntary control of the athlete. At the knee, accessory motions include the cephalic and caudal movement of the patella during flexion and extension, and internal and external rotation of the tibia on the femur that occurs with flexion and extension.[7,19] Joint play is another form of accessory motion; it occurs when the joint is subjected to an external force and as a result motion occurs.

Mobilization of a knee that is restricted owing to soft tissue contracture can be accomplished by specifically applying joint play motions to the restricted soft tissue. In doing so, the therapist is addressing a specific limiting structure rather assaulting the entire joint with a "crank till you cry" technique. Following the release of the soft tissue contracture, accessory motion should improve, and so should total motion.

Cyriax[7] developed a pain-resistance sequence that should be followed when applying any technique for regaining lost motion:

Pain before resistance: do not attempt.

Pain with resistance: only gentle attempts.

Resistance before pain: vigorous exercise tolerated.[7]

For a detailed understanding of joint mobilization techniques, the works of Cyriax and Maitland are recommended; for specific information on mobilization of the knee, the Quillen and Gieck article[19] is recommended. For illustrations of various mobilization techniques, see Figs. 14-1 through 14-4.

Strength

The second goal of rehabilitation is the return of normal strength to the musculature surrounding the knee; included in strength is the return of normal muscular endurance and power. These terms are related but not interchangeable. **Strength** is the force that a muscle can generate; **power** is the amount of force that can be produced per unit of time; and **endurance** refers to the ability of the muscle to produce strength and power over a prolonged period of time.[1,7]

Strength is gained only if the muscle is stressed to the point of overload; the second basic principle of rehabilitation is that healing tissues must never be overloaded. Especially during the early phases of rehabilitation, muscular overload needs to be applied carefully to protect the damaged joint. The recovering knee needs protection and the high-resistance, low-repeti-

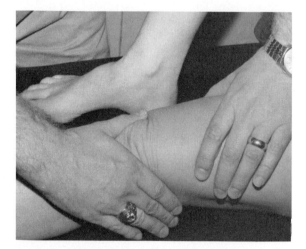

Fig. 14-1. Patella mobilization—superior glide.

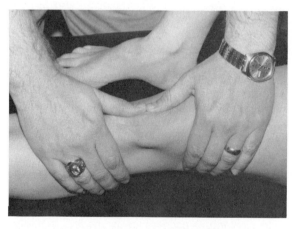

Fig. 14-3. Patella mobilization—lateral glide.

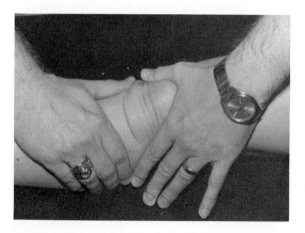

Fig. 14-2. Patella mobilization—inferior glide.

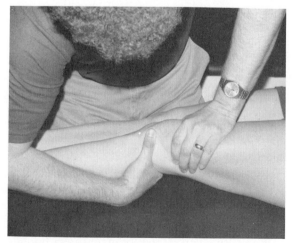

Fig. 14-4. Tibiofemoral mobilization—anterior/posterior glide.

tion program designed to strengthen a healthy knee may compromise the integrity of an injured knee.[15] The strengthening phase of rehabilitation must be gently progressive, and generally it progresses from isometric to isotonic to isokinetic to functional exercise.

Isometric exercise occurs when there is a muscle contraction without joint motion or a change in muscle fiber length. Strength is gained within 10 degrees of the position of the joint during the exercise, and the greatest strength gain occurs if a maximal contraction is held for at least 6 seconds.[1] These exercises are used before and after surgery as a means of muscle education and form the basis for strength training when only a minimal amount of stress is allowed at the healing tissues. They are also employed in the treatment of patellofemoral dysfunction and tibiofemoral arthrosis, both cases where strength is desired but joint irritation needs to be minimized. Recent investigations have looked at the possibility of increasing muscle tension during isometric contraction by using electrical stimulation to the muscle.[8]

Isotonic exercise occurs when a muscle contracts and shortens or lengthens and joint motion results. These classic strengthening exercises were popularized by T. L. DeLorme and involve raising and lowering a weight against the force of gravity. The major disadvantage for this type of exercise is that the muscle can be loaded only to the maximum of the weakest point within the joint's range of motion, hence the development of variable-resistance devices (Nautilus, Eagle, Universal). In theory these devices adjust the resistance to accommodate normal strength variations. Care must be taken in incorporating isotonic exercises 5 to 6 months after surgery because then the damaged ligament is weakest. Isotonic exercise can be performed safely if stressful portions of the range of motion are avoided and appropriate resistance is provided.

Eccentric exercise, a type of isotonic exercise, occurs when a muscle contracts, joint motion occurs, and muscle fibers lengthen. With this type of exercise, the muscle acts as a brake or shock absorber. An example is the action of the quadriceps group on landing from a jump; the muscles slowly lengthen in order to decelerate the body and absorb the shock of landing. Exercises that emphasize eccentric work are important in re-

gaining normal function. Most skilled athletic movements contain eccentric parts, and strength and control must be gained in these movements. Eccentric exercises are very important in regaining hamstring strength and control, and recently they have been described as an effective means of treating patellar-extensor mechanism dysfunction.[16]

Isokinetic exercise occurs when a muscle contracts and the limb moves at a constant velocity even though the resistance may vary. This type of exercise has become available during the last two decades with the development of isokinetic devices (Cybex, Kin Com, Lido, Biodex). This type of exercise offers fast-speed, maximum-resistance exercise, whereas with isometric and isotonic exercise maximum resistance can be achieved only at slow speeds. Isokinetic exercise more closely mimics actual athletic activity. To reduce joint stresses, isokinetic activity usually starts at a higher velocity and gradually progresses to slower speeds. These excellent conditioning exercises are particularly useful in developing power.

Endurance is another component of muscle function that needs to be addressed early in the rehabilitation program because immobilization depletes the type 1 (slow twitch, endurance) muscle fibers of the oxidative enzymes needed for prolonged muscle contraction.[14,15] Any exercises that involve repetitive, high-speed contractions, such as cycling, swimming, and rowing, are effective in maintaining local muscular endurance. These activities should be continued throughout the entire rehabilitation period and, as function improves, be augmented by the repetition of sport-specific activities.

PHASES OF REHABILITATION

The rehabilitation process has been broken into stages by several clinicians,[7,15] as outlined below. Programs for the various knee pathologies can be logically designed with these phases as a guide; then, by assessing the athlete's response to exercise, the sports therapist can safely advance the treatment protocol. The athlete must be closely watched for pain, effusion, changes in motion, and psychological response; such changes must guide the advancement of the rehabilitation process.

PHASE I (maximum protection): Treat the inflammation, achieve primary tissue healing, maintain function; control range of motion.

PHASE II (moderate protection): Tissue maturation, strengthening, endurance, protective development.

PHASE III (minimum protection): Determination of time segment needed for tissue maturation and/or reorientation, light functional activity, skill acquisition.

PHASE IV (advanced rehabilitation): Functional program, return to demanding environment.

PHASE V (maintenance)[7,15]

KNEE INJURY

Injuries to the soft tissues that support the knee occur when these tissues are not able to resist abnormal tension.[10] This abnormal tension develops when the knee is forced through an abnormal motion. The direction of these forces determines which structures within the knee are damaged, and these forces may act in a straight direction (medial, lateral, anterior, or posterior), rotational manner, or in combination.

Anterior Cruciate Ligament

In simple terms, the anterior cruciate ligament (ACL) prevents anterior translation of the tibia on the femur. It works in conjunction with the posterior cruciate ligament to control the gliding and rolling of the tibia on the femur during normal flexion and extension. The twisted configuration of the fibers of the ACL and the shape of the femoral condyles allow for the screw-home mechanism of the knee during the final 20 degrees of extension when the tibia externally rotates on the femur. The ACL is under some degree of tension in all positions of knee motion, with lesser tension present from 20 to 90 degrees.[10,11,20]

With these facts in mind, then ACL rehabilitation should be designed to:

Enhance the ability of the knee to resist anterior and rotational displacement. This need can be addressed by surgical technique and a rehabilitation program that not only strengthens muscles but emphasizes retraining the hamstring group to augment ACL function.

Avoid the ranges of motion where the ACL is under greatest tension. Early in rehabilitation, terminal extension should be avoided.

Most injuries occur from a twisting motion of the knee when the foot is firmly planted. Contact with another athlete is not necessary to cause the injury; simply the rotational force of the body twisting over the fixed limb can focus a damaging rotational force on the knee. The athlete usually reports either hearing or feeling a pop with subsequent swelling within the joint.

In many instances the ACL is injured following the application of an external force to the knee, and this type of trauma may involve numerous structures in the knee. O'Donahue's unhappy triad (ACL, medial collateral ligament, and meniscus) is the classic example. Certainly the more structures damaged, the more complicated the assessment, the surgery, and the rehabilitation.

Following the diagnosis of injury to the ACL, the athlete, the physician, the sports therapist, and the athlete's family are faced with various treatment options. The conservative approach is to allow the acute phase of the injury to pass and then to implement a vigorous rehabilitation program. If normal function apparently cannot be recovered with rehabilitation, that is, the knee remains unstable even with normal strength and hamstring retraining, then reconstructive surgery is considered. For a sedentary individual, this conservative approach may be acceptable, but most athletes prefer a more aggressive approach. Also some surgeons feel that surgery is necessary to prevent the early onset of degenerative changes within the knee.[11]

The medical community is split on the treatment approach for a partially torn ligament. Some feel that a partially damaged ACL is incompetent and that the knee should be viewed as if the ligament were completely gone. Others prefer a prolonged initial period of immobilization and limited motion in hopes that the ligament will heal and remain functional. Clearly the athlete would be wise to seek several opinions before choosing the treatment course.

Successful surgical repair and/or reconstruction of the ACL-deficient knee is dependent upon patient selection.[10] The older and more sedentary individual is usually not an appropriate choice for a major surgical procedure. This individual may not have the inclination or the time for an extensive rehabilitation program and may not be greatly inconvenienced by some degree of knee instability. The ideal patient is a young, motivated, and skilled athlete who is willing to make the personal sacrifices necessary to complete the rehabilitation process successfully.

The surgical approach to ACL pathology is either repair or reconstruction. With a surgical repair, the damaged ligament is sutured if the tear is in the body of the ligament, or the bony fragment is reattached in the case of an avulsion injury. In the case of suturing, the repair may be augmented with an internal splint or an extraarticular reconstruction.

Surgical reconstruction is performed either extraarticular or intraarticular. An extraarticular reconstruction involves taking a structure that lies outside the joint capsule and moving it so that it can affect the mechanics of the knee in a manner that mimics normal ACL function. The iliotibial band is the most commonly used structure. This procedure is effective in reducing the pivot shift phenomenon found in anterior lateral rotational instability but cannot match the normal biomechanics of the ACL.[10,15] Isolated extraarticular reconstructions may be effective in patients with mild to moderate instability. It may also be the treatment of choice for patients who cannot afford the commitment of time and resources for an intraarticular reconstruction.[10] Rehabilitation following an extraarticular reconstruction is aggressive and permits an earlier return to functional activities; however, as an isolated procedure, it is not recommended for high-level athletes.

Intraarticular reconstruction involves placing a structure within the knee that roughly follows the course of the ACL and if successful, functionally replaces the ACL. Patellar tendon grafts are the current state of the art, but research into artificial materials and the use of human allografts is very promising.[10,15,20] Surgical technique is crucial to a successful outcome; improper placement of the tendon graft by only a few millimeters can prevent the return of normal motion. Patient selection is also important for success. It should be reserved for the following special situations:

ACL injury in the highly athletic individual.

Active people with instability and unwillingness to alter their life-styles.

Instability in normal activities.

Recurrent effusions.

Failure at rehabilitation: instability following 6 months of intensive rehabilitation.[10]

In cases of severe injury with extreme instability, both extraarticular and intraarticular reconstruction may be performed, but the rehabilitation process should be dictated by the intraarticular procedure. The rehabilitation should progress slowly; the avoidance of early extension is especially important.

ACL PATELLAR TENDON RECONSTRUCTION

PHASE I (maximum protection): *0 to 3 weeks*

1. Bracing: Between 30 and 60 degrees, locked.
2. ROM: Continuous passive motion as needed, tolerated, and/or ordered. Active motion limited to avoid a full quad contraction.
3. Exercises:
   Quadriceps (quad) sets with brace locked (Fig. 14-5).
   Cocontractions (Figs. 14-6 and 14-7).
   Ankle ROM.
   Patellar mobilizations as tolerated (see Figs. 14-1 to 14-3).
   Contralateral strengthening.
   Electrical stimulation as needed and tolerated; no full quad contraction (see Fig. 14-7).
4. Crutches: Nonweight bearing (NWB) progressing to partial weight bearing (PWB) at 3 weeks.

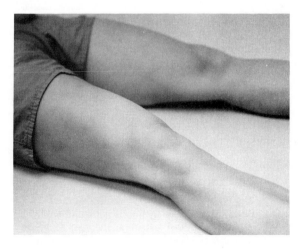

Fig. 14-5. Quadriceps setting at full knee extension.

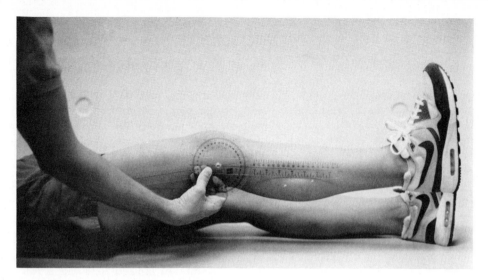

Fig. 14-6. A cocontraction of the quadriceps and hamstring group occurs when leg raising is performed with 10 degrees of knee flexion.

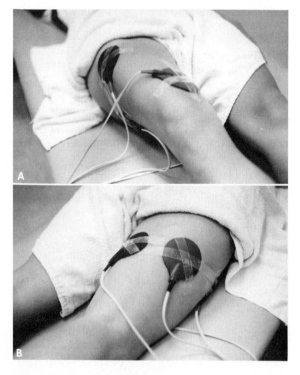

Fig. 14-7. A cocontraction of the quadriceps and hamstring can be initiated by the use of a four-pad configuration during electrical stimulation. **A,** Two pads on the quadriceps. **B,** Two pads on the hamstring.

PHASE II (moderate protection): *3 to 6 weeks*

1. Bracing: Advanced as tolerated toward 90 degrees flexed to 15 degrees extended.
2. ROM:
   Passive, flexion as tolerated to 90 degrees (see Fig. 14-13).
   Active, active assistive, 90 to 45 degrees.
3. Exercises:
   Out of brace.
   Quad sets, cocontractions, submaximal.
   Active flex to 90 degrees.
   Hip flexion.
   Straight leg raising (SLR) 4 planes (Fig. 14-8).
   Begin PRE 90 to 45 quads (Fig. 14-9), standing.
   Hamstring (Fig. 14-10), stationary bicycle, low resistance, low seat.
   Electrical stimulation as needed.
4. Crutches:
   Progress from PWB to FWB by week 6 if strength and ROM allow.

PHASE III (light activity)

1. Bracing: Progress toward bracing for stressful activity only by end of this phase.
2. ROM:
   Flexion to tolerance.
   Allow extension to return gradually, with

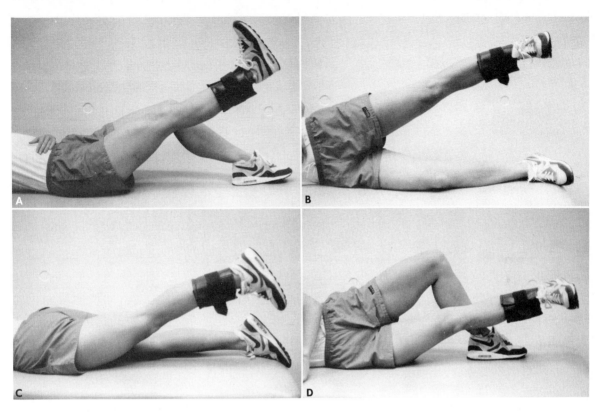

Fig. 14-8. Straight leg raising. **A,** Hip flexion. **B,** Hip abduction. **C,** Hip extension. **D,** Hip adduction.

emphasis placed on assistive motion in the later part of phase 3.

3. Exercises:
   Quad sets, cocontractions, SLR.
   PRE 90 to 45 advance weight.
   PRE hamstrings as tolerated (see Fig. 14-10).
   Tibial rotation, PNF rubber tubing (Fig. 14-11).
   Begin terminal knee extension with closed kinetic chain (Fig. 14-12).
   Stationary bicycle.
   Swimming with no rotational kicking.
   Side step-ups (see Fig. 14-12).
   Isokinetic exercises.
4. Crutches: FWB advancing to functional activities, walking, jogging, running.

PHASE IV (return to activity): *6 to 9 months*

1. Bracing: For stressful activities, use a de-rotational brace (Lenox Hill, CTI, Pro Am).

2. ROM: Flexion normal, extension may still be slightly lacking.
3. Exercises:
   PRE quad, advance to 20.
   PRE ham, progress as tolerated.
   Isokinetic exercises.
   Rotational exercises.
   Progress functional activity level to include activities that mimic sports motions.

Return to activity is based upon isokinetic testing and the successful completion of sport-specific functional tests. Return usually occurs between the ninth and twelfth month after surgery.

PHASE V (maintenance)

Exercises must be performed at least twice a week as long as the patient remains active.*

---

*References 3,4,6,10,15,18,20,21.

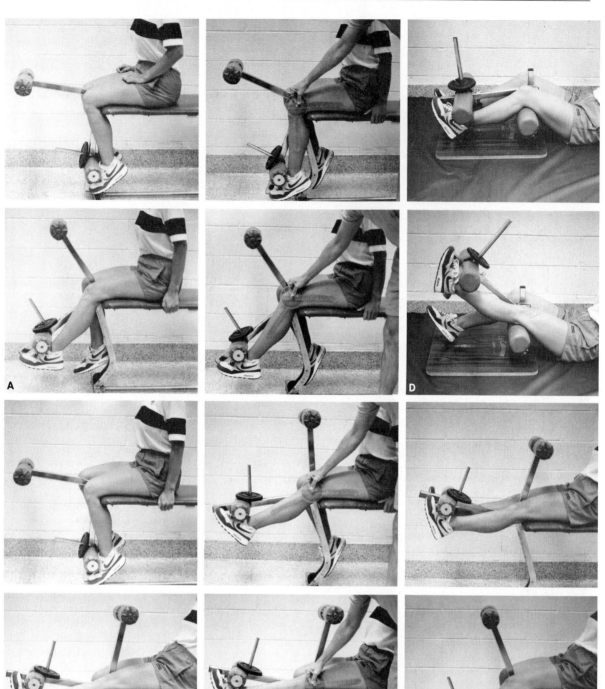

A

B

C

D

E

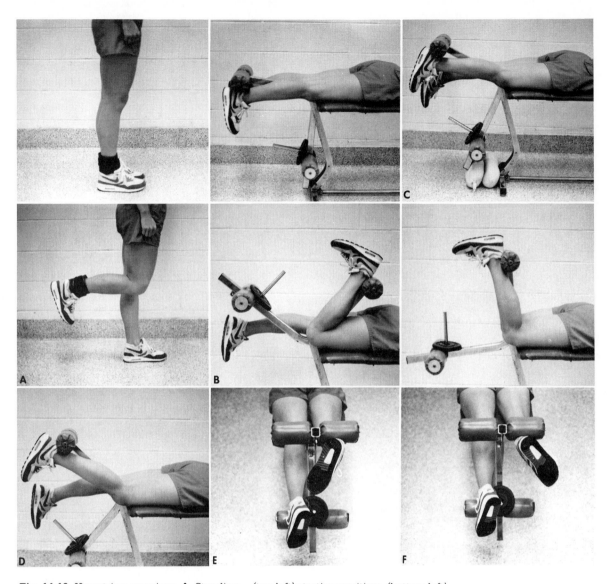

Fig. 14-10. Hamstring exercises. **A,** Standing—*(top left)* starting position; *(bottom left)* stopping position. **B,** Full ROM—*(top middle)* starting position; *(bottom middle)* stopping position. **C,** Extension limited to prevent TKE. **D,** Eccentric exercise—*(center right)* starting position, raise with both legs; *(bottom right)* lower with one leg. **E,** Medial tibial rotation by adjusting foot position during hamstring curls. **F,** Lateral tibial rotation by adjusting foot position during hamstring curls.

Fig. 14-9. Quadriceps exercises. **A,** 90 to 45 degrees—*(top left)* starting position; *(second row left)* stopping position. **B,** Full ROM—*(third row left)* starting position; *(bottom left)* stopping position. **C,** Isometric exercise—*(center top)* at 90 degrees; *(second row center)* at 60 degrees, *(third row center)* at 30 degrees; *(center bottom)* at 0 degrees. **D,** Short arc—*(top right)* starting position; *(second row right)* stopping position. **E,** Eccentric exercise—*(third row right)* starting position, raise with both legs; *(bottom right)* lower with one leg.

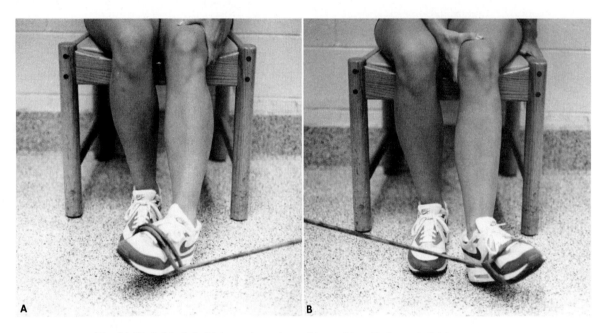

Fig. 14-11. A, Medial tibial rotation using rubber tubing. **B,** Lateral tibial rotation using rubber tubing.

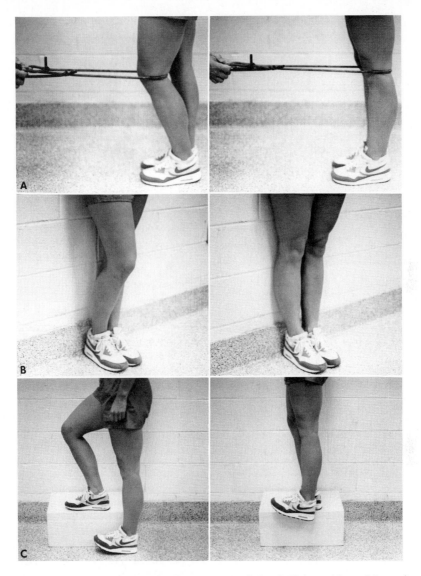

Fig. 14-12. Terminal knee extension—closed kinetic chain. **A,** Using rubber tubing—*(top left)* starting position; *(top right)* stopping position. **B,** Wall standing—*(middle left)* starting position; *(middle right)* stopping position. **C,** Lateral step-ups—*(bottom left)* starting position; *(bottom right)* stopping position.

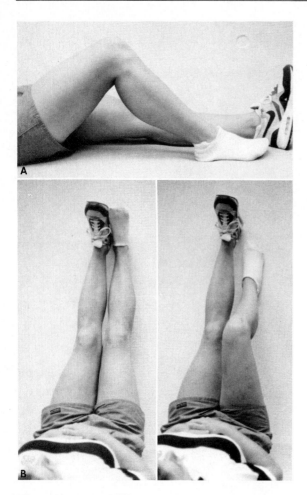

Fig. 14-13. Heel slides. **A,** While the athlete is supine, the heel is moved toward the body. **B,** *(left)* While the athlete is supine, the heel is elevated on the wall; *(right)* gravity assists while the heel is gently moved down the wall.

ACL-DEFICIENT KNEE
PHASE I: *0 to 3 weeks*
1. Bracing: Initially locked between 45 and 90 degrees and advancing toward 90 to 0 degrees by week 3.
2. ROM: As allowed by brace.
3. Exercises:
   Done in brace.
   Heel slides.
   Quad sets, cocontractions.
   Ankle ROM.

Hip flexion extension.
Patellar mobs.
PRE 90 to 45 degrees extension at week 2.
Standing hamstring curls at week 2.
Electrical stimulation as needed.
4. Crutches: PWB.
PHASE II: *3 to 6 weeks*
1. Bracing: 90 to 0 degrees D/C at week 5.
2. ROM: Active out of brace.
3. Exercises:
   Quad sets, cocontractions, SLR.
   Progress PRE 90 to 45 degrees.
   Begin hamstring PRE.
   Stationary cycling.
   Swimming.
   Hip strengthening, all planes.
   Electrical stimulation, as needed.
   90 to 0 degrees extension without weight.
4. Crutches: D/C.
PHASE III: *6 to 9 weeks*
1. Bracing: D/C except for stressful activities; should be fitted for derotational brace for activity.
2. ROM:
   Flexion as tolerated.
   Terminal extension without weight.
3. Exercises:
   PRE 90 to 45 degrees, quads advance.
   PRE hamstring advance.
   TKE closed kinetic chain.
   Rotational exercises—PNF, tibing.
   Step-ups.
   Cycling, swimming.
   Isokinetic exercises, 90 to 45 degrees, with antishear device.
PHASE IV: *9 weeks*
1. Bracing: Derotational for activity.
2. ROM: Assisted as needed.
3. Exercise:
   Progress phase III.
   Begin jogging program, progressing to running, sprinting, cutting, crossovers, and return to sport-specific activity.
   Backward running for hamstring function.
PHASE V (maintenance): Minimum twice per week.*

---

*References, 3,4,6,10,15,18,20,21.

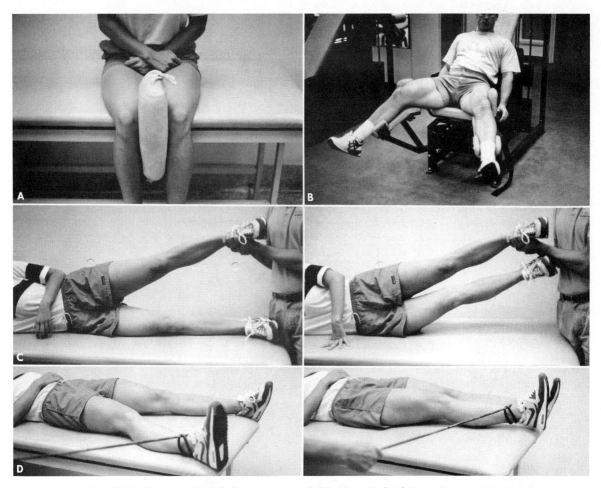

Fig. 14-14. Hip adduction. **A,** Knee squeeze. **B,** Nautilus. **C,** *(left)* Opposite leg elevated; *(right)* involved leg raised to touch contralateral side. **D,** Rubber tubing—*(left)* starting position; *(right)* stopping position.

Posterior Cruciate Ligament

The posterior cruciate ligament (PCL) functions with the ACL to control the rolling and gliding of the tibiofemoral joint. More specifically, the PCL prevents the posterior translation of the tibia on the femur. This activity is evident in the PCL-deficient knee when upon descending an incline the force of gravity works to increase the anterior glide of the femur on the tibia; without the PCL, the femur subluxes on the tibia from midstance to toe off, where the quadriceps are less effective in controlling the anterior motion of the femur on the tibia.[11,15]

The classic mechanism of injury to the PCL is a straight posterior force that drives the tibia posterior on the femur. This injury occurs frequently in auto accidents when the knee crashes into the dashboard and forces the femur forward over the fixed tibia. The PCL is more commonly injured in athletics by extreme valgus or varus stress and by hyperextension of the knee.[5,11,15]

Surgery to reconstruct a PCL-deficient knee may involve a reconstructive procedure that utilizes the medial meniscus, the semitendinous tendon, the tendinous part of the medial gastrocnemius, or the patellar tendon to replace the lost PCL. Rehabilitation following such a procedure must emphasize quadriceps function over the hamstrings.

Medial Collateral Ligament

The medial collateral ligament (MCL) is divided into two parts, the stronger superficial portion and the thinner, weaker "deep" medial ligament or capsular ligament with its accompanying attachment to the medial meniscus. The MCL functions as the primary static stabilizer against valgus stress. In the normal knee, valgus loading is greatest during the push-off phase of gait, when the foot is planted and the tibia externally rotated relative to the femur. The MCL is taut at full extension, begins to relax between 20 and 30 degrees of flexion, and comes under tension again at 60 to 70 degrees of flexion.[11]

The most common mechanism of injury to the MCL is a valgus force upon the slightly flexed knee while the foot is planted.[5,11,15] The treatment of MCL injuries is largely nonsurgical in the case of most grade 1 and 2 tears, and in some cases isolated grade 3 tears may be treated with only immobilization.[15] However, grade 3 injuries that display gross instability and/or the involvement of other structures require surgery. The emphasis for MCL rehabilitation is to protect the knee from valgus stress while the joint heals, which is accomplished by using cast immobilization, cast bracing, splints, functional bracing, and crutch walking. Ranges of motion that stress the MCL should be avoided; early motion is best limited to between 20 and 60 degrees, with care taken to avoid full extension and external rotation of the tibia on the femur.

Lateral Collateral Ligament

The lateral collateral ligament (LCL) functions with the iliotibial band, the popliteus tendon, the arcuate ligament complex, and the biceps tendons to support the lateral aspect of the knee. The LCL is under constant tensile loading, and the thick, firm configuration of the ligament is well designed to withstand this constant stress.[5,11] The incidence of injury to the LCL is much less than either the ACL or the MCL, and

the mechanism is usually a varus stress. A complete disruption of the LCL involves one or both cruciate ligaments.[11,15] Severe injury to the LCL is rare in athletics because most athletic injuries result from a stress placed on the lateral aspect of the knee.[11,15]

Fortunately the lateral aspect of the knee is well supplied with secondary supports that can also provide support for an injured LCL. Except in extreme cases, injuries respond quite well to conservative treatment. The ligament should be protected from varus stress during the recovery phase, and general range-of-motion and strengthening exercises can be initiated as soon as symptoms permit.

CAPSULAR REPAIR: MCL, LCL, CAPSULAR DAMAGE

PHASE I: *0 to 4 weeks* (length determined by the extent of capsular damage).

1. Bracing: Locked at 30 to 60 degrees, if the repair is extensive, progressing toward 90 to 15 degrees for less involved repairs.
2. ROM: As allowed by the brace.
3. Exercises:
   In the brace.
   Quad sets, cocontractions.
   Ankle ROM.
   Hip flexion/extension.
   Patellar mobs.
   SLR.
   Crutches: NWB progressing to touch down.

PHASE II: *4 to 8 weeks*

1. Bracing: Progress flexion; avoid terminal extension.
2. ROM: Flexion to tolerance.
3. Exercises:
   In brace.
   Quad sets, cocontractions.
   PRE quads 90 to 45 degrees sub max.
   PRE hamstrings sub max.
   Bicycle if ROM sufficient.
   For MCL: hip adductor extension, tibial interior rotation; avoid TKE and hip abduction.
4. Crutches: PWB.

PHASE III: *8 to 14 weeks*

1. Bracing: As needed for protection.
2. ROM: Progress toward normal, stress TKE.
3. Exercise:
   Quad sets, cocontractions, SLR—4 planes.
   PRE quads, progress to TKE (see Fig. 14-9).

PRE hamstring progress.
Gastrocnemius strengthening.
Cycling, swimming.
Step-ups.
4. Crutches: FWB.

PHASE IV: *14 weeks to return to activity*
1. Bracing: Protective.
2. ROM: Normal.
3. Exercise: Begin eccentric quad and hamstrings (see Figs. 14-9 and 14-10).
Begin isokinetic quad and hamstrings.
Progress to functional activity.

PHASE V: *Maintenance**
Nonoperative treatment for capsular injuries would begin with phase II of the above protocol.

Meniscal Injury

Injuries to the menisci may be isolated or occur in conjunction with injury to other structures. The injury is caused by either traction or compression force and usually occurs when the knee is flexed and rotated.

The menisci function to aid in joint lubrication; to increase joint congruency, which aids stability; to act as a shock absorber; and to distribute weight-bearing forces.[5,7,14,15] Traditional surgical treatment required the total removal of the damaged meniscus with loss of its functions. With the advent of arthroscopic surgery, the need for total meniscectomy is reduced.

The athlete with a damaged meniscus has three choices: total meniscectomy, partial meniscectomy, and meniscal repair. The outer third of the cartilage is vascular, and, if the damage occurs in this region, repair and healing are possible. If the tear is in the inner two-thirds of the cartilage, then removal of the damaged portion can be accomplished, leaving viable material behind to continue its functions. If the damage is extensive, then total meniscectomy may be required.

Rehabilitation following meniscal repair (accomplished by suturing) requires that joint motion be limited. The menisci move during knee motion, approximately 12 mm, anterior to posterior, with the tibia during flexion and extension; during rotation, they follow the femur.[15]

*References 3,4,6,10,15,18,20,21.

Hence, motion must be restricted to prevent stress at the repair site. Rehabilitation following repair is more prolonged than that following partial or total meniscectomy, where motion does not need to be restricted.

Rehabilitation following arthroscopic surgery for partial or total meniscectomy with no associated capsular damage is rapid, and the likelihood of complications is minimal. Immediate postoperative care consists of wound care for the portal sites, compression to control edema, and a rapid progression of range-of-motion and strengthening exercises.

MENISCAL REMOVAL

PHASE I: Generally not required.

PHASE II: *0 to 10 days*
1. Bracing: Compressive brace for control of swelling.
2. ROM: As tolerated.
3. Exercise:
Quads sets, SLR 4 planes, cocontractions.
Cycling to tolerance.
Add weights to SLR in later stage.
4. Crutches: PWB to FWB quickly.

PHASE III: *10 days to 3 weeks*
1. Bracing: Compressive as needed.
2. ROM: Normal.
3. Exercise:
As in phase 2.
PRE isotonic quads, 90 to 30 degrees, advance to 0 degrees.
PRE isotonic hamstrings.
Isokinetic extension at 3 weeks.
Swimming when wound healing is complete.

PHASE IV: Progress phase III.

MENISCAL REPAIR

PHASE I: *0 to 3 weeks*
1. Bracing: 80 to 30 degrees.
2. ROM: Passive in brace.
3. Exercise:
In brace.
Quad sets, cocontractions.
SLR—3 planes; avoid adduction with medial meniscectomy, abduction with lateral.
Electrical stimulation, as needed.
All exercise in this phase must be submaximal.
4. Crutches: NWB.

PHASE II: *3 to 10 weeks*
1. Bracing: Increase 10 in flexion and extension each week.
2. ROM: Follows bracing toward 0 to 120 degrees at 8 weeks.
3. Exercise:
   Quad sets; SLRs with weight.
   PRE isotonic quads, 90 to 30 degrees.
   PRE isotonic hamstrings at week 6 with limited extension.
   Cycling, swimming.
4. Crutches: PWB at onset, progressing to FWB at end phase.

PHASES III and IV: As in meniscal removal.

Patellofemoral Dysfunction

Disorders of the patellofemoral juncture involve the extensor mechanism of the knee and are the most common cause of knee pain.[16] The extensor mechanism includes the quadriceps group, the patella and its articulating surface, the tendons adjoining the patella, the femur and its articulating surface, the tibial attachments of the patellar tendon, and adjoining soft tissue. Common injuries include patellar subluxation, dislocation, patellofemoral chondrosis (chondromalacia), tendonitis (jumper's knee), and Osgood-Schlatter's disease. Most dysfunction of this region can be traced to anatomic predisposition, and usually pain and dysfunction occur when such predisposition is coupled with acute injury or, more commonly, overuse.

Predisposing factors in patellofemoral dysfunction include:
Patella alta
Lateral patellar tilt
Vastus medialis (VMO) dysplasia
Vastus lateralis (VL) hypertrophy
Extensor mechanism malalignment, femoral neck anteversion, genu valgum, external tibial torsion, genu varum, foot pronation
Increased Q angle (greater than 15 in males, than 20 in females)
Squinting patella
Positive movie sign (increased pain and stiffness with prolonged sitting)[5,9,13-17]

Treating patellofemoral dysfunction requires adjusting these predisposing factors through the use of quadriceps-strengthening exercises, especially the medial aspect; correction of over-

pronation at the foot; bracing to buttress the lateral edge of the patella; and, if needed, lifestyle modification.

Quadriceps strengthening has been the cornerstone of PFD rehabilitation, and two schools of thought exist on the most effective technique to use. The conventional program consists of straight leg raises, quad sets, and short arc exercises in the 30- to 0-degree range.[20,21] This program has been used extensively for years and has met with success. The VMO was thought to be most active in the end of the range, and thus emphasizing short arc quads could enhance VMO function. However, current studies show that the VMO is active throughout the entire range and is counteracted at end range by the strong force of the vastus lateralis.[9,15]

A newer protocol for PFD includes SLR, quad sets, and limited arc exercises from 90 to 40 degrees. By limiting exercise to the 90- to 40-degree range, pain and crepitus are reduced. Several researchers report that the closer the joint comes to terminal extension, the more common are pain and crepitus.[9,15] The sports therapist should adopt a protocol based on clinical judgment, understanding of the individual's problem, and discussion with the physician.

EXTENSOR MECHANISM DYSFUNCTION
TREATMENT GUIDELINES

Nonoperative treatment usually requires minimal or no range-limiting bracing.

Except in extreme cases, treatment can begin while the athlete continues to maintain a low level of activity or phase 3 of the rehabilitation process.

Modalities are used to address any inflammation and pain.

Orthotics should be provided to address any foot dysfunction.

Appropriate footwear should be worn.

A patellar stabilizing brace may be required.

Flexibility of the quads, HS, gastrocnemius, and hip musculature should be addressed.

The activity level must be reduced to below what causes pain.

Exercises to correct any muscle imbalances must not aggravate any symptoms.

Exercises are designed to improve the function of the quad mechanism, with the classic recommendation being short arc quads from 30 to 0 degrees; however, more recently authors are recommending exercise from 90 to 40 degrees.[9,15] Regardless of the approach chosen, exercise within the selected range should not increase the athlete's pain, swelling, or patellofemoral crepitus (see Fig. 14-9).

Especially in the treatment of patellar tendonitis, eccentric exercises should be used, including exercise for the anterior tibialis on the affected side (Fig. 14-15; see Fig. 14-9).[16]

Electrical stimulation and/or biofeedback are helpful in overcoming quadriceps inhibition.

Chondromalacia and Patellofemoral Pain Syndrome

This diagnosis has been applied to any knee problem that causes pain but did not result from a traumatic event. In fact it refers to objective articular cartilage changes and not to general-ized patellar pain. Patellofemoral pain syndrome better describes the problem of many patients with retropatellar pain but no objective find-ings.[16]

Treatment for this syndrome consists of reduction of inflammation with medications and modalities (especially ice), exercises to strengthen the quads, flexibility exercises for the hamstring group to reduce the stress that tight hamstrings can place on the extensor mechanism, patellar bracing, orthotic fabrica-tion, and life-style changes until symptoms clear.

Jumper's Knee

Jumper's knee occurs when chronic inflamma-tion develops in the patella tendon, especially at the distal pole. It usually develops in athletes involved in activities that require repetitive jumping, hence the name. Point tenderness at

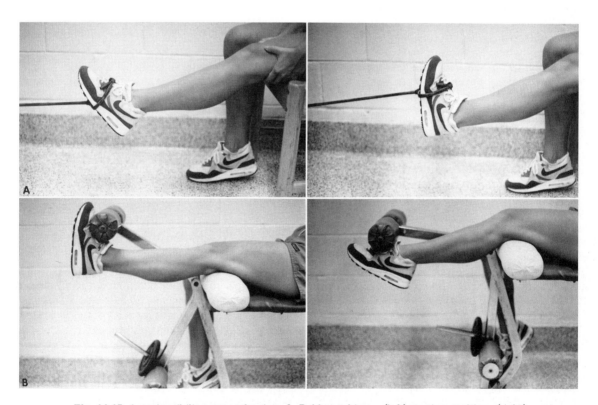

Fig. 14-15. Anterior tibilias strengthening. **A,** Rubber tubing—*(left)* starting position; *(right)* stopping position. **B,** Eccentric, using a Universal bench—*(left)* starting position; *(right)* stopping position.

the inferior pole of the patella is the hallmark of this condition. This condition is felt to be related to the shock-absorbing function that the quadriceps provides upon landing from a jump, an eccentric contraction.[16]

Besides the conventional treatment mentioned for PFD, eccentric strengthening exercises for the quads and the ankle dorsiflexors have shown some success.[16]

Osgood-Schlatter's Disease

This syndrome is characterized by pain and swelling over the tibial tuberosity that increases with activity and decreases with rest. Traditionally Osgood-Schlatter's disease (OSD) was described as either a partial avulsion or an avascular necrosis of the tibial tubercle. Current thinking views it more as an inflammation of a portion of the extensor mechanism, and it is treated as such. It occurs mostly in adolescents, and most sufferers have related extensor mechanism deficiencies that need to be addressed in the treatment program. Especially prominent are quad atrophy and hamstring tightness.[5,16] Treatment is symptomatic, with emphasis placed on icing, quad strengthening, hamstring stretching, and reduction of activity.[5,14]

CONCLUSIONS

Various knee pathologies have been presented, and the treatment of these disorders outlined. The technology relating to sports medicine and the knee in particular is increasing rapidly, and very soon some of the information in this text may be outdated. However, the principles of rehabilitation outlined by the phase concept and the criteria for the safe return to activity should not change. If the sports therapist can couple new techniques and technology with these principles, then good patient care can be assured.

Criteria for Return to Activity

1. Normal ROM.
2. No swelling.
3. No pain or limp with activity.
4. Completion of isokinetic testing: 70 to 80% prior to sprinting and jumping; 80 to 90% prior to agility and sport-specific skills; 90 to 100%

prior to return to competition. The testing should take place at several velocities; recommended are 60–80–240–300.[15]
5. Finally, the athlete must successfully complete a battery of sport-specific functional activities with minimal apparent deficit.

Exercise Protocols

The exercise protocols in this chapter are based on the five-phase approach that was discussed in the text. Below are phases and components.

PHASE I (maximim protection)
Concerns: inflammation, tissue healing
Program emphasis: controlled ROM
PHASE II (moderate protection)
Concerns: tissue maturation, strength and endurance
Program emphasis: crutch walking, low-intensity strengthening
PHASE III (light activity)
Concerns: maturation, return of basic function, skill acquisition
Program emphasis: moderate strengthening, protected activity, protected function
PHASE IV (return to activity)
Concerns: progression of functional activity, reacquisition of skill, return to competition
Program emphasis: advanced rehabilitation, isokinetics, intense strengthening, stressful athletic activities
PHASE V (activity)
Concerns: the weekend athlete, in- or out-of-season activities
Program emphasis: maintenance[3,7,15]

UNC SPORTS MEDICINE / PHYSICAL THERAPY RETURN TO ACTIVITY PROGRESSIVE RUNNING PROGRAM*

The return to activity progressive running program is comprehensive and includes all levels of functions and activities for returning the individual to practice or competition. Each individual under treatment may begin at a different place in this progression and may progress at a more rapid pace than if each step were followed. The sports therapist responsible for the rehabilitation plan should make those decisions based on the evaluation and goals of the individual. This document should be used as a guideline.

Beginning Criteria

Before beginning any return to running activity, several criteria must be met:

1. Patient must have full range of motion (ROM).
2. Patient must be able to ambulate without a limp.
3. Patient must be able to walk straight ahead 100 yards without any increased discomfort, swelling, or pain.
4. Patient must show 70% quad strength of the unaffected leg or lift 25 to 30 pounds on the weight machine.
5. Patient's physician feels the repair or healing is strong enough to stand increased stress at this time.
6. If any swelling occurs after full weight bearing, walking, or running, patient must back off until swelling has decreased.

If all of the above criteria are met, a light program of walking may begin.

Cardiovascular Conditioning

Cardiovascular endurance is maintained throughout the rehabilitation and return to running program. These activities should be started at appropriate stress levels for the patient's condition, and pulse rate should be monitored for maintenance of adequate conditioning stress. Several alternate activities may be substituted for running to maintain cardiorespiratory endurance:

1. Biking or swimming with unaffected limb and/or arms for a 10-minute duration, progressively increasing time to 20 to 30 minutes.
2. May progress to swimming, running in an aquavest, or kickboarding (depending on injury).
3. May substitute rowing, biking, or ergometer workouts. Workouts should be structured to maintain or improve cardiorespiratory condition on a sport-specific basis. These workouts continue throughout the progression. As running conditioning workouts are achieved, the alternate workouts can then gradually be replaced by running workouts.

Walking to Jogging

1. Walk forward; start with a quarter-mile; slowly increase speed and distance to one mile.
2. Walk backwards and sidestepping two 20-yard intervals, progressing to 40-yard intervals each quarter-mile. If no increased swelling or pain occurs with walking, then athlete may progress to a light jog.
3. Jog at a comfortable pace on straightaway on track and then walk turns; progress to eight laps.
4. Straight ahead light jogging on level surface, walking one lap and then jogging one complete lap; jog-walk turns on six laps; progress to jogging eight complete laps. The athlete who can jog without a limp may then progress. If pain or swelling occurs, consult sports therapist.
5. Progress to fast jog, walking curves.
6. Progress to jogging turns by adding turns on one lap. Increases may be on a daily basis, or the progression can be done more slowly by completing several exercise bouts at the same level without pain or swelling before increasing another lap.
7. When jogging four laps in one direction, reverse directions of laps, running two laps in each direction and then switching.

Jogging to Running

1. Progress from jogging to running the straights of the track and jogging the curves—up to 1.5 to 2 miles.
2. Progress to running on straightaways and curves; reverse directions every two laps. Depending on sport specificity, incorporate backward running on straights from step 5 on.

Running to Sprinting Program

The athlete who can run full speed around the track without a limp may then progress to running patterns:

1. Start running large figure eight patterns the size of a football field, and progress down to 50-yard and then 20-yard diameters (half to three-quarter speed). Gradually increase speed to full speed.
2. Start sprints (half speed) at 20- and 40-yard distances straight ahead. Progress to three-

*Compiled and edited by Sue Harter and Dan Hooker, University of North Carolina Department of Sports Medicine.

quarter speed and full speed.

3. Next, run zigzags (half to three-quarter speed), starting at 15-yard cuts and progressing down to 5-yard cuts.
4. Progress to small figure eights—20-yard diameters to 5 yards.
5. Over 40-yard distance, progress to running and cutting at 45-degree angles, and then running and cutting 90-degree angles. Alternate planting right to left foot. Cutting needs to be attempted in both directions off the injured leg.

Each step should start with half-speed sprint, gradually increasing speed on each repetition; a few full-speed sprints should be included and then speed should be decreased over the last several repetitions.

The surface used should be the one normally used in training, and footwear should be used to control stress. Wear smooth bottomed shoes and progress to cleated shoes. When cleated shoes are added, some portions of the running program should be repeated.

6. Sprint full speed and cut on commands, alternating right to left foot.
7. Incorporate lateral running and cariocas once step 4 is accomplished.

At this point, the athlete should be at 90% of full strength, and sport-specific activities should be incorporated.

1. The athlete should be able to sprint full speed in all activities in all directions.
2. The athlete may begin concentrating on decreasing times.
3. Other activities that may be included are running up and down hills, jumping rope, and playing other sports.

If at any time the activity causes pain, increased edema, or discomfort, stop the activity and consult the sports therapist so the program can be modified.

SUMMARY

1. For a safe and successful knee rehabilitation program, the effects of immobilization must be minimized and the healing tissues must never be overloaded.
2. Intraarticular reconstruction of the torn ACL seems to be the technique currently most widely used; it can tolerate an extremely aggressive rehabilitation program emphasizing hamstring strengthening.
3. Rehabilitation following PCL reconstruction should concentrate on quadriceps strengthening.
4. The emphasis for MCL rehabilitation is to protect the knee from valgus stress by avoiding full extension and external rotation while the ligament heals.
5. The injured LCL depends on a number of lateral stabilizing structures for support and should be protected from varus stress by immobilization.
6. Rehabilitation following meniscal repair requires limiting joint motion and requires more time than arthroscopy for a partial or total meniscectomy.
7. Treatment of patellofemoral dysfunction requires use of quadriceps-strengthening exercises, especially of the medial structures; correction of overpronation of the foot; and possibly bracing the lateral aspect of the patella.

References

1. Basmajian J: Therapeutic exercise, Baltimore, 1978, Williams & Wilkins.
2. Bernhardt D, editor: Sports physical therapy, New York, 1986, Churchill Livingstone.
3. Brewster C, Moynes D, and Jobe F: Rehabilitation for the anterior cruciate reconstruction, JOSPT, 5(3):121-126, 1983.
4. DePalma B and Zelko R: Knee rehabilitation following anterior cruciate injury or surgery, JNATA 21(3):200-206, 1988.
5. Ellison A: Athletic training and sports medicine, 1984, American Academy of Orthopaedic Surgery.
6. Ferguson D: Return to functional activities, Sports Medicine Update 3(3):3-5, 1988.
7. Gould J and Davies G: Orthopaedic and sports physical therapy, St Louis, 1985, The CV Mosby Co.
8. Hartsell H: Electrical muscle stimulation and isometric exercise effects on selected quadriceps parameters, JOSPT 8(4):203-209, 1986.
9. Hughston J, Walsh W, and Puddu G: Patellar subluxation and dislocation, Philadelphia, 1984, WB Saunders Co.
10. Jackson D and Drez D: The anterior cruciate deficient knee, St Louis, 1987, Times Mirror Mosby College Publishing.
11. Jenkins D: Ligament injuries and their treatment, Rockville, Md, 1985, Aspen Publications.
12. Johnson D: Controlling anterior shear during isokinetic knee exercise, JOSPT 4(1):23-31,1982.

13 Kramer P: Patellar malalignment syndrome: rationale to reduce lateral pressure, JOSPT 8(6):301-309, 1986.

14 Kuland D: The injured athlete, ed 2, Philadelphia, 1988, JB Lippincott Co.

15 Mangine R: Physical therapy of the knee, New York, 1988, Churchill Livingstone.

16 Mellion M, editor: Office management of sports injury and athletic problems, Philadelphia, 1987, Hanley and Belfus.

17 Paulos L and others: Patellar malalignment: a treatment rationale, JAPTA 60(12):1624-1632, 1980.

18 Prentice W: A manual resistance technique for strengthening tibial rotation, JNATA 23(3):230-233, 1985.

19 Quillen W and Gieck J: Manual therapy: mobilization of the motion restricted knee, JNATA 23(2):123-130, 1988.

20 Saal J, editor: Physical medicine and rehabilitation: rehabilitation of sports injuries, Philadelphia, 1987, Hanley and Belfus.

21 Torg J, Vesgo J, and Torg E: Rehabilitation of athletic injuries: an atlas of therapeutic exercise, Chicago, 1987, Year Book Medical Publishers.

Rehabilitation of Lower Leg Injuries

15

Rich Riehl

OBJECTIVES

Following the completion of this chapter, the student will be able to:

- Differentiate between anterior and posterior shin splints.

- Understand the concept of eccentric overload as it relates to overuse syndromes.

- Explain why the Achilles tendon is susceptible to overuse conditions.

- Distinguish between retrocalcaneobursitis and Achilles tendonitis.

- Define the five compartments of the lower leg.

- Comprehend the bone remodeling theory as it pertains to stress fractures.

- Design and implement an effective rehabilitation program for any lower leg pathology.

Injuries to the lower leg are common. Brody[3] has reported that approximately 30% of all running injuries involve the lower leg. The appropriate recognition, treatment, and rehabilitation of these injuries is important if the incidence of injuries is to be prevented from rising.

The purpose of this chapter is to present various approaches to rehabilitation that are designed to return the athlete to activity as quickly as possible. So many times sports therapists end up using the same old treatments day in and day out. Although nothing is wrong with that approach the intent of this chapter is to present different ideas that can add a little diversity to the rehabilitation of injuries without compromising the objectives.

RECONDITIONING EXERCISES FOR THE LOWER LEG
Range of Motion

Range-of-motion exercises should be started as early as possible in the rehabilitation process.

Both active and passive movements should be initiated once the pain has been reduced to a tolerable level. Range-of-motion exercises serve many purposes:[22]

Prevent muscle atrophy (active only)
Help align collagen fibers along areas of stress
Restore normal joint motion
Decrease edema and pain
Retard loss of connective tissue tensile strength

Range-of-motion exercises should include not only the ankle joint but also the knee. The gastrocnemius muscle is the only muscle to span two joints in the lower leg. Appropriate stretching of the gastrocnemius requires simultaneous dorsiflexion of the ankle and extension of the knee.

Passive motion exercises should be done initially with the help of the sports therapist, who should perform and instruct the athlete in the proper stretching technique. A towel can be used to help with the passive movements, once the athlete has been shown how to do the exercises properly. Plantar flexion and dorsiflexion, along with inversion and eversion, are the desired movements. The stretching should be done for 30 to 45 seconds and repeated 15 times for each direction. A good approach, initially, would be the appplication of ice massage followed by the stretching exercises, both active and passive movements, and then another ice application.

STRENGTHENING EXERCISES

Isometric exercise is quite useful when an injury is immobilized for a prolonged period of time. Isotonic exercises, by far the most common, can be divided into two types: a concentric contraction and an eccentric contraction. Concentric muscle contractions cause a shortening of the muscle and a decrease in the joint angle; eccentric contractions are a lengthening of the muscle and an increase in the angle of the joint. Eccentric muscle contractions are used for antigravity types of actions. An example is the contraction of the quadriceps muscle when landing from a jump.

The concept of eccentric work is especially important when for lower leg injuries. The etiology of injuries to the tendons and muscles of the lower leg is often a repeated eccentric muscle contraction. Proper rehabilitation of these injuries includes eccentric strength training.

One of the most frequently used isotonic methods of acquiring lower leg strength is through the use of ankle weights. This method allows motion in all four ranges (Figs. 15-1 to 15-4).

A typical program involves three sets of 15 repetitions with a 30- to 45-second rest between sets. The resistance should be determined by athlete discomfort. A mild discomfort during the third set of exercises indicates that the muscles are being properly overloaded. If the pain is severe or absent, then the weight should be changed accordingly. A good starting point is usually 5 pounds.

A similar resistance program can be done with surgical tubing. The tubing is fixed around something sturdy. All four motions (plantar flexion, dorsiflexion, inversion, and eversion) should be worked. The same guidelines outlined for the ankle weights should be followed (Figs. 15-5 to 15-8).

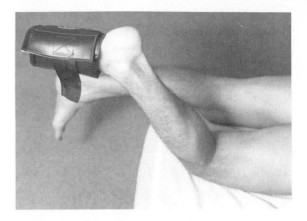

Fig. 15-1. Bent-leg position for plantar flexion strengthening exercises using ankle weights.

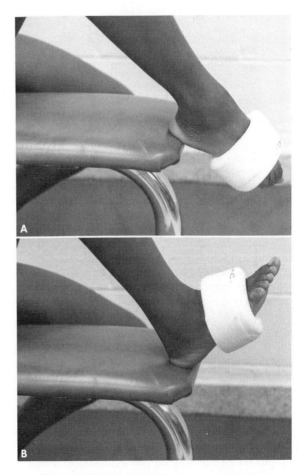

Fig. 15-2. Dorsiflexion strengthening exercises: **A,** starting position; **B,** terminal position.

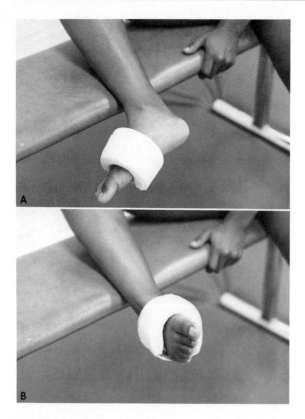

Fig. 15-3. Inversion strengthening exercises: **A,** starting position; **B,** terminal position.

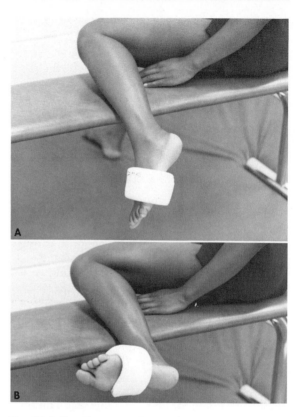

Fig. 15-4. Eversion strengthening exercises: **A,** starting position; **B,** terminal position.

Toe raises also provide an effective method for strength gains. One drawback is that this exercise is done in a single plane of action. Thus it is effective only in strengthening the muscles responsible for plantar flexion. Curwin and Stanish[6] have outlined an eccentric conditioning program using toe raises. The program consists of having the athlete stand on a step, with the ankle in neutral, and then lower the heel until a stretch is felt. This exercise should be done, initially, with both feet at the same time. Three sets of 10 repetitions are performed. The final 10 repetitions should cause mild discomfort, which indicates whether the level is adequate or if the athlete should progress to the next level. The progression is as follows:

1. Weight is supported equally on both feet.
2. Increase shifting of weight to the symptomatic leg.
3. Weight is only on the symptomatic leg.
4. Gradually increase the speed of dropping.

5. Add weight to the shoulders (10% of the body weight at the start).

Pain oftentimes is associated with the early stages of this exercise. This pain should not be alarming because it is an indication that the muscles and tendons are being worked.

Another variation of strengthening is grasping small objects with the toes and moving them from one place to another. The object can be anything from marbles to rocks to scraps of tape. The heel should remain stationary during this exercise. Start by making three different piles of the object, pick up one object and move it to another pile, and continue rotating the objects among the different piles. Two sets of 50 are a desired workout.

Isokinetic programs are extremely useful in improving strength gains because maximal resistance can be attained throughout the entire range of motion. Specific protocols for rehabilitation are quite varied. The speed of contraction

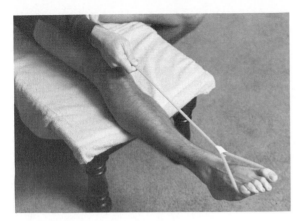

Fig. 15-5. Plantar flexion strengthening exercises using rubber tubing.

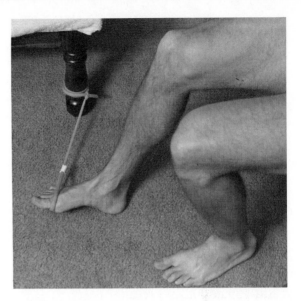

Fig. 15-7. Inversion strengthening exercises using rubber tubing.

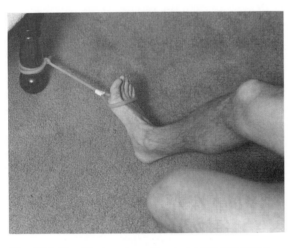

Fig. 15-6. Dorsiflexion strengthening exercises using rubber tubing.

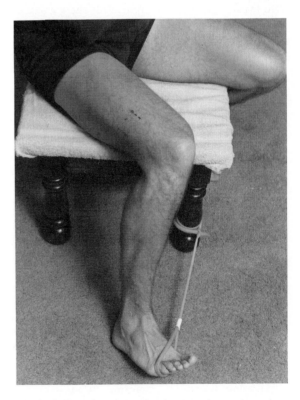

Fig. 15-8. Eversion strengthening exercises using rubber tubing.

should be changed during the workout to provide both muscular endurance and power. Three speeds commonly used are 180, 270, and 300 degrees per second. Plantar flexion and dorsiflexion are the most frequently used exercises. Inversion and eversion should also be done if the equipment has the capability.

Isokinetic machines do have their disadvantages: they are inconvenient for exercising more than one joint; the setup is often time-consuming; eccentric contractions are not possible, except in the most sophisticated equipment; and, finally, the equipment is usually quite expensive. If the isokinetic equipment is available under the proper supervision, however, then it should be utilized because the benefits far outweigh the drawbacks.

CARDIOVASCULAR FITNESS

The athlete's cardiovascular fitness must be maintained while the lower leg is rehabilitated. Athletes are often concerned that they will lose their fitness level during their rehabilitation. The sports therapist is often challenged to supply cardiovascular work that provides a good workout without compromising the healing process. Several ideas that have gained widespread acceptance are stationary bicycling and swimming.

Stationary bicycles are a very effective means of cardiovascular fitness. A variety of workouts can be done, including interval training, sprints, or slow long distance. This exercise is usually well received by athletes because it oftentimes mimics their normal workouts.

Swimming also provides an excellent workout. A good guideline when establishing swimming workouts is to use a 4 to 1 ratio with running distances. Every quarter-mile swum is the equivalent of 1 mile run.[10]

The use of a swimming pool need not be limited to swimming. One type of exercise that is gaining popularity is running in water, either running in the shallow end or using a flotation device to keep the athlete above the waterline while in the deep end. The athlete can simulate sport-specific running patterns without placing the extremities in a weight-bearing position.

The importance of maintaining an athlete's cardiovascular fitness cannot be overstated. Deterioration of the athlete's fitness level delays return to full activity and may put the athlete at risk for reinjury.

RESTORATION OF SMOOTH, COORDINATED MOVEMENT

Restoration of smooth coordination is a vital part of any rehabilitation program. An athlete must be able to perform sport-related functional activities prior to return to competition. Proprioception and sport-specific skill testing are the two primary objectives during this phase.

Proprioception—the body's awareness of where the extremities are in space at any moment in time—is often disrupted following injury. Proper joint proprioception can be restored with a teeter board. Many variations and foot placements can be done. Plantar flexion-dorsiflexion, inversion-eversion, single leg, and both legs should be worked. The number of combinations is limited only by the sports therapist's imagination. A good progression is:

1. Two-footed, front to back.
2. Two-footed, side to side.
3. Two-footed, front to back with legs staggered.
4. One-footed, front to back.
5. One-footed, toe in.
6. One-footed, toe out.

The athlete need not master each level before proceeding to the next. This progression lists the easiest exercises first and then proceeds to the more difficult ones. Athletes should challenge themselves to see how long they can maintain their balance. A progression would be to have the athletes close their eyes while performing the exercises.

Sport-specific skills should be performed prior to the athlete's return to activity. These skills involve running, jumping, cutting, kicking, and throwing. This chapter does not detail a progression for each skill. Common sense should dictate the progression. A conservative approach is better than an aggressive approach.

MAINTENANCE

The rehabilitation program should not be discontinued once the athlete has returned to competition. A proper maintenance program includes stretching and strengthening the affected body parts. Most lower leg injuries need a continuing flexibility program for the Achilles tendon because of the increased workloads placed on the posterior musculature.

Strenthening programs also should be continued. Calf muscles strengthen with the exercise demands placed on them, but light ankle weights should be used as a supplement. The athlete should concentrate on inversion and eversion and on both eccentric and concentric contractions.

INJURIES TO THE LOWER EXTREMITY

A common misconception is that all lower leg pain should be termed *shin splints*. The AMA defines *shin splints* as "pain and discomfort in the leg from running on hard surfaces or forcible excessive use of the foot flexors; the diagnosis should be limited to musculotendinous inflammation, excluding a fatigue fracture or ischemic disorder."[1] This definition might be an accurate definition of one type of lower leg injury, but it by no means includes all forms of lower leg pathology. All lower leg pain is not produced by shin splints. This chapter provides enough information to differentiate between various lower leg pathologies and then explains proper rehabilitation methods.

Achilles Tendonitis

Achilles tendonitis is a common disorder of the lower extremity. James and others[12] have documented that 11% of all running injuries can be attributed to Achilles tendonitis. Achilles tendonitis is an overuse type of injury. A typical runner who jogs 1 mile has 1,500 heel strikes.[25] With such a high demand placed on the posterior musculature and Achilles tendon, how an overuse condition can develop should be apparent.

The Achilles tendon is the common tendon of the gastrocnemius and soleus muscles. The primary action is plantar flexion. These muscles account for 95% of the muscular activity during plantar flexion.[13] A unique characteristic of the tendon is its rotatory component. The tendon has lateral rotation as it descends toward its insertion on the calcaneus. This region, 2 to 5 centimeters above the calcaneus, is also the area of poorest blood supply.[14] This combination of factors has led researchers to believe that this region is the most frequently injured. Several researchers have documented that the pain associated with Achilles tendonitis is located in this area.[5,15]

The Achilles tendon, similar to most tendons, has a very low metabolic rate,[21] which may be significant during the recovery phase of injury. The decreased metabolism delays the healing rate and could account for the prolonged rehabilitation often needed with Achilles tendon injuries.

These various anatomical factors are important considerations when examining the etiologies of Achilles tendonitis. The underlying mechanism is that "the tensile strength of the tendon is inadequate to enable it to meet the demands."[6]

Several etiologies have been associated with the microtrauma produced by eccentric loading of fatigued muscles and the inflexibility of the gastrocnemius-soleus muscle group.[20,25] Clement and others[5] have identified training errors in 75% of all patients who suffered from Achilles tendonitis. These errors include hill training, a sudden increase in mileage, improper warm-up, training on uneven ground, and an increase in intensity.

Hyperpronation is mentioned in 56% of all cases.[5] The rotatory component of the Achilles, as mentioned previously, is accentuated by a foot that hyperpronates and creates snapping action of the tendon that may produce microtears and an inflammatory response.

Poor flexibility and strength of the calf muscles increase the demand placed on the Achilles. If this increased demand is for a prolonged time, it could lead to an inflammatory condition. Achilles tendonitis is likely when any of these factors are present in combination with excessive use of the calf muscles.

CLINICAL FINDINGS. An athlete who is experiencing Achilles tendonitis usually complains of pain in a region 2 to 5 centimeters proximal to the insertion on the calcaneus. The pain increases with activity and subsides with rest. Crepitation is usually present along the Achilles and increases with activity. Poor flexibility of the gastrocnemius-soleus complex is usually apparent.

TREATMENT AND REHABILITATION. The initial concern in treating Achilles tendonitis is to identify which of these factors is causing the problem. Specific changes should be made to prevent further aggravation once the cause is established.

The pain and inflammation of Achilles tendonitis can best be controlled through a modified activity program, cold, and NSAIDs. Severe pain responds best to several days of complete rest.

The use of NSAIDs is beneficial during the early stages of injury. Steroid injections directly into the tendon should be avoided. Several authors have attributed Achilles tendon rupture to steroid injections.[11,26]

Gentle, passive stretching should be begun as soon as the pain allows. An important range-of-motion exercise involves the posterior musculature, specifically the Achilles tendon. The Achilles tendon and gastrocnemius should be stretched in two distinct ways, with the leg straight and then bent at approximately 45 degrees (Figs. 15-9 and 15-10).

The bent-knee method is used to isolate the soleus muscle and allow it to be stretched to a greater degree by putting the gastrocnemius in a relaxed condition. This stretching can also be accomplished with the help of an incline board. This exercise should be done for 1 to 2 minutes at a time three times a day. Again, both straight and bent-leg methods should be used. Ice massage, prior to and following any stretching program, helps to decrease the pain.

Quarter-inch to half-inch heel lifts should be placed in both shoes to help take the stress off the Achilles tendon.[15] Orthotics can be used to correct any biomechanical flaw, which is especially important in a person who hyperpronates.

Strengthening the gastrocnemius and soleus muscles, which is of prime importance, is best accomplished by using an eccentric program, as described on page 317. This exercise increases the strength of the Achilles to the point of returning the athlete to activity.

A stretching program should be continued as well. Ice massage followed by ultrasound can be used quite effectively prior to any exercise. Immediately following exercise the Achilles should be iced for about 20 minutes.

The modified activity program should be continued until the athlete is completely pain free and has good strength and flexibility. Prior to the start of any running, the athlete should be told

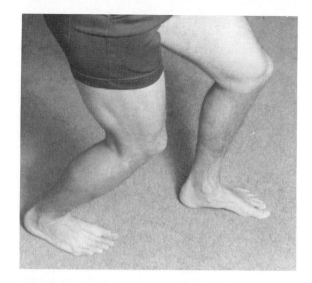

Fig. 15-9. Bent-knee stretch for soleus.

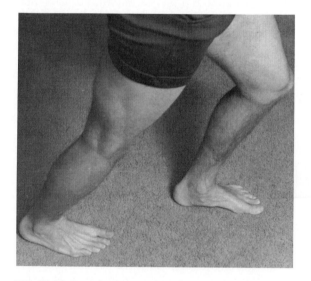

Fig. 15-10. Straight knee stretch for gastrocnemius.

to use walking as an aerobic workout. A walking program serves two purposes. First, it reintroduces the athlete to a weight-bearing form of fitness. Second, emphasis is placed on a proper heel-to-toe gait.

The athlete who has progressed to the point of returning to activity should be monitored and scheduled very judiciously. A progressive running program is an appropriate guideline for return. If pain is felt during the course of the program, the program should be modified to decrease the intensity or duration. Emphasis must be placed on running on flat, soft surfaces. Achilles tendon stretching following the return to activity must be continued.

ACHILLES TENDONITIS TREATMENT

PHASE I

1. Identify etiological factors; biomechanical correction.
2. Ice.
3. Rest.
4. NSAIDs.
5. Non-weight bearing cardiovascular conditioning.

PHASE II

1. Ice massage.
2. Gentle, passive stretching (both straight and bent leg).
3. Ultrasound
4. Heel lifts.
5. Progressive cardiovascular fitness (limited toe push-off).

PHASE III

1. Ice massage.
2. Ultrasound.
3. Stretching.
4. Eccentric strengthening program.
5. Walking, running in the pool.
6. Ice.

PHASE IV

1. Progressive running program.
2. Stretching and strengthening programs.
3. Ice.

Achilles Tendon Rupture

Complete rupture of the Achilles tendon is a relatively uncommon injury in a young, athletic population. The injury is much more frequent with older men who are recreational athletes. Williams[30] has suggested that Achilles tendon ruptures are associated with a previous pathological condition of the tendon. These degenerative changes lead to a weakened area that, if placed under stress, might rupture. The most common site for ruptures is 2 to 6 centimeters proximal to the calcaneus. This area is the same that is associated with Achilles tendonitis, perhaps because of the poor blood supply in that area.[14]

CLINICAL FINDINGS. The two distinct mechanisms for Achilles tendon rupture are a violent dorsiflexion of the foot and a direct blow while the muscle is contracted. Following a complete rupture, the athlete experiences a sudden pain and often an audible snap. The pain often quickly diminishes. This disorder is usually associated with a weakness during push-off.

On exam the sports therapist can note a palpable defect of the Achilles where it has ruptured and an area of marked discoloration that might be distal to the actual site of rupture due to gravitational effects. A positive Thompson test also helps in evaluating this condition.

TREATMENT AND REHABILITATION. The primary objective of treatment is to restore the Achilles tendon to its preinjury strength and flexibility. Immediately following injury, treatment should include ice, compression, elevation, and immobilization. A suspected Achilles tendon rupture should be referred to a physician for accurate diagnosis and care. Whether the best treatment is nonsurgical or surgical intervention is a matter of much controversy.

A conservative nonsurgical approach involves prolonged immobilization. Two months generally provides adequate time for proper healing. A very gradual stretching and strengthening program should follow immobilization. This process is slow and should be undertaken very gradually. Heel lifts should be placed in both shoes to diminish the stress placed on the Achilles tendon.

The athlete may return to activity when full range of motion and strength have been restored. Rehabilitation should be done in a progressive manner with careful monitoring of the athlete's pain and type of activities. In the early stages of return, ballistic types of movements should be avoided to decrease the chance of rerupture.

A conservative approach has several drawbacks. First, the chance of rerupture is quite high, between 22%[11] and 35%.[22] Moreover, the athlete must understand that the rehabilitation process is extremely long.

If surgery is elected, the postsurgical rehabilitation program follows a course similar to the nonsurgical. Following immobilization, usually 6 to 8 weeks, range-of-motion exercises should be initiated. The range of motion, specifically dorsiflexion, should be much easier to attain after surgery than following conservative treatment. A gradual resistive exercise program should be initiated when range of motion is back to normal. The athlete's activity should be monitored following return to sports activity to decrease the chance for rerupture.

ACHILLES TENDON RUPTURE TREATMENT
PHASE I
1. Ice.
2. Compression.
3. Elevation.
4. Immobilization.

PHASE II
1. Conservative: immobilization for 2 to 3 months.
2. Surgical: surgical repair.

PHASE III
1. Heel lifts.
2. Passive and active range-of-motion exercises.
3. Progressive resistance exercises.
4. Ice after workout.

Tennis Leg

The term **tennis leg** is synonymous with a partial tear of the medial head of the gastrocnemius. This injury usually occurs in the sports where a ballistic, side-to-side movement is common. The cause is a sudden overload of the muscle. Abrupt dorsiflexion of the ankle while extending the knee oftentimes produces enough force to cause this overload. The weakest point of the gastrocnemius-soleus complex is the insertion of the medial head of the gastrocnemius into the soleus fascia.[32] This area accounts for the majority of cases of tennis leg.[19]

CLINICAL FINDINGS. An athlete who experiences a tear of the medial head of the gastrocnemius is usually unable to continue activity. On exam the area around the medial head is point tender, discolored, and swollen. A palpable defect is usually present, and pain is present with dorsiflexion.

TREATMENT AND REHABILITATION. Immediate treatment for this injury consists of rest, ice, compression, and elevation. The athlete should use crutches to avoid putting weight on the tennis leg if the injury is severe enough to alter gait. The use of NSAIDs is beneficial during the first

several days following the injury,[4] and heel lifts should be used to relieve stress on the gastrocnemius.

A program of passive and active stretching should be initiated as early as the pain allows. This program should progress to a form of resistive exercise to strengthen the posterior musculature. During this phase, heat treatments can replace cold. Ultrasound may provide a very effective treatment.

Return to activity, as with any injury to the lower leg, should be based on bilateral flexibility and strength measurements. A progressive activity program should be utilized. Any type of ballistic activity may lead to reinjury and should be monitored. A maintenance program of stretching and strengthening should be adhered to following return to activity.

TENNIS LEG TREATMENT
PHASE I
1. Rest.
2. Ice.
3. Compression.
4. Elevation.
5. No weight bearing.
6. Nonsteroidal antiinflammatory medications.

PHASE II
1. Passive range of motion stretching.
2. Active range of motion stretching.
3. Progressive resistance exercises.
4. Heel lifts.
5. Heat, ultrasound.

PHASE III
1. Progressive running program.
2. Maintenance stretching and strengthening.

SHIN SPLINT SYNDROMES

Shin splints are a musculotendinous overuse condition. They generally occur to athletes who are unconditioned and initiate a training program too vigorously. Two distinct shin splint conditions, anterior and posterior, can be differentiated by the location of pain.

Many factors contribute to shin splint syndromes. The three basic causes of shin splints are abnormal biomechanical function, poor conditioning, and improper training methods. They may be present individually or in combination with each other. A proper assessment of these contributing factors not only can help to differentiate between anterior and posterior shin splints but also can help to direct the rehabilitation. If the athlete is allowed to return to competition before the underlying cause of the injury is determined, then the chance of reinjury is significant.

Anterior Shin Splints

Anterior shin splints usually elicit pain and tenderness lateral to the tibia and over the anterior compartment. The muscles that are the most involved are the tibialis anterior, the extensor digitorum longus, and the extensor hallucis longus. The muscles associated with anterior shin splints are active during toe off, heel strike, and the entire swing phase.[28] Anterior shin pain is often a result of hard heel strike, which is caused by a forceful eccentric contraction that helps to decelerate the foot and cushion the impact of the body. As is the basic premise of any overuse type of injury, the muscles are unable to handle the stresses placed upon them. Thus weak foot flexor muscles contribute to this condition. Biomechanical factors also play a role. A person with forefoot varus requires an increase in tibialis anterior activity to help prevent foot slap.[2]

Posterior Shin Splints

Posterior shin splints usually cause pain along the posterior medial border of the lower third of the tibia.[24] This pain is often associated with inflammation of the tibialis posterior, flexor digitorum longus, and flexor hallucis longus. These muscles are active during the first 80% of stance phase.[9] The subtalar joint normally goes from a supinated position at heel strike, to a pronated position during midstance, and then during toe off it returns into supination. A foot that hyperpronates during midstance places a tremendous amount of stress on these muscles.[30] The posterior muscles contract eccentrically to combat this hypermobility. This condition may eventually lead to an inflammatory response of the involved muscles.[18] Training errors, a tight Achilles tendon, and improper footwear in conjunction with a hyperpronating foot can contribute to this type of condition.

Clinical Findings

A thorough history should help to differentiate between anterior and posterior shin splints, but the locations of pain are the best indicator. Anterior shin splints elicit pain lateral to the tibia along the anterior compartment. Posterior shin splints cause pain by the medial border of the lower third of the tibia. This pain is often described as a dull ache that oftentimes increases with the intensity of work. The onset of pain is often associated with constant exercise. Depending on the severity of the condition, pain might be felt only during activity or, in more progressed cases, during inactive times.

The injury is generally quite tender to palpation. In the early stages, tenderness is quite localized, which makes evaluation much easier. A muscle weakness can usually be determined in the affected muscles.

Treatment and Rehabilitation

A thorough history to determine the underlying cause of the condition should be the first step in treatment. More often than not, a biomechanical abnormality is compounded by errors in training.

Treatment for shin splints is basically the same whether the condition is anterior or posterior. As with any overuse condition, the affected muscles must be allowed to rest. Depending on the severity of the pain, this rest period can range from 1 day to many weeks. Ice and NSAIDs are indicated during this time, and any biomechanical abnormality should be corrected.

When the level of pain has decreased to an acceptable level, resistance exercises, including any of the previously mentioned strengthening programs, should be started. Anterior shin splints should emphasize the anterior muscle groups. Athletes with posterior shin pain should work on inversion-eversion exercises done both eccentrically and concentrically.

Therapeutic modalities can be used during this phase. Heat and cold have both been found to be effective methods of treatment. Smith and others[27] have shown that ultrasound, ice, and phonophoresis are all equally effective in terms of treating the pain associated with shin splints.

Modified activity is important. Stationary bicycling (being careful not to push off with the toes) and running in water are excellent alternatives. A progressive running program should be used to return the athlete to activity gradually.

During the course of rehabilitation, a thorough history should be taken. More often than not, a biomechanical abnormality has been compounded by errors in training. These problems must be addressed prior to allowing the athlete to return to competition.

SHIN SPLINT TREATMENT

PHASE I
1. Rest.
2. Ice massage.
3. Nonsteroidal antiinflammatory drugs.
4. Non-weight-bearing cardiovascular training.
5. Biomechanical corrections.
6. Upper body strengthening.

PHASE II
1. Ice.
2. Stretching (both anterior and posterior muscles).
3. Progressive resistance exercises.
4. Heat (ultrasound).

PHASE III
1. Progressive running program.
2. Continued stretching and strengthening.
3. Ice following exercise.

PHASE IV
1. Return to competition.
2. Stretching and strengthening continued.
3. Ice following workout.

RETROCALCANEOBURSITIS

Retrocalcaneobursitis is an inflammatory overuse condition involving the retrocalcaneal bursa. It is located just anterior to the Achilles tendon insertion on the calcaneus. Often it is misdiagnosed as Achilles tendonitis. The two can be differentiated by a careful exam.

Clinical Findings

An athlete who is experiencing retrocalcaneobursitis feels pain and tenderness between the talus and the Achilles tendon. This sensation can help the examiner differentiate between the two structures. Pain associated with retrocalcaneo-

bursitis is not directly on the Achilles, as with tendonitis.

Pain increases with activity and is often accompanied by mild swelling. This condition is usually brought on by an irritation of the shoe heel counter.

Treatment and Rehabilitation

Early treatment measures should be aimed at correcting the irritation caused by the shoe. Raising the heel with the use of lifts and softening the heel counter are both used.

Exercise should be modified to decrease the irritation to the bursa. Ice, phonophoresis with hydrocortisone, and NSAIDs are all effective treatments. Upon return to activity, a well-fitting shoe should be worn to decrease the friction on the bursa.

In extreme cases, surgical intervention might be indicated. An 8-week immobilization period is usually indicated. Following removal of the cast, range-of-motion exercises and a strengthening program should be initiated and continued until strength and flexibility are bilaterally equal.

RETROCALCANEOBURSITIS TREATMENT

PHASE I
1. Ice.
2. NSAIDs.
3. Shoe modification.
4. Correcting any errors in training.

PHASE II
1. Ice.
2. Phonophoresis with hydrocortisone cream.

PHASE III
1. Progressive return to competition.

COMPARTMENT SYNDROMES

Compartment syndromes of the lower leg are a result of an increased compartmental pressure. Among the many factors that can contribute to it are direct trauma, fracture, or muscle hypertrophy. Compartment syndromes can be acute or chronic. The pathology is basically the same, an increase in compartmental pressure, for both acute and chronic syndromes. A chronic compartment syndrome gets better with rest; an acute compartment syndrome gets worse with time.

The lower leg can be divided into five distinct

compartments: the anterior, lateral, superficial posterior, deep posterior, and tibialis posterior. The following structures are contained in each compartment:

Anterior: tibialis anterior, deep peroneal nerve, anterior tibial artery and vein, extensor muscles of the foot and toes

Lateral: superficial peroneal nerve, peroneus longus and brevis muscles

Superficial posterior: soleus muscle, plantaris and gastrocnemius tendons

Deep posterior: flexor digitorum longus, peroneal artery and vein, tibial nerve, posterior tibial artery and vein

Tibialis posterior: tibialis posterior muscle

Acute Compartment Syndrome

Acute compartment syndrome is caused by a sudden trauma that causes swelling within the compartment. The increase in tissue volume within the compartment produces an increase in compartmental pressure that may occlude the blood vessels and produce an ischemic condition. This increased pressure may also produce excessive pressure on the nerves within the compartment that may lead to a neurological deficit. An acute compartment syndrome is considered a medical emergency. Irreversible damage occurs to the structures within the compartment if it is left untreated. Loss of motion is dependent on the severity and length of the condition and can range from complete drop foot (tibialis anterior involvement) to partial limitation of the toe and ankle extensors.

CLINICAL FINDINGS. An athlete who is experiencing an acute compartment syndrome complains of severe pain in the affected muscles. In the case of a traumatic acute compartment syndrome, such as a contusion to the lower leg, pain progresses from a dull aching sensation to a very sharp pain. Passively stretching the affected compartment's muscle group produces an increase in pain.

Local temperature increases, and the area is swollen and feels tense. Paresthesia is often present in the space between the first and second toes with an anterior compartment involvement. Only in extreme cases are distal pulses lost.

TREATMENT AND REHABILITATION. The only effective treatment of acute compartment syndrome is an immediate surgical fasciotomy of the involved compartment. This procedure releases the pressure that has been affecting the tissues within the compartment. Any attempt to treat this condition conservatively only increases the chances for permanent damage to the muscles within the compartment.

Immediately following surgery, the athlete is advised to limit activities and keep the affected leg elevated. Gentle active and passive stretching can be initiated. Ice bags should be applied to the surgical area three to four times a day. Walking can be done as tolerated after the first 2 days.

A more aggressive rehabilitation program should be initiated once the athlete has a full, pain-free range of motion. This program should include Achilles tendon stretching and a manual resistance exercise program. Strengthening programs should not be too aggressive in this phase of rehabilitation. Muscular hypertrophy is contraindicated following fasciotomy. Walking for a longer duration and stationary bicycling should be started and continued in conjunction with a stretching program. A progressive running program should be used as the guideline for returning the athlete to competition.

Chronic Compartment Syndromes

Chronic compartment syndromes (CCS) have also been called *exertional compartment syndrome.* Symptoms of CCS often are produced by exercise or by muscle exertion. Not all individuals who exercise, however, experience CCS. Individual differences in the size of the lower leg musculature and compartmental dimensions justify why some people experience problems and others do not. Detmer[7] has concluded that muscle mass increases by 20% during heavy exercise. The increase in muscle mass may produce an increase in compartmental pressure and in some people may lead to CCS. The increase in pressure may produce a local ischemic condition in the muscle. The ischemic response may produce pain that persists until the compartmental pressure diminishes and normal circulation is sufficient to meet the demands of the working muscles. The pain eventually subsides completely with rest.

Athletes may experience bilateral compartment syndromes. Reneman[23] found that 58 of 61 patients he examined experienced bilateral symptoms. However, the dominant leg usually had more severe symptoms.

CLINICAL FINDINGS. A thorough history helps to determine if a chronic compartment syndrome is occurring. The athlete is usually able to tell an exact time, intensity level, or distance during the workout when the symptoms present themselves. The patient often complains of transient pain with exercise that is described as a deep, cramping feeling. It is oftentimes a bilateral condition. The athlete also complains of a muscle weakness of the affected muscles. If a chronic compartment syndrome is suspected, then diagnosis should be confirmed by comparing compartmental pressure measurements during exercise and rest.

TREATMENT AND REHABILITATION. Conservative treatment of CCS generally does not help alleviate the problem. Rest, ice, stretching, and NSAIDs all have been used with limited success. Remember that pain is a symptom of a pathological condition and not one itself. For athletes who wish to continue at a competitive activity level, therefore, fasciotomy may be the treatment of choice. Rehabilitation following surgical fasciotomy should be the same as was previously described.

COMPARTMENT SYNDROMES TREATMENT (AFTER FASCIOTOMY)

PHASE I
1. Rest.
2. Elevation.
3. Ice 3 to 4 times a day.

PHASE II: *2 to 3 days after surgery*
1. Walking as tolerated.
2. Passive range-of-motion exercises (PROM).
3. Active range-of-motion exercise (AROM).
4. Ice.

PHASE III
1. PROM and/or AROM.
2. Manual resistance (begin with very light work).
3. Bike riding, walking.
4. Ice.

PHASE IV
1. Progressive running program.
2. Stretching.
3. Ice.

STRESS FRACTURES

A **stress fracture** in the lower leg can be defined as a fracture of the tibia or fibula caused by the bones being unable to withstand repeated stress. They are quite common in athletics. McBryde[16] found that 10% of all athletic injuries were stress fractures. Lower leg stress fractures are the most common types. The tibia is the body's primary weight bearer in the lower extremity, and 49% of all stress fractures involve the tibia. The fibula, which plays a lesser role in weight bearing, is only involved in 7 to 10% of the cases.[17]

Stress fractures are very different than acute fractures. Generally no one specific episode of training produces a stress fracture. Frankel[8] has identified four etiological factors associated with stress fractures:

1. Overload placed on bone by continuous muscle contractions
2. Stress distribution in the bone altered by continued activity in the presence of muscle fatigue
3. Change in running surface
4. High repetition of stress, even if the intensity is low

These four factors all place stress on the body, specifically the lower leg. The body's normal response is to adapt to this increased demand. Bone is in a constant state of remodeling that involves removal of old bone and then a replacement of new bone. The sites for this remodeling are based on increased blood flow and specific stress sites. During this remodeling, problems can arise if the stress placed on the body exceeds the recovery time and the body does not have enough time to form new bone. Eventually a weakened area develops that is highly susceptible to a stress fracture.

These overloads are often a result of improper training. Taunton and others[29] have identified the following training errors:

27%—A rapid increase in training
10%—A single severe session
 8%—A rapid increase in mileage
 6%—A sudden increase in hill training
 5%—Faulty footwear
44%—Combination of faulty footwear and training errors

These factors were indicative of all types of stress fractures, not just lower leg. However, a good parallel can be drawn because 52% of the cases examined involved either the tibia or the fibula.

Clinical Findings

Obtaining a careful history is important. Noting type and location of pain and when it occurs can help to differentiate between soft tissue and bony involvement. An athlete with a suspected stress fracture complains of a well-localized pain. Initially this pain occurs only after activity. As the condition progresses, the pain starts earlier, during activity. The intensity of pain is also much greater and lasts for a longer period of time.

On exam some swelling might be present from a local periosteal reaction. Percussion distal to the area of suspected fracture often elicits pain. Suspected stress fractures should be followed up with a bone scan to provide an accurate diagnosis. X-rays at an early stage are often not conclusive.

Treatment and Rehabilitation

The most effective rehabilitation program revolves around a modified activity program. Stress fractures are an overuse syndrome, and the only way they can heal is through rest. In extreme cases, immobilization of the lower leg might be needed. A complete abstention from all activity can be very difficult to enforce. Garrett[10] has suggested that running can be allowed during the healing phase, provided no pain develops. He feels that exercise promotes healing. Alternative methods for aerobic fitness are stationary bicycling, swimming, and running in water.

Relief from the symptoms can be accomplished by rest, ice, and NSAIDs. However, these measures should not mask any pain that the athlete is experiencing because adequate feedback is necessary when the athlete returns to activity.

Strength should be developed in the ankle dorsi and plantar flexors to decrease the stresses placed on the body when the athlete returns to activity. Any biomechanical abnormalities that exist should be corrected with orthotics. Before allowing the athlete to return to preinjury activity levels, a progressive running program should be started. The athlete should also be counseled and monitored about training errors.

STRESS FRACTURE TREATMENT

PHASE I
1. Rest.
2. Biomechanical correction.
3. Alternative cardiovascular training.
4. Bone scan diagnosis.
5. Strengthening of lower leg musculature.
6. Stretching of Achilles tendon.

PHASE II (When fracture is healed)
1. Progressive running program.
2. Ice after workout.

SUMMARY

1. Not all lower leg pain is shin splints.
2. Pain is not a pathological condition in itself.
3. Cardiovascular fitness should be maintained throughout the entire rehabilitation process.
4. Eccentric overloading is a common mechanism with overuse injuries to the lower leg.
5. Biomechanical malalignment should be corrected prior to allowing the athlete to return to activity.
6. A progressive return to competition should be followed.
7. Upon return to activity, the athlete should continue to work actively on building strength and flexibility.

REFERENCES

1 AMA Subcommittee on the Classification of Sports Injuries: Standard nomenclature of athletic injuries, Chicago, 1966, American Medical Association.
2 Andrews JR: Overuse syndromes of the lower extremity, Clin Sports Med 2:137, 1983.
3 Brody DM: Running injuries. In Nicholas JA and Hershmann EB, editors: The lower extremity and spine in sports medicine, St Louis, 1986, Times Mirror/Mosby College Publishing.
4 Calabese LH and Rooney TW: The use of non-steroidal antiinflammatory drugs in sports, Physician Sports Med 14:89–97, 1986.
5 Clement DB, Taunton JE, and Smart GW: Achilles tendinitis and peritendinitis: etiology and treatment, Am J Sports Med 12(3):179–184, 1984.
6 Curwin S and Stanish WD: Tendinitis: its etiology and treatment, Lexington, Mass, 1984, Collamore Press.

7   Detmer DE: Chronic leg pain, Am J Sports Med 8:141–144, 1980.

8   Frankel VH: Editorial comment, Am J Sports Med 6:396, 1978.

9   Friedman MA: Injuries to the leg in athletics. In Nicholas JA and Hershmann EB, editors: The lower extremity and spine in sports medicine, St Louis, 1986, Times Mirror/Mosby College Publishing.

10 Garrett WE: Personal communication, 1985.

11 Jacobs D and others: Comparison of conservative and operative treatments of Achilles tendon rupture, Am J Sports Med 6:107, 1978.

12 James SL, Bates BT, and Osternig LR: Injuries to runners, Am J Sports Med 6:40–50, 1978.

13 Jesse J: Hidden causes of injury, prevention and correction for running athletes and joggers, Pasadena, Calif, 1977, The Athletic Press.

14 Lagergren C and Lindholm A: Vascular distribution: the Achilles tendon, Acta Chir Scand 116:491, 1958.

15 Leach RE, James S, and Wasilewski S: Achilles tendinitis, Am J Sports Med 9:93–98, 1981.

16 McBryde AM: Stress fractures in athletics, Am J Sports Med 3:212–217, 1975.

17 Matheson GO and others: Stress fractures in athletics: a study of 320 cases, Am J Sports Med 15:46–57, 1987.

18 Michael RH and Holder LE: The soleus syndrome: a cause of medial tibial stress (shin splints), Am J Sports Med 13:87–94, 1985.

19 Millar AP: Strains of the posterior calf musculature (tennis leg), Clin Sports Med 2:175, 1983.

20 O'Connor P and Kersey RD: Achilles peritendinitis, Ath Train 15:159–166, 1980.

21 Peacock EE: A study of the circulation in normal tendons and healing grafts, Ann Surg 149:415, 1959.

22 Persson S and Wredmark T: The treatment of total rupture of the Achilles tendon by plaster immobilization, Int Orthop 3:149–152, 1979.

23 Reneman RS: The anterior and lateral compartment syndrome of the leg due to intense use of muscles, Clin Orth Related Research 113:69, 1975.

24 Scheuch PA: Tibialis posterior shin splints: diagnosis and treatment, Ath Train 19:271–274, 1984.

25 Shields CL: Achilles tendon injuries and disabling conditions, Physician Sports Med 10:77–84, 1982.

26 Skeoch DU: Spontaneous partial subcutaneous rupture of the tendon Achilles: review of the literature and evaluation of 16 involved tendons, Am J Sports Med 9:20, 1981.

27 Smith W, Winn F, and Parette R: Comparative study using four modalities in shinsplint treatments, J Ortho Sports Phys Ther 8:77–80, 1986.

28 Subotonick SI: Podiatric sports medicine, Mt Kisco, NY, 1975, Futura Publishing Co.

29 Taunton JE, Clement DB, and Webber D: Lower extremity stress fractures in athletics, Physician Sports Med 9:77–86, 1981.

30 Viitasalo JT and Kvist M: Some biomechanical aspects of the foot and ankle in athletics with and without shin splints, Am J Sports Med 11:125–130, 1983.

31 Williams JGP: Achilles tendon lesions in sport, Sports Med 3:114–135, 1986.

32 Zarins B and Ciullo JV: Acute muscle and tendon injuries in athletics, Clin Sports Med 2:175, 1983.

Rehabilitation of Ankle Injuries

16

Stewart L. (Skip) Hunter

OBJECTIVES

Following completion of this chapter, the student will be able to:

- Identify types of ankle sprains and the mechanisms of injury.

- Identify the stages of rehabilitation for the ankle.

- Discuss the various treatment options available for each of the stages of rehabilitation.

- Discuss criteria for return to activity following ankle injury.

The most frequently injured part of the musculoskeletal system is the lateral ankle.[2,8] The turned ankle is the second greatest cause of days lost from work.[7] Management of these injuries ranges from no treatment to surgical repair and reconstruction. Rehabilitation techniques are varied and the equipment utilized may be as simple as a $1 piece of tubing or as sophisticated as a $50,000 isokinetic device.

MECHANISMS OF INJURY

Injuries to the ligaments of the ankle may be graded so that grade 1 is mild, grade 2 is a greater ligamentous disruption, and grade 3 is a complete tear.[8]

Injuries to the ligaments of the ankle may also be classified according to the site of occurrence. The lateral ankle sprain is by far the most common. The anterior talofibular ligament is the weakest of the three lateral ligaments. Its major function is to stop forward subluxation of the talus. It is injured in an inverted, plantar-flexed, and internally rotated position.[21,40] The calcaneofibular and posterior talofibular ligaments are commonly involved in lateral sprains as the force of the injury is increased and the mechanism is slightly altered. Increased inversion force is needed to tear the calcaneofibular ligament. Because the posterior talofibular ligament prevents posterior subluxation of the talus, it is injured in severe injuries such as complete dislocations.[3]

The medial ankle sprain is less common than the lateral ankle sprain. More often it may involve a fracture avulsion of the tibia before the deltoid ligament tears.[5] Although eversion sprains are uncommon, their severity is such that this category of sprain may take longer to heal than the simple lateral sprain.[32]

The tibiofibular ligaments are stronger and less prone to injury than the other ligaments of the ankle.[44] This ligament extends between the tibia and fibula up the leg as the interosseous ligament. These ligaments are torn with increased rotational force and are often torn in conjunction with a severe sprain of the medial and lateral ligament complexes. Sprains of the tibiofibular and interosseous ligaments are extremely hard to treat and often take months to heal.

TREATMENT AND REHABILITATION OF ANKLE SPRAINS
Phase I (Early Phase)

During the initial phase of ankle rehabilitation, the major goal is reduction of postinjury swelling, bleeding, and pain and the protection of the already healing ligament. All initial treatment should be directed toward limiting the amount of swelling. Initial management includes protection, rest, ice, compression, and elevation.

PROTECTION. The injured ligament must be maintained in a stable position so that healing can occur. In the past, this objective was accomplished by casting until the acute effects of the sprain were over. Recent literature suggests that limited stress on the ankle may promote faster and stronger healing.[3,33] These studies found that protected motion facilitated proper collagen reorientation and thus increased the strength of the healing ligament.

Several appliances are available to accomplish this early protected motion. Quillen[34] recommends the ankle stirrup, which allows motion in the sagittal plane while limiting movement of the frontal plane and thus avoids stressing the ligaments through inversion and eversion (Fig. 16-1). Several commercially available braces accomplish this goal and also apply cushioned pressure to help with edema.[39] When a commercially available product is not feasible, a similar protective device may be fashioned from thermoplastic materials such as Hexalite or Orthoplast (Fig. 16-2).

The open Gibney taping technique also accomplishes this early medial and lateral protection while allowing plantar flexion and dorsiflexion. It also is an excellent edema control mechanism (Fig. 16-3).

Early application of these devices allows early ambulation. Partial weight bearing with crutches helps control several complications to healing. Muscle atrophy, proprioceptive loss, and circulatory stasis are all reduced when even limited weight bearing is allowed. Weight bearing also inhibits contracture of the tendons, which may lead to tendonitis. For these reasons, early ambulation, even if only TWB (touchdown weight bearing), is essential.

REST. In the early phase of rehabilitation, caution should be taken against vigorous exercise. The studies cited previously show that a healing

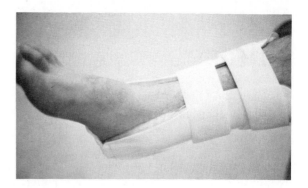
Fig. 16-1. Commercially available Aircast ankle stirrup.

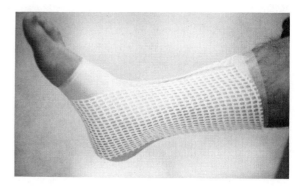
Fig. 16-2. Molded hexalite ankle stirrup.

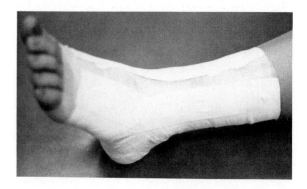
Fig. 16-3. Correctly done open Gibney tape.

ligament needs a certain amount of stress in order to heal properly.

Contralateral exercises may be performed to obtain cross-transfer effects on the muscles of the injured side.[24] Isometric exercises may be performed very early in dorsiflexion, plantar flexion, inversion, and eversion. The athlete should hold these for a 6 to 8 count in all of the major movements of the ankle. These types of exercises may be performed to prevent atrophy without fear of further injury to the ligament. Active plantar flexion and dorsiflexion may be initiated early because they also do not endanger the healing ligament as long as they are done pain free. An excellent method is two sets of 40 of active plantar flexion and dorsiflexion while the athlete is iced and elevated. Inversion and eversion are to be avoided, as they might initiate bleeding and further traumatize ligaments.

ICE. The use of ice on acute injuries has been well documented in the literature. Ice has received attention not only as an aid in acute situations but also for continued use in chronic conditions. The initial use of ice has its basis in constricting superficial blood vessels to prevent hemorrhage. Long-term benefits may be from reduction of pain and spasticity.[23] Garrick[14] suggests the use of ice for a minimum of 20 minutes once every 4 waking hours. Ice should not be used longer than 30 minutes, especially over superficial nerves such as the peroneal and ulnar nerves. Prolonged use of ice in such areas may produce transient nerve palsy.[10]

One of the most frequently asked questions in sports medicine is "When do I use ice, and when do I use heat?" Current literature suggests that ice can be used during all phases of rehabilitation.[25] The sooner it is started, the more effective it is.[18] Ice can certainly do no harm if used properly, but heat if applied too soon following injury may lead to increased swelling.

The author believes that ice should be used as a rehabilitative tool until the process plateaus. At that point the sports therapist may elect to change to heat in an effort to progress the rehabilitative process. Often the switch from ice to heat cannot be made for weeks or months.

COMPRESSION. Ice alone is apparently not as effective as ice used in conjunction with compression.[38] Many devices are available that apply external compression to the ankle to re-

duce swelling. Most of these use either air or cold water within an enclosed bag to provide pressure to reduce swelling. The most commonly used device of this type is the intermittent air compression device (Fig. 16-4).

Several methods may be used to control edema when the patient is away from the treatment area. An Ace wrap can prevent or control swelling. It should be applied evenly, wrapping distally to proximal with enough force so that it does not fall. Uneven pressure or uncovered areas over any part of the extremity may allow the swelling to accumulate.

Open Gibney taping may be applied under an Ace wrap to provide additional support. Care should be taken not to compartmentalize this treatment by placing tape across the top and bottom of the open area of the open Gibney (Fig. 16-5). In cases of severe swelling, tissue may be forced through this compartmental window and cause damage to the skin. As swelling begins to reduce, a bulky dressing may be taped closed with several layers of prewrap or gauze with tape lightly applied over the top. To add more compression, a horseshoe-shaped pad of felt may be inserted under the wrap over the area of maximum swelling.

Electrical stimulation has been used to help control edema. Michlovitz and others[29] used high-voltage pulsed galvanic stimulation at varying pulse rates in conjunction with ice. Although descriptive data indicated some pain relief, the addition of electrical stimulation to the treatment protocol made no significant difference in the amount of acute edema in the first 3 days.

ELEVATION. Elevation is an essential part of edema control. Pressure in any vessel below the level of the heart is increased, which may lead to increased edema.[6] Several publications have stated that any treatment done in the dependent position allows edema to increase.[29,37] Elevation allows gravity to work with the lymphatic system rather than against it and decreases hydrostatic pressure to decrease fluid loss and also assist venous and lymphatic return through gravity.[6]

An attempt should be made to do treatments in the elevated position rather than the gravity dependent position. Patients should be asked to maintain an elevated position as often as possible during the early phase of rehabilitation.

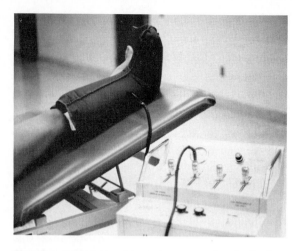

Fig. 16-4. Jobst intermittent air compression device for control of edema.

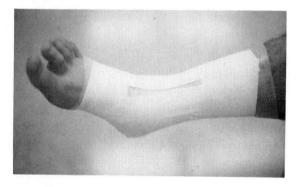

Fig. 16-5. Do not close the open Gibney tape.

OTHER TREATMENT. Cardiorespiratory conditioning should be maintained during the entire rehabilitation process. Pedaling a stationary bike such as an Airdyne or UBE with the hands provides excellent cardiovascular exercise without placing stress on the ankle. Swimming can also be beneficial as long as it is pain free.

SUMMARY OF TREATMENTS FOR PHASE I

1. *Protection:* Air or gel casts, open Gibney taping, self-made hexalite splints
2. *Rest:* Crutches with partial weight bearing, isometric exercises progressing to isometric inversion-eversion exercises with active plantar flexion and dorsiflexion.
3. *Ice:* Ice may be used throughout the entire rehabilitation process, although heat may be substituted when progress is not noted with ice.
4. *Compression:* Intermittent compression devices may be used in conjunction with ice and electrical stimulation. An Ace wrap, open Gibney taping, or closed taping using a bulky dressing can reduce edema.
5. *Elevation*

Phase II (Rehabilitation Phase)

The end of the early protective phase and beginning of the rehabilitation phase is marked by two events: (1) Swelling stops increasing and (2) pain lessens, indicating that the ligaments have reached that point in the healing process at which they are not in danger from minimal stress.

The purpose of this phase of rehabilitation is to increase motion and strength. This increased activity should aid circulation and help eliminate residual inflammatory agents.

RANGE OF MOTION. In the early stages of the rehabilitation phase, inversion and eversion should be minimized. Light joint mobilization concentrating on dorsiflexion and plantar flexion should be started first. It can be accomplished by manual joint mobilization in the anterior-posterior direction (Fig. 16-6) or through exercises such as dorsiflexion stretches with a towel (Fig. 16-7) and standing toe stretches for plantar flexion (Fig. 16-8). Both exercises may be done while ice is being applied. Athletes are encouraged to do these slowly, without pain, and to use high repetitions (two sets of 40). A wedge board may be beneficial for range of motion as well as a beginning exercise for proprioception. These exercises should at first be done seated (Fig. 16-9).

As tenderness over the ligament decreases, inversion-eversion exercises may be initiated in conjunction with plantar flexion and dorsiflexion exercises. Early exercises include pulling a towel from one side to the other by alternately inverting and everting the foot (Fig. 16-10) and alphabet drawing in an ice bath, which should be done in capital letters to ensure that full range is utilized. A wedge board may be turned so that inversion-eversion is the primary movement (Fig. 16-11). These exercises may be supplemented with a seated biomechanical ankle platform

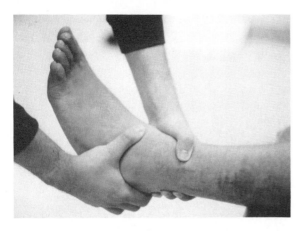

Fig. 16-6. Manual joint mobilization technique.

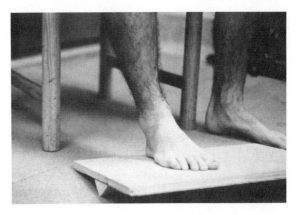

Fig. 16-9. Seated wedge board for plantar flexion and dorsiflexion.

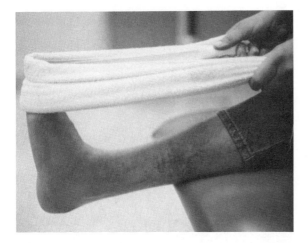

Fig. 16-7. Towel stretch for dorsiflexion.

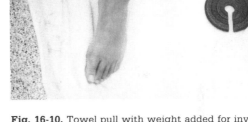

Fig. 16-10. Towel pull with weight added for inversion and eversion.

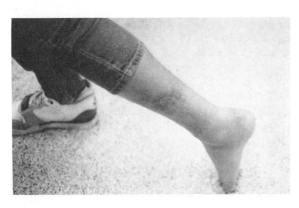

Fig. 16-8. Toe stretch for plantar flexion.

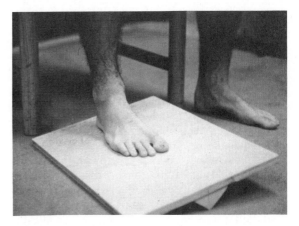

Fig. 16-11. Seated wedge board for inversion and eversion.

(BAP) board technique by rotating the foot through its entire range both clockwise and counterclockwise for two sets of 20 repetitions (Fig. 16-12).

A wedge-BAPS board exercise should follow a progression. Initially the athlete should start in the seated position with a wedge board in the plantar flexion-dorsiflexion direction. As pain decreases and the ligament healing progresses, the board may be turned in the inversion-eversion direction. As the athlete performs these movements easily, a seated BAPS board may be used for full range-of-motion exercises. When seated exercises are performed with ease, standing balance exercises should be initiated. They may be started on one leg standing without a board. The athlete then supports weight with the hands and maintains balance on a wedge board in either plantar flexion-dorsiflexion or inversion-eversion. Next, hand support may be eliminated while the athlete balances on the wedge board. The same sequence is then used on the BAPS board. The BAPS board is initially used with assistance from the hands. Then balance is practiced on the BAPS board unassisted.

Each time a BAPS board is used, the progression should start with a small ball and finish with a larger ball before moving to the next step.

Vigorous heelcord stretching should be initiated as soon as possible (Fig. 16-13). McCluskey and others[26] found that the heelcord acts as a bowstring when tight and may increase the chance of ankle sprains.

The author advocates that athletes have available something on which the foot can rest to stretch the heelcords, perhaps at a location where they stand during the day, such as by the phone, in front of a mirror, or in front of the sink, to ensure that they stretch at least a few minutes each day.

STRENGTH. Isometrics may be done in the four major ankle motion planes, frontal and sagittal. They may be accompanied early in the rehabilitative phase by plantar flexion and dorsiflexion isotonic exercises, which do not endanger the ligaments. They may be done with a device as simple as an ankle weight or as sophisticated as an isokinetic device. As the ligaments heal further and range of motion increases, strengthening exercises may be begun in all planes of

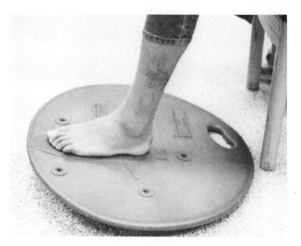

Fig. 16-12. Seated BAPS board.

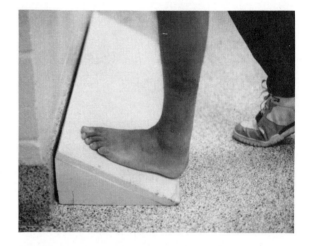

Fig. 16-13. Heelcord stretching using an incline board.

motion (Fig. 16-14). Pain should be the basic guideline for deciding when to start inversion-eversion isotonic exercises. Light resistance with high repetitions has fewer detrimental effects on the ligaments (two to four sets of 10 repetitions).

Tubing exercises and ankle weights around the foot are excellent methods of strengthening inversion and eversion. Tubing has advantages in that it may be used both eccentrically and concentrically (Fig. 16-15). Isokinetics have advantages in that more functional speeds may be obtained (Fig. 16-16). Care must be taken when

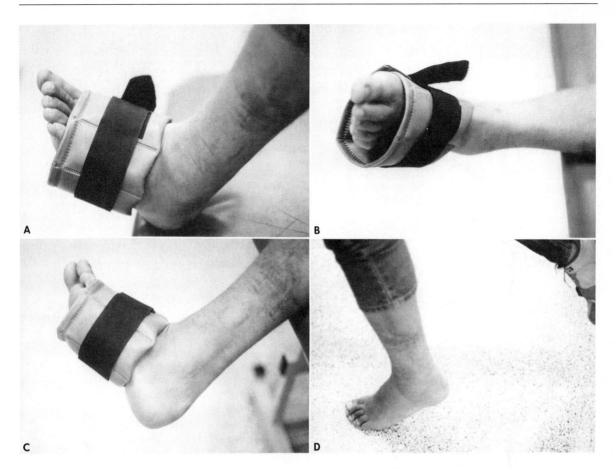

Fig. 16-14. A, Isotonic strengthening of dorsiflexion using an ankle weight; **B,** isotonic strengthening of inversion using an ankle weight; **C,** isotonic strengthening of eversion using an ankle weight; **D,** isotonic strengthening of plantar flexion using toe raises.

exercising the ankle in inversion and eversion to avoid tibial rotation as a substitute movement. Have the athlete palpate the tibial tubercle to ensure that the proper movement is occurring.

PROPRIOCEPTION. The role of proprioception in repeated ankle trauma has been questioned.[4,11,13,31] The literature suggests that proprioception is certainly a factor in recurrent ankle sprains. Rebman[35] reported that 83% of his patients experienced a reduction in chronic ankle sprains after a program of proprioceptive exercises. Glencross and Thornton[16] found that the greater the ligament disruption, the greater the proprioceptive loss. Early weight bearing has previously been mentioned as a method of re-

ducing proprioceptive loss. During the rehabilitation phase, standing on both feet with closed eyes with progression to standing on one leg is an exercise to recoup proprioception. This exercise may be followed by standing and balancing on a BAPS board, which should be done initially with support from the hands. As a final-stage exercise, the athlete can progress to free standing and controlling the board through all ranges (Fig. 16-17).

OTHER TREATMENT. As noted in Chapter 17 the foot and ankle function together very closely. As the foot pronates or supinates, the ankle also rotates with the leg.[9,30] Orthotic therapy following an ankle sprain has proved very helpful in

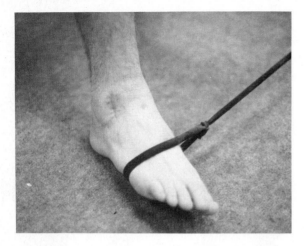

Fig. 16-15. Ankle-strengthening technique using rubber tubing.

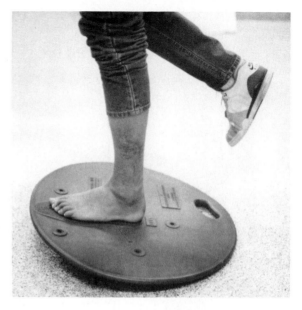

Fig. 16-17. Strengthening while free standing on a BAP board.

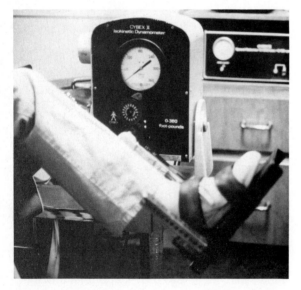

Fig. 16-16. Isokinetic strengthening using an isokinetic device.

lessening pain.[41] The author feels that this is particularly helpful following interosseous and medial sprains.

SUMMARY OF TREATMENTS FOR PHASE II

1. Range-of-motion exercises beginning with plantar flexion and dorsiflexion may be initiated early. As swelling and pain decrease, inversion and eversion may be started with manual mobilization, active exercises, or devices such as a BAPS board.
2. Strengthening may be begun as isometrics with a progression to isotonic or isokinetics as pain decreases.
3. Proprioceptive exercises may be begun early in phase II to limit proprioceptive loss.
4. Orthotic therapy may be of benefit for certain sprains.

Phase III (Return to Activity)

Estimates are that 30 to 40% of all inversion injuries result in reinjury.[11,19,20,28,36] In the past, athletes were simply returned to sports once the pain was low enough to tolerate the activity. Thanks to pioneers such as Donley, this procedure has been replaced by a gradual return to practice through a functional progression.[22] The actual process of "return to activity" is started day 1 after the injury with conditioning exercises and continued strength training on the unaffected joints. This practice not only keeps the athlete physically ready for return but also fosters a healthy mental attitude.

Stationary bicycling is a good way to maintain fitness. For lower extremity injuries that may cause pain with regular bicycling, an upper extremity ergometer is recommended. If nothing else is available, place a stationary bike on a table and have the athlete pedal it with the hands rather than the legs. Running in a pool, using a float vest, or just swimming is also good cardiovascular exercise.

As the athlete begins to progress functionally so that stress on the ankle is tolerated, several measures may be taken to protect the ankle further. Although taping does not appear to interfere with motor performance,[12,26] it does have a stabilizing effect on unstable ankles.[15,42,43] McCluskey and others[26] suggest taping the ankle and also taping the shoe onto the foot to make the shoe and ankle function as one unit. High-topped footwear may further stabilize the ankle.[17] If cleated shoes are used, cleats should be outset along the periphery of the shoe to provide stability.[26]

The athlete should have complete range of motion and 80 to 90% of preinjury strength before considering a return to the sport. This return should include a gradual progression of functional activities that slowly increase the stress on the ligament. The specific demands of each individual sport dictate the individual drills of this progression. Functional progressions may be as complex or simple as needed. The more severe the injury, the more the need for a detailed functional progression. The typical progression begins early in the rehabilitation process as the athlete becomes partially weight bearing. Full weight bearing should be started when ambulation is performed without a limp.

Running may be begun as soon as ambulation is pain free. Pain-free hopping on the affected side may also be a guideline to determine when running is appropriate. A method that allows early running is pool running. The athlete is placed in the pool in a swim vest that supports the body in water. The athlete then runs in place without touching the bottom of the pool. Proper running form should be stressed. Eventually the athlete is moved into shallow water so that more weight is placed on the ankle as running is performed. Progression is to running on a smooth, flat surface, ideally a track. Initially the athlete should jog the straights and walk the curves and then progress to jogging the entire track. Speed may be increased to a sprint in a straight line.

The cutting sequence should begin with circles of diminishing diameter. Cones may be set up for the athlete to run figure eights as the next cutting progression. The predetermined crossover or sidestep is next.[1] The athlete sprints to a predesignated spot and cuts or sidesteps abruptly. When this progression is accomplished, the cut should be done without warning on the command of another person.

The exercise progression begins with plantar flexion-dorsiflexion exercises and gradually involves inversion-eversion also. The BAP board exercises progress from sitting to standing. Jumping and hopping exercises should be started on both legs simultaneously and gradually reduced to only the injured side.

The athlete may perform on different levels for each of these functional sequences. One functional sequence may be done at half speed while another is done at full speed. An example of this is the athlete who is running full speed on straights of the track while doing figure eights at only half speed.

Once the upper levels of all the sequences are reached, the athlete may return to limited practice, which may include early teaching and fundamental drills. Finally, if full practice is tolerated without insult to the injured part, the athlete may return to competition.

SUMMARY OF TREATMENTS FOR PHASE III
1. Exercises to maintain fitness are continued in this phase.
2. Functional exercises are performed that are specific toward returning the athlete to the individual sport.

SUMMARY
1. Ankle sprains are very common. Lateral sprains are more common than medial sprains. Medial and interosseous sprains are usually more severe than lateral sprains.

2. Inversion sprains usually involve the lateral ligaments of the ankle, and eversion sprains frequently involve the medial ligaments of the ankle. Rotational injuries often involve the tibiofibular and interosseous ligaments and may be very severe.
3. Treatment of ankle sprains may be divided into an early phase, a rehabilitation phase, and a return to activity phase.
4. The early phase of treatment uses PRICE. **Protection** and **rest** include a gradual increase in stress on the healing ligament through protected weight bearing. **Ice** should be used until progress reaches a plateau. At that time heat may be initiated to see if progress resumes. **Compression** and **elevation** are essential components in reducing and preventing swelling.
5. The rehabilitative phase begins as swelling and pain lessen. The purpose of this phase is to increase strength and range. Joint mobilization, towel exercises, wedge boards, BAPS boards, tubing, and isokinetic devices may be used to accomplish this purpose. Proprioceptive exercises should be begun during this phase.
6. The return to activity phase is actually begun immediately after the injury. Conditioning exercises that do not involve the injured extremity are started as soon as possible. Before returning to the sport, the athlete should be taken through a gradual functional progression, including drills that involve cutting and mimic the sport.

REFERENCES

1 Andrews JR and others: The cutting mechanism, Am J Sports Med 5:111–121, 1977.
2 Bosien WR, Staples OS, and Russell SW: Residual disability following acute ankle sprains, J Bone Joint Surg 37A:1237, 1955.
3 Bostrum L: Treatment and prognosis in recent ligament ruptures, Acta Chir Scand 132:537–550, 1966.
4 Burgess PR and others: Signalling of kinesthetic information by peripheral sensory receptors, Ann Rev Neurosci 5:171–187, 1982.
5 Calliet R: Foot and ankle pain, Philadelphia, 1968, FA Davis Co.
6 Canoy WF: Review of medical physiology, ed 7, Los Altos, Calif, Lange Medical Publications, 1975.
7 Choi J: Acute conditions incidence and associated disability, Vital Health Statistics 120:10, 1978.
8 Cutler JM: Lateral ligamentous injuries of the ankle. In Hamilton WC, editor: Lateral ligamentous injuries of the ankle, New York, 1984, Springer-Verlag.
9 Donatelli R: Normal biomechanics of the foot and ankle, J Ortho Sports Phys Ther 7:91–95, 1985.
10 Drez D, Faust D, and Evans P: Cryotherapy and nerve palsy, Am J Sports Med 9:256–257, 1981.
11 Freeman M, Dean M, and Hanhan I: The etiology and prevention of functional instability at the foot, J Bone and Joint Surg (Br) 47:678–685, 1965.
12 Fumich RM and others: The measured effect of taping on combined foot and ankle motion before and after exercise, Am J Sports Med 9:165–169, 1981.
13 Garn SN and Newton RA: Kinesthetic awareness in subjects with multiple ankle sprains, J Am Phys Ther Assoc 68:1667–1671, 1988.
14 Garrick JG: When can I . . . ? A practical approach to rehabilitation illustrated by treatment of an ankle injury, Am J Sports Med 9:67–68, 1981.
15 Garrick JG and Requa RK: Role of external supports in the prevention of ankle sprains, Med Sci Sports 5:200, 1977.
16 Glencross D and Thornton E: Position sense following joint injury, J Sport Med Phys Fitness 21:23–27, 1981.
17 Hirata I: Proper playing conditions, J Sports Med 4:228–234, 1974.
18 Hocutt JE and others: Cryotherapy in ankle sprains, Am J Sports Med 10:316–319, 1982.
19 Isakov E and others: Response of the peroneal muscles to sudden inversion of the ankle during standing, Int J Sports Biomech 2:100–109, 1986.
20 Itay S and others: Clinical and functional status following lateral ankle sprains: followup of 90 young adults treated conservatively, Orthop Rev 11:73–76, 1982.
21 Kelikian H and Kelikian AS: Disorders of the ankle, Philadelphia, 1985, WB Saunders Co.
22 Kergerris S: The construction and implementation of functional progressions as a component of athletic rehabilitation, J Ortho Sports Phys Ther 5:14–19, 1983.
23 Klafs CE and Arnheim DD: Modern principles of athletic training, ed 2, St Louis, 1965, The CV Mosby Co.
24 Klein KK: A study of cross transfer of muscular strength and endurance resulting from progressive resistive exercises following surgery, J Assoc Phys Mental Rehab 9:5, 1955.
25 Kowal MA: Review of physiological effects of cryotherapy, J Ortho Sports Phys Ther 5:66–73, 1983.
26 McCluskey GM, Blackburn TA, and Lewis T: Prevention of ankle sprains, Am J Sports Med 4:151–157, 1976.
27 Mandelbaum BR and others: Collegiate football players with recurrent ankle sprains, Phys Sports Med 15:57–61, 1987.
28 Mayhew JL and Riner WF: Effects of ankle wrapping on motor performance, Ath Train 3:128–130, 1974.
29 Michlovitz S, Smith W, and Watkins M: Ice and high voltage pulsed stimulation in treatment of acute lateral ankle sprains, J Ortho Sports Phys Ther 9:301–304, 1988.
30 Morris JM: Biomechanics of the foot and ankle, Clin Orthop 122:10–17, 1977.

31 Nawoczenski DA and others: Objective evaluation of peroneal response to sudden inversion stress, J Ortho Sports Phys Ther 7:107–119, 1985.

32 Nicholas JA and Hershman EB: The lower extremity and spine in sports medicine, St Louis, 1986, Times Mirror/Mosby College Publishing.

33 Noyes FR: Functional properties of knee ligaments and alterations induced by immobilization: a correlative biomechanical and histological study in primates, Clin Orthop 123:210–243, 1977.

34 Quillen S: Alternative management protocol for lateral ankle sprains, J Ortho Sports Phys Ther 12:187–190, 1980.

35 Rebman LW: Ankle injuries: clinical observations, J Ortho Sports Phys Ther 8:153–156, 1986.

36 Sammarco JG: Biomechanics of foot and ankle injuries, Ath Train 10:96, 1975.

37 Sims D: Effects of positioning on ankle edema, J Ortho Sports Phys Ther 8:30–33, 1986.

38 Sloan JP, Guddings P, and Hain R: Effects of cold and compression on edema, Physician Sports Med 16:116–120, 1988.

39 Stover CN and York JM: Air stirrup management of ankle injuries in the athlete, Am J Sports Med 8:360–365, 1980.

40 Tippett SR: A case study: the need for evaluation and reevaluation of acute ankle sprains, J Ortho Sports Phys Ther 4:44, 1982.

41 Tropp H, Askling C, and Gillquist J: Prevention of ankle sprains, Am J Sports Med 13:259–266, 1985.

42 Vaes P and others: Comparative radiologic study of the influence of ankle joint bandages on ankle stability, Am J Sports Med 13:46–49, 1985.

43 Vaes P and others: Comparative radiologic study of the influence of ankle joint bandages on ankle stability, Am J Sports Med 7:110–114, 1985.

44 Yablon IG, Segal D, and Leach RE: Ankle injuries, New York, Churchill, 1983.

Rehabilitation of Foot Injuries

17

Stewart L. (Skip) Hunter

OBJECTIVES

Following completion of this chapter, the student will be able to:

- Discuss the actions of the subtalar and midtarsal joints.
- Define **pronation** and **supination.**
- Discuss the effect the position of the midtarsal joint may have on the forefoot.
- List the causes of pronation.
- Discuss the effect of forefoot varus and valgus on the foot and lower extremity.
- Describe the biomechanical examination of the foot.
- Discuss the methods by which a pronator may be recognized.
- Describe the three types of orthotics.
- Describe an orthotic fabrication.
- Discuss shoe selection in terms of pronation and supination.
- Discuss the problems associated with the foot and the treatment options for each.

Rehabilitation of injuries to the foot requires not only a proper knowledge of therapeutic modalities and exercises but also an understanding of foot biomechanics. Biomechanical understanding leads to a treatment that addresses not only the symptoms of an injury but also the underlying cause.

The foot must possess many functional components in order to function properly. It must be rigid enough to provide a lever upon which the body propels itself. Conversely, it must be adaptive enough to accommodate uneven surfaces and absorb shock during gait. To accomplish both of these tasks, the foot stays in a constant state of change during gait.[31]

The two major joints that determine the func-tional stability of the foot are the subtalar joint and the midtarsal joint.

THE SUBTALAR JOINT

The subtalar joint consists of three articulations between the talus and the calcaneus.[28] Supination and pronation are the normal movements of the subtalar joint through which it acts as a torque convertor to translate leg rotation into the foot as pronation-supination.[32,36] These movements are triplanar movements, that is, movements in all three planes that occur simultaneously.[9,21,24] In weight bearing, supination consists of the talus abducting and dorsiflexing on the calcaneus while the calcaneus inverts on the talus. Without weight bearing, supination consists of the calcaneus inverting as the talus adducts and plantar flexes. The foot itself moves into adduction, plantar flexion, and inversion in supination.[9] These movements are exactly the opposite in pronation. The foot everts, abducts, and dorsiflexes. In weight bearing, the talus adducts and plantar flexes while the calcaneus everts on the talus. Without weight bearing, the calcaneus everts as the talus abducts and dorsiflexes.[9,21]

THE MIDTARSAL JOINT

An old axiom in rehabilitation is that for distal mobility proximal stability is necessary. The function of the midtarsal joint is a prime example.

The midtarsal joint consists of two distinct joints: the calcaneocuboid and the talonavicular joint. The midtarsal joint depends mainly on ligamentous and muscular tension to maintain position and integrity. Midtarsal joint stability is directly related to the position of the subtalar joint. As the subtalar joint is supinated, the talus abducts and dorsiflexes, which raises the level of the talonavicular joint superior to that of the calcaneocuboid joint and allows lesser surface areas of both joint articulations to become congruous.[28] Also the long axes of the joints become more oblique. Both allow less motion to occur at this joint. With pronation, the talus adducts and plantar flexes and makes the joint articulations of the midtarsal joint more congruous. The long axes of the talonavicular and calcaneocuboid joints are now more parallel and thus allow more motion. The resulting foot is often referred to as a "loose bag of bones."[9,28]

As the midtarsal joint becomes more mobile or less mobile, it affects the distal portion of the foot due to the articulations at the tarsal-metatarsal joint. As more motion is allowed at the midtarsal joint, the lesser tarsal bones, particularly the first metatarsal and first cuneiform, become more mobile. These bones comprise a functional unit known as the **first ray.** With pronation of the midtarsal joint, the first ray is more mobile due to its articulations with that joint. One of the original descriptions was Morton's paper describing the now classic Morton's toe.[23] The first ray is also stabilized by the attachment of the peroneus longus tendon, which attaches to the

base of the first metatarsal. The peroneus longus tendon passes laterally around the base of the lateral malleolus and then through a notch in the cuboid to cross the foot to the first metatarsal. The cuboid functions as a pulley to increase the mechanical advantage of the peroneal tendon. Stability of the cuboid is essential in this process. In the pronated position, the cuboid loses much of its mechanical advantage as a pulley, and therefore the peroneal tendon no longer stabilizes the first ray effectively. This condition creates hypermobility of the first ray and increased pressure on the other metatarsals. Calloses under the metatarsal heads of the second and third toes are common in pronators for this reason.

These pronators often wear out the front of the running shoe under the second metatarsal (Fig. 17-1). Shoe wear patterns are commonly misinterpreted by athletes who think they must be pronators because they wear out the back outside edges of their heels. Actually, most people wear out the back outside edges of their shoes. Just before heelstrike, the anterior tibialis fires to prevent the foot from slapping forward. The anterior tibialis not only dorsiflexes the foot but also slightly inverts it, hence the wear pattern on the back edge of the shoe. The key to

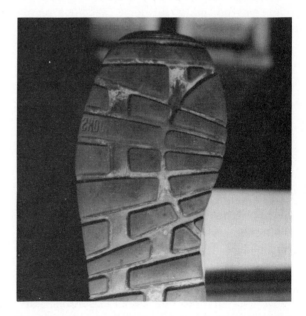

Fig. 17-1. Front forefoot of a running shoe showing the typical wear pattern of a pronator.

inspection of wear patterns on shoes is observation of the heel counter and the forefoot. Many pronators have bunions. As the hypermobility of the first ray occurs, the metatarsal heads splay apart, and the tendons attached to the toe continue to pull in a straight line. This process is one method by which a bunion is formed.

CAUSES OF PRONATION

Most of these pronatory motions occur as compensatory mechanisms for abnormal osseous relationships in the foot. Many of these deformities are the result of faulty rotation of the limb during embryology.[21] Root and others list six congenital defects of the foot that may cause pronation: (1) forefoot varus, (2) plantar flexed fifth ray, (3) fore-foot valgus, (4) lateral instability during propulsion caused by a plantar flexed fifth ray, (5) rearfoot varus, and (6) ankle joint equinus.[28]

Forefoot Varus and Valgus

Forefoot varus has been identified by Subotnick as the leading cause of pronation.[30] Its effect on the proximal foot and extremity are shown in Fig. 17-2.

Forefoot valgus causes the foot to become rigid as the midtarsal joint becomes more oblique. This foot is a poor shock absorber and may also contribute to an increased incidence of lateral ankle sprains as the foot rolls out.[32] Forefoot varus and valgus are discussed further in the examination section of this chapter.

EXAMINATION

Neutral subtalar position. The athlete should be prone with the distal third of the leg hanging off the end of the table (Fig. 17-3). A line should be drawn bisecting the leg from the start of the musculotendinous junction of the gastrocnemius to the distal portion of the calcaneus[33] (Fig. 17-4). With the athlete still prone, the sports therapist palpates the talus as the forefoot is inverted and everted. One finger should palpate the talus at the anterior aspect of the fibula and another finger at the anterior portion of the medial malleolus (Fig. 17-5). The position at which the talus is equally prominent on both sides is considered neutral subtalar position.[15] Root and others[28] describe this as the position of the subtalar joint

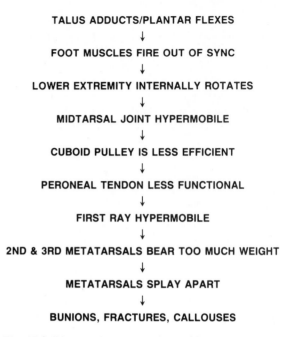

TALUS ADDUCTS/PLANTAR FLEXES
↓
FOOT MUSCLES FIRE OUT OF SYNC
↓
LOWER EXTREMITY INTERNALLY ROTATES
↓
MIDTARSAL JOINT HYPERMOBILE
↓
CUBOID PULLEY IS LESS EFFICIENT
↓
PERONEAL TENDON LESS FUNCTIONAL
↓
FIRST RAY HYPERMOBILE
↓
2ND & 3RD METATARSALS BEAR TOO MUCH WEIGHT
↓
METATARSALS SPLAY APART
↓
BUNIONS, FRACTURES, CALLOUSES

Fig. 17-2. Diagram illustrating the problems associated with forefoot varus.

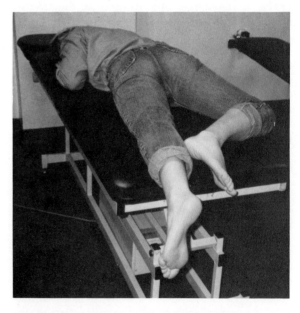

Fig. 17-3. Examination position for neutral position.

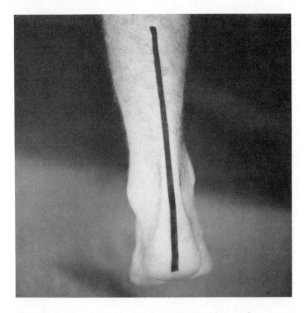

Fig. 17-4. Line bisecting the gastrocnemius and posterior calcaneus.

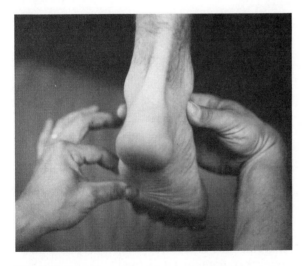

Fig. 17-5. Palpation of the talus to determine neutral.

where it is neither pronated or supinated. It is the standard position in which the foot should be placed in order to examine deformities of the foot.[24] In this position, the lines on the lower leg and calcaneus should form a straight line. Any variance is considered to be a rearfoot valgus or varus deformity. The most common deformity of the foot is a rearfoot varus deformity.[22] A deviation of 2 to 3 degrees is normal.[35]

Another method of determining subtalar neutral involves the lines that were drawn previously on the leg and back of the heel. With the athlete prone, the heel is swung into full eversion and inversion, with measurements taken at each. Angles of the two lines are taken at each extreme. Neutral position is considered two-thirds away from maximum inversion or one-third away from maximum eversion. The normal foot pronates 6 to 8 degrees from neutral.[28] For example, from neutral position a foot inverts 27 degrees and everts 3 degrees. The position at which this foot is neither pronated nor supinated is that point at which the calcaneus is inverted 7 degrees.

Forefoot-rearfoot relationship. Once the subtalar joint is placed in neutral, mild dorsiflexion should be initiated while observing the metatarsal heads in relation to the plantar surface of the calcaneus. Forefoot varus is an osseous deformity in which the medial metatarsal heads are inverted in relation to the plane of the calcaneus (Fig. 17-6). Forefoot varus is the most common cause of excessive pronation, according to Subotnick.[30] Forefoot valgus is a position in which the lateral metatarsals are everted in relation to the rearfoot (Fig. 17-7). These forefoot deformities are benign in a non-weight-bearing position, but in stance the foot or metatarsal heads must somehow get to the floor to bear weight. This movement is accomplished by the talus rolling down and in and the calcaneus everting for a forefoot varus. For the forefoot valgus, the calcaneus inverts and the talus abducts and dorsiflexes. McPoil and others[22] report that forefoot valgus is the most common forefoot deformity in their sample group.

Minimal osseous deformities of the forefoot have little effect on the function of the foot. When either forefoot varus or forefoot valgus is too large, the foot compensates through abnormal

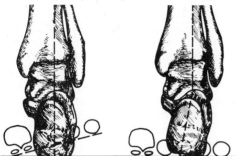

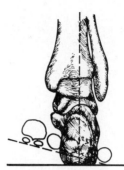

A   NEUTRAL   WEIGHT-BEARING

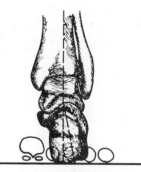

A   NEUTRAL   WEIGHT-BEARING

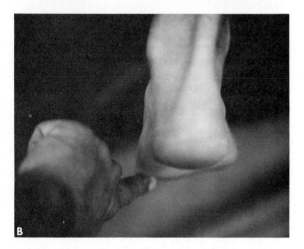

Fig. 17-6. Forefoot varus: **A**, right foot; **B**, left foot.

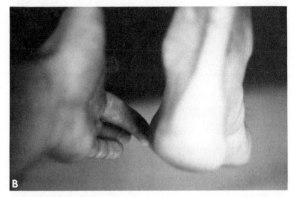

Fig. 17-7. Forefoot valgus: **A**, right foot; **B**, left foot.

movements in order to bear weight.

Extrinsic Factors

Several structural deformities originating outside the foot itself also require compensation by the foot in order for a proper weight-bearing position to be attained. Tibial varum is the common bowleg deformity.[21] The distal tibia is medial to the proximal tibia[11] (Fig. 17-8). This measurement is taken weight bearing with the foot in neutral.[35] The angle of deviation of the distal tibia from a perpendicular line from the calcaneal midline is considered tibial varum.[11]

Tibial varum increases pronation to allow proper foot function.[4] At heel strike the calcaneus must evert in order to attain a perpendicular position.[32]

Ankle joint equinus is another extrinsic deformity that may require abnormal compensation. It may be considered an extrinsic or intrinsic problem.

During normal gait, the tibia must move anterior to the talar dome.[21] Approximately 10 degrees of dorsiflexion is required for this movement[32] (Fig. 17-9). Lack of dorsiflexion may cause compensatory pronation of the foot with resultant foot and lower extremity pain. Often this lack of dorsiflexion is the result of tightness of the posterior leg muscles. Other causes include forefoot equinus, in which the plane of the forefoot is below the plane of the rearfoot.[32] It occurs in many high-arched feet. This deformity has the effect of requiring more ankle dorsiflexion. When enough dorsiflexion is not available at the ankle, the additional movement is required at other sites, such as dorsiflexion of the midtarsal joint and rotation of the leg.

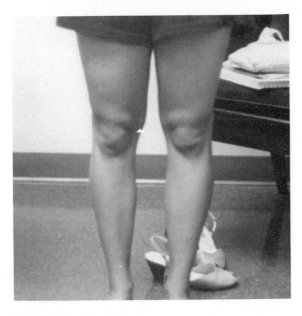

Fig. 17-8. Bowleg deformity.

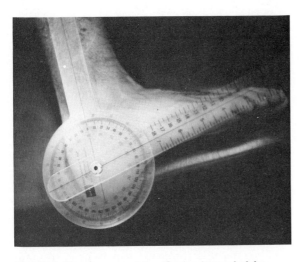

Fig. 17-9. Ten degrees of dorsiflexion is needed for proper ambulation.

IDENTIFICATION OF PRONATORS

An accurate biomechanical analysis of the foot and lower extremity should identify those deformities that require abnormal compensatory movements. Several extrinsic keys may be observed that indicate pronation.[28] Excessive eversion of the calcaneus during the stance phase indicates pronation (Fig. 17-10). Excessive or prolonged internal rotation of the tibia is another sign of pronation. This internal rotation may cause increased symptoms in the shin or knee, especially in repetitive sports such as running. A lowering of the medial arch accompanies pronation. It may be measured as the navicular differential,[8] the difference between the height of the navicular tuberosity from the floor in a non-weight-bearing position versus a weight-bearing position (Fig. 17-11). As previously discussed, the talus plantar flexes and adducts with pronation. It may be seen as a medial bulging of the talar head (Fig. 17-12). This same talar adduction causes increased concavity below the lateral malleolus in a posterior view as the calcaneus everts[21] (Fig. 17-13).

ORTHOTICS

Almost any problem of the lower extremity appears at one time to have been treated by orthotic therapy. The use of orthotics in control of foot deformities has been argued for many years.*

The normal foot functions most efficiently when no deformities are present that predispose it to injury or exacerbate existing injuries. Orthotics are used to control abnormal compensatory movements of the foot by "bringing the floor to the foot."

The foot functions most efficiently in neutral. By providing support so that the foot does not have to move abnormally, an orthotic should help prevent compensatory problems. For problems that have already occurred, the orthotic provides a platform of support so that soft tissues can heal properly without undue stress.

Basically there are three types of orthotics:[18,32]

1. Pads and soft flexible supports of felt (Fig.

---

*References 2,6,7,12,15,27,30,32,36.

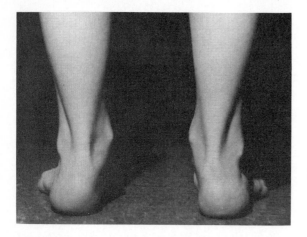

Fig. 17-10. Eversion of the calcaneus indicating pronation.

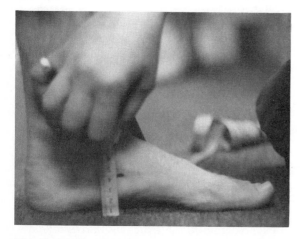

Fig. 17-11. Measurement of the navicular differential.

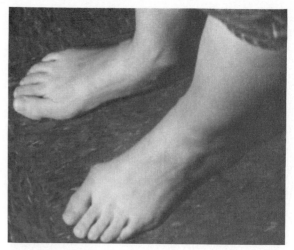

Fig. 17-12. Medial bulge of the talar head indicating pronation.

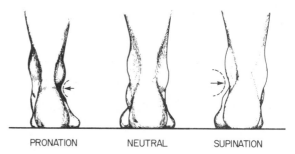

PRONATION   NEUTRAL   SUPINATION

Fig. 17-13. Concavity below the lateral malleolus indicating pronation.

17-14). These soft inserts are readily fabricated and are advocated for mild overuse syndromes. Pads are particularly useful in shoes such as spikes and ski boots that are too narrow to hold orthotics.

2. Semirigid orthotics made of flexible thermoplastics, rubber, or leather (Fig. 17-15). These orthotics are prescribed for athletes who have increased symptoms. These orthotics are molded from a neutral cast. They are well tolerated by athletes who require speed or jumping in their sports.

3. Functional or rigid orthotics are made from

hard plastic and also require neutral casting (Fig. 17-16). These orthotics allow control for most overuse symptoms.

Despite arguments in the literature, the author has found orthotic therapy to be of tremendous value in the treatment of many lower extremity problems. This view is supported in the literature by several clinical studies. Donatelli and others[10] not only found that 96% of their patients reported pain relief from orthotics but that 52% would not leave home without the devices in their shoes. McPoil and others[20] found that orthotics were an important treatment for valgus forefoot deformities only. Riegler[26] reported that 80% of his patients experienced at least a 50%

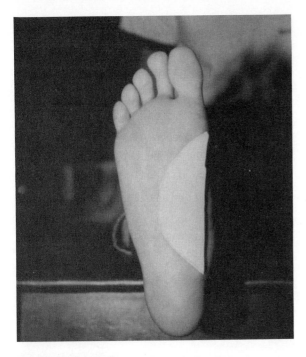

Fig. 17-14. Felt pads.

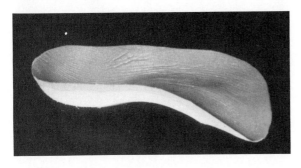

Fig. 17-15. Semirigid orthotics.

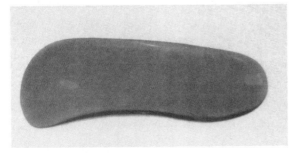

Fig. 17-16. Hard orthotic.

improvement with orthotics. This same study reported improvements in sports performance with orthotics. Hunt[14] reported decreased muscular activity with orthotics.

Orthotic Fabrication

Many sports therapists make a neutral mold, put it in a box, mail it to an orthotic laboratory, and several weeks later receive an orthotic back in the mail. Others like to complete the entire orthotic from start to finish, which requires a much more skilled technician than the mail-in method as well as approximately $1,000 in equipment and supplies. The obvious advantage is cost if many orthotics are to be made.

No matter which method is chosen, the first step is the fabrication of the neutral mold, done with the patient in the same position used to determine subtalar neutral. Once subtalar neutral is found, three layers of plaster splints are applied to the plantar surface and sides of the foot (Fig. 17-17). Subtalar neutral is maintained as pressure is applied on the fifth metatarsal area in a dorsiflexion direction until the midtarsal joint is locked (Fig. 17-18). This position is held until the plaster dries. At this point the plaster cast may be sent out to have the orthotic made or it may be finished (Fig. 17-19). If it is mailed out, the appropriate measurements of forefoot and rearfoot positions should be sent, along with any extrinsic measurements.

If the orthotic is to be fabricated in-house, the plaster cast should be liberally lined interiorly with talc or powder. Plaster of paris should then be poured into the cast to form a positive mold of the foot (Fig. 17-20).

Many different materials may be used to fabricate an orthotic from the positive mold. The author uses eighth-inch Aliplast (Alimed Inc., Boston) covering with a quarter-inch Plastazote underneath. A rectangular piece of each material large enough to encompass completely the lower third of the mold is cut. These two pieces are placed in a convection oven (Fig. 17-21) at approximately 275° F. At this temperature the two materials bond together and become moldable in about 5 to 7 minutes. At this time the orthotic materials are removed from the oven and placed on the positive mold (Fig. 17-22). Ideally a form or vacuum press should be used to form the orthotic to the mold.

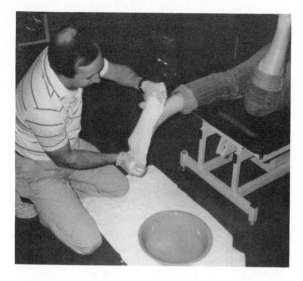

Fig. 17-17. Three layers of plaster form neutral mold.

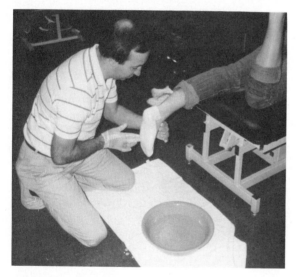

Fig. 17-18. Mild pressure over the fifth metatarsal to lock the midtarsal joint.

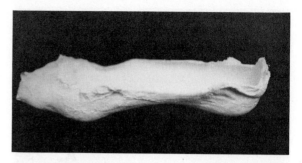

Fig. 17-19. Neutral mold.

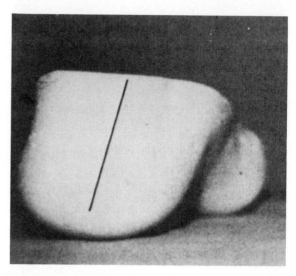

Fig. 17-20. Positive mold.

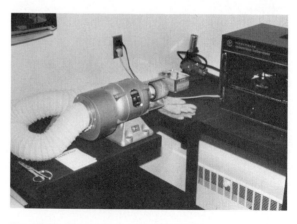

Fig. 17-21. Convection oven and grinder.

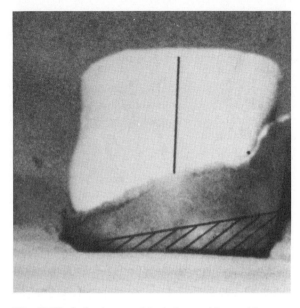

Fig. 17-22. Orthotic material on the positive mold.

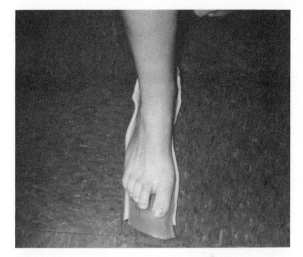

Fig. 17-23. Orthotic mold under the foot with patient sitting.

Once cooled, the uncut orthotic is placed under the foot as the athlete sits in a chair (Fig. 17-23). Excess material is then trimmed from the sides of the orthotic with scissors. Any material that can be seen protruding from either side of the foot should be trimmed (Fig. 17-24) to provide the proper width of the orthotic. The length should be trimmed so that the end of the orthotic bisects the metatarsal heads (Fig. 17-25). This style is slightly longer than most orthotics are made, but the author has found that this length provides better comfort.

Next a third layer of medial Plastazote may be glued to the arch to fill that area to the floor.

Grinding begins with the sides of the orthotic, which should be ground so that the sides are slightly beveled inward (Fig. 17-26) to allow better shoe fit. The bottom of the orthotic is leveled so that the surface is perpendicular to the bisection of the calcaneus. Grinding is continued until very little Plastazote remains under the Aliplast at the heel. The forefoot is posted by selectively grinding Plastazote just proximal to the metatarsal heads. Forefoot varus is posted by grinding more laterally than medially. Forefoot valgus requires grinding more medially than laterally. The final step is to grind the distal portion of the orthotic so that only a very thin piece of

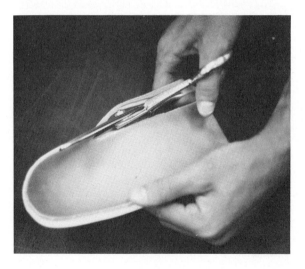

Fig. 17-24. Trim excess material from orthotic.

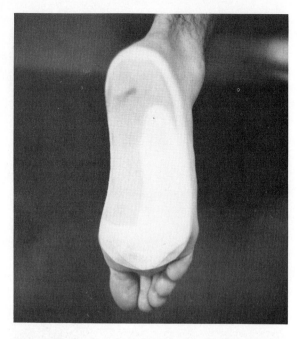

Fig. 17-25. The length of the orthotic should bisect the metatarsal heads.

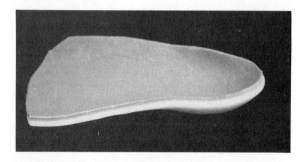

Fig. 17-26. Sides of the orthotic should be beveled inward.

Aliplast is under the area where the orthotic ends. This prevents discomfort under the forefoot where the orthotic stops. If the athlete feels that this area is a problem, a full insole of Spenco or other material may be used to cover the orthotic to the end of the shoe to eliminate the drop off sometimes felt as the orthotic ends.

Time must be allowed for proper break-in. The athlete should wear the orthotic for 3 to 4 hours the first day, 6 to 8 hours the next day, and then all day on the third day. Sports activities should be started in the orthotic only after it has been worn all day for several days.

SHOE SELECTION

The shoe is one of the biggest considerations in treating a problem of the foot. Even a properly made orthotic is less effective if placed in a poorly constructed shoe.

As noted, pronation is a problem of hypermobility. Pronated feet need stability and firmness to reduce this excess movement. Research indicates that shoe compression may actually increase pronation versus a barefoot condition.[1] The ideal shoe for a pronated foot is less flexible and has good rearfoot control.

Conversely, supinated feet are usually very rigid. Increased cushion and flexibility benefit this type of foot. Several construction factors may influence the firmness and stability of a shoe. The basic form upon which a shoe is built is called the *last*.[1] The upper is fitted onto a last in several ways. Each method has its own flexibility and control characteristics. A slip-lasted shoe is sewn together like a moccasin (Fig. 17-27) and is very flexible. Board lasting provides a piece of fiberboard upon which the upper is attached (Fig. 17-28), which provides a very firm, inflexible base for the shoe. A combination-lasted shoe is boarded in the back half of the shoe and slip lasted in the front (Fig. 17-29), which provides rearfoot stability with forefoot mobility. The shape of the last may also be used in shoe selection. Most pronators perform better in a straight-lasted shoe,[1] that is, a shoe in which the forefoot does not curve inward in relation to the rearfoot.

Midsole design also affects the stability of a shoe. The midsole separates the upper from the outsole.[5] Ethylene vinyl acetate (EVA) is one of the most commonly used materials in the midsole.[25] Often denser EVA, which is colored differently to show that it is denser, is placed under the medial aspect of the foot in order to control pronation (Fig. 17-30).

In an effort to control rearfoot movement, many shoe manufacturers have reinforced the heel counter both internally and externally, often in the form of extra plastic along the outside of the heel counter[19] (Fig. 17-31).

Other factors that may affect the performance

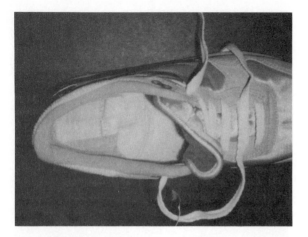

Fig. 17-27. Slip-lasted shoe.

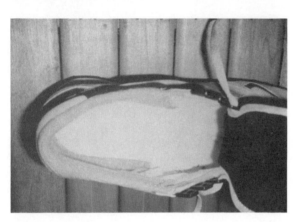

Fig. 17-28. Board-lasted shoe.

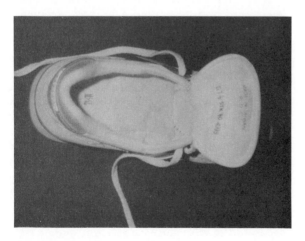

Fig. 17-29. Combination-lasted shoe.

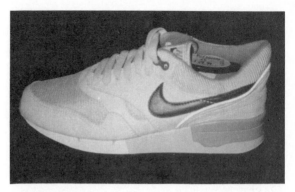

Fig. 17-30. EVA in a midsole.

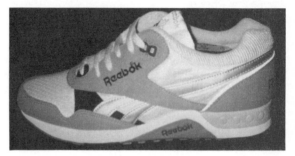

External heel counter.

of a shoe are the outsole contour and composition, lacing systems, and forefoot wedges.

PATHOLOGIES OF THE FOOT

Many of the problems of the foot are biomechanically related. The symptoms of these biomechanical problems may be shown in the foot or lower extremity. Even trauma-induced injuries to the foot may be treated by orthotic therapy as well as modalities and exercises.

Bunions

A bunion is a deformity of the head of the first metatarsal in which the large toe takes a valgus position[17] (Fig. 17-32). Many bunions are the result of a biomechanical fault that causes a hypermobility of the first ray segment. Often a neutral orthotic that increases the weight-bearing properties of the first ray significantly reduces the symptoms and progressions of a bunion.[32]

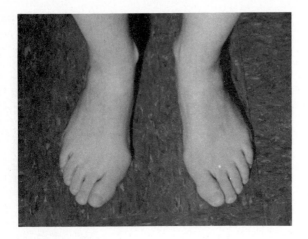

Fig. 17-32. Bunion.

Shoe selection may also play an important role in the treatment of bunions. Shoes of the proper width cause less irritation to the bunion area, especially if exostosis is involved from a chronic bunion. Local therapy including moist heat, soaks, and ultrasound may alleviate some of the acute symptoms of a bunion. Protective devices such as wedges, pads, and tape can also be used.[17]

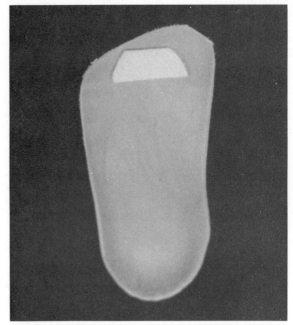

Fig. 17-33. Metatarsal bar.

Neuroma

A neuroma is a neuromatous mass about the nerve sheath of the common plantar nerve as it divides into the two digital branches to adjacent toes. It occurs most commonly between the metatarsal heads and is the most common nerve problem of the lower extremity. A neuroma may occur in any metatarsal space, but the most common site is the third interspace.[32] Orthotic therapy is essential to reduce the shearing movements of the metatarsal heads. To increase this effect, often a bar is placed just proximal to the metatarsal heads in an attempt to have these splay apart with weight bearing (Fig. 17-33). It may decrease pressure on the affected area. The author has used phonophoresis with hydrocortisone with some success in symptom reduction. Shoe selection also plays an important role in treatment of neuromas. Narrow shoes, particularly women's shoes that are pointed in the toe area and certain men's boots, may squeeze the

metatarsal heads together and exacerbate the problem. A shoe that is wide in the toe box area should be selected. A straight-laced shoe often provides increased space in the toe box.[29]

Turf Toe

Turf toe is a hyperextension injury of the great toe, either from repetitive overuse or trauma.[34] Many of these injuries occur on unyielding synthetic turf, although it can occur on grass also. The author believes that many of these injuries occur because artificial turf shoes often are more flexible and allow more dorsiflexion of the great toe. Some shoe companies have addressed this problem by adding steel or other materials to the forefoot of their turf shoes in order to stiffen them. Flat insoles that have thin sheets of steel under the forefoot are also available. When commercially made products are not available, a thin, flat piece of Orthoplast may be placed under the shoe insole or may be molded to the foot.[34] Taping the toe to prevent dorsiflexion may be done separately or with one of the shoe stiffening suggestions (Fig. 17-34).

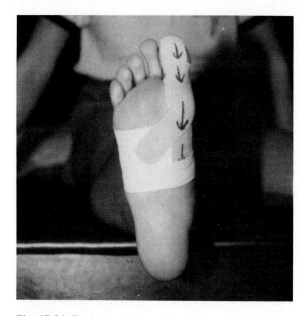

Fig. 17-34. Turf toe taping.

Modalities of choice include ice and ultrasound. One of the major ingredients in any treatment for turf toe is rest. The athlete should be discouraged from returning to activity until the toe is pain free.

Plantar Fasciitis

Heel pain is a very common problem in the athletic and nonathletic population. This phenomenon has been blamed on several etiologies, including heel spurs, plantar fascia irritation, and bursitis. Plantar fasciitis is a catchall term that is commonly used to describe pain in the proximal arch and heel.

The complaints are similar: pain in the medial arch and medial distal heel early that moves to a more central or lateral distribution in the late course of the problem. This pain is particularly troublesome upon arising in the morning or upon bearing weight after sitting for a long period. Orthotic therapy is very useful in the treatment of this problem. The author has found that soft orthotics in combination with exercises can significantly reduce the pain level of these patients.

A soft orthotic works better than a hard orthotic. An extra-deep heel cup should be built into the orthotic. The orthotic should be worn at all times, especially upon arising from bed in the morning. Always have the athlete step into the orthotic rather than ambulating barefooted. When soft orthotics are not feasible, taping may reduce the symptoms. A simple arch taping or alternative taping often allows pain-free ambulation.[38]

Vigorous heelcord stretching should be used, along with an exercise to stretch the plantar fascia in the arch. The old-fashioned exercise of rolling the arch over a rolling pin accomplishes this. The athlete should be cautioned not to roll over the heel area, which usually exacerbates the problem. Another stretch is the use of the "windless" mechanism by controlled dorsiflexion of the talocrural joint and extension of the MP joints. Exercises that increase dorsiflexion of the great toe also may be of benefit to this problem.

Cuboid Subluxation

Another problem that often mimics plantar fasciitis is cuboid subluxation. Pronation and trauma have been reported to be prominent causes of this syndrome.[37] This displacement of the cuboid causes pain along the fourth and fifth metatarsals as well as over the cuboid. The author has found this problem often refers pain to the heel area as well. Many times this pain is increased upon arising after a prolonged nonweight-bearing period. Dramatic treatment results may be obtained by manipulation to restore the cuboid to its natural position. The manipulation is done with the athlete prone (Fig. 17-35). The plantar aspect of the forefoot is grasped by the thumbs with the fingers supporting the dorsum of the foot. The thumbs should be over the cuboid. The manipulation should be a thrust downward to move the cuboid into its more dorsal position. Often a pop is felt as the cuboid moves back into place. Once the cuboid is manipulated, an orthotic often helps to support it in its proper position.

Tarsal Tunnel Syndrome

The tarsal tunnel is a loosely defined area about the medial malleolus that is bordered by the lanciniate ligament, which binds the tibial nerve.[13] Pronation, overuse problems such as tendonitis,

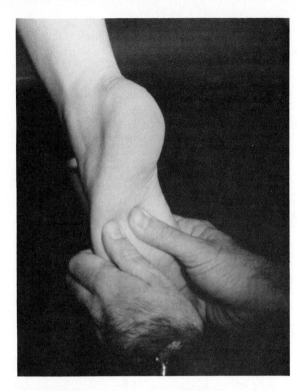

Fig. 17-35. Prone position for cuboid manipulation.

and trauma may cause neurovascular problems in the ankle and foot. Symptoms may vary, with pain, numbness, and paresthesia reported along the medial ankle and into the sole of the foot.[3] Tenderness may be present over the tibial nerve area behind the medial malleolus. Neutral foot control may alleviate symptoms in less involved cases. Surgery is often performed if symptoms do not respond to conservative treatment or weakness occurs in the flexors of the toes.[3]

SUMMARY

1. The foot changes in gait to provide for forward movement, adapt to uneven terrain, and absorb shock.
2. The subtalar and midtarsal joints contribute significantly to the stability of the foot. Dysfunction at either joint may have a profound effect on the foot and lower extremity.
3. Certain intrinsic and extrinsic deformities may cause dysfunction at the subtalar and midtarsal joints.

4. Examination of the foot should focus on intrinsic and extrinsic deformities of the foot.
5. Pronators may be identified by several extrinsic keys.
6. Orthotics may be of great benefit in the treatment of biomechanical problems of the foot and leg. Neutral casting is essential for the production of an orthotic whether it is to be produced in-house or by someone else.
7. Shoe selection is an important parameter in the treatment of foot problems. Various shoe components may dictate the type of foot that a shoe best suits.
8. Of the many possible pathologies in the foot, many may be treated by orthotic therapy as well as by modalities and exercise.

REFERENCES

1 Baer T: Designing for the long run, Mech Eng, pp 67–75, Sept 1984.
2 Bates BT and others: Foot orthotic devices to modify selected aspects of lower extremity mechanics, Am J Sports Med 7:338, 1979.
3 Birnham JS: The musculoskeletal manual, 1982, Academic Press.
4 Brody DM: Techniques in the evaluation and treatment of the injured runner, Orthop Clin North Am 13:541, 1982.
5 Brunwick T and Wischnia B: Battle of the midsoles, Runners World, p 47, April 1987.
6 Cavanaugh PR and others: An evaluation of the effects of orthotics force distribution and rearfoot movement during running. Paper presented at the meeting of the American Orthopedic Society for Sports Medicine, meeting, Lake Placid, N.Y., 1978.
7 Collona P: Fabrication of a custom molded orthotic using an intrinsic posting technique for a forefoot varus deformity, Physical Therapy Forum 8(5):3, 1989.
8 Delacerda FG: A study of anatomical factors involved in shinsplints, J Ortho Sports Phys Ther 2:55–59, 1980.
9 Donatelli R: Normal biomechanics of the foot and ankle, J Ortho Sports Phys Ther 7:91–95, 1985.
10 Donatelli R and others: Biomechanical foot orthotics: a retrospective study, J Ortho Sports Phys Ther 10:205–212, 1988.
11 Giallonardo LM: Clinical evaluation of foot and ankle dysfunction, Phys Ther 68:1850–1856, 1988.
12 Gill E: Orthotics, Runners World, pp 55–57, Feb 1985.
13 Hoppenfield S: Physical examination of the spine and extremities, New York, 1976, Appleton-Century-Crofts.
14 Hunt G: Examination of lower extremity dysfunction. In Gould J and Davies G, editors: Orthopedic and sports physical therapy, vol 2, St Louis, 1985, The CV Mosby Co.
15 James SL: Chondromalacia of the patella in the adolescent. In Kennedy SC, editor: The injured adolescent, Baltimore, 1979, Williams & Wilkins.

16 James SL, Bates BT, and Osternig LR: Injuries to runners, Am J Sports Med 6:43, 1978.

17 Klafs CE and Arnheim DK: Modern principles of athletic training, ed 5, St Louis, 1981, The CV Mosby Co.

18 Lockard MA: Foot orthoses, Phys Ther 68:1866–1873, 1988.

19 McPoil TG: Footwear, Phys Ther 68:1857–1865, 1988.

20 McPoil TG, Adrian M, and Pidcoe P: Effects of foot orthoses on center of pressure patterns in women, Phys Ther 69:149–154, 1989.

21 McPoil TG and Brocato RS: The foot and ankle: biomechanical evaluation and treatment. In Gould J and Davies G, editors: Orthopedic and sports physical therapy, St Louis, 1985, The CV Mosby Co.

22 McPoil TG, Knecht HG, and Schmit D: A survey of foot types in normal females between the ages of 18 and 30 years, J Ortho Sports Phys Ther 9:406–409, 1988.

23 Morton DJ: Foot disorders in general practice, JAMA 109:1112–1119, 1937.

24 Oatis CA: Biomechanics of the foot and ankle under static conditions, Phys Ther 68:1815–1821, 1988.

25 Pagliano JN: Athletic footwear, Sports Med Digest 10:1–2, 1988.

26 Riegler HF: Orthotic devices for the foot, Orthop Rev 16:293–303, 1987.

27 Rogers MM and LeVeau BF: Effectiveness of foot orthotic devices used to modify pronation in runners, J Ortho Sports Phys Ther 4:86–90, 1982.

28 Root ML, Orien WP, and Weed JH: Normal and abnormal functions of the foot, Los Angeles, 1977, Clinical Biomechanics Corp.

29 Sims DS, Cavanaugh PR, and Ulbrecht JS: Risk factors in the diabetic foot, Phys Ther 68:1887–1901, 1988.

30 Subotnick SI: The flat foot, Physician Sports Med 9:85–91, 1981.

31 Subotnick SI: The running foot doctor, Mt Vias, Calif, 1977, World Publications.

32 Subotnick SI and Newell SG: Podiatric sports medicine, Mt Kisko, N.Y., 1975, Futura Publishing Co.

33 Tiberio D: Pathomechanics of structural foot deformities, Phys Ther 68:1840–1849, 1988.

34 Visnich AL: A playing orthoses for "turf toe," Ath Train 22:215, 1987.

35 Vogelbach WD and Combs LC: A biomechanical approach to the management of chronic lower extremity pathologies as they relate to excessive pronation, Ath Train 22:6–16, 1987.

36 Williams JGP: The foot and chondromalacia—a case of biomechanical uncertainty, J Ortho Sports Phys Ther 2:50–51, 1980.

37 Woods A and Smith W: Cuboid syndrome and the techniques used for treatment, Ath Train 18:64–65, 1983.

38 Zylks DR: Alternative taping for plantar fasciitis, Ath Train 22:317, 1987.

Index

A

AAROM; *see* Active-assisted range of motion

ABCs of emergency care, 92

Abdomen, life-threatening injury and, 92

Abdominal muscle, 266

Abuse of drugs, testing for, 148

AC; *see* Acromioclavicular joint

Acceptance, phases of injury and, 111-112

Accessory motion, 65, 66

Ace wrap
   ankle compression and, 333
   elbow injuries and, 234
   initial management of injuries and, 14

Acetaminophen, 140, 141, 143

Achilles tendon
   neurology and, 161
   retrocalcaneobursitis and, 326
   rupture of, 323-324
   tendonitis and, 321-323
   third-degree strain and, 10

Acid, lactic, 10

ACL; *see* Anterior cruciate ligament

Acromioclavicular joint, 207-208

ACTH; *see* Adrenocorticotropic hormone

Actin filament, 36

Active motion
   low back examination and, 156-158
   lower leg reconditioning and, 316-317
   off-field evaluation protocol and, 103
   painful arc and, 63

Active range of motion; *see* Range of motion

Active-assisted range of motion, 29

Active-assisted wrist extension, 253

Acustim (electroacutherapy), 124

Acute compartment syndrome, 327

Acute injury, 132-134

Adenosine triphosphate, 55-56

Adhesion, ligamentous, 64

Adhesive capsulitis, 224-225

Adipose tissue
   energy source and, 56
   tissue type of, 3

Adrenocorticotropic hormone, 124

Aerobic activity, examples of, 57
   metabolism and, 56

Afferent fiber, 123

Age
   Achilles tendon rupture and, 323
   anterior cruciate ligament and, 298-299

Age—cont'd
   impeded healing and, 20
   maximal heart rate and, 53-54, 57-58
   muscle strength and, 37-38

Agonist muscle, 49, 51

Agonist pattern, 69-70

Air compression, Jobst intermittent, 334

Airway, life-threatening injury and, 92

AL; *see* Anatomic limit of motion

Alcohol, respiratory tract and, 144

Aliplast mold, orthotics and, 349

Alka-Seltzer, 146

Allergy
   cryotherapy and, 130
   diarrhea and, 146
   drugs affecting respiratory tract and, 143-144

Anaerobic glycolosis, 56

Anaerobic metabolism, 56

Analgesia
   common, 140-141
   hyperstimulation, 124
   infrared modalities and, 129-130

Anatomic limit of motion, 66-67

Anesthetic, local, 125

Anger, phases of injury and, 111

Angioedema, 143

Angle, joint; *see* Joint angle

Ankle, 331-341
   mechanisms of injury and, 331
   sprains and, 332-340
      elevation and, 14
      phase I of rehabilitation and, 332-334
      phase II of rehabilitation and, 334-338
      phase III (return to activity) and, 338-339

Ankle extensor, 327

Ankle joint equinus, 346

Ankle stirrup, 332

Ankle weight, 317-318

Ankylosing spondylitis, 166

Antacid, 145-146

Antagonist muscle, 49, 51

Antagonist pattern, 70

Anterior compartment, 327

Anterior cruciate ligament, 298-301, 306

Anterior inferior iliac spine, 269

Anterior instability, glenoid labrum tear and, 215

Anterior shin splint, 325

Anterior superior iliac spine
   hip pointer and, 265-268
   low back examination and, 155
Anterior talofibular ligament, 331; *see also* Ankle
Anterior tibialis, 343-344
Anterior view, low back examination and, 155-156
Antibiotic medication, 147
Antidiarrheal medication, 146
Antiemetic, 146
Antihistamine, 141, 143-144
Antiinflammatory drug
   common, 140-141
   elbow injuries and, 235
Antipyretic, 140-141
Antitussive, expectorants and, 144-145
Anxiety, injury and; *see* Psychology
Apprehension test, 104
Approximation, proprioceptive neuromuscular facilitation
     and, 72
Arc, painful, 103
Arm, 10; *see also* Elbow; Hand; Shoulder; Wrist
AROM; *see* Active range of motion
Arterial spasm, 130
Artery, radial, 57
Arthritis, osteoarthrosis and, 12
Arthrokinematic principles, 65
Arthroscopic shoulder reconstruction, 214
Arthrosis, osteoarthrosis and, 12
ASIS; *see* Anterior superior iliac spine
Aspirin
   coagulation and, 140
   tenosynovitis and, 11
Assessment-reassessment, low back and, 152, 153
Asthma, 143, 145
Asymmetrical spinal musculature, 155
Athlete/sports therapist relationship, 115-116
ATP; *see* Adenosine triphosphate
Atrophy
   high-frequency AC current and, 125
   impeded healing and, 19
Autogenic inhibition
   proprioceptive neuromuscular facilitation and, 69-70
   stretching and, 51
Automatic reflex joint control, 240
Avulsion fracture
   characteristics of, 7
   femoral fractures and, 285
   hamstring injuries and, 279-280
Axillary nerve contusion, 227-228

B

Back, low; *see* Low back
Baking soda, 145, 146
Ballistic stretching, 49-50, 51
Bandage, Ace; *see* Ace wrap
Bankart lesion, 215, 216
Bankart procedure, 211
Banned substance, 148

BAPS board, 336, 337, 338
Barbell, 40-41
Basal metabolic rate, 26
Baseball
   hamate injury and, 252
   sport-specific exercise and, 254, 257
Bath, contrast, 130
Benzonatate, 144
Berger's adjustment technique, 45, 46
Beta-endorphin, 124
Bicarbonate of soda, 145
Biceps tendon, 218-219
Bicipital tendonitis, 223
Bicycle, stationary
   ankle rehabilitation and, 334, 339
   interval training and, 58
   lower leg rehabilitation and, 320
Bilateral compartment syndrome, 327-328
Bilateral exercise, shoulder reconditioning and, 194
Bladder, low back examination and, 154-155
Bleeding
   common analgesics and, 140
   contusion and, 12
   severe bursitis and, 273, 274
Blocker, H1/H2 receptor, 143
Blood
   coagulation and, 15, 140
   oxygen transport and, 52-53
   pooling of, 14
   tissue type of, 3
Blood pressure
   cardiac output and, 55
   strength training and, 40
   thermotherapy and, 130
Blood supply
   cardiac output and, 54, 55
   cryotherapy and, 130
   epithelial tissue and, 3
   hand injuries and, 255
Blood vessel, oxygen transport and, 52-53
Blowout fracture, 6
BMR; *see* Basal metabolic rate
Board, wedge, ankle rehabilitation and, 334, 335, 336
Bobath method three, 70
Body, mind and; *see* Psychology
Body composition, preparticipation examination and,
     90-91
Body size, sexual differences and, 46-47
Body weight
   low back examination and, 154-155
   maximal oxygen consumption and, 53
   Sander's program and, 44, 45
Bone
   calcium supplementation and, 145
   characteristics and types of, 5-6
   constant remodeling of, 328
   cuboid, 343
   flexibility and, 47

Bone—cont'd
    healing of, 20-21
    osteoarthrosis and, 12
    periosteum and, 127
    tissue type of, 3
Bone scan, stress fractures of lower leg and, 329
Bone spur, 12-13
Bosworth screw fixation, shoulder sprains and, 208
Boutonniere deformity, 255, 260
Bowel, low back examination and, 154-155
Bowleg deformity, 346, 347
Boxer's fracture, 258
Brace, ankle, 332
Brachial plexus, 228
Brainstem, pain control system and, 124
Breathing, life-threatening injury and, 92
Bronchial muscle, drugs and, 143
Bronchial obstruction, drugs for, 145
Bronchodilator, asthma and, 145
Bruise; *see* Contusion
Brunnstrom Method 4, 70
Bunion, 353-354
    pronation and, 344
Bursa, characteristics of, 11; *see also* Bursitis
Bursitis
    hip and thigh injury and, 273-275
    ice and, 14
    musculoskeletal injuries and, 11-12
    piriformis syndrome sciatica and, 270
    shoulder and, 224
Butterfly exercise, 198
Buttocks
    low back examination and, 153
    piriformis syndrome sciatica and, 270, 272

C

Calcaneocuboid joint, 343
Calcaneofibular ligament, 331
Calcaneus
    Achilles tendon rupture and, 323
    pronation and, 344-345
    subtalar joint and, 342-343
Calcium
    flexibility and, 47
    supplementation of, 145
Calcium deposit, 12
Calf, assessing sciatica and, 272
Calisthenics, 58
Caloric intake, 26
Cancellous bone, 5
Cancer, low-power laser and, 131-132
Cane exercise, shoulder reconditioning and, 194
Capillary, muscle strength and, 38-39
Capsular pattern of motion, 64
Capsule
    collateral ligament and, 308-309
    endpoint pain and, 63
    flexibility and, 47

Carbohydrate, nutrition and, 26
Carbonated soda, nausea and, 146
Cardiac muscle, characteristics of, 3
Cardiorespiratory system
    ankle rehabilitation and, 334
    endurance and, 52-58
    preparticipation examination and, 88
Cardiovascular fitness
    lower leg rehabilitation and, 320
    progressive running program and, 313
Carpal tunnel syndrome, 251
Cartilage
    hyaline, 8
    osteoarthrosis and, 12
    tissue type of, 3
Cast, orthotics and, 349, 350
Cathartic drug, 146-147
CCS; *see* Chronic compartment syndrome
Cellular permeability, 128, 130
Central nervous system, skeletal muscles and, 36
Cervical region, preparticipation examination and, 88-89
Change-of-pace activity, Fartlek and, 59
Checkrein taping, wrist injury and, 252
Chemical change, iontophoresis and, 125
Chest, life-threatening injury and, 92
Chiropractic, manual therapy and, 65
Chloride ion, iontophoresis and, 125
Chondromalacia, 310, 311
Chopping, upper trunk movement and, 81, 82
Chronic compartment syndrome, 327-328
Chronic injury, rehabilitation of, 134-135
Cimetidine, 146
Circuit training, 58-59
Circulation
    elbow injuries and, 234
    infrared modalities and, 129-130
    life-threatening injury and, 92
    medical galvanism and, 125
Clavicle fracture, 215-217
Clicking, passive motion and, 103
Climate, impeded healing and, 20
Closed fracture, 6
Close-packed position, joint and, 63
Clothing and injury prevention, 26-27
Coach
    stress and, 108-109
    support for rehabilitation and, 116; *see also* Psychology
Coagulation
    aspirin and, 140
    inflammation and, 15
Cocontraction, quadriceps and hamstring and, 299, 300
Codeine, antitussives and expectorants and, 144
Codman's pendulum exercise, 192-193
Cold; *see also* Ice
    clinical uses of, 129-130, 131
    elbow injuries and, 233-234
Cold allergy, cryotherapy and, 130

Cold pack, indications/contraindications and, 137
Cold weather, injury prevention and, 26-27
Cold whirlpool, acute injury and, 133, 134
Collagen
  ankle healing and, 332
  connective tissue and, 3
  healing of, 20
  low-power laser and, 131
Collateral ligament
  finger injuries and, 258
  knee injury and, 308-309
Comminuted fracture, characteristics of, 6, 7
Communication between physician and sports therapist,
      294-295
Compact bone, types of bone and, 5
Compartment syndrome, 326-328
Competition, fear of; see Psychology
Compound fracture, 6
Compression
  acute injury and, 133-134
  ankle rehabilitation and, 333
  elbow injuries and, 234
  hip pointer and, 266
  initial management of injuries and, 14
  injury prevention and, 30
  intermittent, 130-131
    indications/contraindications and, 137
  meniscal injury and, 309-310
  trochanteric bursitis and, 274
Computerized tomography scan, low back examination and,
      155
Concentric contraction
  eccentric contraction versus, 317
  isotonic exercise and, 40-41
  wrist rehabilitation and, 253
Conditioning
  prevention of injury and, 24
  shin splints and, 324-326
Congenital defect, foot pronation and, 344
Congestion, decongestants and, 144
Connective tissue
  flexibility and, 47
  musculoskeletal system and, 2, 3
Constipation, drugs affecting gastrointestinal tract and,
      145-147
Continuous training, cardiorespiratory endurance and, 56-57
Contraction
  concentric/eccentric, 40-41
  motion assessment and, 63
  off-field evaluation protocol and, 103
  quadriceps and hamstring, 299, 300
  resistive motion and, 103
  skeletal muscles and, 36
Contract-relax, proprioceptive neuromuscular facilitation
      and, 50, 73-74
Contralateral exercise, cross-transfer effect and, 333
Contrast bath, cryotherapy and, 130

Contusion
  axillary nerve, 227-228
  hip pointer as, 265-268
  iliac spine and, 269
  lumbosacral injury and, 164
  musculoskeletal injuries and, 12
  quadriceps, 289-292
  shoulder joint and, 207-208
Coordination
  drugs affecting respiratory tract and, 144
  lower leg rehabilitation and, 320
Coping with injury, 117-120; see also Psychology
Copper, iontophoresis and, 125
Cortical bone, 5
Corticosteroid, impeded healing and, 19
Coughing, 143, 144-145
Counter, heel
  rearfoot movement and, 352, 353
  retrocalcaneobursitis and, 326
Crepitation, Achilles tendonitis and, 321
Crepitus
  clicking sound and, 103
  tenosynovitis and, 11
Cross-country running, Fartlek and, 59
Crossbridge, skeletal muscle contraction and, 36
Crossover, ankle return to activity and, 339
Cross-transfer effect, ankle rehabilitation and, 333
Cruciate ligament
  anterior, 298-301, 306
  posterior, 307-308
Cryotherapy; see also Ice
  acute injury and, 132-133
  elbow and, 233-234
  hand and, 260, 261
  indications/contraindications and, 137
  infrared modalities and, 129-130
CT scan; see Computerized tomography scan
Cuboid bone, midtarsal joint and, 343
Cuboid subluxation, 355
Curling dumbbell, wrist flexion and, 251
Curve, strength-duration, 122-123
Cutting sequence, ankle and, 339

D

Daily adjusted progressive resistive exercise, 45
DAPRE; see Daily adjusted progressive resistive exercise
De Quervain's tenosynovitis, 250
Decongestant, common medications and, 144
Deep posterior compartment, 327
Degenerative joint disease, shoulder and, 217-218
Dehydration, vomiting and diarrhea and, 146
DeLorme's program, strength training and, 44
Deltoid contusion, shoulder joint and, 207-208
Denial, phases of injury and, 111
Depolarization of nerve fiber, 122-123
Depression, phases of injury and, 111; see also Psychology
Derangement, noncapsular pattern of motion and, 64

Deviation exercise, wrist rehabilitation and, 254, 255
Dexamethasone, elbow injuries and, 235
Dexterity exercise, 261-262, 263
Dextromethorphan, 144
Diagonal pattern, proprioceptive neuromuscular facilitation and, 74-80
Diarrhea, drugs affecting gastrointestinal tract and, 145-146
Diathermy
    acute injury and, 134
    electrical current and, 125-127
    shortwave/microwave, 137
    ultrasound versus, 128
Diet; see Nutrition
DIP; see Distal interphalangeal joint
Diphenhydramine, antitussives and expectorants and, 144
Directional shear, elbow injuries and, 236
Disability, predicting, 93
Discoloration
    Achilles tendon rupture and, 323
    contusion and, 12
Disk
    low back examination and, 153-154
    lumbosacral injury and, 165
    sciatica and, 272
Dislocation
    finger and, 259
    glenohumeral, 209-214
    osteoarthrosis and, 13
    subluxations and, 7-8
Distal interphalangeal joint, 254-255
    fingers and, 260, 261
    splint and, 258
Distraction technique, low back rehabilitation and, 162
DJD; see Degenerative joint disease
Documentation, subjective objective assessment plan and, 104-105
Dorsiflexion
    Achilles tendon rupture and, 323
    ankle rehabilitation and, 333, 334, 335
    causes of pronation and, 346, 347
    lower leg conditioning and, 317, 319
    plantar fasciitis and, 355
    rearfoot-forefoot relationship and, 345-346
    shoe wear patterns and, 343-344
    tennis leg and, 324
Drop finger, 255
Drop foot, 327
Drowsiness, drugs and, 144, 146
Drug
    administering versus dispensing of, 147-148
    antiinflammatory, 140-141
    common, 140-147
        diarrhea and, 146
        drowsiness and, 144, 146
        gastrointestinal tract and, 145-147
        elbow injuries and, 235
        iontophoresis and, 125

Drug—cont'd
    low back examination and, 154-155
    nonsteroidal antiinflammatory drug and; see Nonsteroidal antiinflammatory drug
    record keeping and, 148
    steroidal
        elbow injuries and, 235
        hip pointer and, 266
    tenosynovitis and, 11
    ultrasound and, 128
    vasodilating, 125
Drug abuse, testing for, 148
Dumbbell weight
    isotonic exercise and, 40-41
    wrist rehabilitation and, 253, 254, 255
        flexion and, 251
Dutoit staple capsulorrhaphy, 211
Dynamometer, hand, 262

E
Eccentric exercise
    isotonic exercise and, 40-41
    knee rehabilitation and, 297
    lower leg conditioning and, 317-320
    patellofemoral dysfunction and, 303, 311
    wrist rehabilitation and, 253
Edema
    ankle and, 332-334
    decongestants and, 144
    hand and, 260, 261
    ice and, 14
    impeded healing and, 19
    intermittent compression and, 130-131
    medical galvanism and, 125
    sympathomimetic drugs and, 145
    thermotherapy and, 130
Education
    commitment to rehabilitation and, 117
    injury prevention and, 26
Effusion, synovial, 13
Elastic wrap, injuries and, 14
Elastin, connective tissue and, 3
Elbow, 232-248
    end-feel and, 103, 104
    inflammation and, 232-235
    medication and, 235
    muscular strength and, 37
    musculotendinous unit injuries and, 235-246
        joint mobilization and, 238-240
        laxity and, 240-244
        motion restrictions of, 235-236
        soft tissue mobilization and, 236
        stretching and, 236-237, 238-239
        throwing and tennis protocols and, 245-246
    upper-quarter screening and, 94, 95
    wrist and, 253-254

Electrical stimulating current
  acute injury and, 133, 134
  ankle compression and, 333
  anterior cruciate ligament patellar tendon and, 299, 300
  indications/contraindications and, 137
  intermittent compression and, 131
  pain control and, 124
  rehabilitation and, 121-127
Electroacupuncture, 124
Electroacutherapy, 124
Electrolyte, dehydration and, 146
Electromagnetic device, diathermy and, 126, 127
Electrostatic device, diathermy and, 126, 127
Elevation
  ankle and, 333
  elbow and, 234
  initial management of injuries and, 14-15
  injury prevention and, 30
Emergency care
  acute compartment syndrome and, 327
  on-field evaluation and, 91-93
Emergency medical technician, on-field evaluation and, 91
Emission, low-power laser and, 131
Emotion
  goals of rehabilitation and, 32-33
  injury and; see Psychology
Emotive imagery rehearsal, 115
Empty can raise exercise, 201
EMT; see Emergency medical technician
End feel, evaluation and, 103, 104
  elbow injuries and, 242
β-endorphin, pain control system and, 124
Endpoint, range of motion, 47
  abnormal, 64
Endurance
  cardiorespiratory, 52-58
    energy systems and, 55-56
  definition of, 296
  muscle reconditioning and, 35-47; see also Strength
  shoulder and, 204
  strength versus, 46-47
Energy, high versus low output and, 55-56
Enkephalin, pain control system and, 123, 124
Epicondylitis, 245
Epithelial tissue, 1-3
Equipment, injury prevention and, 26-27; see also Specific
    types of equipment
Ergometer
  ankle rehabilitation and, 339
  interval training and, 58
Ethylene vinyl acetate, midsole production and, 352, 353
EVA; see Ethylene vinyl acetate
Evaluation process, 87-106
  documentation and, 104-105
  initial, 27-31
  off-field, 93-104
    protocol for, 101-104
    quarter screening and, 93-100
  on-field, 91-93

Evaluation process—cont'd
  preparticipation examination and, 87-91
    injury prevention and, 24-25, 26
Eversion, ankle and, 333
Examination; see Evaluation process
Exercise; see also Specific types of exercise
  ankle and, 333
  contralateral, 333
  hand and, 261-262, 263
  initial evaluation and, 27-31
  knee and, 312-314
  low back and, 163
  resistance
    shin splints and, 325-326
    wrist and, 253
Exertional compartment syndrome, 327-328
Expectorant, 144-145
Extensibility, skeletal muscles and, 36
Extension
  active-assisted wrist, 253
  diagonal patterns and, 78, 79-80
  low back examination and, 156-157
Extensor
  ankle and toe and, 327
  hand injuries and, 254-255
  patellofemoral dysfunction and, 310-311
  tenosynovitis and, 250, 251
Extensor digitorum longus, 325
Extensor hallucis longus, 325
Extraarticular lesion, 64
Extraarticular reconstruction, 299
Extremity, lower; see Lower extremity
Extremity, upper, proprioceptive neuromuscular facilitation
    patterns and, 74-78; see also Specific parts of body
Eye, low-power laser and, 131-132

F

Facet syndrome, 154
Facilitation, proprioceptive neuromuscular, 69
Family history, preparticipation examination and, 88; see
    also Evaluation process; History
Fartlek, cardiorespiratory endurance and, 59
Fasciculus; see Muscle fiber
Fasciotomy, 327, 328
Fast contractile velocity spectrum program, 203-204
Fast-speed program, shoulder and, 203-204
Fast-twitch muscle fiber, 5
  slow-twitch versus, 36-37
Fat
  adenosine triphosphate and, 55-56
  diathermy and, 126
  flexibility and, 47
  ice and, 14
  infrared modalities and, 129-130
  nutrition and, 26
  preparticipation examination and, 91
  ultrasound and, 128

Fatigue
  maximal oxygen consumption and, 55
  muscle soreness and, 10
FCU; *see* Flexor carpi ulnaris
FCVSP; *see* Fast contractile velocity spectrum program
FDA; *see* Food and Drug Administration
FDP; *see* Flexor digitorum profundus
FDS; *see* Flexor digitorum superficialis
Fear of injury; *see* Psychology
Female athlete, sex distinctions and; *see* Sex difference
Femur
  hip and thigh injury and, 285-286
  posterior cruciate ligament and, 307
Fever, common analgesics and, 140
Fiber, muscle
  characteristics of, 5
  strength and splitting of, 36-37, 38
Fiber, nerve, 122-123
Fibrillation, osteoarthrosis and, 12
Fibroblast, connective tissue and, 3
Fibroplasia, 15, 17, 19
Fibroplastic stage, 133-134
Fibula, stress fractures of lower leg and, 328
Finger
  boutonniere deformity and, 255, 260
  drop, 255
  ligament injuries and, 256, 258
  mallet, 255, 258, 260
  tenosynovitis and, 11
Finger splint, 262-263
First aid, 13-15
First ray, midtarsal joint and, 343
First-degree sprain, 8
First-degree strain, 9
Fitness level
  alternative activities and, 11
  preparticipation examination and, 91
Flexibility; *see also* Range of motion
  Achilles tendonitis and, 321
  circuit training and, 58
  definition of, 48
  hand and, 260-261
  preparticipation examination and, 88-89
  reconditioning and, 47-52
  static and dynamic, 48
  stretch and, 52
  wrist and, 253, 254
Flexion
  diagonal patterns and, 78, 79-80
  low back examination and, 156, 157, 160
  plantar
    ankle and, 332-333, 334, 335
    lower leg conditioning and, 317-320
  wrist rehabilitation and, 253-254
Flexor carpi ulnaris, 250-251
Flexor digitorum profundus, 255-256, 260, 261
Flexor digitorum superficialis, 261

Flexor group, elbow, 232
Flexor mechanism
  hand injury and, 255-256
  wrist tendinitis, 250-251
Flow of blood; *see* Blood supply
Fluid; *see also* Edema
  bursitis and, 11-12
  common analgesics and, 140
  decongestants and, 144
  dehydration and, 146
  intermittent compression and, 130-131
  nausea and, 146
Food, peristalsis and, 147
Food and Drug Administration, regulation of lasers and, 131
Foot, 342-357
  midtarsal joint and, 343-344
  orthotics and, 347-352
  pathologies of, 353-356
  pronated
    causes of, 344-346
    low back examination and, 155
  pronator identification and, 347
  sciatica and, 272
  shoe selection and, 352-353
  subtalar joint and, 342-343
Footwear; *see* Shoe
Forearm, wrist rehabilitation and, 253-254
Forefoot equinus, 346
Forefoot valgus/varus, 344-346
Forefoot-rearfoot relationship, 345-346
Fracture
  avulsion, 279-280, 285
  classifications of, 6-7
  compartment syndrome and, 326-328
  femoral, 285-286
  hand and, 258-259
  healing of, 20-21
  humerus and neck, 217
  inferior ramus and, 276
  lower leg and, 328-329
  lumbosacral injury and, 164, 166
  osteoarthrosis and, 12
  vertebral, 269
  visual inspection and, 101
  wrist and, 251-252
Free weight, isotonic exercise and, 40-41
Friction, bursa and, 273
Friction massage, elbow injuries and, 236
Frostbite, cryotherapy and, 130

G

Gaenslen's sign, low back palpation and, 160
Gait
  hip pointer and, 266
  sciatica and, 272
Gallium arsenide laser, 131
Galvanism, medical, 122-127

Gamekeeper's thumb, 258
Gas, blockage of ultrasound and, 128
Gastric discomfort, 140
Gastrocnemius
  Achilles tendonitis and, 321, 322
  partial tear in, 324
  preparticipation examination and, 89
  pronation and, 344-345
Gastrointestinal tract, drugs and, 142, 145-147
Gate control theory
  infrared modalities and, 129
  pain and, 123
Gel, ultrasound and, 128
Gibney taping, ankle and, 332
Girdle exercise, shoulder, 227
Gland, pituitary, pain control and, 124
Glenohumeral joint
  dislocation of, 209-214
  mobilization of, 190-192
Glenoid labrum tear, 215
Gliding, 65, 67
Glucose, 55-56
Glycogen, 55-56
Glycolosis, anaerobic, 56
Goal setting, psychology and, 119-120; *see also* Psychology
Goals of rehabilitation, 25-33
  short-term, 30-31
Golf
  De Quervain's tenosynovitis and, 250
  sport-specific exercise and, 254, 257
  wrist flexion and, 251
Golgi tendon organ, 51, 69, 70
Goniometer
  assessing flexibility and, 48, 49
  preparticipation examination and, 89
  small-amplitude movements and, 66
Gordon's *Teacher Effectiveness Training*, 114
Grade-point average of athlete, 117
Grade-three injury, anxiety and, 115-116
Granulation tissue, healing and, 19
Green-stick fracture, 6, 7
Grip strength, 262
Groin strain, 276-278

H

H1/H2 receptor blocker, respiratory tract and, 143
Hamate, wrist injury and, 252
Hamstring
  flexibility and, 47
  healing period and, 10
  hip and thigh and, 279-284
  knee injury and, 303
  Osgood-Schlatter's disease and, 312
  piriformis syndrome sciatica and, 269-270
  preparticipation examination and, 89, 90
  proprioceptive neuromuscular facilitation and, 50
  quadriceps and, 299, 300

Hamstring—cont'd
  strain and, 280-284
Hand
  injuries and, 254-259
  rehabilitation of, 259-263
  upper-quarter screening and, 94, 96
Hand dynamometer, 262
Hay fever, 144
Healing, phases of, 15-20
Heart
  cardiorespiratory system and, 53-55
  isometric exercise and, 40
  oxygen transport and, 52-53
Heart rate
  continuous training and, 57
  Karvonen equation and, 58
  maximal, 53-54
Heat
  acute injury and, 134
  clinical uses of, 129-130
  diathermy and, 126-127
  injury prevention and, 26-27
  loss of, 140
  shin splints and, 325
  ultrasound and, 127-128
Heavy metal ion, iontophoresis and, 125
Heel
  anterior shin splints and, 325
  plantar fasciitis and, 355
  trochanteric bursitis and, 273
Heel counter
  rearfoot movement and, 352, 353
  retrocalcaneobursitis and, 326
Heel lift, Achilles tendon and, 322, 323
Heelcord stretching, ankle and, 336
Helium-neon laser, 131
Hemarthrosis
  finger ligament injuries and, 256
  hand rehabilitation and, 260, 261
  osteoarthrosis and, 13
Hematocrit, cardiorespiratory endurance and, 55
Hemoglobin, cardiorespiratory endurance and, 55
Hemorrhage
  healing of bone and, 20
  ice and, 14
    ankle rehabilitation and, 333
  impeded healing and, 19
Hexalite, ankle stirrups and, 332
High school athlete, preparticipation examination and, 91
Hill training, stress fractures and, 328-329
Hill-Sachs lesion, 215, 216
Hip adductor strain, 276-278
Hip and thigh, 265-293
  bursitis and, 273-275
  contusion and, 12
  femoral fractures and, 285-286
  hamstring and, 279-284
  hip dislocation and, 278-279

Hip and thigh—cont'd
  hip pointer and, 265-268
  iliac spine and, 268-269
  myositis ossificans and, 292
  osteoarthrosis and, 13
  piriformis syndrome sciatica and, 269-270, 272-273
  preparticipation examination and, 89, 90
  pubic injury and, 275-278
  quadriceps contusion and, 289-292
  quadriceps muscle strain and, 286-289
  sciatica and, 272
Hip flexor strain, 276-278
Hip pointer, 265-268
Histamine
  inflammation and, 15
  respiratory tract and, 141, 143-144
History; *see also* Evaluation process
  hip pointer and, 266
  low back examination and, 152-154
  off-field evaluation protocol and, 101
  preparticipation examination and, 88
  stress fractures of lower leg and, 329
  trochanteric bursitis and, 274
Hives, cryotherapy and, 130
Hold-relax technique, proprioceptive neuromuscular facilita-
        tion and, 50, 74
Hopping, ankle and, 339
Hot whirlpool, 137
Hughston exercise program, shoulder and, 198, 199,
        200
Humerus fracture, 217
Humidity, impeded healing and, 20
Hunting response, cryotherapy and, 130
Hyaline cartilage, 8
Hydrochloric acid, antacids and, 145
Hydrocodone, antitussives and expectorants and, 144
Hydrocollator, 137
Hydrocortisone, 326
Hydrotherapy, infrared modalities and, 129
Hydroxide salt, antacids and, 145
Hypermobility
  physiological versus accessory motion and, 65
  valgus stress and, 242
Hyperpronation, Achilles tendonitis and, 321
Hyperstimulation
  infrared modalities and, 129
  pain control system and, 124
Hypertrophic scar, 19
Hypertrophy, muscle
  compartment syndrome and, 326-328
  strength and, 37-38
Hypochondria, 120-121; *see also* Psychology
Hypomobile joint, physiological versus accessory motion
        and, 65
Hypothalamus
  common analgesics and, 140
  infrared modalities and, 129

I
Ibuprofen, 140
Ice
  ankle rehabilitation and, 333, 334
  elbow injuries and, 233-234
  elevation and, 14
  hip pointer and, 266
  indications/contraindications and, 137
  initial management of injuries and, 14
  injury prevention and, 30
  muscle soreness and, 10, 13
  nausea and, 146
  posterior superior iliac spine contusion and, 269
  shin splints and, 325
  stress fractures of lower leg and, 329
  trochanteric bursitis and, 274
  wrist rehabilitation and, 252-254
Idiopathic pain, lumbosacral injury and, 165-166
Iliac spine
  direct blow to, 265-268
  hip and thigh injury and, 268-269
  superior, 155
Iliopectineal bursitis, 274-275
Iliotibial band, 89, 90
Illness, mental; *see* Psychology
Imagery, emotive, 115
Immersion, ultrasound and, 128
Immobilization; *see also* Individual injuries
  Achilles tendon rupture and, 323
  anterior cruciate ligament and, 298-299
  bone fracture and, 7
  hand and, 259, 260
  healing of bone and, 21
  high-frequency AC current and, 125
  knee strengthening and, 297
  medial collateral ligament and, 308
Impacted fracture, characteristics of, 6, 7
Impingement
  painful arc and, 104
  shoulder inflammation and, 221-223
Implant, metal, 126, 128
Inactivity, flexibility and, 47
Incontinence, low back examination and, 155
Indigestion, drugs and, 145-146
Inert tissue
  motion assessment and, 63
  off-field evaluation protocol and, 103
Infection
  antibiotic medications and, 147
  impeded healing and, 19
  iontophoresis and, 125
  medical galvanism and, 125
Inferior iliac spine, 269
Inferior ramus, fracture of, 276
Inflammation
  Achilles tendonitis and, 322
  acute injury and, 133-134

Inflammation—cont'd
  drugs affecting respiratory tract and, 143
  elbow injuries and, 232-235
  ice and, 14; *see also* Ice
  low back examination and, 154
  low-power laser and, 131
  mucous linings and, 145
  phases of healing and, 15, 16
  shoulder complex and, 220-225
  tendonitis and, 11
  tenosynovitis and, 11
  thermotherapy and, 130
  wrist and, 249-254
Infrared lamp
  indications/contraindications and, 137
  rehabilitation and, 128-130
Inhibition
  autogenic/reciprocal, 51
  proprioceptive neuromuscular facilitation and, 69
Injury
  acute, 132-134
  chronic, 134-135
  prevention of, 24-27
Innominate, anterior/posterior torsion of, 155
Intermediate muscle fiber, characteristics of, 5
Intermittent compression, 134
  indications/contraindications and, 137
Intermittent training, disadvantages of, 57
Internal derangement, noncapsular pattern of motion and, 64
Internal injury, posterior superior iliac spine contusion versus, 269
Interosseous ligament, ankle injuries and, 331
Interpersonal relationship, athlete/sports therapist and, 115-116
Interphalangeal joint, finger injuries and, 256
Interval training, cardiorespiratory endurance and, 58
Inversion
  ankle rehabilitation and, 333
  population, 131
Involuntary muscle, characteristics of, 3
Ion transfer, 125
Iontophoresis
  chemical changes and, 125
  electrical current and, 122
Irradiation, muscle strength and, 71
Irrational thinking, injury and, 112-114; *see also* Psychology
Ischemia
  compartment syndrome and, 327
  muscle soreness and, 10
Ischemic Volkmann's contracture, 234
Ischial bursitis, 274
  piriformis syndrome sciatica and, 270
Ischial tuberosity, 279-280
Isokinetic exercise
  elbow joint laxity and, 241, 242
  knee strengthening and, 297
  lower leg strengthening and, 319-320

Isokinetic—cont'd
  shoulder and, 201-204
Isometric exercise
  ankle rehabilitation and, 333, 336-337
  elbow joint laxity and, 241
  hamstring contraction and, 50
  hand dynamometer and, 262
  knee rehabilitation and, 297
  lower leg and, 317
  shoulder and, 194-196
  strength improvement and, 39-40
  trauma and, 40
Isotonic exercise
  ankle rehabilitation and, 336, 337
  knee rehabilitation and, 297
  lower leg and, 317
  shoulder and, 197-201
  strength training and, 40

J

Jammed finger, 256, 258
Jersey finger, 256
Jobst intermittent air compression, 131
  ankle edema and, 334
Jogging, cardiorespiratory endurance and, 59
Jogging to running, progressive running program and, 313
Joint
  ankle rehabilitation and, 334, 335
  calcaneocuboid, 343
  cryotherapy and, 130
  degenerative disease of, 217-218
  elbow, 244, 246
    laxity and, 240-242
    muscular strength and, 37
    musculotendinous unit injury and, 238-240
  lower leg coordination and, 320
  midtarsal, 343-344
  mobilization of
    manual therapy and, 65-67
    shoulder and, 189-192
  proximal interphalangeal, 256
  sternoclavicular injury and, 209
  structure of, 8
  subtalar, 342-343
  synovial, 64
  talonavicular, 343
  tibiofemoral, 307
  ulnohumeral, 232
Joint angle
  isometric exercise and, 39
  isotonic exercise and, 41-42
  muscular strength and, 37, 38
Joint capsule, 47
Joint compression injury, elbow and, 234
Joint equinus, ankle, 346
Jumper's knee, 310, 311-312

Jumping
    ankle return to activity and, 339
    energy systems and, 55-56

K

Kaolin, diarrhea and, 146
Karvonen equation, maximum heart rate and, 57-58
Kehr's sign, life-threatening injury and, 92
Keloid, impeded healing and, 19
Kernig's sign, low back palpation and, 160
Kinesiology, elbow injuries and, 234
Kirshner wiring, shoulder rehabilitation and, 208
Knee, 294-315
    anterior cruciate ligament and, 298-301, 306
    apprehension test and, 104
    chondromalacia and, 311
    evaluation checklist and, 102
    general principles and, 295-297
    illustrated exercises and, 302-305
    jumper's, 311-312
    lateral collateral ligament and, 308-309
    ligament sprains and, 8-9
    medial collateral ligament and, 308
    meniscus and, 309-310
    Osgood-Schlatter's disease and, 312
    osteoarthrosis and, 13
    patellofemoral dysfunction and, 310-311
    phases of rehabilitation and, 297-298
    posterior cruciate ligament and, 307-308
    progressive rehabilitation exercises and, 28
        running program and, 312-314
Knight's DAPRE program, strength training and, 44, 45,
        46
Knott and Voss Method 14, proprioceptive stimulation and,
        70; *see also* Proprioceptive neuromuscular facilita-
        tion

L

Lactic acid
    anaerobic glycolosis and, 56
    muscle soreness and, 10
Laser, 131-132
    acute injury and, 133
    definition of, 131
    indications/contraindications and, 137
Lasèque's sign, low back palpation and, 160
Lateral ankle; *see* Ankle
Lateral collateral ligament, knee injury and, 308-309
Lateral compartment, compartment syndrome and, 327
Lateral epicondylitis, 245
Lateral view, low back examination and, 155
Lateral-distal carpal row, 251-252
Laxative, 146-147
Laxity
    elbow and, 240-244
    on-field evaluation and, 93
Leg; *see also* Lower extremity
    length of, low back examination and, 155

Leg—cont'd
    raising of
        knee injury and, 300, 301
        low back palpation and, 160
    sex differences and, 47
Legal problem, rehabilitation and, 120
Lesion
    Bankart, 215, 216
    differentiating, 64-65
    extraarticular, 64
    Hill-Sachs, 215, 216
    pain and, 62-63
Leukocyte, 15
Lever, muscular strength and, 37
Life-threatening injury, 92
Lifting, upper trunk movement and, 81, 82
Ligament
    ankle, 331
    anterior cruciate, 298-301, 306
    endpoint pain and, 63
    flexibility and, 47
    hand injuries and, 256, 258
    lateral collateral, 308-309
    medial collateral
        joint laxity and, 240-241, 242
        knee injury and, 308
    on-field evaluation and, 92-93
    posterior cruciate, 307-308
    sprains and, 8-9
    tissue type of, 3
    wrist and, 251, 252
Ligamentous adhesion, 64
Light, laser, 131
Light amplification of stimulated emissions of radiation; *see*
        Laser
Lightning, injury prevention and, 26-27
Liver, glucose storage and, 56
Local anesthetic, iontophoresis and, 125
Long-distance running, 55-56
Long-term goals of rehabilitation, 31, 32
Low back, 150-185
    examination and, 152-161
    lumbosacral injuries and, 164-166
    manual therapy and, 161-163
    palpation and, 158, 159-160
    phases of, 166-169, 170-182
    repetitive movement and, 157-158
    statistics on, 150-151
    symptoms and time of day and, 154
Lower extremity, 316-330
    cardiovascular fitness and, 320-321
    compartment syndromes and, 326-328
    coordination and, 320
    injuries to, 321-324
    low back examination and, 153
    maintenance and, 320-321
    orthotics and, 348-349
    preparticipation examination and, 89, 90

Lower extremity—cont'd
 proprioceptive neuromuscular facilitation patterns and,
   74-75, 78-80
 reconditioning exercises for, 316-317
 retrocalcaneobursitis and, 326
 shin splint syndromes and, 324-326
 strengthening exercises for, 317-320
 stress fractures and, 328-329
Lower leg; see Lower extremity
Lower-quarter screening, 96-100
Low-power laser, 131-132
 acute injury and, 133
 indications/contraindications and, 137
L-S; see Lumbosacral injury
Lumbosacral injury, 163, 164-166
 nerve root and, 158
Lung, 52-53
 volumes and capacities of, 55
Lymph, tissue type of, 3

M

MacQueen's technique of strength training, 44
Magnesium ion, iontophoresis and, 125
Magnetic field, diathermy and, 126-127
Maitland's five grades of motion, 66, 67
Malingering, rehabilitation and, 120-121; see also Psychology
Malleolus, medial, tarsal tunnel syndrome and, 355-356
Mallet finger, 255, 258, 260
Manual joint mobilization, ankle and, 334, 335
Manual resistance, opposition exercise and, 262-263; see
   also Hand
Manual therapy, 62-86
 contraindications and, 67-68
 low back rehabilitation and, 161-163
 mobilization techniques and, 65-67
 motion assessment and, 63-65
 musculoskeletal dysfunction and, 62-63
 physiological versus accessory motion and, 65
 proprioceptive neuromuscular facilitation and, 68-84; see
   also Proprioceptive neuromuscular facilitation
Massage
 elbow injuries and, 236
 low back and, 163
Maturation stage
 acute injury and, 134
 phases of healing and, 18, 19
Maximal oxygen consumption, 52-53
McKenzie extension exercise, 163
MCP; see Metacarpal phalangeal joint
Medial ankle sprain, 331; see also Ankle
Medial collateral ligament
 joint laxity and, 240-241, 242
 knee injury and, 308
Medial malleolus, 355-356
Medical galvanism, 122-127
 electrical current and, 125
Medical history; see History

Medical technician, emergency, 91
Medication; see Drug
Melzak and Wall's gate control theory of pain, 123
Meniscectomy, 309
Meniscus
 knee injury and, 309-310
 ligament sprains and, 8
MENS; see Microamperage electrical nerve stimulation
Mental health; see Psychology
Metabolism
 Achilles tendonitis and, 321
 aerobic versus anaerobic, 56
 basal metabolic rate and, 26
Metacarpal phalangeal joint, 255, 260, 261
Metal implant, 126, 128
Metal ion, iontophoresis and, 125
Metatarsal head, 354
Microamperage electrical nerve stimulation, 122
Microorganism, low-power laser and, 131
Microwave diathermy
 indications/contraindications and, 137
 shortwave diathermy versus, 126-127
Midtarsal joint, 343-344
Mileage, stress fractures of lower leg and, 328-329
Mind, body and; see Psychology
Mineral, nutrition and, 26
Mineral oil, ultrasound and, 128
Mobilization technique
 contraindications to, 67-68
 manual therapy and, 65-67
 shoulder joint, 189-192
Modesty, off-field evaluation protocol and, 101
Modified Bristow, 211, 212-213
Mold, orthotics and, 349, 350
Moodiness, injury and; see Psychology
Morton's toe, 343
Motion; see also Range of motion
 accessory, 66
 acute compartment syndrome and, 327
 agonist/antagonist muscle groups and, 69-70
 ankle healing and, 332
 assessment of, 63-65
 capsular/noncapsular pattern of, 64
 five gradations of, 66
 lower leg rehabilitation and, 320
 off-field evaluation protocol and, 102-104
 painful arc and, 63
 physiological versus accessory, 65
 resisted, 64-65
Motion sickness, 143, 144
Motor neuron
 electrical stimulation of, 124-125
 proprioceptive neuromuscular facilitation and, 69-70
Motor unit, skeletal muscles and, 36
Mucous lining, sympathomimetic drugs and, 145
Muscle
 abdominal, 266
 agonist versus antagonist, 49, 69-70

Muscle—cont'd
   anatomy and physiology of, 35-37
   biceps, 12
   bronchial, 143
   characteristics of, 3
   elasticity of, 36
   elbow injuries and, 242-244
   electrical current and, 122-127
   flexibility and, 47-52
   glucose storage and, 56
   healing of, 21
   hypertrophy and, 326-328
   infrared modalities and, 129-130
   length of, 37, 38
   quadriceps, 12
      hip and thigh injury and, 286-289
   reconditioning and, 35-47; see Reconditioning
   sexual differences and, 46-47
   shoulder rehabilitation and, 218
   size of, 38-39
   skeletal, 35-37
   soleus, 321, 322
   soreness and, 10
   strain and, 9-10
   tissue of, 2, 3-5
Muscle fiber
   characteristics of, 5
   slow- versus fast-twitch, 36-37
   strength and splitting of, 36-37, 38
Muscle relaxant, oral, 143
Muscle spasm
   impeded healing and, 19
   theory about, 10
Muscle spindle, 51, 69
Muscle-bound person, 52
Muscle-tendon unit, off-field evaluation protocol and,
      103
Musculoskeletal system, 1-23
   bone healing and, 20-21
   bursitis and, 11-12
   contusion and, 12
   dislocations and subluxations and, 7-8
   fractures and, 6-7
   healing process and, 15-20
   initial management of injuries and, 13-15
   ligament sprains and, 8-9
   manual therapy and, 65
   muscle injury and, 21
   muscle soreness and, 10
   muscle strains and, 9-10
   nerve tissue regeneration and, 21
   osteoarthrosis and, 12-13
   pathophysiology of injury and, 6-13
   preparticipation examination and, 88
   tendon healing and, 20
   tendonitis and, 10-11
   tenosynovitis and, 11
   tissue types and, 1-6

Musculotendinous unit injury, elbow and, 235-246
   chronic laxity and, 242-244
   joint laxity and, 240-242
   joint mobilization and, 238-240
   motion restrictions of, 235-236
   soft tissue mobilization and, 236
   stretching and, 236-237, 238-239
   throwing and tennis protocols and, 245-246
Myelin, nerve tissue and, 5, 21
Myocardium, blood flow to, 55
Myofilament, muscle contraction and, 36, 39
Myosin filament, muscle contraction and, 36
Myositis ossificans
   contusion and, 12
   hip and thigh injury and, 292

N

Naproxen, elbow injuries and, 235
Narcotic drug, antitussives and expectorants and, 144; see
      also Drug
Nasal membrane, drugs affecting, 143
Nausea
   cryotherapy and, 130
   drugs affecting gastrointestinal tract and, 142, 145-147
   drugs affecting respiratory tract and, 141, 143-144
Nautilus, range of movement and, 41-42, 46
Neck
   fracture of, 217
   passive flexion and, 160
   proprioceptive neuromuscular facilitation patterns and,
      81, 84
Necrosis of skin, hand and, 255
Negative thinking, 107-108
   rehabilitation and, 114-115; see also Psychology
Negative Thomas test, 90
Nerve
   axillary contusion of, 227-228
   characteristics of, 2, 5
   depolarization of, 122-123
   electrical current and, 122-124
   ice and, 14
   lumbosacral root of, 158
   regeneration of, 21
   sciatic, 269-270, 272-273
Neurology, low back palpation and, 160-161
Neuroma, metatarsal heads and, 354
Neuromuscular system
   paralysis and, 50
   strength and, 37
Neuron; see also Nerve
   characteristics of, 5
   proprioceptive neuromuscular facilitation and, 69-70
Neutral mold, orthotics and, 349, 350
Neutral subtalar position, 344-345
Nociceptive input, transcutaneous electrical nerve stimula-
      tion and, 122-123, 124
Noncapsular pattern of motion, 64

Noncontractile structure, off-field evaluation protocol and, 103

Non-life-threatening injury, on-field evaluation and, 92-93

Nonnarcotic drug, antitussives and expectorants and, 144

Nonsteroidal antiinflammatory drug (NSAID)
  Achilles tendonitis and, 322
  elbow injuries and, 235
  ibuprofen and, 140, 141, 143
  retrocalcaneobursitis and, 322
  shin splints and, 325
  stress fractures of lower leg and, 329

Nonthrust technique, low back rehabilitation and, 161

Nose drops, 144

NSAID; see Nonsteroidal antiinflammatory drug

Nucleus, Raphe, pain control system and, 124

Numbness, tarsal tunnel syndrome and, 355-356

Nutrition
  impeded healing and, 20
  injury prevention and, 25-26

O

Ober test
  low back palpation and, 160
  preparticipation examination and, 89, 90

Oblique fracture
  characteristics of, 6, 7
  finger injuries and, 259

Obstruction, bronchial, 145

Off-season conditioning
  Fartlek and, 59
  prevention of injury and, 24, 25

Olecranon bursa, 12

On-field evaluation, preparticipation, 91-93

Open fracture, 6

Open Gibney taping, ankle and, 332

Organ injury, posterior superior iliac spine contusion versus, 269

Orthoplast
  ankle stirrups and, 332
  shoe insole and, 354

Orthotics, 347-352
  Achilles tendonitis and, 322
  ankle sprains and, 337-338
  foot injuries and, 347-352
  patellofemoral dysfunction and, 310
  plantar fasciitis and, 355
  stress fractures of lower leg and, 329

Oscillation, elbow injuries and, 236

Oscillatory valgus stress, 242, 243

OSD; see Osgood-Schlatter's disease

Osgood-Schlatter's disease, 310, 312

Osseus deformity, forefoot and, 345-346

Osteitis pubis, 275-276

Osteoarthrosis, musculoskeletal injuries and, 12-13

Osteoblast, bone fracture and, 7

Osteochondritis dissecans, 13

Osteopathic medicine, 65

Osteophytosis, 12-13

Overexertion; see Overuse

Overflow effect, muscle strength and, 71

Overload; see also Overuse
  knee rehabilitation and, 296-297
  stress fractures of lower leg and, 328-329

Overpressure, low back examination and, 157, 158

Overuse
  Achilles tendonitis and, 321-323
  bursitis and, 273
  chronic injury and, 134, 135
  compression wrap and, 14
  isometric exercise and, 40
  muscle soreness and, 10
  musculoskeletal injuries and, 11
  retrocalcaneobursitis and, 326
  shin splints and, 324-326
  wrist injuries and, 249-252

Oxford technique of strength training, 44

Oxygen
  cardiorespiratory endurance and, 52-53
  preparticipation examination and, 91

Oxygen tension, impeded healing and, 20

P

Pad, orthotic, 347-348, 349

Padding, contusion and, 12

Pain; see also Specific injury
  active range of motion and, 63
  acute injury and, 132-133
  attitude toward, 109; see also Psychology
  commitment to rehabilitation and, 116-117
  compartment syndrome and, 327-328
  compression and, 14
  electrical current and, 122-127
  end feel, 242
  gate control theory of, 123
  ice and, 14; see also Ice
  idiopathic, 165-166
  infrared modalities and, 128-130
  life-threatening injury and, 92
  low back examination and, 153-154
  low-power laser and, 131
  mobilization technique and, 66-67
  muscle soreness and, 10
  musculoskeletal dysfunction and, 62-63
  negative thoughts and, 114-115; see also Psychology
  off-field evaluation and, 93-94
  sciatica and, 272
  shin splints and, 324-326
  thermotherapy and, 130
  trochanteric bursitis and, 274

Painful arc
  musculoskeletal dysfunction and, 63
  passive motion and, 103

Palmar intracapsular ligament, 251, 252

Palpation
  hamate injury and, 252
  hip pointer and, 266
  low back examination and, 155, 158-161
  off-field evaluation protocol and, 101-102
  posterior superior iliac spine and
    contusion and, 269
    low back examination and, 155
  shin splints and, 325
  trochanteric bursitis and, 274
  wrist flexion and, 251
Par cours, 59
Paraffin, hand rehabilitation and, 260, 261
Paralysis, proprioceptive neuromuscular facilitation and, 50
Paramedic, on-field evaluation and, 91
Paresthesia
  acute compartment syndrome and, 327
  carpal tunnel syndrome and, 251
  low back examination and, 153-154
  tarsal tunnel syndrome and, 355-356
Passive motion
  cuboid subluxation and, 355, 356
  low back examination and, 158-161
  lower leg reconditioning and, 316-317
  off-field evaluation protocol and, 103
  painful arc and, 63
Passive range of motion
  assessment of, 63-64
  rehabilitation goals and, 29
Patella
  anterior cruciate ligament and, 296, 299
  glides and mobilization of, 296
  neurology and, 161
Patellofemoral dysfunction, 310-311
Patrick's test, low back palpation and, 160
Pectin, diarrhea and, 146
Pelvic level, low back examination and, 155
Pepto-Bismol, 146
Periosteum, ultrasound and, 127
Peristalsis, 147
Permeability, cellular, 128, 130
Personal relationship, athlete/sports therapist and, 115-116
Personality, injury and; see Psychology
Phalanx fracture, 258-259
Pharmacology, 139-149; see also Drug
  common medications and, 140-147
  drug testing and, 148
Phonophoresis
  hydrocortisone and, 326
  shin splints and, 325
  ultrasound and, 128
Physical conditioning, prevention of injury and, 24
Physical examination, preparticipation, 24-25
Physiological motion
  accessory motion versus, 65
  five gradations of, 66
PIP; see Proximal interphalangeal joint

Piriformis syndrome sciatica, hip and thigh and, 269-270, 272-273
Pituitary gland, pain control and, 124
PL; see Point of limitation
Plantar fasciitis, 355
Plantar flexion
  ankle rehabilitation and, 332-333, 334, 335
  lower leg conditioning and, 317-320
Plantar wart, 125
Plantar-flexion-dorsiflexion exercise, 339
Plastazote mold, orthotics and, 349, 351
Plaster cast, orthotics and, 349, 350
Platelet
  common analgesics and, 140
  inflammation and, 15
Playing environment, injury prevention and, 26-27
Plexus, brachial, 228
PNF; see Proprioceptive neuromuscular facilitation
Point of limitation, anatomic motion and, 66-67
Pooling of blood, elevation and, 14
Popping sound, grade V mobilization technique and, **66**
Population inversion, low-power laser and, 131
Position coach, stress and, 108-109
Positive mold, orthotics and, 349, 350, 351
Posterior Bankart lesion, 215, 216
Posterior cruciate ligament, 307-308
Posterior instability, glenoid labrum tear and, 215
Posterior shin splint, 325
Posterior superior iliac spine
  contusion and, 269
  palpation and, 155
Posture
  hip pointer and, 266
  off-field evaluation protocol and, 101
  posterior superior iliac spine contusion and, 269
  sciatica and, 272
Power, definition of, 296
Power lift, 40
Pregnancy, low-power laser and, 131-132
Preparticipation examination, 87-91
Prepatellar bursa, 12
Prepubescent athlete, 91
Pressure, blood; see Blood pressure
Prevention of injury, 24-27
PRICE (protection, restricted activity, ice, compression, **and** elevation), rehabilitation goals and, 30
Progressive resistance exercise, wrist rehabilitation **and,** 253
Progressive running program
  acute compartment syndrome and, 327
  knee rehabilitation and, 312-314
  shin splints and, 326
PROM; see Passive range of motion
Pronation
  cuboid subluxation and, 355
  foot and, 344-346, 347
  low back examination and, 155
  shoe selection and, 352

Pronation—cont'd
  shoe wear patterns and, 343-344
  subtalar joint and, 342-343
Pronation-supination exercise
  elbow joint laxity and, 241, 242
  wrist rehabilitation and, 254
Proprioception
  ankle trauma and, 337, 338
  lower leg coordination and, 320
Proprioceptive neuromuscular facilitation
  elbow injuries and, 236, 237
  eleven principles of, 71-73
  flexibility and, 49
  manual therapy and, 68-84
    basic principles of, 71-73
    neurophysiological basis of, 69-70
    patterns of, 74-84
    rationale for use of, 70-71
    strengthening and, 73
    stretching and, 73-74
  neurophysiological basis of, 51
  piriformis syndrome sciatica and, 272
  shoulder and, 197
  stretching and, 50, 51-52
Protection, injury prevention and, 26-27
  PRICE and, 30
Protein
  collagen as, 3
  nutrition and, 25-26
  ultrasound and, 128
Proximal control, elbow joint laxity and, 241, 242
Proximal interphalangeal joint
  finger injuries and, 256
  hand injuries and, 254-255, 260, 261
PSIS; see Posterior superior iliac spine
Psychology, 107-120
  athlete/sports therapist relationship and, 115-116
  career goals and, 108, 117
  coping with injury and, 117-119
  emotional self control and, 114-115
  injury-prone athlete and, 108-111
  irrational thinking and, 112-114
  phases of injury and, 111-112
  rehabilitation and, 32-33
    discipline and, 116-117
    personnel and, 121
    problems with, 120-121
Pubescent athlete, 91
Pubic injury, 275-278
Pulley exercise, 193-194
Pulse duration, transcutaneous electrical nerve stimulation
    and, 123-124
Pulse rate, cardiorespiratory endurance and, 57-58
Push-relax sequence, proprioceptive neuromuscular facilita-
    tion and, 50
Putti-Platt procedure, glenohumeral subluxation and disloc-
    cation and, 211, 213-214

Q

Q angle, trochanteric bursitis and, 273
Quadriceps muscle
  contusion and, 12, 289-292
  hamstring and, 299, 300
  hip and thigh injury and, 289-292
    strain and, 286-289
  knee injury and, 302
  Osgood-Schlatter's disease and, 312
  patellofemoral dysfunction and, 303, 310
Quarter screening, off-field evaluation and, 93-100

R

Racquetball, extensor mechanism tenosynovitis and, 250
Radial artery, pulse rate and, 57
Radial extensor tendon, 250, 251
Radiography, scaphoid fracture and, 251
Radiohumeral joint, 239, 240
Rain, injury prevention and, 26-27
Range of motion
  active/passive, 63-64
  active-assisted, 29
  ankle and
    rehabilitation and, 334-336
    return to activity and, 339
  anterior cruciate ligament and, 298-299
  anterior superior iliac spine injury and, 266
  hand and, 259-263
  high-frequency AC current and, 125
  improving, 47-52
  knee rehabilitation and, 295-296
    medial collateral ligament and, 308
  lower leg and, 316-317
  lower-quarter screening and, 96-100
  musculotendinous unit injury, elbow and, 235-246; see
    also Musculotendinous unit injury, elbow and
  on-field evaluation and, 93
  painful arc and, 103
  preparticipation examination and, 88-89
  rehabilitation goals and, 29
  shoulder complex and, 192-194
  static stretching and, 51-52
  ultrasound and, 128
  upper-quarter screening and, 93-94
  wrist and, 252-254
Raphe nucleus, pain control and, 124
Ray, first, midtarsal joint and, 343
Raynaud's phenomenon, 130
Rearfoot varus deformity, 345
Rearfoot-forefoot relationship, 345-346
Receptor, stretch reflex and, 69
Receptor blocker, H1/H2, 143
Reciprocal inhibition
  proprioceptive neuromuscular facilitation and, 69-70, 71
  stretching and, 51
Reconditioning, 34-61
  cardiorespiratory endurance and, 52-58

Reconditioning—cont'd
  flexibility and, 47-52
  strength and endurance and, 35-47; *see also* Strength, reconditioning and
  stretch and flexibility relationship and, 52
Record keeping, importance of, 148
Recovery from injury, mental state and; *see* Psychology
Recreational drug, testing for, 148
Reflex control, elbow joint laxity and, 240, 241-242
Rehearsal of emotive imagery, reducing anxiety and, 115
Reinjury
  ankle rehabilitation and, 338-339
  mental attitude and, 113-114; *see also* Psychology
Relaxation, attitude toward injury and, 114; *see also* Psychology
Relax-hold technique, proprioceptive neuromuscular facilitation and, 50
Repetition of exercise
  endurance training and, 46
  interval training and, 58
  strength training and, 44
Repetitive movement; *see* Overuse
Rescue squad, on-field evaluation and, 91-93
Resistance exercise, shin splints and, 325-326
Resisted motion
  assessment of, 64-65
  off-field evaluation protocol and, 103-104
Respiratory tract, drugs affecting, 141, 143-145
Rest period, interval training and, 58
Resting pulse, Karvonen equation and, 58
Retrocalcaneobursitis, lower leg injuries and, 326
Retropatellar pain, 311
Return to activity program
  ankle rehabilitation and, 338-339
  knee rehabilitation and, 312-314
Reverse Hill-Sachs lesion, 215, 216
Rheumatoid condition, cryotherapy and, 130
Rhinitis, drugs affecting respiratory tract and, 143
Rhythmic stabilization, proprioceptive neuromuscular facilitation and, 73
Rifle exercise, shoulder reconditioning and, 194
Rigid orthotic, 348, 349; *see also* Orthotics
Rolling, accessory motions and, 65, 67
ROM; *see* Range of motion
Rood Method 28, proprioceptive stimulation and, 70
Rotation
  limb, 344
  low back examination and, 157, 158-160
Rotator cuff, shoulder rehabilitation and, 219-220
Rubber band, finger resistance and, 262, 263
Rubber tubing, ankle rehabilitation and, 336-337, 338
Rules of game, goals of rehabilitation and, 32
Running
  knee rehabilitation and, 312-314
  long-distance, 55-56
    Fartlek, 59
  progressive program for; *see* Progressive running program

Running—cont'd
  trochanteric bursitis and, 273-274
Running in water
  ankle rehabilitation and, 339
  lower leg rehabilitation and, 320
  shin splints and, 326
Running surface, stress fractures and, 328
Running to sprinting, 313-314
Rupture
  Achilles tendon, 323-324
  strain versus, 255

S

Sacral nerve root, 158
Sacroiliac, 154
Safety, injury prevention and, 26-27
SAID principle (specific adaptations to imposed demands), 31, 32
Salary, feared loss of, 108
Salicylate; *see* Aspirin
Salt, hydroxide, antacids and, 145, 146
Sander's program for strength training, 44, 45
Scan, bone; *see* Bone scan
Scaphoid, wrist and, 251-252
Scapula, neck injury and, 228
Scar tissue
  flexibility and, 47
  healing process and, 15-19, 20
  hypertrophic, 19
  iontophoresis and, 125
  ultrasound and, 128
Schwann cell, regeneration of nerve tissue and, 21
Sciatic nerve, piriformis muscle and, 269-270, 272-273
Scissoring, elbow injuries and, 236
S-D curve; *see* Strength-duration curve
Second-degree sprain, 8-9
Second-degree strain, 9-10
Self image, injuries and; *see* Psychology
Semirigid orthotic, 348, 349; *see also* Orthotics
Sensation, testing for, palpation and, 161
Sensory nerve, electrical current and, 122-124
Separation of tissue, impeded healing and, 19
Set, interval training and, 58
Sex difference
  body composition and, 91
  cardiac output and, 55
  muscle strength and, 37-38, 46-47
  piriformis syndrome sciatica and, 269
  trochanteric bursitis and, 273
Shear, directional, elbow injuries and, 236
Shin splint
  definition of, 321
  lower leg injuries and, 324-326
Shoe
  ankle rehabilitation and, 339
  artificial turf, 354
  foot rehabilitation and, 352-353
  neuroma and, 354

Shoes—cont'd
  orthotics and, 352-353; *see also* Orthotics
  stress fractures and, 328-329
  wear patterns of, 343-344
Shoe heel counter, retrocalcaneobursitis and, 326
Shortwave diathermy
  indications/contraindications and, 137
  microwave diathermy versus, 126-127
Shoulder, 186-231
  elbow joint laxity and, 240-241, 242
  Kehr's sign and, 92
  rehabilitation programs and, 207-229
    axillary nerve/neuropathy and, 227-228
    biceps tendon dislocation and, 218-219
    brachial plexus and, 228-229
    clavicle fractures and, 215-217
    contusions and, 207-208
    degenerative joint disease, 217-218
    glenohumeral dislocations and subluxations and, 209-214
    glenoid labrum tear and, 215
    inflammation and, 220-225
    muscular strains and, 218
    rotator cuff and, 219-220
    sprains and, 208-209
    thoracic outlet syndrome and, 225-227
    winging scapula and, 228
  rehabilitation techniques and, 187-206
    endurance programs and, 204
    functional progressions and, 204-206
    isokinetic exercises and, 201-204
    isometric exercises and, 194-196
    isotonic strengthening exercises and, 197-201
    joint mobilization and, 189-192
    proprioceptive neuromuscular facilitation and, 197
    range-of-motion exercises and, 192-194
    stretching techniques and, 187-189
    surgical tubing/thera-band exercises and, 196-197
  upper-quarter screening and, 94, 95
SI; *see* Sacroiliac
Sidestep, ankle return to activity and, 339
Silicone splint, scaphoid fracture and, 252
Simple fracture, 6
Sit-and-reach test, preparticipation examination and, 89, 90
Size, body, sexual differences and, 46-47
Skeletal muscle; *see also* Muscle
  anatomy and physiology of, 35-37
  characteristics of, 3
Skier's thumb, 258
Skin
  characteristics of, 1-3
  electrical current and, 122-127
  flexibility and, 47
  iontophoresis and, 125
  low back palpation and, 158
  necrosis and, 255
Skinfold measurement, preparticipation examination and, 90-91

Sleeping position, low back examination and, 154
Slow reversal technique, 73
Slow reversal-hold technique, 73
Slow reversal-hold-relax technique, 50, 74
Slow-twitch muscle fiber
  fast-twitch fiber versus, 36-37
  type one, 5
Slump test, low back palpation and, 160
Smooth muscle, characteristics of, 3
SOAP notes; *see* Subjective-objective assessment plan, documentation and
Soda, baking and carbonated, gastrointestinal tract and, 145, 146
Sodium bicarbonate, gastrointestinal tract and, 145
Soft tissue
  definition of, 1
  mobilization of, 236
Soleus muscle
  Achilles tendonitis and, 321, 322
  preparticipation examination and, 89
Spasm
  ankle rehabilitation and, 333
  arterial, 130
  muscle
    impeded healing and, 19
    soreness and, 10
  proprioceptive neuromuscular facilitation and, 69
Specific adaptations to imposed demands, goals of rehabilitation and, 31, 32
Spin movement, accessory motions and, 67
Spinal cord
  enkephalins and, 123
  life-threatening injury and, 92
  musculature and, 155
  proprioceptive neuromuscular facilitation and, 69-70
  stenosis and, 154-155
Spindle, muscle, stretch reflex and, 51, 69
Spine
  anterior superior iliac, 155
  iliac, 268-269
  life-threatening injury and, 92
  posterior superior iliac, 155
  upper-quarter screening and, 93-94
Spiral fracture, characteristics of, 6, 7
Splint
  finger
    hand injury and, 255, 258
    protection and, 262-263
  plaster, 349, 350
  shin, 324-326
  silicone, 252
Spondylolisthesis
  low back examination and, 154
  lumbosacral injury and, 164-165
Spondylolysis
  low back examination and, 154
  lumbosacral injury and, 164

Spongy bone, types of bone and, 5
Spontaneous emission, low-power laser and, 131
Sports therapist
    communication between physician and, 294-295
    motives for career as, 121
    relationship with athlete and, 115-116
Sprain
    ankle, 14
    ligament, 8-9
    lumbosacral injury and, 164
    shoulder joint, 208-209
Sprinting, energy systems and, 55-56
Spur
    bone, 12-13
    plantar fasciitis and, 355
Squash, hamate injury and, 252
Squat, isometric exercise and, 40
Staple capsulorrhaphy, Dutoit, 211
Static flexibility, 48
Static stretching
    flexibility and, 49, 50
    Golgi tendon organs and, 51
    range of motion and, 51-52
Stationary bicycle
    ankle rehabilitation and, 334, 339
    interval training and, 58
    lower leg rehabilitation and, 320
Stenosing tenosynovitis, De Quervain's, 250
Stenosis, spinal, 154-155
Sternoclavicular joint injury, 209
Steroidal drug; see also Drug
    elbow injuries and, 235
    hip pointer and, 266
Stimulating current, electrical, 121-127
Stirrup, ankle, 332
Stoved finger, 256, 258
Straight leg raising
    knee injury and, 300, 301
    low back palpation and, 160
Strain
    groin, 276-278
    hamstring tendon, 284
    hip adductor versus hip flexor, 276-278
    quadriceps muscle, 286-289
    rupture versus, 255
    shoulder muscles and, 218
Strength
    Achilles tendonitis and, 321
    age and, 38
    ankle rehabilitation and, 334-338
    circuit training and, 58-59
    definition of, 296
    elbow and, 240-241, 242
    endurance versus, 46-47
    flexibility and, 52
    hand, 261-262, 263
    high-frequency AC current and, 125

Strength—cont'd
    leg, 47
    preparticipation examination and, 89
    proprioceptive neuromuscular facilitation and, 73
    quadriceps, 303, 310
    reconditioning and
        factors determining, 37-38
        methods of improving, 39-47
        physiology of, 38-39
        skeletal muscle contraction and, 35-37
    sexual differences and, 46-47
    wrist rehabilitation and, 253-254
Strength curve, 37, 38
Strength-duration curve, 122-123
Stress
    ankle healing and, 332
    antidiarrheal medications and, 146
    elbow and, 234
    injury and; see Psychology
Stress fracture
    characteristics of, 7
    femoral, 285
    lower leg, 328-329
    lumbosacral injury and, 164
Stress test, on-field evaluation and, 92
Stretch and flexibility, relationship of, 47, 48-50, 52
Stretch reflex
    muscle strength and, 37
    proprioceptive neuromuscular facilitation and, 69
Stretching
    Achilles tendonitis and, 322-323
    low back rehabilitation and, 164
    musculotendinous unit injury and, 236-237, 238-239
    plantar fasciitis and, 355
    proprioceptive neuromuscular facilitation and, 73-74
    shoulder rehabilitation and, 187-189
Striated muscle, characteristics of, 3
Stroke volume, maximal heart rate and, 54
Subacromial bursa, bursitis and, 12
Subacute joint, elbow injuries and, 244, 246
Subcutaneous contusion, hip pointer as, 265-268
Subcutaneous fat, preparticipation examination and, 91
Subjective-objective assessment plan, documentation and, 104-105
Subluxation
    cuboid, 355
    dislocations and, 7-8
        glenohumeral, 209-214
    osteoarthrosis and, 13
Subtalar joint
    foot and, 342-343
    orthotics and, 349, 350
    pronation and, 344-345
Sulindac, elbow injuries and, 235
Superficial posterior compartment, 327
Superior iliac spine, 268, 269
Supination
    elbow injuries and, 243

Supination—cont'd
  subtalar joint and, 342-343
Supination-pronation exercise, wrist rehabilitation and, 254
Supraspinatus tendonitis, 221-223
Surgical tubing exercise
  lower leg conditioning and, 317, 318-319
  shoulder and, 196-197
Swelling; *see also* Individual injuries
  acute injury and, 132-133
  drugs affecting respiratory tract and, 143
  initial management of injuries and, 13-15
  intermittent compression and, 130-131
  muscle soreness and, 10
  off-field evaluation protocol and, 101
  on-field evaluation and, 93
  thermotherapy and, 130
  visual inspection and, 101
Swimming
  ankle rehabilitation and, 334, 339
  energy systems and, 55-56
  lower leg rehabilitation and, 320
Sympathomimetic drug, asthma and, 145
Synovial joint
  capsular pattern of motion and, 64
  ligament sprains and, 8
Synovial sheath
  bursitis and, 12
  osteoarthrosis and, 13
  tenosynovitis and, 11
Synthetic turf, turf toe and, 354-355

T

Talofibular ligament, ankle injuries and, 331; *see also* Ankle
Talonavicular joint, midtarsal joint and, 343
Talus
  retrocalcaneobursitis and, 326
  subtalar joint and, 342-343
Taping
  ankle rehabilitation and, 332, 339
  De Quervain's tenosynovitis and, 250
  palmar checkrein, 252
  turf toe and, 354, 355
Tarsal tunnel syndrome, 355-356
Teacher Effectiveness Training (Gordon's), 114
Teeter board, joint proprioception and, 320
Temperature, body
  dehydration and, 146
  electromagnetic energy and, 126-127
  ultrasound and, 127-128
Tendon
  Achilles rupture and, 323-324
  biceps, 218-219
  hand injuries and, 254-256
  healing of, 20
  muscle, 36
  patellar, 296, 299
  radial extensor, 250, 251
  tissue type of, 3

Tendon—cont'd
  wrist injuries and, 249-251
Tendon organ, Golgi, 51
Tendonitis, 223-224
  Achilles, 321-323
  bicipital, 223
  ice and, 14
  musculoskeletal injuries and, 10-11
  supraspinatus, 221-223
Tennis
  De Quervain's tenosynovitis and, 250
  elbow injuries and, 245
Tennis leg, 324
Tenosynovitis
  De Quervain's, 250
  ice and, 14
  musculoskeletal injuries and, 11
TENS; *see* Transcutaneous electrical nerve stimulation
Tension oscillation, elbow injuries and, 236
Terminal knee extension, 305
Terrain, Fartlek and, 59
Testing for drug abuse, 148
Testosterone, sexual differences and, 46-47
Thalamus, aspirin and, 140
Thera-Band exercise, shoulder and, 196-197
Therapeutic exercise, 27-31; *see also* Reconditioning
Therapist, sports; *see* Sports therapist
Therapy, types of, 121-138; *see also* Reconditioning
  acute injury and, 132-134
  chronic injury and, 134-135
  electrical stimulating currents and, 121-127
  exercises and, 27-31
  indications/contraindications and, 135, 136
  infrared modalities and, 128-130
  intermittent compression and, 130-131
  low-power laser and, 131-132
  ultrasound and, 127-128
Thermoplastic material, ankle protection and, 332
Thermotherapy
  acute injury and, 134
  diathermy and, 126-127
  indications/contraindications and, 137
  infrared modalities and, 129, 130
  shin splints and, 325
  ultrasound and, 127-128
Thigh; *see* Hip and thigh
Third-degree sprain, 9
Third-degree strain, 10
Thompson test, Achilles tendon rupture and, 323
Thoracic outlet syndrome, 225-227
Throat, antitussives and expectorants and, 144-145
Thromboplastin, inflammation and, 15
Throwing
  elbow injuries and, 245
  shoulder rehabilitation and, 204-206
Thrust technique, low back rehabilitation and, 161-162
Thumb
  De Quervain's tenosynovitis and, 250

Thumb—cont'd
    hand injuries and, 258
    opposition exercise and, 262-263
Thumb spica, 250
Tibia, stress fractures of lower leg and, 328
Tibial rotation, knee injury and, 301, 304
Tibial varum, pronation and, 346, 347
Tibialis anterior
    shin splints and, 325
    shoe wear patterns and, 343-344
Tibialis posterior compartment, 327
Tibiofemoral joint, 307
Tibiofibular ligament, 331
Timing
    interval training and, 58
    on-field evaluation and, 92
    proprioceptive neuromuscular facilitation and, 72
Tissue repair, phases of, 19
Toe
    acute compartment syndrome and, 327
    ankle rehabilitation and, 335
    lower leg conditioning and, 317-320
    Morton's, 343
    turf, 354-355
Toe box, shoe width and, 354
Topical drug, ultrasound and, 128
Torsion of innominate, low back examination and, 155
Touchdown weight bearing, ankle rehabilitation and, 332-333
Towel stretch, ankle rehabilitation and, 334, 335
Trabecula, types of bone and, 5
Trachea, antitussives and expectorants and, 144
Traction
    manual therapy and, 67
    meniscal injury and, 309-310
    proprioceptive neuromuscular facilitation and, 72
Trainer-therapist; see Sports therapist
Training
    circuit, 58-59
    continuous, 56-57
    improper, 324-325
    injury prevention and, 26-27
    interval, 58
Transcutaneous electrical nerve stimulation, 122-124
Translation, accessory motions and, 67
Transverse fracture
    characteristics of, 6, 7
    finger injuries and, 259
Trochanter level, low back examination and, 155
Trochanteric bursitis, 273-274
Trunk
    active motion and, 156-157
    proprioceptive neuromuscular facilitation patterns and, 81-83
Tubing, rubber
    ankle rehabilitation and, 336-337, 338
    lower leg conditioning and, 317, 318-319
Tunnel syndrome, tarsal, 355-356

Turf toe, 354-355
TWB; see Touchdown weight bearing

U

UBE; see Upper body ergometer
Ulnar collateral ligament, 258
Ulnar deviation of wrist, 250
Ulnohumeral joint, 232, 238
Ultrasound, 127-128
    acute injury and, 134
    hip pointer and, 266
    indications/contraindications and, 137
    posterior superior iliac spine contusion and, 269
    shin splints and, 325
    turf toe and, 354-355
Ultraviolet, indications/contraindications and, 137
University of North Carolina return to activity program, 312-314
Upper body ergometer, 204, 205
Upper extremity, proprioceptive neuromuscular facilitation patterns and, 74-78
Upper-quarter screening, 93-96

V

Valgus stress
    elbow injuries and, 242
    forefoot, 344-346
    knee injury and, 308
Valsalva effect, 40
Varus stress
    deformity of rearfoot, 345
    forefoot, 344-346
    knee injury and, 308
Vascular system
    diathermy and, 126
    drugs affecting respiratory tract and, 143, 144
Vascularization, low-power laser and, 131
Vasoconstriction, ice and, 14
Vasodilation
    common analgesics and, 140
    cryotherapy and, 130
    iontophoresis and, 125
Velocity spectrum program, shoulder and, 202-204
Verbal command, proprioceptive neuromuscular facilitation and, 72
Vertebral fracture, 269
Vibrational energy; see Ultrasound
Visual inspection; see Evaluation
Visual rehearsal, reducing anxiety and, 115
Visual stimulus, proprioceptive neuromuscular facilitation and, 72
Vitamins, 26
Volkmann's contracture, 234
Voluntary muscle, characteristics of, 3
VO_{2max} (Maximal oxygen consumption), 52-53
Vomiting; see Nausea

W

Walking to jogging, progressive running program and, 313
Wall finger-walking exercise, 193
Wand exercise, 194
Warm whirlpool
    hand rehabilitation and, 260, 261
    wrist rehabilitation and, 253
Wart, plantar, iontophoresis and, 125
Water, expectorants versus, 144
Weather, injury prevention and, 26-27
Weaver-Dunn procedure, 208
Wedge board, 334, 335, 336
Weight, ankle, 317-318
Weight, body
    low back examination and, 154-155
    maximal oxygen consumption and, 53
    Sander's program and, 44, 45
Weight bearing
    phase I ankle rehabilitation and, 332-333
    proprioceptive loss and, 337, 338
Weight distribution, low back examination and, 155
Weight training
    circuit and, 58
    dumbbell and, 253, 254, 255
    extensor mechanism tenosynovitis and, 250
    flexibility and, 52
    isotonic exercise and, 40-41
    muscular strength and, 37-38
        endurance versus, 46
    sex differences and, 46-47
    strength versus endurance and, 46

Wheel exercise, shoulder reconditioning and, 194
Whirlpool
    cold, 133, 134
    warm
        hand rehabilitation and, 260, 261
        indications/contraindications for, 137
        wrist rehabilitation and, 253
Winging scapula, neck injury and, 228
Wiring, Kirshner, shoulder rehabilitation and, 208
Woman, sex distinctions and; *see* Sex difference
Work load, cardiorespiratory endurance and, 55, 56
Work period, interval training and, 58
Wrap
    ankle compression and, 333
    initial management of injuries and, 14
Wrist
    elbow joint laxity and, 240-241, 242
    injuries and, 249-252
    tennis and, 245
    upper-quarter screening and, 94, 96
Wrist flexor mass, elbow injuries and, 232

X

X-ray
    contusion and, 12
    dislocation and subluxation and, 7-8
    low back examination and, 154-155
    stress fracture and, 7

Z

Zinc, iontophoresis and, 125